Breastfeeding
Pure & Simple

Breastfeeding
Pure & Simple

Gwen Gotsch

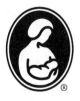

La Leche League International
Schaumburg, Illinois

Revised edition, January 2000
Second Printing, June 2000
First edition, January 1994; July 1997
©2000, 1993 La Leche League International
Cover photos: David C. Arendt
Cover and book design: Digital Concepts, LLC
Printed in the USA
All Rights Reserved
Library of Congress 99-068033
ISBN 0-912500-59-X

*This book is dedicated to the staff,
present and past, at La Leche
League International Headquarters;
people whose commitment to helping
mothers and babies has made a
difference in the lives of families
around the world.*

Contents

Acknowledgements

This book is based on the experiences of many thousands of women who have shared their breastfeeding stories with each other in the years since La Leche League's founding in 1956. They have helped to build a tradition of breastfeeding knowledge from which families all over the world benefit. My special thanks go to the following individuals who worked on this book: David Arendt for the design and and for his patience in taking photographs; Kim Cavaliero for the title; Bill Sears, Jan Riordan, Betty Crase, and Marijane McEwan, for reading the manuscript; Elayne Shpak for typing; Lon Grahnke for perspectives on fathering; and Judy Torgus, who came up with the idea for this book, asked me to write it, and nagged me cheerfully until it was finished.

Gwen Gotsch

Photo Credits

David Arendt, front cover, pages 1, 3, 9, 11, 13, 25, 26, 27, 28, 29, 30, 31, 32, 48, 59, 62, 65, 69, 73, 75, 78, 79, 81, 82, 85, 89, 94, 101

JJ Anderson, pages 5, 90, 105, 107

Mary Ann Cahill, page 7

Medela, Inc., page 14

Darrell Rideout, page 17, 21

Mary Joan Deutschbein, page 23

Judy Torgus, pages 19, 37

Dariuz Michalowski, page 35

Jean Hoelscher, Association for Breastfeeding Fashions, pages 41, 83, 103

Paul Torgus, page 44, (Sketches)

Cindi Salazar, pages 45, 66

Pascale, page 54

Dale Pfeiffer, page 93

Eleanor Randall, page 70

Sharon Kay, page 72

Lon Grahnke, page 99, back cover

Foreword

Twenty-five years ago I knew little about breastfeeding, and I didn't think it made much difference. In medical school the baby feeding lectures were mainly recitations of the contents of the formula can. I was fresh out of school and into pediatric practice when my first breastfeeding patient told me she hadn't experienced a let-down yet; I thought she meant postpartum depression. Now, after twenty years of pediatric practice and being in the supporting role as my wife, Martha, breastfed all eight of our children, I am happy to report: breastfeeding does matter.

There will be times when mothers feel that breastfeeding is all giving, giving, giving. This is true early on in the breastfeeding relationship. Babies are takers, and parents are givers. But in our breastfeeding experience we have learned to appreciate the concept of mutual giving—the more you give to your baby, the more the baby gives back to you. When a mother breastfeeds her baby, she gives nourishment and comfort. The baby's sucking, in turn, stimulates the release of hormones that further enhance mothering behavior.

Another dividend to expect is mutual sensitivity. Breastfeeding helps you become more sensitive to your baby and helps your baby become more sensitive to you. This sensitivity helps breastfeeding mothers make the right choice at the right time when confronted with the daily "What do I do now?" baby-care decisions. The connected pair mirror each other's feelings. Baby learns about himself through mother's eyes. The mother reflects the baby's value to her, and therefore to himself. Breastfeeding helps mothers click into these feelings earlier and maintain them longer.

Everything a breastfeeding mother needs to know is concisely found in Breastfeeding *Pure & Simple*. This little book with lots of information will help newborns and new mothers get connected and stay connected. As an author myself, I truly enjoyed how Gwen Gotsch has masterfully presented so much information in so few pages. This book is indeed a testimony to the axiom, "Good things come in small packages."

Both novice breastfeeding mothers and professionals who offer breastfeeding advice will find this book a pleasure to read and a valuable lactation resource.

William Sears, MD
Clinical Assistant Professor of Pediatrics
University of Southern California
School of Medicine

Chapter One

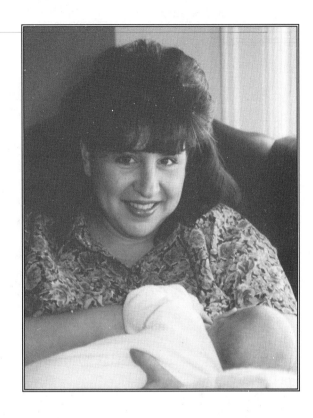

Breastfeeding in Today's World

Mothers agree, it's worth it.

Breastfeeding your baby requires some effort, but it definitely has its rewards. A healthy, thriving baby is one of the payoffs; a real sense of accomplishment for mother is another. Many a breastfeeding mother over the years has paused to gaze at her bright-eyed three- or four-month-old nursling, so much bigger now than at birth, and smiled proudly to herself while thinking, "I did that. My body nourished that baby."

Breastfeeding makes sense—human milk is the perfect food for babies. It contains all the nutrition babies need, along with protection from infection and disease. It comes from the same warm maternal body that nourishes the baby in the womb, holds and soothes the newborn in tender embraces, and helps the growing infant feel secure while getting to know an exciting but sometimes overwhelming new world. Mother's milk is there, warm and sweet and waiting, in response to baby's need for food and comfort.

Breastfeeding is not all romance. It may be natural, but breastfeeding a baby, like mothering, is an art, a skill that requires learning and practice. The mother and baby teach each other during the first days and weeks, and more discoveries follow as the months go by. Some lessons are learned quickly. Others take a little longer. Problems are solved more easily within a supportive environment; nevertheless, many mothers breastfeed successfully on their own.

This book is an introduction to the art of breastfeeding. It tells you what you need to know to get off to a good start and to continue nursing your baby through the first several months of life. It also tells you something about feelings that go along with breastfeeding and how to overcome common problems. With support and accurate information, breastfeeding can be a happy, treasured experience for both baby and mother.

Why mothers breastfeed

For many families, breastfeeding is the natural thing to do; they prefer an "all natural" product over one concocted in a factory. Human milk has been tested by time over thousands of years, and its special properties cannot be duplicated by infant formula. Babies who are breastfed have significant nutritional, immunological, and psychological advantages.

Human milk is the nutritional standard against which infant formula is measured, but it has properties that make it far superior. The composition of human milk is always changing to meet the changing needs of the developing infant. The first milk, a thick yellowish substance called colostrum, is high in protein, low in fat, and contains a high concentration of immune factors, which may be especially important to the baby in the first days of life outside the womb. As the mother's breasts begin to make more milk, the concentrations of protein and immune factors gradually decrease and levels of fat, lactose, and total calories increase. As the baby gets older, milk composition varies less, but it will change again during weaning. One study found that an older baby, who is nursing more for comfort than nutrition, receives a greater concentration of immune factors; breastfeeding continues to play a role in protecting the weaning child from disease.

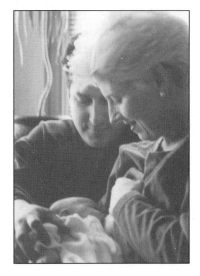

Breastfeeding protects against infection

The list of protective factors in human milk is a long one, and scientists are only beginning to unravel the mysteries of how they all work together to protect the baby from infection. Meanwhile, studies comparing groups of breastfed and formula-fed babies clearly show that breastfed babies have fewer and less severe problems with diarrhea, respiratory infections, ear infections, and other common diseases. Breastfed babies are much less likely to end up in the hospital with a serious illness. They are also less likely to become victims of Sudden Infant Death Syndrome (SIDS).

Each mother's milk helps to protect her baby from whatever illness is going around.

One especially interesting feature of breastfeeding's immunological benefits is the way each mother's milk helps to protect her baby from whatever illness is going around. When the mother is exposed to bacteria or a virus, her more mature immune system quickly produces antibodies that are transferred to the baby through the milk. This is important, because young infants cannot muster the same level of defense against infection as adults. It's also a reminder to breastfeeding mothers and those who advise them: if a mother is feeling ill, coming down with a cold or flu, she should not stop nursing or even hesitate to breastfeed her baby. Her milk will not harm her baby; in fact, it will help the baby fight off the infection.

Human milk provides ideal nutrition

Breastfed babies generally need to be fed more often than formula-fed babies. One reason for this is that human milk is very well suited to the baby's digestive system and is digested very quickly. The protein is made up of 60 percent whey proteins and 40 percent casein proteins; this makes a very soft curd that is easy and efficient to digest. (Cow's milk contains only 20 percent whey proteins and 80 percent casein.) The fat in human milk is also highly digestible because of the enzyme lipase, which keeps the fat globules small and totally digestible. Since fat is the major source of energy for infants, its easy availability is important to growth.

Besides fat and protein, the other major components of human milk are water and lactose, or milk sugar. Human milk provides all the water that infants need. Even in very warm, dry climates, breastfed babies do not need supplementary bottles of water.

Human milk provides all the nutrients that infants need.

All the vitamins, minerals, and trace elements that babies need to grow, develop, and stay healthy can be found in human milk. Iron levels are low, but the iron is absorbed and used far more efficiently than that in iron-fortified formula. Breastfed babies do not need iron supplements. And the vitamins in human milk meet all of baby's needs. Some physicians recommend vitamin D supplements for breastfed babies, but these are not usually necessary.

Science is just beginning to investigate the many ways in which human milk affects babies' development. Studies have found that longer periods of breastfeeding are associated with higher scores on IQ tests and other measures of intellectual development. While heredity and environment also influence how smart a child turns out to be, researchers now believe that at least some of the intellectual benefits of breastfeeding come from nutrients in human milk that contribute to optimal brain development.

Besides delivering the right balance and the right types of fats and proteins, human milk also contains various enzymes and hormones. Some of these aid infant digestion, and others promote the development of different parts of the body. These highly specialized functions cannot be duplicated by infant formula.

Breastfeeding brings mother and baby closer together

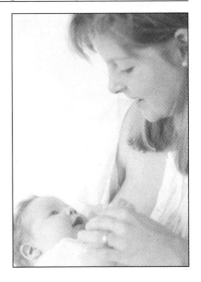

Breastfeeding is an undeniably different experience from bottle-feeding. The breastfed baby is pulled close against the mother, touching her warm, smooth skin. The nipple is soft and pliable; it is shaped by baby's mouth. The baby sucks at his own rate, and the sucking determines how fast the milk flows and when the feeding is over. A hungry baby will suck eagerly until his tummy is full. A baby who is upset may suck more for comfort, and the small amounts of milk he receives, plus the rhythm of his suck, will lull him into a more peaceful state. Whether mother is gazing into baby's eyes or talking, reading, or watching television during a feeding, her body is actively present for her baby. Feeding is always associated with the warmth and security that is mother.

Breastfed babies make their mothers feel special.

Babies let their mothers know how much they enjoy nursing: they wriggle with delight, they smile, they coo, they play games, they fall blissfully asleep. They make their mothers feel important, special, and capable. Frequent nursing sessions, following the baby's cues, help mothers learn to understand their baby's behavior and become flexible about meeting baby's needs. Prolactin and oxytocin, the hormones that regulate milk production and release, also produce feelings of calm, relaxation, and love. Both baby and mother benefit from the feelings of closeness that come from breastfeeding.

Breastfeeding is practical

Breastfeeding is also cheap, convenient, and good for the environment. It costs $20 to $30 a week to buy infant formula in the United States, but human milk is free, and available from mother instantly anywhere. With breastfeeding, there's no need to mix formula or worry about how many bottles to bring along on an outing, how to keep them cold, or how to warm them when you need them. Human milk doesn't pollute the environment—its production and distribution systems don't require electrical energy, throwaway packaging, cross-country shipping, or cows that produce excess methane gas.

Breastfeeding gives busy mothers many chances during the day to sit down and rest for a while, or to read books or play games with baby's older sibling. Nighttime feedings are simple, and nursing will often put mother as well as baby back to sleep quickly. While critics of breastfeeding like to point out that breastfeeding is "inconvenient" or "difficult in today's busy world," experienced breastfeeding mothers often feel that the best thing about breastfeeding is its simplicity and convenience.

Confidence: What breastfeeding mothers need most

Breastfeeding involves a mother's heart and mind as well as her body, and gaining confidence is an important part of learning to nurse her baby. But sometimes confidence in breastfeeding can be hard to come by.

Several generations ago mothers didn't turn to books for advice about breastfeeding. They learned about nursing their babies from seeing other women breastfeed healthy, thriving infants, and they learned from other women's problems, too. Almost everybody breastfed, because babies who were "hand-fed" on animal milk or other concoctions often didn't survive.

Today, fortunately, artificial feeding is not so dangerous, as long as a mother has access to clean water, fuel, and affordable supplies of infant formula (conditions that are difficult to meet in many parts of the world). But even though human milk remains the standard for infant feeding, artificial feeding has become a common and well-established part of today's baby culture. The decorations, cards, and wrappings at baby showers picture bottles along with all the other

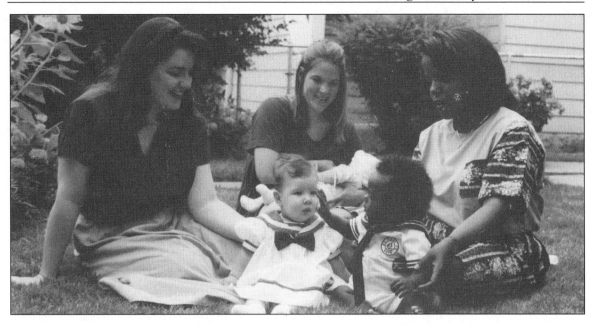

equipment every baby "requires." Infant formula is advertised on television, and breastfeeding women find coupons for formula in their mailbox, right about the time when babies experience growth spurts and mothers may have doubts about their milk supply. Hospitals may even send formula samples home with breastfeeding mothers—implying that breastfeeding may not succeed. Is it any wonder that new mothers have doubts and anxieties about breastfeeding?

Breastfeeding really does work, and in most circumstances, it's surprisingly simple. Confidence in breastfeeding will come with experience. However, most of today's soon-to-be mothers were not breastfed as babies, and unless they have friends who are nursing babies, they may never have gotten a close look at a baby latched onto a breast and actively sucking. But there are ways to gain experience with breastfeeding before your baby is born. Learning about breastfeeding, seeking out health-care providers who have confidence in breastfeeding, and talking to experienced, successful nursing mothers will help a mother gain confidence in her ability to breastfeed her baby.

Breastfeeding is not difficult or complicated, but it does take some practice for mothers and babies to become skilled at it. The problems that women sometimes encounter with breastfeeding can be solved, and deserve to be. Most of them are not medical problems at all, but are the result of misunderstanding the needs of mothers and babies. The answer to breastfeeding problems is seldom a bottle of formula; the best solution is the telephone—a call to someone knowledgeable about breastfeeding.

La Leche League International

La Leche League offers the kind of support that many women feel is essential to breastfeeding success. For more than thirty-five years, La Leche League has been learning about breastfeeding from mothers and the people who assist them and has been sharing this knowledge with other mothers and with health professionals all over the world. La Leche League's mother-to-mother support and its practical approach to parenting have enabled millions of women to enjoy breastfeeding and mothering their babies.

Problems that women encounter with breastfeeding deserve to be solved.

La Leche League Leaders are available by phone to answer questions about breastfeeding. They are all experienced nursing mothers who have been accredited by La Leche League International. Written materials, workshops, conferences, and networking with other Leaders have prepared them to give you the information you need, to help you explore options for solving problems, and to offer the encouraging words you need to hear. If you have a breastfeeding question a La Leche League Leader can't answer herself, she can use LLLI's vast network of resources to find out what you need to know. From fussy babies, critical relatives, and dwindling milk supplies to going back to work or needing to take medication, breastfeeding dilemmas are La Leche League's business.

Local La Leche League Groups offer monthly meetings at which expectant and new mothers gather along with experienced breastfeeding mothers and the Group's Leaders. They discuss the how-to's, the whys, the what-not-to-do's of breastfeeding and talk of their own experiences. Mothers can speak frankly about difficulties they're having with nursing or with the day-to-day stresses of motherhood. They can be assured of responses that are not only full of helpful ideas but are also warmly supportive of every mother's efforts to do the very best for her own baby and family.

To find a La Leche League Group in your area, call La Leche League International Headquarters at 1-800-LA LECHE or 847-519-7730. The staff there can provide you with names and phone numbers of La Leche League Leaders near you. They'll also be happy to send you an LLLI Catalogue and other information. You may also find information about La Leche League meetings listed in your local newspaper or posted in your doctor's office, or your childbirth educator may be able to refer you to a local LLL Group. If you use the Internet, go to LLLI's website at http://www.lalecheleague.org for lots of helpful information about breastfeeding and about La Leche League Leaders and Groups in your area.

Support is crucial to new mothers. Your partner, your friends, your family will play important roles, caring for you and encouraging you as you learn to breastfeed and mother your baby. La Leche League can provide an added boost, especially if you should run into an unusual problem or if the people closest to you understand little about breastfeeding. There are few things mothers find as reassuring as talking to another mother who has had similar experiences.

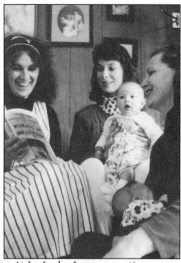

At La Leche League meetings you find mothers helping other mothers with information and confidence-building support.

Chapter Two

Getting Ready

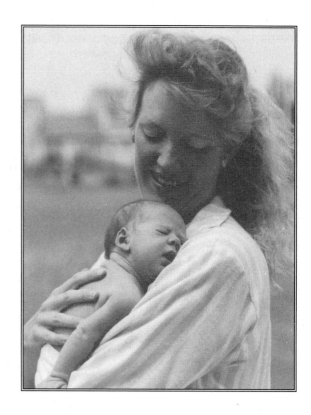

All through pregnancy, a woman's body prepares for breastfeeding.

Her breasts enlarge and may feel tender as the milk-making structures inside of them grow. The areola, the pigmented area around the nipple, darkens, and the nipples may become more erect and protruding. The Montgomery's glands, the pimply bumps around the nipple, secrete a substance that lubricates the nipples and protects them. Sometime in the second trimester, the breasts begin producing colostrum, the first milk that is especially high in antibodies. Some women notice small amounts of colostrum leaking from their breasts late in pregnancy.

All these changes take place whether or not a mother plans to breastfeed. So the most important part of getting ready to breastfeed is done naturally and automatically. And really, beyond this, little preparation is needed.

However, adding a new baby to your life is a big change and a challenge. Knowing what to expect and being prepared can ease the way.

Breast and nipple care

As you look ahead to breastfeeding, you may begin to think of your breasts in a new way. From the time when a girl's figure changes to that of a woman's, breasts are an important part of her body image and her feminine identity. Some women like their breasts and some don't; some are comfortable handling them and others aren't. Some women are anxious about breastfeeding while others feel more confident.

Thinking of breasts as functioning organs, a source of nourishment and nurture for an infant, can seem odd, even scary, at first. Women wonder if their breasts will make enough milk, how the baby will get the milk out of there, and whether their breasts, changed by pregnancy, will ever be the same again. Discovering after the baby is born that the whole process really does work can be an awesome experience, one that gives a woman a new appreciation of her body and her breasts.

Breasts and nipples come in many sizes and shapes. Breast size has no effect on a woman's ability to produce milk for her baby. Small breasts contain plenty of milk-producing glands; larger breasts contain more fatty tissue—which has no influence on lactation.

Buying bras

Whether or not to wear a bra is up to you. Some women are more comfortable without one. Pregnancy alters the size, shape, and firmness of breasts, regardless of whether or not a woman goes on to breastfeed. Heredity and gravity influence breast contours far more than wearing or not wearing a bra.

You'll probably find that you need a larger bra size during pregnancy. It makes sense to buy bras with cups that open so you can use them later when you're nursing. You may need bras that are larger still during the first weeks after your baby is born. Shop for nursing bras during the last few weeks of pregnancy, but buy only two or three at first. If you find a particular style comfortable, you can get more later. There should be extra room in the cup and an extra row of hooks in the back to allow for breast enlargement. The fastener on the cup should be easy to open and close with one hand, while the other arm holds the baby. Bras should be comfortable; they shouldn't pinch or bind. Be especially careful with underwires, which can obstruct the flow of milk if they don't fit properly.

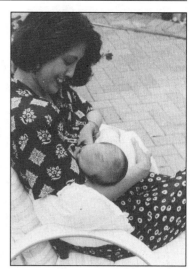

Bras and breast pads (used by some women to absorb milk leakage) should allow air to circulate to the nipples. This helps prevent chapping and soreness. All-cotton materials are best; avoid bras and pads with plastic linings.

Breast surgery

Previous breast surgery can affect breastfeeding if milk ducts or major nerves have been severed. In some types of breast reduction surgery, the ducts are cut; this can prevent the milk from reaching the nipple during breastfeeding. Breast implants themselves don't usually present problems for breastfeeding, but sometimes nerves or ducts are cut during breast augmentation surgery. Checking with the surgeon can help clarify exactly what was done, but the only way to find out for sure if breastfeeding will work in a given situation is to go ahead and give it a try, paying close attention to the basics: positioning and latch-on, frequent feedings, and signs that the baby is getting enough milk.

Nipple preparation

Years ago, doctors, nurses, and even breastfeeding advocates prescribed all kinds of regimens to help pregnant women "toughen" their nipples ahead of time, in order to avoid soreness during breastfeeding. Happily, those days are gone. Experts now agree that most sore

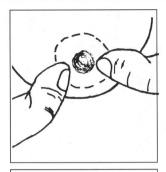

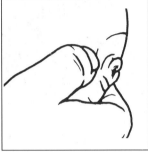

To check for inverted nipples, compress the areola an inch behind the base of the nipple. It should protrude rather than cave in.

Breast shells can correct inverted nipples.

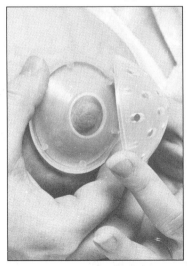

nipples are the result of babies being poorly positioned at the breast during feedings or not sucking effectively, and that you really can't toughen up a nipple anyway. Nipples are supposed to be pliable and sensitive.

Most mothers don't need to do anything special to prepare their nipples for breastfeeding. Pregnant and nursing women should avoid using soap on their nipples—you don't want to wash away the natural oils that keep the skin supple. It isn't necessary, but it won't hurt to use a lotion or moisturizer on the nipples, as long as it's applied sparingly. Modified lanolin (sold under the brand name of Lansinoh®) is a good choice and can also be used after the baby arrives.

Inverted nipples

Flat or inverted nipples can make latching on to the breast more difficult for the baby; babies usually find it easier to grasp a nipple that protrudes from the breast. Checking for inverted nipples during pregnancy can help you anticipate and prevent breastfeeding problems. To determine if your nipples are flat or inverted, gently compress the areola about an inch behind the base of the nipple. A flat nipple cannot be compressed outward and does not protrude when stimulated. An inverted nipple caves in when the areola is compressed. Your nipples are not identical; a woman may have one nipple that is very inverted while the other may be only slightly inverted or have no problem at all.

Nipples invert because tiny bands of tissue connect them to the inside of the breast, but a healthy baby who sucks well can latch on even to a breast with an inverted nipple. Eventually, baby's sucking will stretch these bands and the nipple will protrude. It really isn't necessary to do anything special during pregnancy to treat inverted nipples. There is no evidence that special exercises or other techniques that stretch the nipple at its base have any effect.

Some mothers may choose to use breast shells during pregnancy to encourage their nipples to protrude. These lightweight plastic cups are worn inside a bra. An inner ring, worn next to the skin, applies gentle pressure on the areola, causing the nipple to protrude through the center. The outer cup holds the bra away from the nipple, for comfort. You wear the breast shells for a few hours a day at first and gradually increase the time you use them. They are not noticeable under clothing. After the baby is born, the shells can be worn before feedings to help the nipple protrude. Breast shells are also called breast shields, milk cups, breast cups, or Woolwich shields.

If wearing breast shells doesn't appeal to you, don't worry about not using them. The best remedy for flat or inverted nipples is a healthy newborn with a good suck. If you're concerned that your baby may have trouble latching on to your breast, you may want to do what you can to minimize the drugs he is exposed to during labor. Some can affect infant sucking in the first days after birth.

After the birth, careful attention to how the baby is positioned at the breast and lots of opportunities for practice enable most full-term healthy babies to latch on and draw out flat and inverted nipples with their sucking. If it's difficult to get your baby to latch on to the breast after birth, ask for help from the hospital's lactation consultant or an experienced nurse. A breast pump or special suction device can also be used to draw out an inverted nipple before feedings.

Inverted nipples need not prevent a mother from breastfeeding.

If you have questions about inverted nipples, or if you're not sure if you have inverted nipples, talk to a La Leche League Leader, board certified lactation consultant, doctor, or midwife with some knowledge of breastfeeding. Many professionals who provide health care for pregnant women routinely check for inverted nipples when doing breast exams. If you have questions about getting started breastfeeding, talk to a La Leche League Leader.

Choosing health care providers

Most doctors nowadays agree with the maxim that "breast is best," but not all of them have learned enough about breastfeeding to be helpful to nursing mothers. Many physicians–even pediatricians–have been taught little or nothing about breastfeeding techniques in the classroom or lecture hall. Many of those who do know the ins and outs of breastfeeding have learned on the job, from watching other knowledgeable health workers, from talking to experienced nursing mothers, or from nursing their own babies.

Physicians who are knowledgeable and enthusiastic about breastfeeding are a blessing to nursing mothers. They help them off to a good start and encourage them to continue. Hospitals with "baby-friendly" routines also make a difference. Studies have shown that breastfeeding rates vary greatly, depending on the hospital staff's attitude toward breastfeeding.

Choosing health-care providers may seem like a daunting task, and the number of eligible candidates may be limited by things beyond your control—for example, geography or the provisions of your health insurance plan. Still, making inquiries, interviewing, and stating your needs ahead of time will help you establish a good relationship with your physician, one that may be very important in the months to come.

There are many ways to find a doctor who suits your needs. Ask around—most people are happy to tell you about their physician. Talking to other mothers at La Leche League meetings is one way to find out about doctors who are supportive of breastfeeding. Calls to local hospitals or area medical societies will also yield names. Your obstetrician or midwife may be able to recommend colleagues who are supportive of breastfeeding.

To find out more about a doctor, call his or her office. The staff there can answer basic questions about office hours, procedures for calling after hours, back-up, professional credentials, hospital affiliation, insurance, and fees. When you've narrowed down the field to just a few names, call and make an appointment to talk with the doctor. Some physicians will give you a free consultation; others may charge a fee.

Make a list of questions to ask at the interview. Don't expect to get them all into the conversation. More important than covering every possible contingency is finding someone with whom you can communicate, who shows genuine respect and interest in your needs and choices, and whose basic philosophy of child-bearing and child-rearing is compatible with yours. Finding a physician who is flexible and willing to work with you to solve a problem is more important than finding one who knows all the "right" answers.

Baby doctors

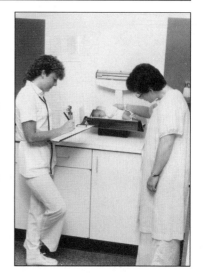

Pediatricians and many family physicians care for infants and children. Besides being available in case of serious illness, they provide well-baby checkups, immunizations, reassurance, and answers to questions about everything from sniffles and rashes to infant behavior, development, and parenting skills.

Look for a physician who shows genuine respect for your choices.

When interviewing potential doctors for your baby, you'll want to inquire about their feelings about breastfeeding. However, it's more important to ask what percentage of babies in the practice are breastfed, and for how long. How many mothers use supplements? When and how does the physician recommend weaning? Were the doctor's own children breastfed? What will the doctor do to help you get off to a good start at breastfeeding in the first days after birth? Following up with these kinds of questions will reveal more about a physician's support for nursing mothers than a simple "How do you feel about breastfeeding?" Ask also about office staff, since you may have as much contact with these people as with the doctor. Do any staff members have a special interest in helping nursing mothers? What are their qualifications and experience?

You may find a supportive, knowledgeable physician on the first try, or you may not find such a creature at all in your community. Let your doctor know what you need and why. Remember that many physicians have learned about breastfeeding from mothers in their practices. Your enthusiasm and knowledge about breastfeeding may rub off on your doctor.

Hospitals and birth attendants

In the first 24 to 48 hours after the birth of a baby, hospital routines loom large in the day and nighttime life of a nursing mother. Breastfeeding gets off to the best start when mother and baby can be together early and often, preferably all the time. New babies need to nurse frequently, but at unpredictable intervals. This is easier to do in hospitals where the baby stays with the mother 24 hours a day or when mother and baby return home soon after the birth. Rules and routines that keep mother in one room and baby in the nursery for specified times of the day interfere with the natural rhythms of breastfeeding and with the mother and baby getting to know one another.

Ideally, hospital staff will not only allow, but also encourage a breastfeeding mother to keep her baby at her side and nurse frequently, following the baby's cues. Keeping baby close also guards against the possibility that nursery staff will give the baby bottles of formula or water or offer a pacifier, all of which can interfere with breastfeeding.

To learn more about a hospital's breastfeeding policies, call and arrange to talk with the head nurse of the birth and postpartum unit. Many hospitals have lactation consultants on staff who can provide hands-on help at early feedings along with specialized assistance if problems develop. Ask if an LC is available and what her credentials are. The letters IBCLC after her name indicate that she has accumulated many hours of experience and has passed a certifying exam.

Breastfeeding women benefit from positive experiences with labor and birth; the feeling that you've managed well and have been treated with respect during the challenges of birthing carries over into your self-

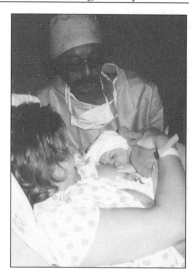

confidence as a mother. While some difficult situations call for all the medical help that modern obstetrics can muster, much of the technology associated with birth in the hospital can hinder a mother in her efforts to give birth naturally. And many of the medications given to mothers in labor and delivery alter infant sucking behavior for several days after birth.

Learn about birth, medical interventions, and ways to cope with contractions by taking childbirth education classes and by reading a variety of books. (The bibliography at the end of this book lists several books on pregnancy and birth.) Discuss your plans for the birth with your care provider. Sometimes it's a good idea to put it all down in writing and ask the doctor to sign the birth plan. You can then take copies to the hospital and refer staff members to your agreement with your doctor if they propose to do something you don't want. You might also want to get orders ahead of time from your baby's doctor, specifying that your baby is to be breastfed frequently and is not to be given formula or water in the nursery.

Of course, you don't have to have a "perfect" birth for breastfeeding to succeed. Breastfeeding will work, even if there are unforeseen complications or you have a cesarean or you and your baby are separated for a time after birth. You can't control everything that happens, even under the best of circumstances. But you can know that once your baby is in your arms, you are just exactly what he needs.

Adjusting your lifestyle

After your baby arrives, you'll be spending lots of time with him, holding him, rocking him, nursing him. Prenatal visions of spotless housekeeping, time for hobbies, and gourmet cooking, all accomplished while the baby takes long naps, will fade into the reality of full-time baby care. There may not be much time for anything else. Life will settle into manageable routines eventually, but the first weeks postpartum go by in a blur for many new families.

Anticipating your after-baby needs can smooth the

transition from one way of life to another. Don't plan on tackling big projects during your baby's first months. If there's heavy cleaning or a decorating project that needs attention, volunteer efforts that demand your time, or a job-related deadline that must be met, plan on getting the work done well ahead of your due date. Give yourself the luxury of devoting as much attention as you desire to your new baby. Stock up on groceries, and cook and freeze meals ahead of time. Clean closets, and give some thought to what you can wear in those first weeks after birth, when your waistline is not yet back to normal and two-piece outfits are handiest for nursing.

If parents, in-laws, or friends offer to help in the days and weeks postpartum, ask them to see to it that you and your family are fed and have clean clothes and a relatively neat environment. Let them know that what you'll need the most is someone to take care of you so that you can take care of and get to know your baby. Tell potential helpers about your plans to breastfeed, and let them know that their support is important to you.

Your helpers should take care of you so that you can care for the baby.

Returning to work

Employers, understandably, want to know if and when mothers will be returning to work after their babies are born. Although it takes some determination, you can continue to breastfeed even if you and your baby are separated during an eight-hour workday. Both you and your baby will benefit, however, from as much time off as possible after the birth, to allow breastfeeding to become well established and to get to know one another.

The strength of your feeling for your baby after he's born may surprise you. Leaving him with a substitute caregiver will be difficult–for you and for him. Babies need to be able to count on their mother's presence to develop to their fullest potential.

If possible, it's wise not to make a firm commitment about your return to work until after the baby is born. After you've had a chance to adjust to being his mother, you can shape your plans according to your baby's needs. Studies have found that part-time

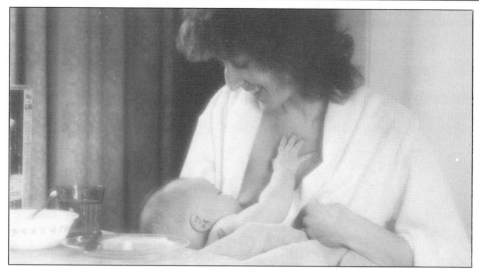

employment is more conducive to continued breastfeeding than working 40 hours a week, and that delaying the return to work by several months also makes breastfeeding easier.

If full-time mothering is possible for you (or you and your partner can find a way to make it possible), give that choice serious consideration. Many psychologists believe that a secure attachment between mother and baby is critical to the child's self-image and ability to form relationships later on. (See the bibliography at the end of the book for more on this subject.)

Staying home

For many women, having their first baby, or sometimes their second, marks a transition into being at home full-time, after having worked for a number of years. Even when you've looked forward to enjoying full-time mothering, the adjustment will take time. Your new lifestyle will bring new demands, a need to find ways of managing your time, even the need to make new friends. Whether your time at home is a maternity leave or the beginning of a new life as a full-time mother, build in plans for taking care of yourself. The quiet moments of rest that come with breastfeeding will help you to find time to read, enjoy some television, converse with your family and friends, or just think and dream. This special time will never come again. Enjoy.

Chapter Three

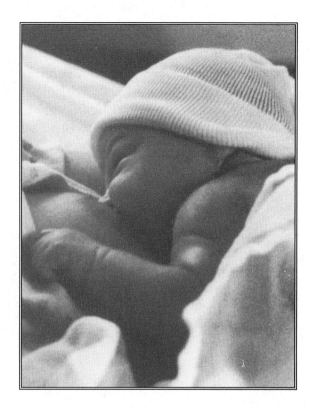

Off to a
Good Start

First breastfeedings are wonderful, exciting, and sometimes a bit awkward.

Babies know a lot about nursing right from the start. Even so, they need some guidance from their mothers—who are learning themselves. Some babies nurse like pros at the very beginning; others may be more tentative in the first few days. You may feel clumsy or inexperienced during these initial feedings, but you and your baby will soon get accustomed to each other.

Newborns, new mothers, and nursing

Babies are born with reflexes that help them learn to feed at the breast. Touch their cheeks and they turn their heads, searching for a nipple. Their mouths open wide, ready to grasp the breast, and once they have latched on, they suck and swallow readily. They even know when their tummies are full and it's time to let go.

Mothers' bodies also react by reflex. Once the placenta is delivered, levels of estrogen and progesterone fall, allowing the hormone prolactin to stimulate plentiful milk production in the breasts within two or three days. This is often referred to as the milk "coming in," and can be quite dramatic. From this point on, the law of supply and demand regulates milk production: the more the baby sucks and the more milk that is removed from the breast, the more milk the mother's body will make.

When the baby is put to the breast, the mother's system releases another hormone, oxytocin, which causes tiny muscles to squeeze the milk out of the cells high in the breast where it is made, forcing it down the milk ducts toward the nipple. This is called the milk-ejection reflex or the let-down. Oxytocin also causes the uterus to contract, helping it return to its non-pregnant size more quickly. These contractions, while beneficial, may be noticeably uncomfortable for a few days, especially with second or subsequent births. Do some deep breathing or try another relaxation technique if these "afterpains" trouble you. You might also talk to your doctor or midwife about using a non-aspirin pain reliever.

Breastfeeding soon after birth

A newborn's first hour or so after birth is spent in quiet alertness, a state where her body is calm and all her energy is focused on seeing and hearing. Newborns in the quiet alert state gaze into adult faces and respond to their mother's voice, already deeply familiar to them from the months spent inside her body. This special time should not be wasted on hospital routines that separate

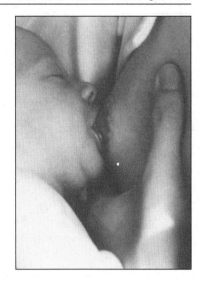

babies from parents. Unless there is a problem requiring immediate attention, newborn babies belong with their mothers. Eyedrops (which temporarily blur infant vision), baths, and exams can wait until parents and baby have had time to become acquainted. Mother's body will keep baby warm, and medical personnel can observe mother and baby without coming between them.

Mothers and babies are often ready to nurse soon after birth, during those magical moments when mother holds the tiny infant who has just emerged from her body. A newborn baby placed on her mother's chest, skin-to-skin, will seek the nipple, nuzzle it, lick it, and very likely latch on and suck. These first attempts at breastfeeding soothe newborns and warm them. They also reassure mothers and help control postpartum bleeding, thanks to the effects of oxytocin on the uterus.

Your partner or one of your care providers can lend a hand with these first attempts at nursing. You may need help getting the baby in a comfortable position at the breast. Don't worry too much about getting everything just perfect at first. Now is a time to relax and enjoy your baby after the hard work of giving birth.

A newborn baby will seek the nipple, latch on, and suck.

Some babies may not be interested in breastfeeding at this time; they may be preoccupied with all the new sensations of life outside the womb. In some cases, mother and baby may be too tired from the work of the delivery; after both have had a good rest they will be ready to begin nursing.

Talk to your birth attendant ahead of time about keeping baby close to you in the first hours after birth and about breastfeeding then. Even if you have a cesarean, it should still be possible for you to share some or all of this special time with your baby.

Getting baby started at the breast

You and your baby will get lots of practice at breastfeeding in the first weeks after birth. It's important to get it right. Expert breastfeeders—babies of five or six

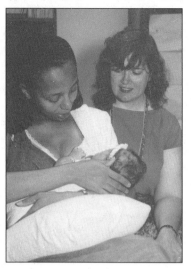

These mothers are using pillows to bring their babies up to the level of their breasts.

Their babies are lying on their sides, tummy to tummy with their mothers, pulled in close for breastfeeding.

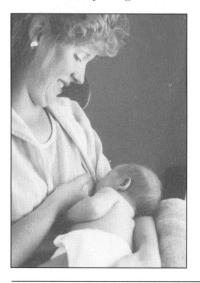

months of age—can nurse efficiently in just about any position, even while wriggling around. But at first, while your baby is learning what to do, you will need to pay careful attention. How you are sitting or lying, how you hold your baby, and how you offer the breast all affect the position of the baby's mouth on the breast as she nurses. Not getting latched on properly can lead to sore nipples for mother, poor weight gain for baby, and frustration for everyone.

Early breastfeedings work best if the baby is alert and calm. Take a few minutes to soothe a fussy baby or wake a sleepy one before you offer the breast.

To wake a sleepy baby gently, lay her along your forearms, facing you at a right angle to your body, and slowly bring her to a more upright position. You can repeat this up-and-down motion while you talk to her and call her name. When she opens her eyes, try to get her to look at you; dim the lights so that she can keep her eyes open comfortably. If the room is not cold or drafty, undress her down to her diaper. Babies nurse better when they are not too warm, and skin-to-skin contact with mother is very stimulating. A lightweight receiving blanket tucked around both of you will keep her cozy.

Positioning the baby

When you and your baby are ready to nurse, the first thing to do is make sure that you are comfortable. Use pillows to support your back so that you can sit up straight or lean back at a slight angle. Place one or two pillows on your lap to bring the baby's mouth up to the level of your nipple. A pillow can also help support your elbow. You should not have to lean over your baby to nurse her, nor should you be leaning way back. It's usually easier to breastfeed in a straight, comfortable chair with arms than sitting up in a hospital bed. If you're not very tall, a footstool or a few big books under your feet can help you sit straighter and more comfortably. If you're sitting in bed, bend your knees and support them with a pillow to help straighten your back and shoulders.

Hold your baby on her side, her head at the inside of your elbow, her neck and shoulders supported along your forearm, and your hand at her buttocks. Her head, neck, and body should be in a straight line. Pull her in close; you and she should be tummy-to-tummy. Your baby should not have to turn her head to take the breast. (It's very hard to swallow with your head turned sideways—try it!) Her bottom arm can nestle into your abdomen, or extend back around your waist, whichever is more comfortable.

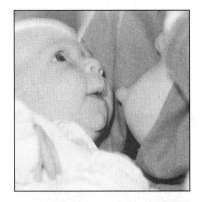

Hold your breast with your hand in the shape of a C, fingers underneath, thumb on top, well back from the areola. Cup your breast gently, don't squeeze and distort its shape. If you have large breasts, try using a rolled-up towel or receiving blanket underneath to help support the breast. If your breasts are small, you may not need to support them at all once the feeding is underway.

Latching on and sucking

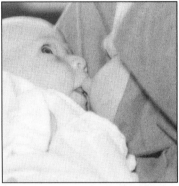

Tickle the baby's lips lightly with your nipple to encourage her to open wide. As she opens her mouth wide, quickly pull her in close to take the breast. The nipple should be far back in her mouth, and she should take at least an inch of the areola as well. The tip of her nose should be touching the breast. Even when pulled in this close, she will not have trouble breathing; babies' noses are turned up and their nostrils flare out just so they can breathe while breastfeeding. The baby's chin should also touch the breast, and her lips should be flanged outward.

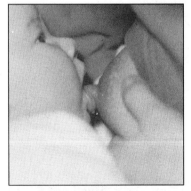

Proper positioning of the baby at the breast and the baby's mouth on the breast help her to compress the milk ducts under the areola and obtain the most milk. Good positioning also protects mother's nipple. Breastfeeding should not hurt. Sore nipples are caused by friction—the baby's tongue or gums rubbing the sensitive skin of the nipple during sucking. If the nipple is far enough back in the baby's mouth, it is away from all the movement that can cause damage.

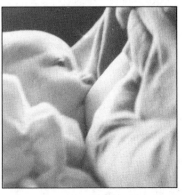

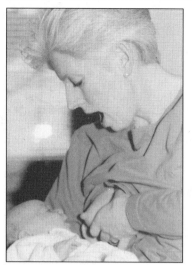

*Say "Open" to encourage your baby
to open her mouth wide
like a yawn.*

Problems? Try again

Don't worry if your baby doesn't latch on at the first try. Stay calm, and try again. If the baby is sucking only on the end of the nipple, press down a bit on the breast tissue or put your finger into the corner of the baby's mouth to break the suction and take the baby off. Check the baby's position and yours, and then offer the breast again. Don't let the baby suck only on the nipple—you'll soon get sore.

Some babies need some encouragement to get them to open their mouths wide. Try saying "open" as you open your own mouth; newborn babies can imitate adult facial expressions and learn to associate a word with an action. Your baby will latch on better and nurse more efficiently if you can teach her to take a large portion of the breast all at once, rather than slurping the nipple into a half-open mouth with two or three sucks.

If the baby starts to get upset before she has latched on properly, take a few moments to calm her down. Put her up on your shoulder, rub her back, walk around the room, and when she is ready, try again to put her to the breast. She can't learn what to do if she is crying. You'll find that she's easier to comfort if you catch her before she totally goes to pieces.

If you, too, are becoming very frustrated, get some help—someone to soothe the baby while you take some deep breaths or walk away for a few minutes. Your helper can also arrange pillows for you, get you a glass of water or juice, hold a tiny hand that gets in the way, or help you anticipate just the right moment to pull the baby close to the breast to get her latched on.

Signs of effective sucking

Once the baby is latched on, she will start to suck. The first rapid sucks stimulate your let-down reflex; after the milk lets down, the rhythm will change to slow, even sucks with swallowing after every two or three sucks. Some women feel a tingling sensation in their breasts with the let-down, while others do not. However, the change in the rhythm of the baby's sucking indicates for certain that the reflex is operating.

When the baby is sucking well, you will see her ears (or her temples) wiggle as her lower jaw moves to compress the areola and release the milk. A baby who is latched on and sucking well should not slip off the breast easily. Some babies nurse best if mother is quiet and distractions are kept to a minimum. Others—at least in the first days—may need some encouragement to stick with it. Your voice and your touch can keep baby alert and breastfeeding until her tummy is full.

When to stop

Babies can decide for themselves when they're finished nursing or when they're ready to switch to the other breast. Limiting breastfeedings to five or ten or twenty minutes a side does not prevent sore nipples, and it can cause other problems. Let your baby nurse as long as she likes on the first side. When she has had enough she'll let go of the breast on her own.

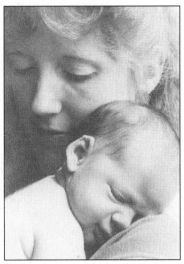

This baby is obviously satisfied and has a full tummy.

When your baby comes off the breast, burp her gently. If you place her on your shoulder to burp, her tummy should rest on your shoulder bones to encourage the air to come up. You can also place her in a sitting position to burp, with one hand supporting her chest, neck, and chin and the other patting or rubbing her back. If the bubble comes up in a minute or so, fine; if not, don't worry about it unless your baby seems uncomfortable. Not all babies need to be burped after breastfeeding.

Offer the baby the other breast, and let her nurse as long as she likes—until she lets go of the breast, or drifts off to sleep. If she nurses for only a short time on the second breast, be sure to start the next feeding on this same side.

If your baby falls asleep at the second breast, don't wake her to burp her. In fact, this is a good time to doze off yourself. If you and baby are well supported, snuggled into pillows, you don't need to worry about dropping her. Just enjoy the chance to relax.

If the baby's sucking slows nearly to a stop and she seems to be drifting off to sleep without having nursed long enough (a total of ten to twenty minutes of

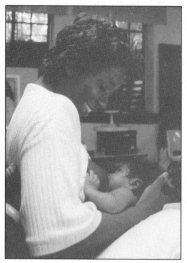

The football hold: The baby is bent at the hips and her feet are up, not pushing against the back of the chair.

The mother's hand controls the back of the baby's head.

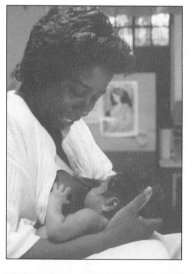

active sucking, with swallowing), you can take her off the breast and use a burping session or a diaper change to rouse her enough to nurse some more.

To release the suction, press down on your breast, slide a clean finger into the baby's mouth, or pull down gently on her chin. Don't "pop" the baby off the breast without breaking the suction first. It will hurt!

Other positions for breastfeeding

The cradle hold described above is not the only way to hold a breastfeeding baby. Sometimes there are reasons for choosing another position—the football (or clutch) hold or the transitional hold.

When using the football hold, again start by making sure that you are comfortable, your back and shoulders well supported by pillows. The baby faces you, and your hand supports her head and neck. Your baby's body is tucked under your arm, to the side, and her bottom rests on pillows that are high enough to bring her up to the level of the breast. Use your other hand to support and offer the breast, waiting for the baby's mouth to open wide and then pulling her head in close. In the football hold, it is easier to see the baby latch on to the breast, and you can provide continuous gentle support on the back of the head to help keep the baby's head in position. Once the baby is latched on and nursing well, you can settle back comfortably into the pillows. If the hand and arm holding the baby begin to get tired, you can slide another pillow or folded receiving blanket underneath for support. Or you can place your foot on a footstool or a low table and use your thigh to prop up your arm.

The transitional hold is useful when babies need extra help latching on. It is similar to the cradle hold, except that your arms exchange jobs. If you are nursing on the left breast, the right arm and hand hold the baby and the left hand supports the breast. Use pillows behind you for comfort and pillows in your lap to bring the baby up to the breast. The baby is turned on her side, tummy-to-tummy with you, and your hand supports the back of her head and neck as she latches on and sucks. As with the football hold, you can apply gentle support to help keep her latched on and nursing. Use a folded blanket or a small pillow under your hand or forearm if they begin to tire.

For some babies, the feeling of mother's hand on the back of the head or mother's fingers near their cheeks is too stimulating. The feel of skin on skin confuses them, and they turn their heads from side to side toward the hand, searching for a nipple. A receiving blanket or a cloth diaper placed between your hand and the baby's head will solve the problem.

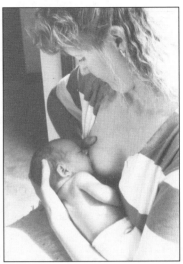
Transitional hold

Breastfeeding while lying down

Nursing while lying down has helped many a tired mother get the rest she needs. It's also a great way to soothe babies off to sleep, or to nurse at night with minimal interruption of your sleep.

You can make yourself comfortable lying on your side with a pillow behind your lower back, pillows under your head, and perhaps a pillow under the knee of your upper leg. Your body is not perpendicular to the bed; instead, you lean back slightly into the pillow behind you. (This is also a comfortable sleeping position for late in pregnancy.)

Your baby is on her side, facing you, mouth at the level of your nipple, and pulled in very close. Your forearm and the crook of your elbow support her back, shoulders, and neck—much as they do in the cradle hold, only lying down. Use your other hand to support and offer the breast, encouraging your baby to open wide and latch on. If you (and your baby) prefer, you can put the baby down on the bed and tuck your arm up under your head, using a folded blanket, towel, or pillow to keep the baby positioned on her side.

To nurse from the other breast, hold the baby on your chest, roll over, and reposition yourself. Or you can continue lying on the same side and roll your body toward the bed to offer the top breast. This second method is more likely to work if your baby is a little older and more adept at latching on.

Some babies catch on to lying-down nursing right from the start; others may need to grow a bit before it works well. Even if you feel awkward at first, keep trying; it's a skill worth mastering.

Pull baby close to you to nurse lying down.

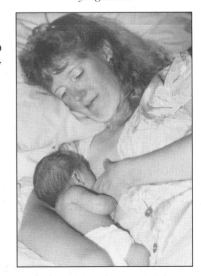

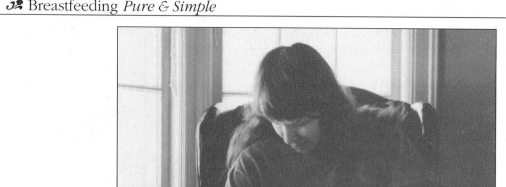

Worrying about getting it right

All these instructions about positioning your baby at the breast can make breastfeeding sound tricky and complicated. As with many other things, it takes a lot more time to explain how to breastfeed your baby than to do it. Putting the baby to the breast quickly becomes second nature for most mothers and babies.

Seeing breastfeeding in action can be a more effective way to learn than reading about what to do. Attending La Leche League meetings gives you an opportunity to observe other breastfeeding mothers and babies. Videos about breastfeeding can also be helpful, although it's best to stick with materials available from breastfeeding advocates, such as La Leche League, rather than free tapes distributed to new mothers from formula companies.

If you and your new baby are experiencing problems getting started at the breast, don't give up—get to work. Most latch-on and sucking problems improve within a few days with patience and persistence. The longer you wait, the longer it can take to teach a baby to nurse efficiently. Use the basic principles described above, and look to the next chapter for further suggestions. Call a La Leche League Leader, or if you're in the hospital, ask to see the lactation consultant or a nurse with experience helping breastfeeding mothers. With a little help, you and your baby will soon work things out.

No bottles, frequent breastfeeding

Most newborns will breastfeed eight to twelve times every twenty-four hours. These feedings will not be at regularly scheduled intervals. If your baby is rooming-in with you, you can offer to nurse her whenever she seems hungry or fretful. You'll soon learn to read her cues, whatever they are—a fist in the mouth, an open mouth searching for a nipple, restlessness, a certain cry.

Newborns breastfeed for lots of reasons besides hunger. Cuddling close to mother's breast and sucking rhythmically help babies get themselves under control when the sights and sounds of the big world threaten to overwhelm them. Go ahead and offer the breast if your baby seems fussy, even if it has been only ten or twenty minutes since she last nursed. Think of it as your baby's dessert. The comfort of breastfeeding and a little more milk may be just what she needs to fall asleep. Many mothers find that breastfeeding for another few minutes is a lot easier than walking the floor with a fussy baby.

Newborns will breastfeed eight to twelve times in twenty-four hours.

Frequent breastfeedings in the early days benefit both mothers and babies. The baby gets lots of colostrum, the first milk that is especially rich in antibodies. Frequent feedings help the baby pass meconium, her first stools, more quickly, which helps to prevent jaundice. These early feedings are also a good opportunity for the baby to master latching-on and sucking before the mother's milk becomes more plentiful and feeding at the breast may be somewhat more challenging. Mothers, too, gain confidence with frequent early breastfeedings; they're reminded of how important they are to their newborns. Frequent breastfeedings bring in the full milk supply sooner and help prevent problems with engorged and painful breasts. Also, nursing helps the uterus return to its pre-pregnant size more quickly.

If your baby is staying in the hospital nursery, ask that she be brought to you whenever she awakens or any time that she cries. Be very specific about asking that she be brought to you during the night for feedings. Tell the nurses that you want to be awakened and that you don't want your baby given bottles "so that mother can get her rest." Taping a "no bottles, no pacifier" sign to the baby's crib informs anyone who might be caring for your baby of your wishes.

Risks of giving bottles and formula

Breastfeeding newborns don't need supplementary bottles of formula or glucose water. Sugar water will not "wash out the jaundice," nor is it needed for preventing hypoglycemia in healthy babies; frequent feedings at the breast will help your baby avoid both of these problems. Supplements interfere with the supply and demand principle that regulates how much milk the mother produces. A baby with a tummy full of artificial formula or water may not be willing to nurse at the breast again for several hours. The mother's body reacts to the lowered demand for breast milk by producing less. If the baby then gets even more supplemental formula or water, the mother's milk supply dwindles still further, and mother and baby are on the road to early weaning.

The artificial nipples screwed onto those bottles can also cause lots of problems with breastfeeding in the early days. It doesn't matter if the nipple's attached to a bottle of formula or water, to a bottle of expressed breast milk, or to a pacifier—sucking on an artificial nipple is different from sucking at the breast. Many babies can become confused if they are asked to learn how to do both at the same time, at least in the beginning. They try to nurse at the breast as if they were sucking at a rubber nipple. It doesn't work, and mother and baby both get very frustrated. Nursing at the breast isn't really harder than feeding from a bottle; studies have shown that bottle-feeding is actually more physiologically stressful than breastfeeding. But breastfeeding does require a certain finesse.

Even if you will be returning to work or want your baby to take an occasional bottle when you are separated, it's better to wait until four to six weeks of age—when the baby has mastered breastfeeding and your milk supply is well established—before introducing an artificial nipple. You may have heard that it can sometimes be difficult to get an older breastfed baby to accept a bottle, but there are ways to overcome this problem, if you should face it in the future. With some very young babies, even one experience with a bottle or pacifier is enough to cause breastfeeding problems that can lead to early weaning.

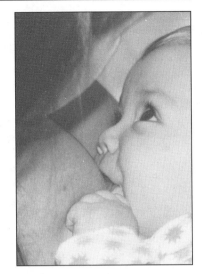

If your baby does get some bottles in the first few days, for whatever reason, all is not lost. Many babies have no trouble switching from breast to bottle. However, you have no way of knowing before giving that bottle whether or not it will cause problems for your baby. It's better to avoid the risk and get breastfeeding off to a good start. The next chapter has suggestions for what to do about nipple confusion.

Supplemental bottles of formula also carry the risk of allergies. Soy formula as well as cow's milk formula can cause allergic reactions, especially when given to a baby only a day or two old. Your baby's delicate digestive system can be overwhelmed by foreign foods, even if the manufacturing process has "humanized" them. Authentic human milk protects babies' immature immune systems and prepares them gradually for the introduction of other foods.

Engorgement

Overly full, engorged breasts can be a problem in the early days of breastfeeding, as your milk supply adjusts to the baby's demand. Nursing the baby frequently is the best way to relieve engorgement, and get your body tuned in to your baby. Use warm moist washcloths applied to the breast for a few minutes before feedings to help get the milk flowing, and try gentle breast massage as well. Cold compresses (crushed ice in a plastic bag or even a bag of frozen vegetables) will reduce swelling and pain between feedings. Don't put the ice bag directly on the breast; use a cloth or towel to protect the skin. You can also use a pump or try hand expression for a few minutes to soften the breasts when the baby won't nurse or to make it easier for the baby to latch on at the beginning of feedings. While you don't want to stimulate your breasts to produce more milk, it is important to relieve the pressure and prevent the possibility of plugged ducts.

Getting enough?

When you're breastfeeding, it's surprisingly simple to tell if your baby is getting enough milk. True, you can't count the ounces as they're going in, but you can keep track of what's coming out the other end.

Once your milk "comes in," your baby should have five or six wet diapers a day if you're using disposables, or six to eight wet cloth diapers daily. After the black, tarry meconium has been cleared from their system, young breastfed babies will have two to five bowel movements every twenty-four hours; these will be loose and unformed, possibly seedy. They will be yellow to yellow-green or tan in color, with only a mild odor, as long as the baby is getting only human milk. Some babies have small bowel movements after nearly every feeding. In the early weeks, frequent bowel movements are a sign that the baby is getting plenty of the hindmilk, the milk far up in the breast that is released by the let-down reflex. This milk is higher in fat, and it's full of the calories that babies need to grow.

If your baby has plenty of wet diapers and bowel movements, there's no need to worry about whether she is getting enough milk. What comes out must have gone in! After six weeks of age, older breastfed babies' bowel movements may be several days apart, with no signs of constipation.

If your new baby is not having enough wet diapers and bowel movements within a day or two of your milk coming in, you need to take action. Read more about weight gain problems in the next chapter, and call a La Leche League Leader for help with figuring out ways to get your baby to breastfeed better. Most breastfeeding problems improve quickly with a few days of patient, persistent attention.

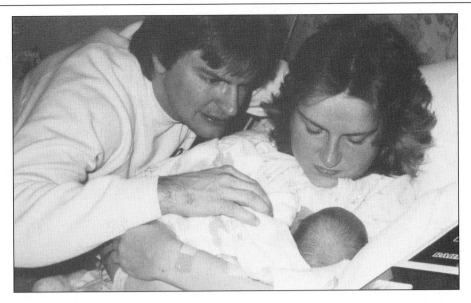

Breastfeeding after a cesarean

Breastfeeding works for mothers who have given birth by cesarean, too. All the same principles apply. Once the placenta is removed from the uterus during the surgery, the hormonal process that stimulates milk production goes to work, and the milk becomes more plentiful within a few days. In the meantime, frequent nursing and lots of contact with your baby will help get breastfeeding off to a good start.

Depending on the reasons for the operation, the type of anesthetic used, and the availability of assistance, you may be able to hold and nurse your baby right on the operating table or in the recovery room. Your partner or a nurse can help you position the baby at the breast or just hold and stroke her and talk to her. If you have had regional, rather than general anesthesia, this is a good time to get to know your baby, before the effects of the medication wear off and you begin to feel discomfort. General anesthesia can leave you feeling groggy and disoriented and not yet ready to take in the idea of having a new baby, but as soon as you are feeling alert, ask for your baby to be brought to you to nurse.

Many hospitals routinely provide for early contact between mothers and babies after cesareans; in others, you will have to ask to see your baby and keep her close. If you know ahead of time that your baby will be born by cesarean, you can plan ahead for these important hours by discussing your needs with your doctor and the hospital staff. If your cesarean is not planned, you or your partner can still request that mother and baby be kept together as much as possible, as long as both are doing well.

Breastfeeding positions after cesarean surgery

Positioning yourself for breastfeeding may take some care in the first day or two after surgery. For some mothers, the side-lying position works well after a cesarean. Begin with the bed flat and the side railings up. Grasp the railings to help yourself roll carefully onto your side. Besides using pillows to support your head, back, and upper knee, use a small pillow or a folded towel over your abdomen to protect your incision from baby's sudden movements. Your partner or a nurse can help you position the baby and switch sides when it's necessary. After a day or two, you'll be able to hold the baby to your chest and, keeping your feet flat on the bed, turn your hips a little at a time to roll over and move the baby to the other side.

Other mothers find it easier to get their babies latched on to the breast if they are sitting up. You will be more comfortable sitting in a chair than trying to sit up straight in bed. Be sure to place pillows in your lap, to protect your incision as well as to bring the baby up to breast height. You might also need a pillow behind your lower back. The football hold will keep baby off your lap entirely, if that seems necessary.

You'll want to breastfeed your baby frequently, following her cues, with no supplements and no pacifiers. Ask that she be brought to you whenever she awakens or seems hungry or fussy, even at night. Rooming-in is possible after a cesarean, particularly if your partner or another helper can be with you to help with diaper changes and feedings. Hospital personnel can fill in if your helper can't be present all the time.

Medications and complications

Most medications given routinely after cesareans are compatible with breastfeeding. Sometimes a baby born by cesarean may be drowsy in the early days from the anesthetic or other medications used during labor. This can affect breastfeeding behavior. Most medications given for pain following a cesarean birth do not appear in mother's milk at levels likely to affect the baby, so you should not hesitate to use pain-relieving medication in the days after birth. Breastfeeding will get off to a better start if you are not putting up with a lot of discomfort. Talk to your doctor or to a nurse if you do have concerns about medications or about how your baby is taking the breast.

Women who've had cesareans are more likely to run a low fever in the days after birth. This should not lead to routine separation of the mother and the baby. Some fevers are the result of swelling in the breast tissue that accompanies the rapid increase in milk production a few days after birth. If the doctor wants to isolate you from other patients because of the possibility of infection, ask that you and your baby be isolated together. Washing your hands before holding your baby will prevent any infection from spreading.

A cesarean delivery may not be the birth you looked forward to during your pregnancy, and you may need time to grieve over what was supposed to have been and to adjust to what actually happened. These feelings of loss or anger can be hard for you and others to acknowledge at the same time that you are rejoicing over your new baby. Find someone with whom you can talk about your feelings–a friend, your partner, perhaps a nurse with a knack for listening. Hospital personnel or your local La Leche League Leader may be able to refer you to a nearby cesarean support group.

Spend lots of time touching and holding and admiring your baby. These kinds of positive interactions with your baby will help to heal many of the negative feelings that can arise from an unplanned cesarean birth. Go easy on yourself. Each of us is trying hard to do the best she can, but we can't control everything that happens in our lives. Even if you and your baby are separated in the first hours or days after birth, you'll have plenty of time to spend together breastfeeding and just enjoying one another in the months to come.

Chapter Four

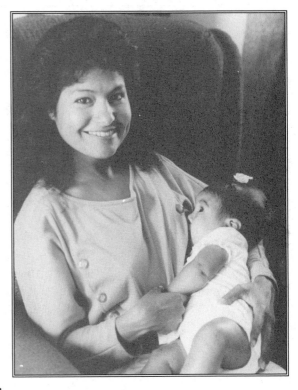

Solving Problems

Difficulties with breastfeeding are not unusual and can have many causes.

Mothers should not blame themselves for problems that occur. Many are the result of a lack of information or poor advice. In other cases, the baby's behavior is part of the problem. It may take time for even a mother who has nursed previous children to learn how best to nurture, understand, and breastfeed this particular baby.

Most breastfeeding problems improve within a day or two. The best solutions are ones that keep mother and baby working together. Temporary weaning or giving supplementary bottles seldom solves the problem, but these things do interfere with the mother's milk supply, the baby's sucking skills, and the developing interdependent relationship of mother and nursling. It's important to be sure that baby is getting enough to eat, but if the baby does need additional nutrition, supplements can be given in ways that don't interfere with breastfeeding.

Don't let breastfeeding problems, which may last only a few days, keep you from enjoying months of nurturing your child at the breast. But don't just endure any difficulties that come your way, hoping things will get better. Figure out what's wrong and why, and take some action. Get help if you need it, from a La Leche League Leader or a lactation consultant–someone with experience in helping mothers succeed at breastfeeding. Not only will you solve the problem; in the process, you'll also get to know your baby better and grow to feel more confident as a mother.

Why nipples get sore

The good news is it shouldn't hurt to breastfeed. Nevertheless, many new mothers do experience some nipple soreness in the early days, while they and their babies are working out some of the finer points of latching onto and sucking at the breast. If your nipples are sore, not only will you want to find ways to ease the pain, but you'll also want to try and determine what's causing the discomfort, so that you can fix it and stop dreading the next nursing.

The most frequent cause of sore nipples is the baby not taking enough of the breast tissue into his mouth while nursing. Babies should feed from breasts, not just nipples. They need to take at least an inch of the areola, the pigmented area behind the nipple, as well as the nipple itself. Otherwise, the nipple, with its tender skin and sensitive nerve endings, ends up in the front of the baby's mouth, where his gums and tongue can rub against the same sore spot with every suck.

If the baby takes more of the breast tissue into his mouth, the nipple will end up farther back where it can't get hurt. The baby will also get more milk more easily, as his gums and tongue compress the milk sinuses (the reservoirs where milk is held) that lie directly underneath the areola. You can locate the milk sinuses by trying to express milk by hand from the breast. Cup your hand around your breast with your fingers behind the nipple. Press your hand back in toward your chest while squeezing your fingers together on the breast. When you see milk spurt from the nipple, you'll know you've found the milk sinuses; you'll notice that they are an inch or so behind where your nipples hurt. This is where the baby's gums should be during feedings.

Flat or inverted nipples

Flat or inverted nipples may make it more difficult for some babies to latch on to the breast and take in enough breast tissue to nurse efficiently. Try firming up the nipple by rolling it between your fingers before offering the breast to the baby. Wearing breast shells for twenty to thirty minutes before a feeding will also bring the nipple out. If your nipple seems flat because there is a lot of milk in your breasts, gently hand-express some milk before starting the feeding—just enough to soften the nipple and areola. Flat or inverted nipples can also be drawn out by using a breast pump for a few minutes before trying to get the baby latched on.

Try to stay calm and patient as you work with your baby.

Working toward a better latch-on

Gritting your teeth and putting up with pain during feedings is no solution to latch-on problems. The baby becomes accustomed to doing the wrong thing, and sore areas on nipples quickly turn into painful cracks and blisters.

As you work on improving your baby's latching-on skills, try to stay calm and patient. If the baby doesn't get it right on the first attempt, gently take him off the breast and keep working with him until he latches on correctly. If you and your baby are getting more and more frustrated, stop for a while, wait for everyone to calm down, and come back to it again in fifteen or

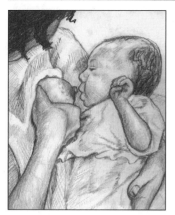

Tickle baby's lips.

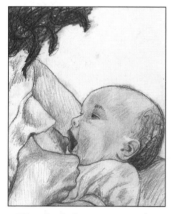

Wait for baby to open wide.

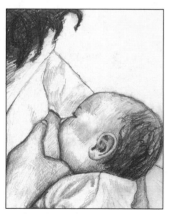

When baby is latched on well, his nose and chin should touch your breast.

twenty minutes. Most babies do catch on within a few days.

Encouraging your baby to latch on better calls for a trip back to the basics. Reread the section on positioning the baby at the breast and latching-on in chapter 3. As you work with your baby, pay careful attention to the following points.

Make sure that you and the baby are well supported, with pillows in your lap and under your elbow all through the feeding; sometimes a baby who has latched on well at the beginning slips down onto the nipple as the feeding goes on and the mother's arm tires. Perhaps you need to be sitting straighter, not leaning back and not hunched over the baby. Remember that you are bringing the baby to the breast, rather than putting the nipple in the baby's mouth as you would with a bottle.

Wait for the baby to open his mouth wide, like a yawn, before pulling him in close to take the breast. Try to anticipate when his mouth will be open the farthest so that it happens just as he takes the breast. Be sure he takes lots of the areola underneath the nipple as well as on top. With some babies, getting that mouth open wide calls for lots of patience. Extending a curved index finger from the hand supporting the breast to firmly push down on the baby's chin can encourage him to open his mouth and keep it open while he latches on and nurses.

The baby's nose and chin should touch the breast as he nurses. If they don't, he has not taken enough of the breast into his mouth. Take him off the breast, and try again.

The baby's lips should be flanged outward. Sometimes a baby sucks his lower lip in as he nurses, and this can cause soreness. If this is the case, you can pull the lip gently outward while the baby sucks, without having to stop the feeding. Also check that the tongue is under the breast, where it belongs, by pulling down gently on the lower lip during nursing. You or a helper should be able to see the tongue resting on the baby's lower gum. If it's not visible, and your nipple hurts, try the latch-on again, making sure that the tongue is down and the baby has opened his mouth very wide as he takes the breast.

Your baby's body should be pulled in close during the entire feeding, his tummy against yours, in both the cradle hold or while nursing lying down. This helps him to stay latched on and suck properly. Be sure to support his head right up at the level of the nipple. Sometimes the football hold or the transitional hold provides better support for babies who need more help in controlling their heads.

When the baby seems overwhelmed by the amount or shape of breast tissue confronting him at the start of a feeding, a technique called the "nipple sandwich" can make latching on easier. This is a slightly different way of supporting the breast while baby latches on. Instead of holding the breast with your hand roundly cupped like a C, flatten the breast tissue somewhat between your thumb above and fingers beneath. Pull back slightly on the tissue to make the nipple protrude. Babies often find it easier to grasp the breast when its shape is compressed like this.

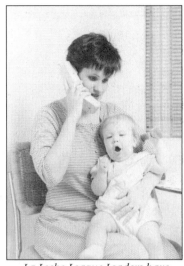

La Leche League Leaders have experience nursing their own babies and can provide the support and information you need.

Call a La Leche League Leader for support and more suggestions about solving latch-on problems. You may be able to get together with her so that she can see what your baby is doing at the breast and help you figure out what to do about it. A lactation consultant or other medical professional with experience helping breastfeeding mothers may also be able to work with you and help you teach your baby to latch on to the breast correctly.

Call a La Leche League Leader for suggestions about latch-on problems.

Soothing sore nipples

The breasts themselves provide an excellent substance for soothing and healing sore or cracked nipples: human milk. Express a little milk after a feeding, spread it over the nipple and areola, and let it air-dry. The milk's anti-bacterial qualities will help the nipples heal.

Keeping the nipples dry between feedings will hasten healing. Leave the cups of your nursing bra open after feedings to allow air to get at the nipples. Try going braless under a soft cotton t-shirt. If you can't bear to have clothing touching your nipples, breast shells with large air holes worn inside a bra can hold the fabric away from tender skin while allowing air to circulate. (A La Leche League Leader can tell you where to purchase these.) Avoid bras and nursing pads that are made from synthetic fibers or that contain a layer of plastic.

Many of the creams and ointments sold for the treatment of sore nipples must be removed before feedings since they are not safe for babies. This can hurt and irritate rather than help. Modified lanolin, sold under the name Lansinoh® for Breastfeeding Mothers, is safe to use on nipples during breastfeeding; it is pure and has nothing in it that could affect the baby. It helps the skin retain its inner moisture, which aids in healing. It also prevents cracks or blisters from forming scabs and keeps the skin soft and pliable. To use it, pat your nipples dry after feeding and apply a small amount to the nipple and areola. Lansinoh® is available from La Leche League International and local La Leche League Groups, as well as in many pharmacies and discount stores.

Breastfeeding while your nipples are sore

Improved positioning and latch-on will usually put an end to sore nipples, but feedings may still be uncomfortable while blistered or cracked nipples heal. Often the most painful part of the feeding is right at the beginning, before the let-down, when the baby is sucking but not getting much milk. Feedings will be easier if you start on the side that is less sore and switch to the more tender side after you notice the baby swallowing more frequently (a sign that the let-down has occurred). If both nipples are very sore, try hand expression or gentle stimulation with a breast pump to trigger the let-down before putting the baby on the breast. Deep breathing and other relaxation techniques from childbirth classes can ease discomfort during the feeding.

Be sure to break the suction before taking the baby off the breast. "Popping" the breast out of the baby's mouth, even just once or twice, can leave nipples hurting for a long time.

Nipple shields, artificial nipples that you place over your own during feedings, are not much help with either sore nipples or latch-on problems. In fact, they usually make things worse. They interfere with the baby learning to latch on and suck correctly, and they decrease the amount of stimulation to the mother's breast, which can affect her milk supply and her let-down reflex. Use of a nipple shield can cause nipple confusion in the same way that other artificial nipples do.

Sore nipples should not go on for days and weeks. Remember, it shouldn't hurt to breastfeed. If your nipples are not improving and feedings are very uncomfortable, get some help in figuring out what's wrong.

Sleepy babies, lazy nursers, and other slow-to-get-started types

Some babies take longer than others in learning to breastfeed effectively. They lose weight in the early days and are slow to regain it. They don't produce six to eight wet cloth diapers (five to six disposables) and two to five bowel movements daily, and hence, don't seem to be getting enough milk. Because of the poor feeding, they are more likely to become jaundiced. Their mothers feel worried and frustrated and don't know what to do. They don't want to give bottles, but breastfeeding does not seem to be working.

There's no need to give up on breastfeeding. These kinds of problems are solvable, often with only a few days of careful attention. It can be hard to muster the will and energy you need to work at breastfeeding during the ups and downs of postpartum adjustments. But if you feel that breastfeeding is important to you and your baby, weeks from now when you have a happy nursing baby, you'll be glad and proud that you made the effort.

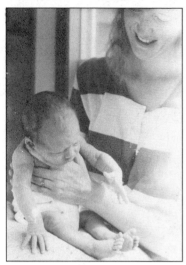

Undress a baby down to his diaper to help him stay awake through feedings.

The sleepy baby

Newborns are often sleepy in the first days after birth, and some babies seem to prefer sleeping to nursing. They don't wake up very often for feedings, or they go right back to sleep after only a few minutes or a few sucks at the breast. They don't produce many wet diapers or bowel movements, and may be slow to gain weight, even after the mother's milk has come in. Sleepiness can result from a difficult labor and birth, from medications used during labor, or from another problem, such as jaundice or prematurity.

Don't just sit back and wait for your sleeping beauty to awaken for feedings. Remember that most newborns nurse at least eight to twelve times in twenty-four hours. If he has slept for more than two or three hours during the day, wake him. It's easiest to do if he's in a light sleep cycle—restless, eyes moving under the eyelids, making sucking movements. Talk to him and try to make eye contact. Hold him in an upright position or bend him at the hips into gentle sit-ups on your lap. Change his diaper, rub his back, wipe his face with a cool, damp cloth—anything that seems to stimulate him.

To prevent a baby from drifting off to sleep too soon during a feeding, switch sides as soon as he begins to lose interest in feeding. This technique is called "switch nursing." When he's no longer swallowing after every one or two sucks, take him off the breast, sit him up, burp him, or change his diaper to wake him up. Then offer the other side. When his nursing slows down again, take him off, rouse him, and go back to the first side. Keep switching back and forth for twenty minutes or so before you let him go back into a deep sleep. Be certain that he latches on well and takes the breast far back into his mouth as he nurses.

The lazy nurser

The lazy nurser seems to nurse all the time and yet is never satisfied. He cries when his mother ends a feeding. His lazy nursing style doesn't stimulate the breast enough to produce let-downs during the feeding, and so he doesn't get the richer, higher calorie milk that will make him feel full. He may produce plenty of wet diapers, but few bowel movements. His mother's milk supply may be dwindling because of his ineffective sucking. He is probably losing weight. The lazy nurser uses only his lips to suck. You won't see his jaw moving or his ears wiggling while he nurses. He may nurse almost continuously and protest being taken off the breast.

The switch nursing technique described above will help the lazy nurser learn to suck better. You may have to switch him as often as every thirty or sixty seconds at first, to keep him sucking well and swallowing regularly. Pay close attention to how he latches on.

Sucking problems

Some babies come off the breast easily while nursing. Some don't use their tongues correctly. Some invent other tricks. These kinds of problems may require assistance from someone who has experience with sucking problems. A La Leche League Leader may be able to provide the help you need, or you may wish to arrange to see a lactation consultant. If the Leader or the LC you contact can't give you the assistance you need, she will know who can. And she will be glad to go on providing support and encouragement while you help your baby learn to breastfeed better.

Pumping and supplementing

Babies who are not breastfeeding well by the third day postpartum need to be evaluated carefully. They may temporarily need more nourishment than they are able to take from the breast. Baby's breastfeeding problems can also cause a decrease in the mother's milk supply. Pumping after feedings and giving the pumped milk to the baby will help the mother's body continue to produce plenty of milk, and the baby will get the best possible nutrition while he is learning to breastfeed better.

Renting an electric pump is well worth the money, especially if you are pumping milk in the early days postpartum, when frequent breast stimulation is important for establishing a good milk supply. (Your health insurance should pay for the pump if your doctor writes orders for it.) The electric pumps available for rental are very efficient, easy to use, and allow you to pump both breasts at once, or pump from one side while the baby is nursing on the other. Some mothers find that hand pumps work well also, but they require more effort from you. You'll need to pump for ten to twenty minutes after each feeding–for as long as the milk is flowing. For more on pumping and storing milk, see the section at the end of this chapter.

The milk you pump after feedings is high in fat and calories, exactly what your baby needs to start growing. Avoid giving it to him in a bottle; artificial nipples usually make breastfeeding problems worse. One alternative to bottle-feeding is cup-feeding. Use a small, flexible plastic cup, one that can be bent or squeezed slightly to form a spout. Support the baby upright in your lap, with a towel or diaper tucked under his chin. Rest the cup on his lower lip and tip it gently so that a few drops flow onto baby's lips. Allow him to sip and swallow the milk at his own pace. You can also use an eyedropper or even a teaspoon to give babies extra milk. Be patient. This can take time, but it really does work. Usually you'll want to give the supplement after the baby nurses. If your baby seems very hungry and irritable, giving him a small amount from the cup before a feeding may settle him down and help him breastfeed better. Experiment and see what works well for your baby.

Supplemental milk can be given using a cup, eyedropper, or teaspoon.

Supplemental milk can also be given at the breast during feedings using a nursing supplementer. These devices have some advantages, especially with sucking problems that take several weeks to resolve. Another alternative is finger-feeding: using a supplementer to give a baby milk as he sucks on an adult finger. A La Leche League Leader or lactation consultant can help you decide which of these techniques will work for you.

If your milk supply is very low and the amount of milk you pump is not enough for your baby's needs, talk to your doctor about other supplements for your baby. Artificial formula can be fed from a cup rather than a bottle. Keep pumping, even if you do need to use a formula supplement for a while; you want to maintain and build up your milk supply so that the milk is there and waiting when the baby's sucking improves.

The pumping and supplementing routine takes a lot of time. For a few days, you may not do much more than pump and feed the baby. Take advantage of friends and family who are willing to fix meals, do laundry, and entertain older children. Set up a breastfeeding center for yourself. Choose a comfortable chair and keep all your equipment nearby, along with clean diapers, a pitcher of water or juice, and comfortable pillows.

Nipple confusion

Feeding at the breast is different from an artificial nipple.

Some people refuse to believe it, but nipple confusion really does happen. When a baby begins to act confused and upset at the breast after receiving one or more bottle-feedings, it may be because the sucking technique that worked with the artificial nipple is not allowing him to get any milk out of the breast. Pacifiers can also contribute to problems with nipple confusion.

Feeding at the breast is different from getting liquid through an artificial nipple. To take the breast, the baby must open his mouth wide; a bottle nipple can be pushed through half-closed lips. The breastfeeding baby uses his gums and his tongue to compress the breast tissue and get the milk out; an artificial nipple requires less participation from the baby. The breastfed baby's lips are flanged out on the breast; with an artificial nipple, the baby purses his lips tightly. Milk flows instantly from a bottle–there's no waiting for the mother's let-down, and when it flows too fast, the baby uses his tongue to block it. This motion, when used at the breast, pushes the mother's nipple right out of the baby's mouth.

One or two bottles are enough to affect some babies' ability to breastfeed. With others, nipple confusion may result from several days of supplemental bottles. In either case, eliminating all artificial nipples is the first step in getting the baby back to breastfeeding. Besides bottle nipples, this means pacifiers and nipple shields, if you have been using them. If your baby has been getting a lot of supplementary formula and your milk supply is low, you'll need to continue giving the supplement using a cup, a bowl, an eyedropper, or a teaspoon. You can also pump after feedings and give your baby this milk as a supplement. You can eliminate the supplement gradually as your baby begins to breastfeed well and his sucking builds up your milk supply. Count the diapers to be sure he's getting enough.

Getting a nipple-confused baby to breastfeed well is largely a matter of patience and persistence. You'll have to work with him as he rediscovers what to do at the breast. Give him lots of skin-to-skin contact and plenty of opportunities for practice. Don't wait for the baby to get very hungry before offering the breast; it's hard for him to learn something new when his mind is on the important business of filling his tummy. Catch him when he's just waking up from a nap, or another time when he's calm. Expressing a little milk onto your nipple may help give him the idea. Encourage him to open his mouth wide by saying "open" and showing him how; even newborns imitate facial expressions. Pay close attention to how he is positioned at the breast and how he latches on. Stimulating your let-down reflex before putting the baby to the breast will assure that his first sucks are well rewarded. Your let-down reflex can be stimulated by expressing some milk, gently rubbing the nipples in a circular motion, taking a warm shower, or even just looking at your baby and smelling his sweet baby smell.

Forceful let-down

Sometimes the milk comes down in such a rush with the let-down that the nursing baby can't keep up with the flow. He may pull away from the nipple or gasp and sputter and swallow a lot of air. He may even start to fuss when put to the breast, because he has come to expect trouble.

Take him off the breast for a minute or so when this happens. The milk flow will slow down, and soon he'll be able to nurse again more easily. You could also position him so that he is nursing "uphill." Use two or three pillows on your lap to raise his head so that he is looking down at the breast while nursing. Leaning way back in a recliner also works well.

A forceful let-down can be caused by an overabundance of milk. If problems like this persist beyond the early weeks, try limiting your baby to one breast at a feeding, at least in the morning and early afternoon when your breasts are more full. If the baby wants to nurse again within the next two hours, offer him the same side he had at the last feeding. For example, use the left breast for feedings between 8 and 10 o'clock, the right breast from 10 till noon, the left breast again from 12 to 2, and so forth. This will help bring your milk supply in line with your baby's needs. Be sure to keep count of wet diapers and stools to be sure that your baby is getting enough milk.

Leaking milk

Leaking milk is a nuisance, but fortunately in most women it is a short-lived problem, limited to the early weeks of breastfeeding. Some women leak milk from one breast while the baby nurses at the other. Others leak when their breasts become overly full between feedings or when the baby's cries or some other stimulus triggers the let-down reflex.

You can stop leaking by applying gentle pressure to the nipples. To do this subtly, fold your arms over your chest and press in. However, leaking is a signal that it's time to breastfeed the baby, and if possible, this is what you should do.

Nursing pads in your bra will absorb the milk. You can buy cloth pads that can be washed and used over and over again, or you can make them from folded handkerchiefs or cloth diapers. Disposable pads with

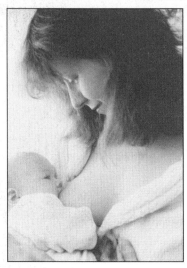

plastic liners will protect your clothes from wetness. They will also prevent air from getting to your nipples, which can cause soreness, so don't use them all the time. Wear clothing with prints that will camouflage wetness, or bring along a jacket or sweater. If you leak during feedings, a cloth diaper under the breast will catch the overflow.

Newborn jaundice

Jaundice is common in newborn babies, but it is seldom, if ever, a reason to stop breastfeeding, not even temporarily.

Newborn jaundice is the result of the rapid breakdown of red blood cells in the first days of life. Babies need fewer red blood cells after birth than they did in the womb. As the extra cells are destroyed, a waste product called bilirubin is released into the blood, eventually to be excreted in the baby's stool. When bilirubin is made faster than the baby can eliminate it, the result is jaundice. Bilirubin is a yellow pigment, and an excess of it gives the skin a yellowish cast; the whites of the eyes may also look yellow.

Why does bilirubin reach higher levels in some infants? Sometimes jaundice is the result of blood or liver problems or an infection. If bilirubin levels rise quickly in the first day or two of life, your physician will do further testing to determine the cause and appropriate treatment. Most of the time, however, jaundice is simply a part of baby's adjustment to life outside mother's body. This kind of jaundice is called physiologic jaundice, because it is part of a normal body process. In physiologic jaundice, bilirubin levels rise slowly, and the yellowish color appears on the third or fourth day of life. The jaundice gradually disappears by itself, although this may take several weeks in some babies.

Physicians disagree about when–or whether–to treat ordinary newborn jaundice. In sick babies or premature infants, very high levels of bilirubin may affect the brain, but there is no decisive evidence that peak bilirubin levels below 20 to 25 mg/dl are harmful to normal, healthy full-term infants with physiologic jaundice. Because jaundice is so common in breastfed infants, some researchers wonder whether it may actually have a beneficial effect.

To bring down bilirubin levels, babies are placed under special lights, a treatment called phototherapy. The lights help break down the bilirubin so that it can be eliminated more quickly. In extreme cases, blood transfusions may be used to lower bilirubin levels.

Phototherapy is complicated and worrisome to parents and can create problems with breastfeeding. It's hard to watch a baby's cues and breastfeed frequently when baby is out of mother's arms in an isolette in the nursery, with patches over his eyes to protect them from the lights. Newer options in phototherapy include having the lights set up in your hospital room or in your home. There is also a device called a Wallaby phototherapy unit, a fiberoptic blanket that wraps around the baby's trunk, making it possible to hold and nurse the baby while treatment continues.

Avoiding jaundice problems

Good breastfeeding practices work to prevent jaundice.

Studies have found a higher incidence of jaundice in breastfed babies, though researchers are still trying to figure out why this is so. Meanwhile, studies have shown that good breastfeeding practices work to lower bilirubin levels. Colostrum, while small in quantity, has a laxative effect. Frequent feedings right from birth stimulate more frequent stools, so that bilirubin can be eliminated more quickly. Infrequent feeding in the early days may contribute to higher bilirubin levels.

If you have a baby whose bilirubin levels are rising, be sure to encourage him to nurse as much as possible. This is easiest to do if the baby is rooming-in with you and stays with you throughout the night. A baby who is not nursing well in the first few days is more likely to have higher bilirubin levels. Wake him during the day, if necessary, so that he nurses at least every two hours. Be sure that he is positioned correctly at the breast and that he is sucking actively for ten to

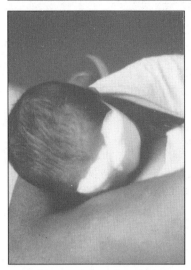

Babies receiving phototherapy still need to breastfeed frequently.

twenty minutes at each feeding. Call a La Leche League Leader or ask to see the hospital's lactation consultant if you need more help.

Exposing the baby's skin to indirect sunlight can also help to bring down bilirubin levels. Undress your baby down to his diaper and place him in a warm room that gets plenty of daylight through the windows. Don't put him directly in the path of sunlight coming in the window and don't take your baby outside into the sun; his newborn skin burns easily.

Water supplements do not help to "wash out" the jaundice. In fact, they can make it worse. They fill up the baby's tummy, making him less eager to nurse at the breast. They are usually given with an artificial nipple, which can lead to sucking problems. And water does nothing to encourage stooling–and that's what gets rid of bilirubin.

If the baby's doctor wants to begin phototherapy, ask about alternatives. Could treatment be delayed another twelve or twenty-four hours, while you nurse the baby more frequently? By then, a blood test may find that the levels are dropping or at least are no longer rising quickly. If phototherapy is necessary, ask about having the lights in your hospital room, or at home if you are about to be discharged. Phototherapy does not have to be continuous to be effective. If the baby must be in the nursery, ask to stay with him there so that you can take him out of the isolette and nurse him as soon as he awakens or whenever he fusses. Frequent feedings are necessary to prevent dehydration when the baby is under the lights. If the baby is not nursing well, you need to be able to keep working with him, even during phototherapy. If supplements are considered necessary, ask that they be given by cup, eyedropper, or syringe, rather than with an artificial nipple.

Breastfeeding mothers may be told that something in their milk is slowing down the baby's elimination of bilirubin and that it is necessary to discontinue breastfeeding or to supplement with infant formula for a day or two. While switching to formula for a short time may make the jaundice disappear sooner, it can be the beginning of the end of breastfeeding. The baby may not take the breast well after being given artificial nipples, and the mother may not have as much milk.

If the mother and baby are already experiencing difficulties with breastfeeding, temporary weaning may make these problems harder to solve. If you do end up having to wean temporarily or give formula supplements for a day or two, you will need to pump at the feeding times when your baby is not nursing. Give the formula using a cup or an eyedropper rather than an artificial nipple to minimize problems with nipple confusion. While the doctor might suggest formula supplements as an alternative to phototherapy, some parents may choose to go ahead with phototherapy while continuing to breastfeed exclusively, since this avoids the risks associated with giving formula.

Jaundice can create a lot of concern for new parents–the treatments along with the condition itself. It's difficult to be a confident breastfeeding mother if a nurse or doctor is suggesting that your baby needs water or formula supplements to bring the bilirubin levels down. You need to stay in touch with the baby's doctor, listen to his or her suggestions, and ask about alternatives. Your desire to continue breastfeeding will influence your doctor's recommendations, so it's important to communicate your preferences clearly. If talking to physicians is difficult for you, practice what you will say ahead of time; write down your questions and the points you wish to make. Seek a second opinion if you need to, from a doctor who is more supportive of breastfeeding. If a baby is otherwise healthy, jaundice should not interfere with getting a good start at breastfeeding.

Illness in mother or baby

Colds and flu come and go in nursing mothers and babies, just as in everyone else. You can and should continue to nurse your baby if you become ill. By the time you actually start feeling sick, the baby has already been exposed to the germs, so breastfeeding is certainly not going to make things any worse. In fact, the antibodies that your body makes to fight the germs will appear in your milk and give your baby an edge in dealing with the bug himself. It's not unusual to find that when a cold or the flu rolls through a family, the nursing baby gets only a mild case, if he gets sick at all.

Sometimes a change in the usual nursing pattern is the first indication a mother has that her baby is ill. Stuffy noses make breastfeeding more difficult. Lying on his side to nurse can be painful for a baby with an ear infection. Your baby's behavior at the breast tells you a great deal about how he's feeling, and continuing to breastfeed will help him feel better.

Babies with tummy-aches may want to breastfeed very often—almost continuously. It's okay to let them do so. Frequent short nursings help prevent dehydration, and all the immunities in human milk will help fight the virus that's causing the problems. There's no need to stop breastfeeding, even for a day or two, if your baby has an upset tummy and diarrhea. Studies have shown that breastfed babies with diarrhea recover more quickly and lose less weight if they are allowed to continue to nurse. They will accept the breast far more readily than any other substance offered to them.

Treat a breast infection with rest, heat, gentle massage, and frequent breastfeeding.

A baby who is vomiting may do best with only a little milk at a time; larger amounts may come right back up. In this situation, try nursing the baby on a fairly empty breast. Pump or hand-express for several minutes before feeding the baby. The slower trickle of milk will be more soothing to his stomach, and he'll be able to nurse for comfort without the upset of another episode of vomiting.

Plugged ducts and breast infections

Tender, sore lumps in the breast are usually plugged ducts. A red, hot, swollen area that is painful to the touch may be a breast infection, especially when accompanied by a fever, achiness, and an all-over tired feeling, like flu. Prompt home treatment can prevent a plugged duct from becoming a breast infection and can keep an infection from developing into an abscess. Three things are needed to get the milk flowing again in the affected area: heat, gentle massage, and frequent breastfeeding.

You can apply heat by taking a warm shower, soaking the breast in a basin or bowl of warm water, or using warm, wet washcloths, a hot water bottle, or a heating pad. While it is warm, massage your breast gently with your fingers and palm, using a circular motion first and then kneading gently from high up in the breast behind the sore spot down toward the nipple. Then put the baby to breast or express some milk with a pump or by hand. You may want to continue to massage above the sore area while the baby is nursing in order to loosen the plug and get the milk moving down the duct.

To keep the breast from becoming too full, breastfeed your baby as often as he is willing to nurse, at least every two hours. Use the heat-and-massage routine before feedings, as much as possible, and breastfeed on the sore side first. Take baby to bed with you for a few hours' nap, or just relax with baby in your arms and feet propped up.

Sometimes a breast infection changes the taste of the milk slightly. If your baby is not cooperating and doesn't want to nurse from the sore breast, start him out on the other side. Once the let-down has occurred slide him over to the affected breast, without changing his body position. You may be able to trick him into taking the breast he thinks he doesn't want.

It's very important to continue breastfeeding when you have a plugged duct or a breast infection. Keeping the breast soft and the milk flowing will prevent the development of an abscess, which may have to be surgically drained. Neither pumping nor hand-expressing is as efficient as your baby when it comes to getting milk out of a breast. Even if you had planned to quit breastfeeding soon, keep nursing frequently at this time and delay weaning until the breast infection has cleared up. You don't have to worry about a breast infection making your baby sick. The antibodies in your milk will protect him.

If you are running a fever and are feeling achy, tired, and miserable, go to bed and rest. If you've had the fever for more than twenty-four hours, call your

Go to bed and rest if you have a breast infection.

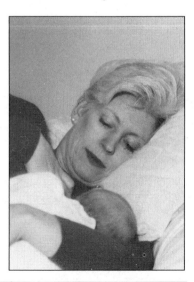

doctor. He or she may want to prescribe an antibiotic—one that's safe for nursing mothers and babies. Be sure to take the medicine for as long as the doctor suggests. Even if you're feeling better, you need to take the full course of the antibiotic in order to wipe out the infection completely.

Give some thought to what may have caused the plugged duct or the breast infection, so that you can avoid a recurrence. A bra that's too tight or one with ill-fitting underwires can block milk ducts. So can pressing on the breast during feedings or sleeping on your stomach. Skipping feedings, going longer between feedings, or having a baby unexpectedly sleep through the night can cause engorgement, which may lead to plugged ducts or breast infections. Latch-on difficulties can also contribute to problems with breast infections, since a baby who is not latched on well cannot get milk out as efficiently.

Breast infections are often a sign that a mother is too busy or is under a lot of stress. In her rush to get things done, she may delay feedings or cut them short, leading to engorgement, plugged ducts, and breast infections. If she's not getting enough rest, isn't taking the time to eat good foods, or is just plain worn out, her body will be less able to fight off illness. A breast infection warns her to slow down and take better care of herself.

Thrush

Thrush is a yeast infection in the baby's mouth. There may be patches of white on the inside of his lips or cheeks or on his tongue or gums. A mild case of thrush seldom bothers babies, but it can spread to mother's nipples and make breastfeeding painful. Sore nipples that appear after several weeks or months of uneventful breastfeeding may be caused by thrush.

Yeast thrives in places that are dark, warm, and moist—like the mouth. Usually there are other "good" bacteria around that keep yeast from multiplying, but sometimes it gets out of control, especially when people take antibiotics. Antibiotics can kill off good bacteria, along with the harmful kind, allowing thrush to take over.

Thrush can turn the nipple and the part of the areola covered by baby's mouth bright pink. The skin may be flaky and dry. It's possible to have thrush on your nipples even if you can't see any signs of it in baby's mouth. Yeast can also cause a red, raised diaper rash on baby's bottom or a vaginal infection in mother.

Your doctor can give you a prescription for medication that will get rid of thrush—a liquid to squirt in your baby's mouth and a cream to put on your nipples. Diaper rashes and vaginal yeast infections should be treated at the same time. Rinsing your nipples with plain water after feedings may also help.

During the time you have thrush on your nipples, any milk you pump should either be used immediately or discarded. Freezing does not kill yeast organisms, and giving the milk to your baby later could start another round of yeast infections for both of you.

How to express and store your milk

Expressing milk from your breasts, whether by hand or with a pump, is a separate skill from breastfeeding a baby, and it takes practice to become good at it. If you get only a teaspoonful of milk the first time you pump, don't jump to the conclusion that you're not making enough milk for your baby. Your body reacts quite differently to a warm and cuddly infant. With practice, you can get better at pumping, if that's what you need to do.

Equipment

There may be only two or three kinds of breast pumps on the shelf at the local pharmacy or discount store, so you may not have much of a choice if that's the only place you shop. A greater variety of pumps is available by mail, on the web, or from local representatives of breast pump companies. (See the resource list in the back of this book for more information.) The type of pump you choose depends on how often you will be using it, how much money you have to spend, and your own preferences. A La Leche League Leader or a lactation consultant who rents and sells pumps can help you choose the best one for you.

Hand-operated pumps work well for many women and are relatively inexpensive ($30 to $50 in the USA). Some can be adapted for use with fully automatic electric pumps. Some hand pumps require two hands to operate, and your hand or arm may tire while using them. Avoid the cheap, bicycle-horn type; it doesn't work well and the rubber bulb can harbor bacteria.

Electric breast pumps are more expensive, but they are often preferred by women who are pumping regularly. Many offer the option of pumping both breasts at the same time, cutting your overall pumping time in half.

Expressing or pumping milk is a skill that takes practice.

Fully automatic hospital-grade pumps are very effective and can be rented at a reasonable rate. If you are pumping to keep up a milk supply for a baby who is not yet breastfeeding, you should use this type of pump. Working mothers might also consider renting one of these pumps.

Other kinds of electric pumps can be purchased for $100 to $300, a worthwhile investment for a mother who is regularly away from her baby. The price of the pump is less than what it would cost to wean to formula. Many of these electric pumps can be used almost anywhere, since they can run on batteries or on an AC or car adapter.

Follow the manufacturer's directions for putting the pump together and cleaning and sterilizing the parts that come in contact with the milk. Many pump parts can be washed in the dishwasher.

Besides a pump, you'll need something to store the milk in. Hard plastic or glass containers do the best job of protecting the milk in the refrigerator or the freezer. Many mothers use the plastic bags that are designed to be used for bottle-feeding. It's wise to double-bag when using these, as they break easily. A more durable plastic bag made especially for storing human milk is available through La Leche League International's Catalogue and from breast pump retailers. These can be attached directly to most pumps, so they're very convenient to use.

How to express milk by hand

Not every breastfeeding mother needs a breast pump. Some mothers discover that hand-expression works very well for them; it's cheap and convenient, especially for women who don't need to express milk very often. Hand-expression is not difficult to learn, but there is a knack to it. Remember that the milk reservoirs are under the areola, behind the nipple. This is where you must apply gentle pressure in order to get the milk out.

A pre-pumping routine will help condition your let-down reflex.

Wash your hands before expressing milk. Place your thumb on top of the breast and your fingers underneath, about an inch to an inch-and-a-half behind the nipple. Don't cup your breast in your hand; instead, the thumb and fingers should be opposite each other with the nipple in between. Push straight back into the chest wall and then roll the thumb and fingers forward as if you were making fingerprints. Repeat this action rhythmically to empty the milk reservoirs. Rotate the hand around the breast and use the other hand as well to reach all the reservoirs. When the flow slows down on one side, switch to the other breast and then back again until you've worked on each side two or three times. Use a wide-mouthed cup or glass to catch the spray.

Avoid squeezing or pulling on the breast; breast tissue is delicate and bruises easily. Be careful not to slide the fingers along the skin as you roll them forward; this can cause skin burns.

Suggestions for pumping

Wash your hands before you pump and have everything you need ready. Moistening your breast with water will create a better seal between the skin and the flange on the pump. Start out at the lowest pressure setting—pumping should not hurt. Pump rhythmically to imitate the way a baby sucks at the breast. Work on one side until the milk flow slows down, then change to the other breast. Switch back and forth until you've pumped each breast two or three times. This should take fifteen to twenty minutes.

But what if you're not getting much milk? The key to pumping or expressing milk successfully is being able to trigger the let-down reflex. A regular place for pumping and a pre-pumping routine will help condition your reflex. Before you start to pump take a few moments to get comfortable and to relax. Close your eyes, take some easy, deep breaths, and think of something pleasant—a mountain stream, a sunny beach. Imagine your baby at your breast and the feel of his skin. If you like, you can gently roll or stroke the nipples with your fingers to help stimulate a let-down.

Massaging your breasts will help you relax before you pump your milk.

Another way to relax before pumping or expressing milk is to massage the breasts. Starting near the armpit, use the fingers to press firmly into the chest wall, using a circular motion. After a few seconds, move to another spot, and repeat the motion. Work around the breast in a spiral until you reach the nipple. Then stroke the breast with a light touch from the top down to the nipple. Lean forward and shake the breasts so that gravity will help release the milk. You can repeat this routine midway through a pumping session to increase the milk flow and stimulate additional let-downs.

When to pump

If you are separated from your baby, you will need to pump about as often as he nurses, at two- to three-hour intervals. If you are expressing milk for an occasional bottle for your baby, try pumping early in the morning, when your baby has not nursed for an hour or two. Most women have more milk early in the day than in the late afternoon or evening. Another strategy is to pump a small amount of milk several times during the day, cool it in the refrigerator, and combine it into one container. If your baby is nearby, try feeding him on one side and pumping or hand-expressing on the other; the baby's nursing will trigger the let-down, and you'll be able to pump more milk.

Storing human milk

The antibacterial factors in your milk help protect it from bacterial contamination during storage. Recent studies have found that it's possible to store human milk in the refrigerator, or even at room temperature, for longer than previously believed. Here are some general guidelines. Human milk can be kept safely:

- at room temperature (66°-72°F; 19°-22°C) for 10 hours after it is expressed;
- in the refrigerator for 8 days (32°-39°F; 0°-4°C);
- in a freezer compartment inside a refrigerator for 2 weeks (temperature varies);
- in a freezer unit with its own door for 3 or 4 months (temperature varies);
- in a deep-freeze (0°F; -19° C) for 6 months or longer.

Frozen milk that has been thawed can be kept in the refrigerator for up to 24 hours, but it cannot be refrozen.

Store milk in clean containers that have been washed in hot soapy water. Leave an inch or so of room at the top, since milk expands when frozen. If you want to add freshly expressed milk to already frozen milk, cool it first in the refrigerator and don't add a greater amount than is already in the freezer container. If you're storing milk in plastic bags, stand the bags up in a heavy plastic container with a lid, rather than putting them in the refrigerator or freezer on their own, where they could easily tear.

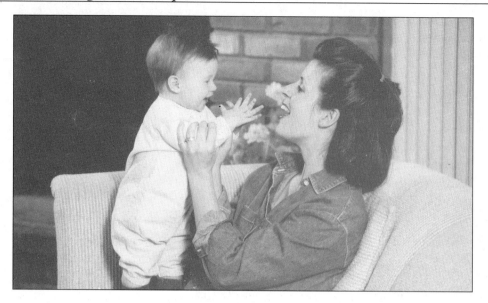

There are very few medical reasons why a baby cannot be breastfed.

Human milk should be thawed under running water, first cool and then gradually warmer until the milk is ready for baby. Gently shake the container before testing the temperature. The milk can also be thawed by placing the container in a pan of water that has been heated on the stove. Human milk should not be heated directly on the stove or in a microwave oven; many of the immunological components can be destroyed if the milk is allowed to get too hot. Uneven heating in a microwave produces "hot spots" that may burn the baby.

When human milk is stored, the fat (or cream) rises to the top, leaving the milk underneath it looking watery or bluish. This is perfectly normal. Cow's milk from the dairy used to do this too, before homogenization was invented. Gently shaking the milk before using it will redistribute the cream.

Special medical situations

There are very few medical reasons why a baby cannot be breastfed. The health benefits of breastfeeding become even more important when mother and baby face special challenges. A mother's desire to breastfeed her baby should be honored, if at all possible, because it is an important part of how she will get to know and feel connected to her child. Breastfeeding matters—for multiple births, for premature infants, for babies with health problems, for mothers who are ill or disabled. Discussing more unusual breastfeeding situations is beyond the scope of this book, but the resource list in the back can direct you to further information. A La Leche League Leader can also help you find out what you need to know and give you the support you need as you learn to breastfeed your baby.

Chapter Five

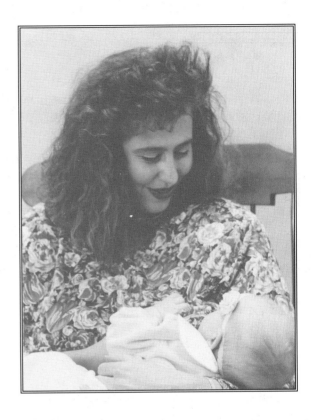

Life with a Breastfed Baby

Babies change their parents' lives forever after—in big ways, of course, and in more mundane matters.

Love, responsibility, concern, pride, uncertainty—these are all a big part of becoming a parent. But you'll also find yourself struggling with issues as basic as getting enough sleep, finding time to eat, and managing to get yourself, the baby, and the diaper bag out of the house with less than two hours of preparation.

Breastfeeding simplifies many of these challenges. It helps build the bond between you and your baby, helps you feel good about yourself as a mother, and provides simple solutions to some practical parenting problems.

Getting enough sleep

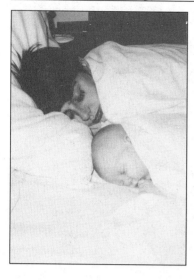

From day one of your baby's life and for months afterward, people will ask you, "Does she sleep at night? Is she sleeping through the night? Can you sleep at night?"

This obsession with sleep is well grounded in most people's experience of new parenthood. It's not easy to recover from the physical stresses and strains of pregnancy and childbirth while caring for a vulnerable, demanding infant who knows nothing about the difference between night and day.

Yet a baby who sleeps no more than a few hours at a stretch is doing what is natural and right for her. She needs frequent feedings to keep her tiny tummy comfortable. Frequent—almost constant—contact with mother assures her that she is safe and warm. Being able to wake easily from sleep may even help protect her from Sudden Infant Death Syndrome, which many experts believe is related to an infant's ability to rouse herself when she needs to take a breath during deep sleep.

How can a mother survive? Sleep when the baby sleeps, whenever it is that the baby sleeps. Take a nap during the day. Even if you've never much cared for daytime naps, you may find that lying down and nursing your baby off to sleep lulls you into slumber as well. During the first weeks of your baby's life, housework, kitchen clean-up, and other nagging tasks are not nearly as important as resting both body and mind.

Napping can be difficult if you have other young children. Perhaps mother, baby, and older sibling can all lie down together, or at least enjoy some quiet time with puzzles, books, or conversation. Or bring some favorite toys into your child-proofed bedroom, close the door, and let your toddler play while you and the baby doze. Even stretching out on the floor and letting your toddler tumble over you for fifteen or twenty minutes can recharge your battery and keep you going until bedtime.

Nighttime feedings

New babies do have to be fed at night, and when your baby is breastfed, this is one job that only you can do. Because human milk is digested so quickly, breastfed babies may awaken more often than artificially fed infants. Research has also found that breastfed infants are older when they finally sleep through the night. Nevertheless, it's possible to breastfeed and get enough sleep.

How? Nursing at night requires nothing more than a mother and a baby and a comfortable place for them to be together. There's no trek down to a cold kitchen for bottles, no waiting to warm the formula while baby howls. You don't need to turn a light on, once the baby can latch on easily. You may not even have to get out of bed, if dad is willing to help out or if baby is already sleeping beside you. You can manage a nighttime breastfeeding without completely waking up, and this makes it much easier to drop back into a sound sleep.

The easiest place to breastfeed at night is in bed, lying down. Once mother gets the baby started, she can doze off, or at least rest while the baby nurses. To switch sides, place the baby on your chest and roll over. (Or, if there's not much room, scoot the baby along the bed underneath you and climb over.) When the feeding is over and baby is again sleeping, you can take her back to her bed or let her sleep next to you until she wakes again to nurse.

You needn't worry about rolling over onto the baby; even while sleeping, mothers are aware of their baby's presence (though you should not sleep with a baby if you are using alcohol, drugs, or medications that alter sleep patterns). Pushing the bed against the wall will prevent baby from rolling out, or you can purchase a guard rail. Be sure that there are no cracks between the mattress and the wall, the bed frame, or the guard rail that could trap baby's head or body. Babies should not sleep on waterbeds, pillows, or other soft surfaces that can obstruct their airway. Mothers and babies have slept together since the human race began. Even if you have some doubts, it's worth a try, at least in the early weeks.

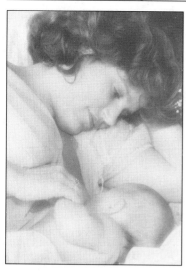

Sleeping together works out well for many breastfeeding mothers and babies, enabling everyone in the family to get enough sleep.

It's a good idea to discuss this idea with your partner if you'd like to try it. You'll need his support. A baby in bed with them does not have to come between parents; baby can sleep next to the wall so that her parents can still cuddle up together. And many parents find that keeping their baby with them at night is another way to enjoy this magical being their love has created. One common worry that goes along with a baby in the parents' bed is finding a place and opportunities for making love. If your baby nurses to sleep in your arms, put her down in her crib or bassinet for the first part of the night, while you and your husband enjoy some privacy. When she wakes you can bring her into bed with you for the remainder of the night. Or you can gently move a sleeping infant from your bed into her crib. Remember, too, that beds are not the only place suitable for having sex.

Sleeping with baby isn't for everyone. Some mothers find that a comfortable easy chair, the kind you can curl up in, works well for nighttime feedings. Others prefer a rocking chair. Keep a warm blanket or afghan nearby to wrap around you and baby when it's chilly. Use pillows in your lap to help support the baby, especially if you doze off. Most babies need to be held a few minutes extra, until they're in a sound sleep, before you can put them down without waking them.

Be flexible about nighttime nursing arrangements. They can change as your baby's, your family's, and your own needs change. You can nurse your baby to sleep in the guest bedroom or on a mattress on the floor, and then sneak away to sleep with your husband. This is sometimes easier than trying to put a baby who has fallen asleep in your arms down into a crib without waking her. Older babies can be moved into their own beds after falling asleep somewhere close to you. Dad can help out by being the one who gets up to bring a crying baby into bed with her parents. Try not to count the hours and minutes of interrupted sleep; becoming obsessed with how much sleep you're not getting will only make you feel more tired.

Babies and toddlers who are accustomed to sleeping with parents do eventually "wean" to a crib or their own bed, and babies and children do eventually stop waking up at night. They will do this at their own pace, with some gentle encouragement and guidance from mother and dad. While some contemporary sleep experts maintain that babies must be taught at an early age to fall asleep by themselves, other experts and many parents believe that good sleep habits are best learned gradually, without conflict and crying, as the child is ready, in a safe and secure environment.

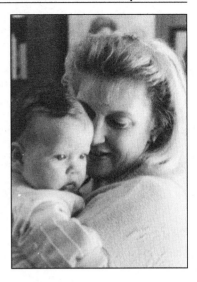

And if you do find yourself awake and unable to go back to sleep while your baby is breastfeeding, make the most of it: Think, plan, meditate—or get yourself a rip-roaring, page-turning paperback novel and indulge. You can always nap tomorrow.

Why is your baby crying?

Babies cry for lots of reasons: hunger, discomfort, loneliness, being tired, feeling out of control. What you do about your baby's crying is more important than whether or not you understand exactly what it's all about. Pick her up, cuddle her, walk her, rock her, offer the breast. Change her diaper if she's wet. Swaddle her in a blanket if she's flailing about; she's used to feeling warm and enclosed from her months in the womb. Quiet singing or talking may calm her, or she may prefer gentle jiggling or patting that starts out fast and slows as she settles down. Putting her in a baby carrier (either a front pack or a sling) while you do housework or go for a walk is another way to soothe her. If one thing doesn't work, stay calm and try another.

Babies learn that they can make things happen in the world when someone responds to their cries. They discover that they can trust their own feelings and perceptions, because caregivers take them seriously when they express their needs. As parents help them regain control, babies get into the habit of feeling happy. The more you soothe and carry your baby in the early weeks, the more content she will be later on. Don't be afraid to hold her much of the time. You can't spoil a tiny baby. In fact, "spoiling" her now will make her easier to live with as time goes on.

Don't hesitate to offer to nurse your baby when she's upset. Breastfeeding is a powerful anti-crying agent. The warm skin contact, the familiar feel-good position, and the rhythmic sucking motion will help the baby relax and feel calm again. A baby who sucks for comfort usually doesn't get much milk. If you're worried about over-feeding and spitting up, offer the least-full breast, the one the baby nursed from most recently; the milk flow will be slower.

Some babies cry more than others. Fussy or colicky babies are hard on parents' nerves and on their confidence. It's difficult to feel like a good mother or father when your baby is howling and nothing you do seems to help. But stand by your baby. Even if she goes on crying, she'll have the security of knowing that someone cares about how she feels. Get some support for yourself—talk to the parents of other fussy babies, attend La Leche League meetings, or read one of the books listed in the bibliography about coping with crying and colic.

Babies learn to trust themselves when someone responds to their cries.

"How often should I nurse this baby?"

Newborn babies breastfeed an average of eight to twelve times a day. That's a fact.

But what does this mean for your baby? How do you know when to feed her? How do you know if she's getting enough? Can she really be hungry just forty-five minutes after the last feeding? Why does it seem as though you're nursing all the time?

Breastfeeding works best when it's done "on demand" or "on cue." This means there is no by-the-clock feeding schedule, and mother must learn to read her baby's behavior. This is easier than it sounds, especially if you can let go of preconceived notions (and the instructions in certain popular books of baby care advice) and get to know your baby as an individual.

Her needs and habits may seem chaotic at first, but after several weeks some kind of pattern will begin to emerge. You and she will both know when she's hungry or when nursing will help to calm her down. In the meantime, go ahead and offer the breast when she fusses or has gone a while without nursing. She'll let you know if she's not interested. "On demand" feeding seldom, if ever, works out to be every three or four hours regularly throughout the day. Babies may learn to sleep longer between feedings at night, but at other times, perhaps in the late afternoon or early evening, they may want to breastfeed very frequently, or be almost continuously attached to the breast. This is normal. Nursing calms frazzled nerves—baby's and mother's.

There will be people who will tell you that a baby who was last fed less than three hours ago "can't possibly be hungry again" and shouldn't be fed yet. They don't realize that human milk is digested very quickly, and baby's tummy may well be feeling empty after ninety minutes or less. In spite of all the trappings of civilization that surround us, human beings are still, biologically speaking, a continuous contact species. This means that infants naturally stay with their mothers and breastfeed frequently, for nourishment and for comfort. If your baby wants to nurse again twenty minutes after the last feeding, go ahead; think of it as the infant equivalent of lingering over coffee and dessert, in the company of someone you love.

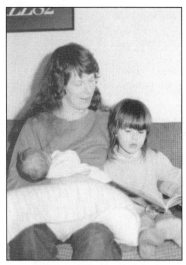

You'll be spending lots of time nursing your baby in the early weeks.

Worries about milk supply

In study after study, not having enough milk is the most frequently given reason for stopping breastfeeding. Oddly, this fear has no real basis in fact. The more your baby nurses, the more milk your body will make. Your breasts can make enough milk for twins, or even triplets, if necessary, as long as they receive enough stimulation from nursing.

So why are so many mothers concerned about milk supply? It seems to go with the job. Lives there a mother anywhere who hasn't at some time or another worried about whether her child was eating enough?

Babies also play a part in creating mothers' concerns about milk supply. When babies fuss at the breast, nurse for a long time, or seem to be nursing more frequently, it's easy to assume there's a problem with the amount of milk available. Actually, these behaviors usually have other explanations. Perhaps the mother's milk is not letting down as quickly as the baby would like, perhaps the baby is tired or overstimulated and needs to suck longer in order to unwind, perhaps baby needs some closeness and cuddling to get her through whatever tensions she's noticing in the world around her, or maybe she isn't feeling well.

Growth spurts

One explanation for an increase in babies' breastfeeding time is that the baby is going through a growth spurt. She is nursing more frequently in order to stimulate the mother's breasts to produce the additional milk needed for rapid growth. Growth spurts seem to occur most often around two to three weeks, six weeks, and three months of age. The baby may want to nurse every hour or so for a day or two, but will eventually taper off and go back to her usual feeding pattern. Relax, put other things aside, and let her nurse. Your body knows what to do. The baby's increased demand and time at the breast will soon boost your milk supply, and things will get back to normal.

Things you shouldn't worry about

Your baby's breastfeeding pattern and your body's functioning change over time. Babies become experts at getting milk out of the breast and may shorten some of their feedings while still getting enough milk. As mother's milk production becomes more efficient and in tune with her baby's needs, her breasts may feel softer and less full between feedings, even though they are making the same or even greater amounts of milk. Leaking becomes less of a problem as time goes on, and this, too, has nothing to do with milk supply. Changes in sensations associated with the let-down reflex—or not feeling a let-down at all—are also perfectly normal.

Someone may suggest that you offer your baby a bottle after nursings—"to see if she's still hungry." This proves nothing about whether your baby is getting enough to eat at the breast; some babies will suck on anything offered to them, regardless of hunger. (The breast is ideal for this kind of sucking, since the baby will receive only a small amount of milk when she sucks for comfort and larger amounts when she's truly hungry.)

Don't be discouraged if you try to pump milk and get only a few drops or a teaspoonful. Your body doesn't respond as well to a pump as it does to your baby. Pumping larger amounts of milk is a skill that comes with practice. How much milk you can express has no relation to how much milk your baby gets while nursing.

The bottom line

As long as your baby is wetting six to eight cloth diapers or five to six disposables every twenty-four hours, along with two to five bowel movements daily, you can be assured that she is getting enough milk. After six weeks, as baby's bladder gets bigger, the number of wet diapers may drop a bit, to five or six for cloth or four or five for disposables. Stool patterns may change as baby matures. Some older breastfed babies may go several days or longer between bowel movements, without showing any signs of constipation, or hard, dry stools. When breastfed babies follow this pattern, the once-every-so-many-days bowel movement will be substantial.

Some cultures have never heard of "not having enough milk."

With breastfeeding, baby's food comes right from mother's body, which can intensify worries about baby getting enough to eat. These concerns may be connected to how you feel about yourself and your body and to social messages that reach you from friends, family, advertising, and the media. In cultures where everyone breastfeeds and there are no alternatives, the idea of not

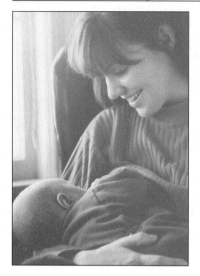

having enough milk for your baby is unheard of. In our culture, where it's assumed that babies eventually will be fed with bottles, every quirk of normal baby behavior gets blamed on breastfeeding.

Weight gain

Just as babies are born in a wide range of sizes, they grow at different rates. As long as your breastfed baby is wetting enough diapers and having regular bowel movements, you can assume that she's growing at the right pace for her. It's impossible to overfeed a breastfed baby.

Slow weight gain in a breastfed baby can sometimes worry mothers and doctors. If everything else checks out okay—wet diapers, enough stools (especially in a baby under six weeks), the baby's general health—she is probably just destined to be a slow gainer, which is fine. Babies don't have to be big to be healthy. Standardized growth charts represent only averages, and the charts currently in use were drawn from populations consisting largely of artificially fed infants. More recent research has found that breastfed babies may gain more slowly than formula-fed infants after the first four months of life. They're destined to be leaner than their bottle-fed counterparts.

Supplementing with formula can lead to the end of breastfeeding.

If you have reason to believe that your baby may not be getting enough milk, take a careful look at her nursing pattern. Is she breastfeeding fewer than 8 to 12 times a day? Is she sleeping long stretches during the day without waking up to nurse? Is she sucking well for only a few minutes at a feeding, then drifting off into leisurely comfort sucking? Do you hear at least ten to twenty minutes of active sucking and swallowing during every feeding? Is she latched on well and sucking effectively? (For more on this, see chapter 4.)

Some simple changes in routine can often improve a baby's weight gain. Offer the breast more frequently. The shorter the time since your baby last breastfed, the higher the fat (and calorie) content of your milk. Don't use a pacifier–let all the baby's sucking be at the breast. Switch sides several times a feeding, if necessary, to keep baby awake and encourage her to nurse longer. If she's nursing actively, allow her to finish one side and get all the high-fat milk from that breast before moving her to the other.

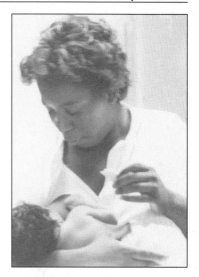

A slow-gaining baby can undermine a mother's confidence. It's easy to assume that there must be something wrong with you, and it can be difficult to figure out what to do if you're feeling worried about your baby or down on yourself. If you're concerned about your baby's growth pattern, talk to a La Leche League Leader or a lactation consultant who can tell you how to build up your milk supply while you teach your baby to breastfeed better. Supplementing with formula is seldom the answer to weight gain problems, although in some situations it may be necessary. Even if your baby needs supplements for a while, with additional information and support, you will soon feel more confident and you will be able to continue nursing your baby.

Early days at home

The responsibility that comes with a new baby is awesome. And it never goes away, even if the two of you are apart. The tie is especially close when you are the food supply as well as the comforter and caretaker. A new breastfed baby changes life at home and away from home.

Your first weeks postpartum may go by in a blur of feeding, changing, holding, and doing the laundry. Mothering your newborn takes up most of your time and energy. Now is the time to let other things slide, to ask for help from others, and to accept any and all offers from friends and relatives who want to lend a hand— with one exception. Helpers can clean your house, bring you meals, or fold the diapers, but you should be the one who cares for the baby. This is your special time to get to know your baby, and you are the expert on what this baby needs. Sensitive helpers will concentrate on taking care of your needs (and dad's, too), and give you the luxury of worry-free time to know and nurse your newborn.

Unfortunately, postpartum helpers are not always sensitive to mothers' real needs, and the baby's own magic is hard to resist. They'll offer to hold the baby—even give her a bottle, so that you can sleep or make dinner. This is not really helpful to you, and you'll need to be ready with tactful ways to channel their energy into other tasks: "Thanks for the offer, but the baby really needs to be with me right now so she can nurse. Could you take care of something else for me? I would feel so much better if the dishes were done. Then you can hold her while she sleeps so I can take a shower."

Showing a new baby off to visitors is part of the fun of having one, but don't fall into the trap of expending all your energy on entertaining, feeding, and cleaning up after guests. Most people are willing to help out, if given some direction. They've been new parents themselves, or at least can recognize that you do need some assistance.

This is your special time to get to know your baby.

Getting back to normal

The excitement from the birth wears away, your baby begins to grow and change, and the fog of the early weeks lifts. Soon you begin to wonder, will I ever get anything done? When will life get back to normal? Why does breastfeeding seem to take so much time?

Whether you're taking off from work on a short maternity leave or you plan to care for your baby full-time for many months to come, the adjustment to being at home all day is not always easy. During pregnancy you may have imagined yourself cleaning closets, wallpapering the bathroom, or having lots of time for hobbies, while baby napped or looked on from his comfy infant seat. Reality looks quite different, and perhaps the only things you manage to keep up with are daytime television shows that you have plenty of time to watch while the baby nurses.

Life at home with a baby is quite different from going out to a job every day. It is much less predictable, with no built-in schedule, no systematic rewards, no paycheck. Even the simplest of housekeeping tasks can seem daunting when you try to tackle it with a baby cradled in one arm—a baby who has told you in no uncertain terms that she does not want to be put down. Experienced mothers and grandmothers looking back on their baby days are quick to remind you to enjoy your baby while you can, because "they grow up so fast." That may be true, but some days seem endless.

How do you keep all the balls in the air as you juggle household chores, time with your husband and older children, the things you want to do for yourself, and your baby's need for nursing and nurturing? The first thing to do is get your priorities in order: people first, things second. Babies and small children can't wait; adults can, if necessary. Reminding yourself of these two principles makes it much easier to decide what to do first when you know you can't do everything.

The adjustment to being home all day is not always easy.

Second, lower your expectations: simple meals, clean clothes (no ironing), and surroundings that are orderly enough to be safe but far short of the perfection captured in photographs for magazines like *House Beautiful.* There will be time to fuss over these things as your children get older. (Really!) Put away the dust collectors. Open up the meals-in-minutes cookbooks. Get a comb-and-go haircut. Wear clothing made of easy-care fabrics or knits.

Third, think creatively about how to get things done. Anything goes! Cook dinner in the morning before baby wakes up and reheat it when it's time to eat. Make enough for several meals of leftovers. Fold clothes while you talk on the phone. Put the baby in the baby carrier while you straighten up and vacuum. At the very least she'll be content to be near you; if you're lucky, the

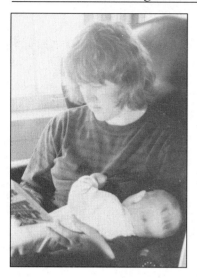

movement and the noise will put her to sleep. Invite grandma or another helper over if you've got a really big job to do; she can hold or play with the baby while you work and carry on with the work when you stop to nurse. Set yourself small tasks: clean one kitchen cupboard today, another next week; embroider tiny holiday ornaments, not full-sized samplers; read short stories or try a new magazine, but stay away from 900-page best-sellers.

Be open and honest about your limitations during the time you have small children. Many people, husbands included, don't realize that taking care of a baby all day is a full-time job. Enlist your partner's support as together you work out a lifestyle for your new family.

Overwhelmed by breastfeeding

When you're the mother of a small, totally dependent and very demanding human being, you can temporarily lose sight of yourself, as you are taken over by your baby's needs. This can be a challenging stage of life, and sometimes it looks as though breastfeeding is part of the problem. But if you're thinking about weaning, or giving regular bottles, think again. What do you expect that weaning will do for you? It won't lessen your baby's need to be held, and it won't make her less demanding. It won't decrease her desire to be with you, and it won't make her sleep through the night. In many ways, switching to formula feeding can make life harder, and you'll miss the ease and simplicity of comforting your baby at the breast. Fatigue is common in mothers of infants, no matter how they are feeding their babies.

If you're feeling restless or listless or burned out by motherhood, take a good look at your own needs. What can you do for yourself to help you feel better? Do you need to get out more? Do you need other adults to talk to during the day? Do you need exercise or clothes that flatter your postpartum figure? Do you need more support from your partner or friends? It's not too hard to solve these problems, and paying some attention to yourself will often improve your outlook on mothering and coping with your baby's need for you.

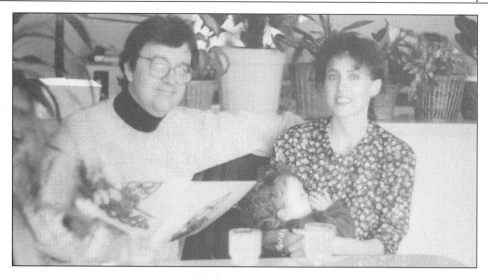

Going out with baby

If you've got places to go and people to see, do it.
Breastfed babies travel easily—just grab some diapers
and go.

But wait! What if your baby needs to breastfeed
while you're out? What do you do then?

Women sometimes hesitate about breastfeeding
away from home, in public places or in the presence of
people outside the immediate family. They've never seen
anyone else do it, or if they have, they may feel that
they're "just not that type." Or their minds keep flashing
back to stories they've heard about nursing mothers
being asked to leave restaurants or department stores.
Such incidents are rare, but they can loom large in the
minds of new mothers.

What is most important here is meeting your
baby's needs. Breastfed babies need to nurse frequently,
and it can be very difficult to bend and squeeze a list of
errands, an afternoon at the park, or an evening out with
your partner into the short span of time between
feedings. Bringing baby along and nursing her wherever
you happen to be makes everything easier. Nurse
discreetly, and you don't have to worry about
disapproving looks. Your baby will be happy and quiet,
and if people do notice, you can take pride in your

decision to give your baby the very best.

Breastfeeding discreetly, so that the breast is not exposed, is a skill that requires the right clothing and some practice. Try it at home in front of a mirror, or ask your partner or friend for a critique. Two-piece outfits where the top is loose and not tucked in to the bottom work best. You can lift the blouse or sweater from the bottom so that the baby can get to the nipple. If the blouse has buttons, unbutton it from the bottom up. The baby covers your midriff, and the top drapes over the breast. Or throw a receiving blanket over the baby's head, your breast, and on up over your shoulder for even better coverage. Sling-type carriers are ideal for discreet nursing; the carrier helps to support the baby and you can pull the fabric up and over the breast while she nurses. A number of mail-order companies sell special fashions for breastfeeding. The clothing—everything from dresses to separates to leotards—has pleats and tucks and openings that are designed to facilitate discreet breastfeeding away from home. (See the appendix for more information.)

Breastfed babies travel so easily. Grab some diapers and go!

Where do you go to nurse the baby at the shopping mall? There are several possibilities. Some restrooms have lounge areas with comfortable seating. These facilities, however, are often used by cigarette smokers, so they're not always the best place for babies, or very pleasant for mothers. If the store is not busy, you may be able to use a dressing room. A comfortable bench along a walkway works well. Or stop at a fast-food restaurant or coffee shop for a drink or a snack, and nurse the baby at a table. The table itself will give you some privacy; you might also want to sit with your back to the rest of the room. (Now is a good time to enjoy meals out in restaurants; it grows more difficult when your baby becomes a toddler.)

Dealing with criticism

Fashions in infant care have gone through many changes in the past century. A generation ago breastfeeding was

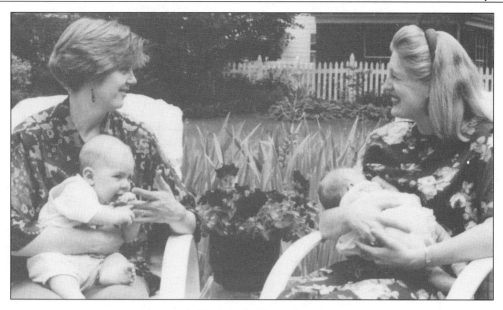

out of style, and as a result, many of the people who feel free to give you baby-rearing advice don't know very much about it. They may even feel very uncomfortable with the idea of feeding a baby at the mother's breast. Their ignorance and defensiveness about breastfeeding can come out as criticism of you.

Feelings run high when childcare choices are the topic of debate, and it can be difficult to tolerate criticism when you're new at mothering and in need of approval. Sometimes just understanding where the other person's attitudes and ideas come from will help defuse the criticism, at least in your own mind. Mothers and mothers-in-law who decided against breastfeeding thirty years ago or who tried and had little success may have complicated feelings about breastfeeding that influence their comments to you. They may genuinely believe that breast milk is inadequate or that "women in our family don't make enough milk." Educating them about breastfeeding's benefits and how it works may help bring them around. You can also reassure these critics that you know they did the very best they could for their babies, just as you are trying to make your own best judgments about how to raise your children. Sometimes the only way to handle critics is to agree to disagree and then move on to other topics which are easier to discuss.

Sometimes you must reconcile yourself to the fact that these particular people are not ever going to see things your way, and no amount of arguing will change their minds. Of course, these are not the people to go to for a sympathetic ear when your baby is nursing non-stop through a growth spurt or is waking up frequently at night for feedings. When you are having problems with breastfeeding, it's best to take them to someone who understands your desire to continue nursing, even when the going is temporarily tough. If you're encountering a lot of criticism of breastfeeding from family or friends, find out about La Leche League meetings in your area, and attend them. This is one place where you can let your hair down about breastfeeding without having somebody suggest formula as the answer to your problems.

Taking care of yourself

While your baby is small and totally dependent on you, taking care of yourself should be a priority. When you're feeling good, you can do a better job of mothering your baby.

What to eat while breastfeeding

You don't have to eat perfectly balanced meals or follow any complicated dietary rules in order to produce enough good quality milk for your baby. Women all over the world make enough milk for their babies on diets ranging from barely adequate to overindulgent. Human milk quality is remarkably consistent, despite variations in mothers' eating habits. While a steady diet of junk food and sweets isn't good for anyone, it won't seriously affect the nutritional value of your milk.

You will probably find that while you are breastfeeding you can eat a little more than you did before you became pregnant without having to worry about gaining weight. A diet that includes lots of fruits, vegetables, and complex carbohydrates (whole-grain bread and cereals, pasta, rice, and beans) will give you the stamina you need to get through the day. Snack on

wholesome healthful foods, and choose water or fruit
juice rather than soda pop, cola, or coffee.

Losing weight

You don't have to wait until your baby weans to lose
extra pounds put on during (or before) pregnancy. Some
women find that they slowly shed weight during the time
they're nursing, without even restricting calories, due to
the extra energy demands of lactation. Be patient—
nursing mothers tend to lose the weight when their
babies are three to six months old.

Even if you want to take some initiative to get the
weight off—or get it off more quickly, it's not a good
idea to go on a quick weight loss diet while
breastfeeding. A drastic drop in your energy intake
mobilizes your body's fat stores, which can
raise the level of environmental
contaminants in your milk. Also, you'll be
tired and crabby, less able to cope with a
demanding infant. Instead, try cutting back
on the amount of fat in your diet—skip the
butter on toast, use fat-free salad dressing,
remove the skin from chicken. Get some
exercise daily; put the baby in the carrier
or stroller and go out for a thirty-to-forty-
minute walk. You can safely and easily
lose two or three pounds a month this way, and never
feel deprived.

Mothers shed weight while they are nursing without restricting calories.

What not to eat

You don't have to give up chocolate or caffeine or even
an occasional glass of wine just because you're
breastfeeding. Most nursing mothers can eat whatever
they like with no effects on their babies. Warnings about
avoiding cabbage, broccoli, chocolate, or other specific
foods are merely old wives' tales.

Sometimes, a particular type of food will bother a
particular baby, perhaps one with a family history of
allergy. A persistent rash or unexplained fussiness may
clear up if mother eliminates milk products or eggs or

another food from her diet. For more information about breastfeeding and food allergies, see the resource list at the end of this book.

While there is currently some controversy about the effects of alcohol on nursing babies, light-to-moderate drinking—a glass of wine with dinner or an occasional beer—has not been shown to be harmful. Larger amounts of alcohol may interfere with the let-down reflex. Being even slightly intoxicated will affect your ability to tune into your baby and care for her needs.

Illicit drugs and smoking

Smoke from parents' cigarettes is hazardous to babies and children. Studies have shown that children of smokers get more colds and are more likely to have other respiratory problems. You can still breastfeed, even if you smoke, but it's a good idea to cut down. Heavy smoking may affect your milk supply, and your baby may gain weight more slowly. The nicotine from cigarettes does appear in human milk, though the levels are low; if you smoke less than a pack a day, the nicotine will probably not affect your baby. In any case, avoid smoking around the baby.

Breastfeeding mothers should not use recreational drugs such as cocaine or marijuana. Cocaine appears in human milk up to sixty hours after use and can cause cocaine intoxication in the breastfeeding baby. The active ingredient in marijuana, THC, is concentrated in milk, lingers for days after the mother's exposure, and can be found in the baby's urine and stools. As with alcohol intoxication, abusing these and other drugs affects the mother's ability to care for her infant.

Medications

Be sure your doctor knows that you are breastfeeding if he or she prescribes any medication for you. Most medications are safe for nursing mothers and babies, though not all physicians are aware of this—especially those who seldom treat nursing mothers. Sometimes the baby's doctor is more familiar with the effects of medication on a breastfed baby than the doctor who is treating you. If you are being advised to wean your baby in order to take medication, tell your doctor that continuing to breastfeed your baby is very important to you. Often, the doctor may be able to prescribe a different medication, or further investigation reveals that the medication is compatible with breastfeeding. Your local La Leche League Leader can help you find information about specific medications that you can share with your doctor.

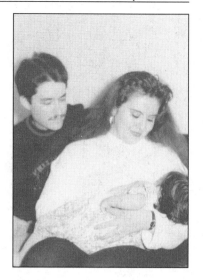

Fathers and their feelings

Fathers may have questions about breastfeeding, so it's helpful for mothers to share what they learn with their partners. Knowing about the benefits will help fathers understand that breastfeeding is worth a little extra effort; seeing that it's possible to nurse a baby in a public place without exposing the breast will ease another common worry. Other frequent concerns include whether demand feeding will "spoil" the baby and how breastfeeding will affect the couple's time together and their sexual relations. Talking these problems over as they occur, or even ahead of time, will enable parents to work together so that everyone's needs can be met.

Many men don't realize that fathers are crucial to breastfeeding success. Emotional support from her partner can help a woman grow more confident as a mother and overcome difficulties she may encounter with breastfeeding. It may seem like a little thing to tell someone "I know you can do it" or "You're so important to our baby" or "I'm proud that you're breastfeeding," but heartfelt comments like these make a new mother's heart soar, and she'll remember them for a lifetime. Watching out for the mother's needs while she nurses the baby can be a father's way of showing his love for both wife and child. Arranging pillows, bringing a glass of water or a snack, giving a back rub, playing with an older child, or just sitting and talking quietly while the baby is nursing can help a mother feel loved and loving. Both father and baby will reap the benefits.

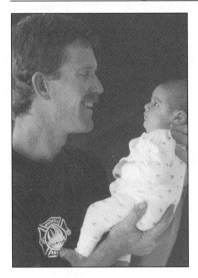

Just like mothers, fathers need to spend time getting to know their babies. Even though the mother is doing all the feeding, there are plenty of baby chores left over for fathers who want to get involved. Bathing, burping, walking, soothing, and nuzzling up to a sleeping baby all have their rewards; fathers don't have to give bottles in order to enjoy their offspring. As time goes on and babies' needs expand from care and comfort to stimulation and excitement, fathers become a major source of just plain fun.

Your sex life

Finding the right time for love-making postpartum isn't always easy. Babies consume lots of time and energy, and fatigue tends to dampen sexual desire. Having a baby brings changes to a couple's relationship, and sexual relations may be affected by the adjustments both father and mother are making to new routines and priorities. It's important to talk about these changes and make an effort to keep the romance alive in a relationship. Sex may not be as spontaneous as it once was—you may have to plan ahead, sneak around a bit, and be prepared to take a break if the baby wakes up. But despite these obstacles, postpartum sex can take on a new glow, as the warmth and tenderness parents feel toward their baby spill over into their feelings for each other.

Breastfeeding does affect a woman's sexual response. The same hormone that is responsible for the let-down reflex, oxytocin, is released during arousal, so lactating women may leak milk during sex. Pressing on the nipple may stop the leaking, or keep a towel handy. If you feed the baby or express some milk beforehand you can minimize leaking, if this is a problem for you.

Breastfeeding women may also experience vaginal dryness and discomfort during intercourse. This is related to hormone levels during lactation; it doesn't mean that you're not enjoying your partner's attentions. A longer period of foreplay may help, or try using a lubricant, such as K-Y jelly. Hormone levels may also contribute to decreased desire for sex among some lactating women.

This is only temporary and often improves when the woman's menstrual cycle resumes.

Menstrual cycles and fertility

Breastfeeding suppresses ovulation and menstruation, making it unlikely that a woman will become pregnant again right away. While breastfeeding is not foolproof as a contraceptive, recent research has found a pregnancy rate of only two percent in the first six months postpartum among women who are fully breastfeeding and who are not having periods. This compares favorably to pregnancy rates for many artificial methods of contraception. "Fully breastfeeding" means that the baby receives all, or almost all, of her nourishment at the breast. The baby is fed frequently, including night feedings, rarely gets bottles, and has all her sucking needs met at the breast—no pacifiers.

As your baby starts solids, goes longer between feedings, and sleeps longer at night, the chances of getting pregnant increase, even if your periods have not resumed. Some women ovulate without having a "warning" menstrual period first, especially as the baby gets older, starts solids, or is well on the way to weaning. If your periods have started again, you should consider yourself fertile and take precautions if you don't wish to become pregnant.

Non-hormonal methods of contraception have no effect on breastfeeding; this category includes the diaphragm, cervical cap, condoms, spermicides, the contraceptive sponge, and the copper IUD. The combined oral contraceptive pill may present problems for breastfeeding women; the estrogen component can reduce a mother's milk supply, alter milk composition, and affect infant growth. These effects have not been found with the progestin-only minipill, progestin implants, and injectable forms of progestin. With any type of hormonal contraceptive, small amounts of synthetic hormones appear in the mother's milk, and some experts have expressed concern about possible long-term effects on the baby. You may wish to discuss this with your health-care provider.

Chapter Six

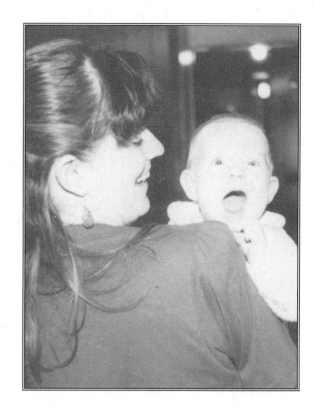

Looking Ahead

Babies change—every day.

Skills replace reflexes, coos and smiles replace the wide-eyed gaze with which newborns once regarded their parents. Growing babies wriggle with anticipation when they know it's time to nurse, and sometimes they stop feeding for just a moment to grin up at mother, as if to say, "Oh, this is *sooo* good." Though mothers may struggle with breastfeeding in the early weeks, they often find that it becomes more rewarding as time goes on— and much easier.

Changing behavior as baby grows

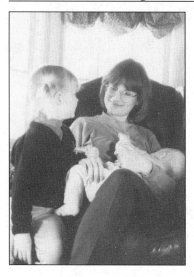

Babies' needs change as they grow. Older breastfed babies may still need to nurse frequently, but not as often as when they were newborns. There will be fussy periods such as late afternoon or early evening, when they seem to nurse all the time, but at other times growing babies may be so involved with playing with daddy, discovering their toes, or watching the shelves go by at the grocery store that they forget about eating, for a little while anyway.

Some babies become so interested in the outside world that it's difficult to get them to settle down and nurse. Feeding them in a quiet, dimly lighted place, at least part of the time, can help, or they may make up for lost time at the breast during the day by breastfeeding more often at night.

Losing interest in nursing?

Babies rarely wean without some help from mother before the age of a year. If a younger baby seems to be losing interest or is refusing to nurse, there may be reasons other than readiness to wean. A stuffy nose makes it difficult to breathe while breastfeeding, so a baby with a cold may fuss at the breast or cut back on feeding time. The doctor may suggest a mild decongestant, or you can use a nasal syringe to clean out mucus from baby's nose. A baby with an ear infection may not want to lie on his side for feedings because it hurts; if you suspect an ear problem, call your doctor. Some babies may change their nursing pattern when they're teething or if their mouths are sore for another reason.

Frequent supplementary bottles are a leading cause of disinterest in breastfeeding. Babies who get bottles regularly may come to prefer them—or at least to expect the breast to act like a bottle. They may complain about having to wait for the mother's let-down to work. As bottles take the place of breastfeedings and the baby nurses less, the mother's milk supply decreases, prompting her to offer more bottles. Soon mother and baby are on the road to weaning, even if this is not what mother had originally intended.

It is possible to build up your milk supply again while gradually cutting out the supplements. The more your baby nurses the more milk you will have. Offer the breast before offering the bottle. Let your baby nurse for comfort even if you don't think he's hungry yet. For a few days, plan on spending much of your time feeding and cuddling, holding and carrying your baby. As your milk supply increases, your baby will take less formula from the bottle, and you can eliminate the bottle feedings one at a time.

If your baby must get bottles regularly because you are working and are separated from him, breastfeeding frequently while you are with him will help keep his interest high. So will skin-to-skin contact and lots of interaction with mother.

Nursing Strike

When a baby who had been breastfeeding well suddenly refuses to nurse at all, it's called a nursing strike. This can be a frustrating, unhappy time for both mother and baby. The reasons for a nursing strike are as individual as the babies involved. You may never know why your baby refuses to nurse, but with persistence and patience on mother's side, most babies will start breastfeeding again in two to four days. Give the baby lots of attention and skin-to-skin contact, so that he remembers how nice it is to be with you. Offer the breast when he's not quite aware that you're trying to feed him—when he's drowsy or just starting to wake up. Try fooling him with a different nursing position. Feed him in a rocking chair or while walking; being in motion may distract him from not wanting to nurse. During the time he's not nursing, you will need to pump or express your milk in order to keep up the supply, and you can give the milk to your baby using a cup.

When a baby goes on a nursing strike or fusses a lot at the breast, it can feel as though he is rejecting you right along with your milk. It's hard not to take it personally. Finding a reason for the refusal to nurse may make it easier to cope with these feelings, but explanations aren't always available. If your baby's breastfeeding behavior has you confused or concerned, call a La Leche League Leader and talk things over with her. She may be able to help you determine what's going on and can give you the support you need in order to figure out what to do.

When your baby gets teeth

Babies can acquire a complete set of teeth—incisors, molars, canines—without their mothers ever feeling a thing during breastfeedings. The tongue covers the lower teeth during sucking; the upper teeth may leave a small mark or indentation where they have been pressed against the mother's soft areola, but this doesn't hurt.

There's no need to quit breastfeeding when your baby gets teeth.

There's no need to quit breastfeeding when your baby gets teeth.

However, some babies do bite, especially when their teeth are new and they're not sure what to do with them. Biting is most likely to occur toward the end of a feeding when the baby is sucking for comfort or playing around.

If your baby clamps down while drifting off to sleep, your main concern is getting your nipple out of his mouth safely. Work your index finger in between his gums and hook it around the nipple as you pull it out; the finger will protect the nipple in case baby clamps down again as he tries to keep the breast in his mouth.

When babies bite for the first time, they can count on a big reaction from you: "Ouch!" This is enough to persuade some not to try it again. Others will go on experimenting. What you do to teach your baby not to bite again depends on his age and his temperament. An older baby may be able to understand that if he bites, mother ends the feeding immediately, and there's no more nursing for a while—perhaps twenty minutes or more. This, along with mother's sudden yell of pain, may be too much for a more sensitive baby to bear, while a younger baby may not be able to understand the relationship between his actions and the consequences.

You can prevent biting from happening by paying close attention to your baby toward the end of the feeding. His behavior at the breast, maybe a certain gleam in the eye, will warn you that he's about to bite, and you can take him off the breast before he has a chance.

Starting solids

Breastfed babies don't need solid foods until sometime around age six months. There are good reasons for waiting this long. Solid foods gradually take the place of milk in the baby's diet. If he fills up on cereal or bananas or carrots, he will not be as hungry and will be less interested in nursing at the breast. As he nurses less, your milk supply will decrease, and your baby may lose interest in nursing sooner than you had planned. Also, solid foods are not as nourishing as your milk. It takes a full and varied diet to supply all the nutrients that children and adults need; a baby's limited intake of solids can not measure up to the complete nutrition available to him in human milk. Thus, early solids replace human milk with less nutritious alternatives.

Early solids replace human milk with less nutritious alternatives.

Allergies are another reason for waiting. Babies are more likely to develop food allergies when they begin solids at an early age. Early solids may also contribute to obesity. Last, but not least, from mothers' point of view, feeding solids to young babies is a messy business. It's much easier when they can sit up on their own and no longer automatically push everything foreign out of their mouth with their tongue.

Why do some advisors recommend solids even before four months of age? There was a time when babies as young as three or four weeks were fed cereal and other solid foods as a sort of nutritional insurance; physicians were reluctant to have babies depend on only one food product–artificial formula–for all their nutritional needs for a long period of time. This fear does not really apply to breastfed babies who are receiving a completely nourishing diet of mother's milk. Then there's the idea that adding cereal to the diet will help baby sleep through the night. Research studies, along with the experiences of many mothers, have shown that this is not true.

Your doctor may suggest you give your baby iron-fortified cereal to prevent anemia. This is not really necessary. Although the amount of iron in human milk is small, it is very well absorbed, and this, together with the iron stores the baby has from birth, is usually sufficient until well past six months of age. If there is any question, a simple blood test can determine if your baby needs an additional source of iron in his diet.

Ready for solids?

Magazine ads and coupons arriving in the mail can make those cute little jars of baby food on the supermarket shelf look very tempting. But it's better to watch your own baby for signs of readiness. You are a better judge of your baby's needs than the companies who are trying to get you to buy their products.

When a baby is truly ready for solids it's hard to stop him from trying them. It becomes challenging to hold him on your lap while you're eating. He grabs for things and is fully capable of dumping your dinner all over the table. He'll watch you eat, following every forkful from plate to mouth with bright attentive eyes. And everything he gets his hands on goes into his mouth.

An increase in appetite is another sign that a baby is ready for solid foods. If a baby who is around six months of age suddenly wants to nurse more frequently, and this goes on for four or five days with no other apparent explanation, he is probably ready for more food. Bring on the solids! If he is much younger than six months, be a little cautious. This change in nursing routine may be just a growth spurt, or the baby may not be feeling well or for some reason may need more of your attention.

Even as your baby begins to eat a wider variety of foods, your milk remains an important part of his diet. It supplies much of the protein and many of the calories and other nutrients he needs each day.

How to begin

A baby's first encounter with solid foods is more like an experiment than a meal. He has a lot to learn about taste, texture, and how to move the food from the front of his mouth to the back and then swallow it. Measure the success of early feedings by how much practice baby gets, not how much food you manage to get into him.

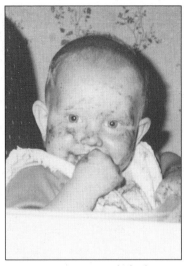

Expect some messes as baby learns to feed himself.

Mashed ripe bananas make an excellent first food; they're sweet and soft and sticky enough to be interesting. You can use fresh bananas right out of the peel; you don't need to depend on jarred baby food for simple, tasty infant meals. If you wait until your baby is about six months old before starting solids, he'll be able to handle a few bumps and lumps. Foods should be soft and mashed, but they don't need to be pureed pudding-smooth or liquefied. Ripe avocado or cooked sweet potatoes also make excellent first foods. Offer only one new food at a time, and wait several days or a week before adding another food. If the baby has an allergic reaction—a rash, diarrhea, upset stomach, stuffy nose— you'll know which food is responsible.

Choose a time when your baby isn't terribly hungry, maybe a half-hour to an hour after he has nursed. Start with a tiny amount of food. (You can increase the portion size gradually as time goes on.) Breastfed babies often feel most comfortable on their mother's lap during these first feedings. You can use a spoon to place the food in your baby's mouth, or try using your finger. You shouldn't have to coax, cajole, or put on a big show to get your baby to eat. If he's not interested, he'll turn his head away, clamp his mouth shut, or spit the food out. Respect his wishes and try again another time. Some breastfed babies aren't much interested in solids until they're seven, eight, or nine months old, and will continue to grow well and stay healthy on breast milk alone.

Preparing nutritious foods for an adventuresome new eater can be a lot of fun. La Leche League's book The Womanly Art of Breastfeeding contains many ideas for fresh, easy foods for growing babies. If you wait until your baby is six months old before you start solids, you'll find that he can soon eat many of the things you prepare for the rest of the family. He may even teach you a thing or two about what's good, and good for you.

Returning to work

Many women continue to breastfeed after they return to jobs outside their homes. They want to maintain the loving feeling of closeness that nursing provides. Even though others may care for the baby and even feed him, only mother can breastfeed; this is a reminder for both mother and baby that their relationship is unique. Reunions at the end of the workday are especially pleasant when the two of you can curl up together on the sofa to nurse and relax before it's time to start dinner or attack the household chores.

The how-to of breastfeeding and working comes down to two issues: how you will keep up your milk supply and how your baby will be fed while you are gone. The way you work these things out will depend on your work and caregiving situations and the age of your baby.

Keeping up your milk supply

Your body will go on making milk while you are away from your baby. If you pump that milk out, your body will make more milk, and the milk you pump can be given to your baby while you're gone. Expressing milk for your baby provides him with the best possible nutrition even when you can't be there to feed him. Pumping will also prevent you from getting plugged ducts or a breast infection.

You'll probably need to pump your breasts every three to four hours while you and your baby are apart. This will depend partly on how often your baby nurses and how soon your breasts begin to feel full. If you're working part-time, four to six hours at a stretch, one pumping session will probably be enough. With an eight-hour work day, you'll need to pump at least twice. Remember to include travel time to and from the job when figuring out how long you'll be away from your baby.

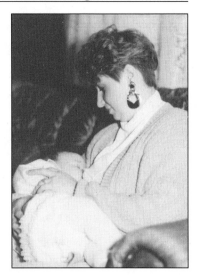

Where to pump can sometimes be a problem. A clean, comfortable private place is nicest; perhaps there's an empty office available, or another empty room with a chair and a lock on the door. Many women have to make do with the bathroom, a toilet stall, or the ladies' lounge, but you may be able to come up with a better alternative with the support of co-workers or your boss. Packing a picture of your baby in the bag with your pump will help your let-down function better no matter where you are.

Pumping requires fifteen to twenty minutes of your lunch time or break. When you're finished pumping you'll probably want to refrigerate the pumped milk or store it in a small cooler. You can take the milk home with you in a cooler at the end of the day, and it can either be given to your baby the next day while you are gone or stored in the refrigerator or freezer for future use. (For help with pumping and guidelines for storing milk, see chapter 4.)

Your co-workers may find the whole idea of pumping milk strange or embarrassing, particularly if you're the first woman at your place of employment to do this. Keep in mind that you're doing this for your baby, and it's important. A sense of humor helps, too. You might even point out to your co-workers that breastfeeding benefits them: your breastfed baby is less likely to get sick, so you are less likely to be absent from the job.

Feeding baby while you're gone

How many bottles and how much milk your baby needs will depend on his age, his feeding habits, and how long you're gone. There are no hard and fast rules. An older baby who can eat solids while away from you might require less; a baby of three or four months who gets nothing but milk may take more. It's a good idea to start pumping at home a few weeks before going back to work. You won't feel as pressured about pumping if there's a supply of milk in the freezer for days when baby's demands are running ahead of what you've supplied. Store the milk in small amounts at first—about two ounces in each container—until you feel more certain about how much milk he'll take at a feeding.

Take the milk to the caregiver's on ice in a cooler. She should store it in the refrigerator (or freezer, if it's already frozen) until feeding time. The baby should get the fresh, refrigerated milk you pumped the day before first and then, if necessary, milk from the freezer. The sitter should warm or thaw the milk gently, holding the bag or container under warm running water.

Many mothers who work continue to breastfeed their babies.

What if the baby won't take the bottle? This is a common worry and occasionally a problem for caregivers. But breastfed babies can be persuaded to take a bottle. Though some people may tell you to introduce bottles early and get the baby accustomed to them right away, it's better to wait until four to six weeks of age, when the baby has mastered nursing at the breast. Giving bottles before that time can lead to nipple confusion, poor nursing at the breast, and early weaning. There's no need to introduce an artificial nipple until about two weeks before you return to work.

Drinking from an artificial nipple is a new skill for your baby, and learning it may require time and patience from caregivers. Someone other than the mother should be offering the bottle; many babies won't accept substitutes when they know the breast is nearby. Don't wait until the baby is desperately hungry to offer the bottle; he's more likely to accept something new when he's relatively calm. Try different positions; some babies like to be held as they would be for breastfeeding while others prefer a totally different posture, facing away from the caregiver or propped against her raised legs. Try different kinds of nipples, with different sized holes.

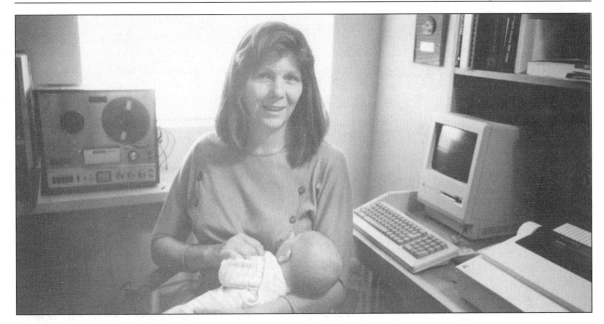

Hold the bottle nipple near the baby's mouth and allow
him to take it rather than pushing it between his lips. Try
warming the nipple before offering it to the baby. And
remember that even very young babies can take milk
from a cup or a spoon, if they decide they will have
nothing to do with bottles for the time being.

Making it work

Juggling a job and a baby is not easy. Here are some
suggestions that may help you along the way.

During the time you are home with your baby,
nurse him frequently. Spend lots of time together
cuddling and playing. Put him in the baby carrier while
you prepare dinner or do laundry. Nursing frequently
while you're together—at night, on weekends—will
encourage your body to keep making lots of milk,
though you may need to pump more often on Monday
or Tuesday to keep up with the increased supply
stimulated by nursing on the weekend.

Some babies react to their mother's being gone
during the day by staying awake longer in the evening
and by waking more often to nurse at night. If you tuck
the baby in bed with you, you can still get the rest you
need; he'll be able to nurse and enjoy the closeness

while you doze. Babies who nurse more frequently at night may sleep more at the caregiver's and need fewer bottles.

Set the alarm fifteen minutes early so that you can breastfeed the baby before you have to get up. This should keep him content while you're getting ready. Then nurse him again once more before you leave.

Choose a caregiver for your baby who understands and supports your desire to continue breastfeeding; your working-and-breastfeeding routine will go more smoothly with this helper's cooperation. Talk to her about breastfeeding's importance for your baby, and tell her what she can do to help you. For example, the caregiver can avoid giving the baby a bottle toward the end of the day, or give only a few ounces of milk, so that your baby is ready to nurse when you arrive.

Some mothers look for childcare near their jobs rather than close to home. They nurse the baby at the caregiver's before going to work and before setting out for home after work. If you have a long commute, this can shorten the length of time you are away from your baby. Sometimes it's possible to go to the caregiver's and nurse the baby on your lunch hour, or even to have the baby brought to you for feedings.

A good breast pump is a worthwhile investment. Many women prefer the ease of using an electric pump; some are battery-operated for use where there are no electrical outlets. It's possible to rent a high-quality electric pump on a long-term basis for a lot less money than it would cost to give your baby formula. These pumps are the most effective at maintaining a milk supply.

Friends may wonder why you "bother" to breastfeed, with all the other demands on your attention. Look to other breastfeeding mothers for support. At La Leche League meetings, you can often meet other women who are combining breastfeeding with employment outside the home.

Supplementing

If you decide that pumping is not for you or that you've pumped long enough, your baby can receive formula supplements when you're not there to nurse him. In babies of four to six months or older, solids can substitute for one or more breastfeedings. You can still continue to breastfeed your baby when you and he are together. Your body will adjust to this new pattern of milk-making, though at first you may need to express some milk while you're at work to relieve fullness. Frequent nursing sessions at home will help keep your baby interested in the breast and remind him that mother is the source of this special food.

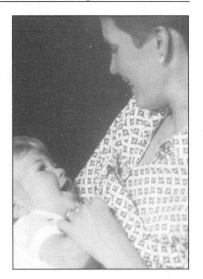

Weaning—or not

How long you breastfeed is up to you and your baby. There's no minimum length of time that you must breastfeed, nor is there a certain age by which a baby must be weaned. A mother can choose to set her own pace for weaning, or she can follow her baby's lead. As long as the baby continues to nurse, the breasts will go on producing nutritious milk that contains valuable immunities.

Weaning is best done gradually, to allow your breasts to adjust to the decreasing demand for milk and to make the change easier on your baby. Stopping breastfeeding "cold turkey" can be very distressing for both mother and baby and can cause plugged ducts or a breast infection. Watch your baby for signs of stress; he'll let you know if weaning is going too quickly for him.

The weaning process begins the first time your baby takes food from a source other than your breast—whether it's formula from a bottle or mashed banana from a spoon. Weaning is the gradual replacement of breastfeeding with other foods and ways of nurturing. Babies who are approaching one year of age and eating a variety of foods may be able to wean directly to a cup; younger babies generally require bottles. Ask your doctor about what kind of nourishment your baby should get in place of your milk.

Eliminate only one nursing session at a time. Offer the bottle or a cup at a time when your baby normally would have nursed. Wait at least two or three days, preferably longer, before you eliminate another feeding. If your breasts feel full from skipping feedings, express a small amount of milk—enough to relieve the pressure and prevent plugged ducts. Within a few days your breasts will be producing less milk and this won't be necessary.

It's easiest to begin by eliminating feeding sessions that are less important to the baby. Be prepared to slow the pace if your baby becomes fussy or clingy, gets ill, or seems to be teething. Naptime, bedtime, and first-thing-in-the-morning feedings are usually the last to go. Take your time with these, especially if you enjoy a bedtime snuggle as much as your baby does.

Weaning sometimes brings feelings of sadness, especially if you have been forced to wean your baby abruptly, for reasons beyond your control. Even for mothers who feel ready for weaning, there may be some sense of loss. Weaning marks the end of a physical oneness with your child, the close of a very special period in your lives. Remember that your baby-child's strong need for your presence continues, even if it is now expressed in other ways.

You can continue to breastfeed as your baby grows.

It's important to be realistic about your expectations for weaning. Stopping breastfeeding does not make mothering any easier or force your child to grow up any faster. Your baby will still demand lots of your attention; supplying this in ways other than nursing can be challenging. Breastfeeding can be a real worksaver when you can count on it as a surefire way of getting a baby to quiet down or sleep. Often there are ways other than total weaning to cope with mothers' feelings of restlessness or being tied down.

If you choose to do so, there's nothing wrong with continuing to breastfeed as your baby grows into toddlerhood. This is the most natural path to follow. Babies who are allowed to wean at their own pace usually continue to nurse well past their first birthday. As they learn to eat other foods and to drink from a cup, breastfeeding becomes more important for comfort and reassurance than for nourishment. These children wean gradually, when they are ready.

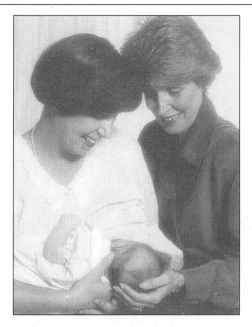

Nursing a toddler is considered unusual in American culture, perhaps because we push our children toward independence at an early age. But in many other cultures around the world, children nurse until two-and-a-half or three years of age or even longer. The idea of breastfeeding a toddler may seem peculiar to you at first; it makes more sense as your baby grows and you see how much nursing means to him.

If you want to know more about natural, baby-led weaning, or about weaning in general, check the resource list in the back of this book, or call a La Leche League Leader. She can help you wean your baby gradually and with love or can give you the support you need if you want to breastfeed longer.

A world of breastfeeding women

Memories of breastfeeding last a lifetime. Studies have shown that women's recall of how long they breastfed is very accurate many years later—a sign of how important a mark nursing a baby has left on their lives. Nourishing a baby at the breast is both profoundly practical and totally astonishing. Enjoy it while it lasts and then treasure the memory as your child grows.

The experience of breastfeeding binds women together, across the barriers of language, culture, and nationality. We can feel a rapport with one another as we seek to give our babies the very best of ourselves. So the next time you see another nursing mother, smile and acknowledge the womanly bond that we all share. Talk about breastfeeding with your friends, join La Leche League, learn about breastfeeding in other parts of the world. If mothers can be more forthright about how wonderful it is to breastfeed and how important it is to babies, we can make this a better world for our children and our grandchildren to come.

Notes

Page 3   Older baby receives greater concentration of immune factors: A.S. Goldman et al., "Immunologic components in human milk during the second year of lactation," *Acta Paediatr Scand* 1983; 722:133-34.

Breastfed babies have fewer illnesses and are less likely to be SIDS victims: American Academy of Pediatrics, Work Group on Breastfeeding, "Breastfeeding and the use of human milk," *Pediatrics* 1997; 100(6):1035-39.

Each mother's milk protects her baby from whatever is going around: R. Garofalo and A. S. Goldman, "Expression of functional immunomodulatory and anti-inflammatory factors in human milk," *Clin Perinatol* 1999; 26(2): 361-77.

Page 4   Nutritional components of breast milk: For a summary of the literature see the chapter "Biochemistry of human milk," in R. Lawrence and R. Lawrence, *Breastfeeding: A Guide for the Medical Profession,* 5th ed., (St. Louis: Mosby, 1999).

Longer periods of breastfeeding are associated with higher scores on IQ tests and other measures of intellectual development: L. Horwood and D. Fergusson, "Breastfeeding and later cognitive and academic outcomes," *Pediatrics* 1998; 101(1):e9.

Enzymes and hormones in human milk: M. Hamosh, "Enzymes in human milk," in *Human Milk in Infant Nutrition and Health,* ed. R. R. Howell et al., (Springfield, IL: Charles C. Thomas, 1986); L. A. Ellis and M. F. Picciano, "Milk-borne hormones: Regulators of development in neonates," *Adv Exp Med Biol* 1991; 262:69-76.

Page 14   Preparing nipples during pregnancy is not necessary: MAIN Trial Collaborative Group, "Preparing for breastfeeding: Treatment of inverted and non-protractile nipples in pregnancy," *Midwifery* 1994; 10:200-14.

Page 18   Hospital routines affect breastfeeding success: G. Nylander et al., "Unsupplemented feeding in the maternity ward: positive long-term effects," *Acta Obstet Gynecol Scand* 1991; 70:205-9.

Page 20   Part-time employment and delaying the return to workmake breastfeeding easier: K. G. Auerbach and E. Guss, "Maternal employment and breastfeeding: A study of 567 women's experiences," *Am J Dis Child* 1985; 138:958-60.

Page 29   Babies decide for themselves when they have finished a feeding: M. W. Woolridge, "Do changes in pattern of breast usage alter the baby's nutrient intake?" *Lancet* 1990; 336:395-97.

Page 34   Frequent feedings help prevent jaundice and hypoglycemia: D. Tudehope et al., "Breastfeeding practices and severe hyperbilirubinaemia," *J Paediatr Child Health* 1991; 27:240-44; J. M. Hawdon et al., "Patterns of metabolic adaptation for preterm and term infants in the first neonatal week," *Arch Dis Child* 1992; 67:357-65.

Bottle-feeding is more physiologically stressful than breastfeeding: P. Meier, "Bottle and breast feeding: Effects on transcutaneous oxygen pressure and temperature in small preterm infants," *Nurs Res* 1988; 37:36-41.

Page 35   Risk of allergy from supplemental formula: A. Host, "Importance of the first meal on the development of cow's milk allergy and tolerance," *Allergy Proc* 1991; 12:227-32.

Page 42   Sore nipples caused by baby not taking enough breast tissue: N. Mohrbacher and J. Stock, >THE BREASTFEEDING ANSWER BOOK (Schaumburg, IL: La Leche League International, 1997, rev. ed., 388-91).

Page 43   Additional material on sore nipples and latch-on and sucking problems can be found in S. M. Maher, *An Overview of Solutions to Breastfeeding and Sucking Problems* (Schaumburg, IL: La Leche League International, 1988); in N. Mohrbacher and J. Stock, THE BREASTFEEDING ANSWER BOOK (Schaumburg, IL: La Leche League International, 1997, rev. ed., 52-72); and in materials by Chele Marmet and Ellen Shell from the Lactation Institute in Encino, California.

Page 46   Modified lanolin helps skin retain moisture and aids healing: D. A. Sharp, "Moist wound healing for sore or cracked nipples," BREASTFEEDING ABSTRACTS 1992; 12:19.

Page 54   Physicians disagree about when to treat newborn jaundice: For a review of the research and treatment recommendations see T. B. Newman and M. J. Maisels, "Evaluation and treatment of jaundice in the term newborn: A kinder, gentler approach," *Pediatrics* 1992; 89:809-18.

           Frequent breastfeeding keeps bilirubin levels within the normal range: L. Gartner, "Neonatal jaundice," *Pediatr Review* 1994; 15(11):422-32.

Page 63   This technique for hand-expressing was developed by Chele Marmet. For more details, see *Manual Expression of Breast Milk–Marmet Technique* (Schaumburg, IL: La Leche League International, 1989).

Page 65   Guidelines for storing human milk: J. Barger and P. Bull, "A comparison of the bacterial composition of breast milk stored at room temperature and stored in the refrigerator," *Int J Childbirth Educ* 1987; 2:29-30; R. Sosa and L. Barness, "Bacterial growth in refrigerated human milk," *Am J Dis Child* 1987; 141:111-12; A. Pardou et al., "Human milk banking: Influence of storage processes and of bacterial contamination on some milk constituents," *Biol Neonate* 1994; 65: 302-09.

Page 66   Human milk should not be heated in a microwave oven: R. Quan et al., "Effects of microwave radiation on anti-infective factors in human milk," *Am J Dis Child* 1987; 89:667-69.

Page 70   Being able to wake easily related to a lower risk of SIDS: S. Mosko, C. Richard, and J. McKenna, "Infant arousals during mother-infantbed sharing: Implications for infant sleep and sudden infant death syndrome research," *Pediatrics* 1997; 100(5):841-49.

Page 71   Breastfed babies were older before they slept through the night: M. F. Elias et al., "Sleep/wake patterns of breast-fed infants in the first 2 years of life," *Pediatrics* 1986; 77:322-29; J. Eaton-Evans and A. E. Dugdale, "Sleep patterns of infants in the first year of life," *Arch Dis Child* 1988; 63:647-49.

Page 75   Not having enough milk most frequent reason for stopping breastfeeding: P. D. Hill, "The enigma of insufficient milk supply," *MCN* 1991; 16:313-15; C. Hillervik-Lindquist, "Studies in perceived breast milk insufficiency," *Acta Paediatr Scand* 1991; suppl 376:6-27.

Page 78   Breastfed babies gain more slowly after four months: K. Dewey and M. J. Heinig, "Are new growth charts needed for breastfed infants?" Breastfeeding Abstracts 1993; 12:35-36; K. G. Dewey et al., "Breastfed infants are leaner than formula-fed infants at one year of age: The DARLING study," *Am J Clin Nutr* 1993; 57:140-45.

Page 86   Human milk quality is remarkably consistent despite variations in mother's eating habits: See "Diet and dietary supplements for the mother and infant." in R. Lawrence and R. Lawrence, *Breastfeeding: A Guide for the Medical Profession,* 5th ed., (St. Louis: Mosby, 1999).

Page 87   Weight loss in breastfeeding women tends to occur from 3-6months postpartum. See "Lactation and postpartum weight loss" in M.Heinig et al., *Mechanisms Regulating Lactation and Infant Nutrient Utilization,* 1992; 30:397-400.

Page 88   Heavy smoking may affect your milk supply: F. Vio et al., "Smoking during pregnancy and lactation and its effects on breast-milk volume," *Am J Clin Nutr* 1991; 54:1011-16.

Page 89   Most medications are safe for nursing mothers and babies: For an extensive referenced list of drugs compatible with lactation see the statement from the American Academy of Pediatrics Committee on Drugs, "Transfer of drugs and other chemicals into human milk," *Pediatrics* 1994; 93(1):137-50; C. Howard and R. Lawrence, "Drugs and breastfeeding," *Clin Perinatol* 1999; 26(2):447-78.

Page 91   Pregnancy rate of only two percent in the first six months postpartum among women who are fully breastfeeding: K. Kennedy et al., "Consensus statement on the use of breastfeeding as a family planning method," *Contraception* 1989; 39:477-96.

            Effects of hormonal methods of contraception on breastfeeding: World Health Organization (WHO) Task Force, "Progestogen-only contraceptives during lactation: I. Infant growth, II. Infant development," *Contraception* 1994; 50:35-68.

Page 107   Women's recall of how long their children breastfed is very accurate: L. J. Launer et al., "Maternal recall of infant feeding events is accurate," *J Epidemiol Commun Health* 1992; 46:203-6.

Resources

Breastfeeding

THE WOMANLY ART OF BREASTFEEDING, Sixth Revised Edition
(Schaumburg, IL: La Leche League International, 1997).
LLL's classic with everything you need to know about nursing
your baby.

So That's What They're For! Breastfeeding Basics
by Janet Tamaro
(Holbrook, MA: Adams Media Corporation, 1996). A light-
hearted approach to the questions mothers are sometimes
afraid to ask.

HOW WEANING HAPPENS by Diane Bengson
(Schaumburg, IL: La Leche League International).
Helps mothers understand that weaning is a natural process
and does not have to be a stressful event for
mother or child.

MOTHERING YOUR NURSING TODDLER by Norma Jane Bumgarner
(Schaumburg, IL: La Leche League International, 1999).
Information and insights into the joys and challenges of
nursing a toddler.

Eat Well, Lose Weight While Breastfeeding by Ellen Behan
(New York: Villard Books, 1992). Nutrition, dieting, and
exercise for breastfeeding mothers.

Baby's First Solid Foods by Debbie Boehle
(Schaumburg, IL: La Leche League International, 1993).
Pamphlet with ideas for nutritious first foods.

A Mother's Guide to Milk Expression and Breast Pumps
by Nicole Bernshaw
(Schaumburg, IL: La Leche League International, 1991).
Pamphlet with information on types of pumps and how to use
them effectively.

Working and Breastfeeding

Nursing Mother, Working Mother by Gale Pryor
(Boston, MA: Harvard Common Press, 1997).

Staying at Home

Sequencing by Arlene Rossen Cardozo, PhD
(Minneapolis, MN: Brownstone Books, 1986).

Being There: The Benefits of a Stay-at-Home Parent
by Isabelle Fox (Hauppauge, NY: Barrons, 1996).

Crying Babies

THE FUSSY BABY by William Sears
(Schaumburg, IL: La Leche League, International, 1985).

Crying Babies, Sleepless Nights by Sandy Jones
(Boston, MA: Harvard Common Press, 1992).

Parenting the Fussy Baby and High Need Child
by William Sears and Martha Sears
(Boston, MA: Little, Brown and Company, 1996).

Sleeping with Your Baby

NIGHTTIME PARENTING by William Sears
(Schaumburg, IL: La Leche League International, 1999).

The Family Bed by Tine Thevenin
(Wayne, NY: Avery Publishing, 1987).

Pumps and Other Equipment

Many kinds of breast pumps, along with breast shells and nursing supplementers, are available from La Leche League International. Call 1-800-LA LECHE to receive a Catalogue. Or call 847-519-9585 to place an order using Visa or MasterCard.

The following companies have electric breastpumps for rent through local representatives, who may also have manual pumps, breast shells, and nursing supplementers available for sale. To find out who to contact in your community write or call:

Hollister, Inc.
2000 Hollister Drive
Libertyville, IL 60048
(800) 323-4060 USA
(800) 263-7400 Canada
www.hollister.com

Medela, Inc.
P.O. Box 660
McHenry, Illinois 60051 USA
(800) 435-8316
www.medela.com

Wallaby Phototherapy Unit
Fiberoptic Medical Product
Suite 300, Commerce Plaza
5100 Tilghman St.
Allenstown, Pennsylvania 18104 USA

Clothes for Breastfeeding Women

Motherwear
Box 927LLL
Northhampton, Massachusetts 01061 USA
(800) 950-2500
www.motherwear.com

Motherhood Nursing Wear
(800) 4MOM2BE
www.motherhoodnursing.com

Index

About La Leche League

La Leche League International offers many benefits to breastfeeding mothers and babies. Local La Leche Groups meet monthly in communities all over the world, giving breastfeeding mothers the information they need and the opportunity to learn from one another. La Leche League Leaders, women who have nursed their own babies and who have met accreditation requirements, are only a phone call away. They provide accurate information on breastfeeding problems and can lend a sensitive ear to women with common new mother worries. You don't have to be a La Leche League member to contact a Leader or attend Group meetings. However, members receive added benefits. They receive LLLI's bimonthly magazine, NEW BEGINNINGS, which is filled with breastfeeding information, stories from nursing mothers, tips on discipline and common toddler problems, and news about breastfeeding from all over the world. Members also receive a 10% discount on purchases from LLLI's extensive Catalogue of carefully selected books, tapes, pamphlets, pumps, and other products for families. Members may also borrow books from local Group libraries. Membership is $30 a year in the USA and helps to support the work of local LLL Groups as well as LLL projects all over the world. You can pay your dues to the LLL Group in your area or directly to LLLI.

For more information on a Group and Leaders near you, call 1-800-LA LECHE. (In Canada, call 1-800-665-4324 or 613-448-1842.) You can also visit our award winning website at www.lalecheleague.org for more information about LLLI and resources for breastfeeding support. In addition to finding information on membership or a Group near you, you can also find links to Group pages in the USA and all around the world. You can learn about the history of La Leche League International, browse the LLLI Catalogue, get answers to frequently asked questions, or peruse a collection of articles and selected passages from LLLI publications. The website also offers information and schedules for online LLL meetings as well as information on upcoming educational opportunities offered by LLLI.

ORDER FORM

La Leche League International

P.O. Box 4079, Schaumburg, IL 60168-4079 USA

To order by phone, call (847) 519-9585, fax (847) 519-0035 on line www.lalecheleague.org
e-mail: lllhq@llli.org/or orderdepartment@llli.org

METHOD OF PAYMENT

o Check or money order payable to LLLI.

o Visa   o Master Card

SIGNATURE_____

QUANTITY		TOTAL
	The Womanly Art	
	So That's What They	
	How Weaning Happen	
	Mothering Your Nursing	
	Eat Well, Lost Weight While	
	Baby's First Solid Food	
	A Mother's Guide to Milk Expres	
	Sequencing	
	Being There: The Benefits of a Stay-a	
	Nursing Mother, Working Mother	
	The Fussy Baby	
	Crying Babies, Sleepless Nights	
	Parenting the Fussy Baby and High Need Child	.95
	Nighttime Parenting	$9.95
	The Family Bed	$9.95
	LLLI Catalogue	Free

SHIPPING & HANDLING	
up to $4.99	$2
$5.00- 19.99	$4.25
$40.00-59.99	$6.50
$60.00-79.99	$7.25
$80.00-109.00	$8.00
$110.00 and up	7%

Subtotal _____
CA and Illinois ass 7.75% Sales Tax _____
Shipping & Handling _____
LLL Membership $30 _____
Membership Discount 10% _____
Total _____

SHIP TO:

name _____   phone _____

street address _____   state/province _____

zip/postal code _____   country _____

12/99

FOURTH EDITION

DEATH
Current Perspectives

John B. Williamson
Boston College

Edwin S. Shneidman
University of California at Los Angeles

Mayfield Publishing Company
Mountain View, California
London • Toronto

To Bette and Jeanne

Library of Congress Cataloging-in-Publication Data
Death : current perspectives. — 4th ed. / [edited by] John B.
  Williamson, Edwin S. Shneidman.
     p.   cm.
   Includes bibliographical references and index.
   ISBN 1-55934-011-8
   1. Death—Psychological aspects.   2. Terminally ill—Psychology.
 3. Suicide.   4. Bereavement—Psychological aspects.   I. Williamson,
 John B.   II. Shneidman, Edwin S.
 BF789.D4D38   1995
 155.9'37—dc20   94-25375
                                                          CIP
                                                          AC

Manufactured in the United States of America
10 9 8 7 6 5 4

Mayfield Publishing Company
1280 Villa Street
Mountain View, CA 94041

Sponsoring editor, Franklin C. Graham; production editor, George Calmenson; manuscript editor, Sonsie Conroy; text designer, Wendy Calmenson; cover designer, Susan Breitbard; cover image, © True Redd. The text was set in 10.5/12.5 Bembo by Wilsted & Taylor and printed on Ecolocote by Malloy Lithographing, Inc.

IF THE PREVIOUS THREE EDITIONS were psychological, literary, and philosophical, this fourth edition is—in addition to being all of these—now more sociological, anthropological, and historical. There are more changes in this edition than there were in the last two. We broadened the scope by adding an editor. Overall, the revision reflects an effort to present a more balanced and comprehensive survey of contemporary death and dying.

John Williamson is a sociologist with a background in gerontology, and Edwin Shneidman is a thanatologist with a background in psychology. Although there is an appropriate focus on psychology and sociology, we both have a strong commitment to an interdisciplinary approach to the study of thanatology. Contributors also include ethicists, philosophers, anthropologists, historians, physicians, nurses, social critics, and writers.

Another change in this volume is reflected in the numbers: 36 of the 43 selections are new. As a result, this edition has a fresh and contemporary feel. The pieces that are retained have, in their authors, a comfortable and familiar ring: Gorer, Becker, Glaser and Strauss, Sudnow, C. S. Lewis, Elie Wiesel, and Bertrand Russell.

Although we have replaced a substantial proportion of the readings in the previous edition, we have retained the spirit by providing a mix of the best of the classical and the best of the contemporary literature. We have sought to profit from the comments and suggestions made about the previous editions in the interest of improvement, currency, and comprehensiveness. We have sought to provide exposure to the most important issues and ideas relating to death and dying as well as giving exposure to those authors who are responsible for much of the literature that has had the greatest impact on the field in recent years. Our goal is to present this material in one handy volume that will be of interest to the undergraduate student, the professional, and the concerned layperson. What was written in the preface of the first edition (1976) in large measure is true for this edition: "The essential aim in assembling this volume is to provide a representative sample of recent and contemporary writings on the myriad aspects of death and dying."

This anthology is designed to provide the instructor with a great deal of flexibility. Those who want to emphasize psychological issues will be able to do so, those who want to emphasize sociological issues will be able to do so. Similarly, those who want to emphasize ethical issues will also be able to do so. But in each case we would hope that the instructor also has a commitment to an interdisciplinary approach to the study of thanatology.

In addition to a number of thoughtful essays, readers will be exposed to studies based on empirical data obtained using a variety of different methodologies; some emphasize quantitative approaches (for example, survey research or aggregate data), and some emphasize qualitative approaches (for example, social history or intensive interviews). Instructors will have freedom with respect to which methodologies to emphasize and with respect to how much emphasis to place on the classical statements (selections by Emile Durkheim, Geoffrey Gorer, Erich Lindemann, and Maria Nagy) as opposed to contemporary cutting-edge articles published during the late 1980s and early 1990s.

Many people have helped to make this volume possible. We want to thank two librarians who have been particularly helpful in connection with this project, Shari Grove of Boston College and Judith Harding of the National Center for Death Education at Mt. Ida College. Both were very helpful to our efforts to locate material for this book. We want to thank Bette Johnson, Maureen Eldredge, Eunice Doherty, and Roberta Negrin for their contributions. We also want to thank those who served as outside reviewers in connection with this project, including: Charles A. Corr, Southern Illinois University at Edwardsville; Patrick Vernon Dean, Director, Milwaukee Bereavement Center, Inc.; Rita S. Santanello, Belleville Area College; Sharon Scholl, Jacksonville University; and Robin Moremen Uili, Northern Illinois University. There are also many of the staff at Mayfield Publishing Company we want to acknowledge. We want to thank Frank Graham for bringing the two of us together to do this project and for his expert guidance and support throughout. We want to thank Andrea Sarros, Pamela Trainer, Carol Zafiropoulos, Linda Toy, and Jonathan Silvers, all at Mayfield, for their contributions. Sonsie Conroy did an excellent job with the copyediting.

Special thanks to David Karp for reminding us that people on their death beds never say they wish they had spent more time at the office and to Charlie Derber who seems determined to prove this adage wrong.

CONTENTS ❧

Introduction ❧

PERHAPS THE SINGLE MOST IMPRESSIVE FACT about death today—independent of the unchangeable truth that death can never be circumvented—is how much (and in how many different ways) various aspects of death and dying are currently undergoing dramatic changes. Nowadays, there are many breezes in the thanatological wind.[1] We are experiencing a cultural revolution in many areas of our lives. In the last short generation, dozens of our folkways (in dress, behavior, civility, morality, sexuality) and even some of our mores have been changed, often in breathtaking ways. The ethics, sociology, psychology, and morality of death have not been exempt from these culture-wide changes. This book attempts to reflect these changes in relation to death—changes that have led us to new, and often startling, insights into the very process of dying; into the intricate interactions between the dying and those who care for them; into the impact of death on those left behind; and even into the need for reexamining such fundamental questions as, when death occurs and when death should occur.

In order to place these current trends in thanatology in context, this volume examines death from many perspectives, ranging from cultural strategies for dealing with death as a philosophical concept to individual tactics for dealing with death as an inevitable reality.

What will be discussed here are the threads of change that weave through the various chapters and constitute some of the more important developments in the current thanatological scene.

Consider this paragraph:

"Haul in the chains! Let the carcass go astern!" The vast tackles have done their duty. The peeled white body of the beheaded whale flashes like a marble sepulcher; though changed in hue, it has not perceptibly lost anything in bulk. It is still colossal. Slowly it floats more and more away, the water around it torn and splashed by the insatiate sharks, and the air above vexed with rapacious flights of screaming fowls, whose beaks are like so many insulting poniards in the whale. The vast white headless phantom floats further and further from the ship, and every rod that it so floats, what seem square roods of sharks and cubic roods of fowls, augment the murderous din. For hours and hours from the almost stationary ship that hideous sight is seen. Beneath the un-

1

clouded and mild azure sky, upon the fair face of the pleasant sea, wafted by the joyous breezes, the great mass of death floats on and on, till lost in inifinite perspectives.[2]

What is to be especially noted in this superlative passage is the breathtaking shift in mood between the first eight sentences and the last—from horror and rapaciousness to the most pacific calm. Such a combination of opposites is called an *oxymoron*. The best-known examples of oxymorons in the English language are from *Romeo and Juliet*: ". . . Feather of lead, bright smoke, cold fire, sick health," and, of course, ". . . Parting is such sweet sorrow." We have dwelled on the subject of oxymorons because it so aptly describes death in our time. Death is oxymoronic: a paradox made up of contrasting values, opposite trends, and even contradictory facts.

We live in an oxymoronic century. At the same time that we have created the most exquisitely sophisticated technological procedures for saving lives one at a time, we have also created lethal technological devices of at least equal sophistication, with the capacity of exterminating millions at a time, of expunging cultures, of jeopardizing time itself by not only erasing the present but also threatening the future—what Melville, in *White Jacket*, called ". . . the terrible combustion of the entire planet." On the one hand, marvelous devices for emergency surgery, organ transplantations, and medical procedures linked to recent advances in biotechnology promise life; on the other hand, the proliferation of nuclear weapons, communal conflict around the world, and the poverty, drugs, guns, and hopelessness in many of America's inner cities promise death.

We live in paradoxical times. There has been more killing by the state than ever before: over 110 million deaths since 1900 due to deliberate famines, planned starvations, police and government executions, and brutish wars by Elliot's (1972) estimate and over 142 million by Rummel's (1992) estimate; at the same time, there has been no century where so much effort has been put into saving individual lives and increasing the general life span.

Even the scientific marvels of our age for saving individual lives are part of the oxymoronic nature of death in our times, for they exist side by side with the frustrating and unfulfilled promises of medicine to save us for the dread maladies of heart disease and cancer. It has been referred to as "the mirage of health" and as "the mythology of American medicine." We have been over-promised in part because we have over-sought. But great strides have been made: in the United States, life expectancy has been extended 29 years since 1900, from 47 years to 76 years in 1990 (World Bank, 1992). However, it is important to note that this remarkable increase has been due not so much to medicine's miracles for adults as to everyday public health practices in the areas of infant mortality (reduced from 150 to 9 per 1,000 births in this century), sanitation, immunization, and environmental control—unpretentious activities when compared with the dramatic surgical and medical cures that can increase the life span of a relatively few specially selected individuals. The elimination of diphtheria, scarlet fever, and typhoid fever, and the reduction of mortality from tuberculosis have been much more effective in increasing general longevity than heart transplants and bypass surgery.

Conquering the causes of death over the age of 40—cancer and cardiovascular disease—will do relatively little to increase life expectancy. The elimination of deaths due to all forms of cancer would increase life expectancy in the United States by about 3 years and the elimination of all deaths due to cardiovascular diseases would add only 9.8 years. Why? Those who would have died of these conditions will eventually die of something else. As the death rates due to certain diseases decrease, those due to other causes will increase due to what is called multiple-cause mortality (Siegel, 1993). Probably the most significant changes in mortality are to be found less in medical and hospital care than they are in health education: by instituting voluntary and controllable changes in our routine daily patterns of eating, exercising, and smoking (Kurzweil, 1993).

Today the great change seems to lie in improving the kinds of lives we lead. It seems more important than extending life by a year or two to enhance the quality of those 70 or 80 years by elevating the current level of our common courtesy, moral rights, education, employment, and contentment. This refocusing on the quality, rather than the quantity, of life has profound implications for our changing views on death and for our treatment of the dying.

Certainly one of the most refreshing currents in the changing thanatological wind is the increasing emphasis on a humanistic approach to death—an approach that seems to parallel the humanistic trends in other sectors of society today. This new approach is seen, for example, in an increasing concern that the dying individual live as fully and as richly as possible until death and that communications with the dying person be tailored to specific human needs, and in the recognition of a need for special therapies to help those who have suffered the loss of someone close. Indeed, this humanistic trend in the treatment of the dying and those immediately affected by death is causing a complete reexamination of the premises on which we have traditionally based our views of death and dying.

A very impressive aspect of thanatology in the current scene is the dynamic and changing nature of its vital issues. A few years ago there was a great deal of debate about the relative merits of active voluntary euthanasia and of rational suicide; while this debate continues, it seems also to have evolved into the more recent debate over assisted suicide. Some say assisted suicide is a form of rational suicide; others consider it, as it is currently being practiced, as basically a form of voluntary active euthanasia. If, as it has been said, war is too important to be left to generals, then is a life too precious (or too miserable) to be left solely to the judgment of doctors? Should a weakened citizen, too ill to kill himself or herself, have the right to say, "Enough!" And, considering what we read and know of occasional heinous derelictions in some nursing homes, what are the chances, without any opportunity for redress, of abuses in the practice of voluntary euthanasia? For young readers especially, these questions may become real issues before their time to die.

Another important current trend is related to the rapid pace of advances in biotechnology, medical technology, and the costs associated with therapies linked to some of these advances. The use of a new machine or a new procedure may double the medical costs associated with the final months or years of life, but may yield a substantial benefit for only 5% of those who make use of this machine or procedure. In an era of limited health care resources, it may not make budgetary sense to turn routinely to such procedures; but if it is you or your parent or your child who has a life-threatening condition, that cost/benefit ratio will look quite different. The ethics of the allocation of health care resources promises to be an issue of increasing importance in the years ahead, especially in light of recent health care legislation.

One additional current trend can be mentioned. Today there is a new permissiveness regarding death, almost an urgency to speak and to think about it. In this century death has become, as Gorer (1965) says, the new pornography: a subject banned from polite society and social discourse. Yet, in the last 25 years or so there has been a spate of books on death; death has become a respectable field of inquiry and death has become an acceptable topic of study in the college curriculum.

The cultural revolution that we are experiencing today is effecting sweeping changes in the pattern and texture of our lives, changes that are now reaching to the very threshold of our deaths. The scope and impact of these changes concerning death are the central concerns of this book.

References

Eliot, G. (1972). *Twentieth century book of the dead*. New York: Ballantine Books.

Kurzweil, R. (1993). *The 10% solution for a healthy life*. New York: Crown.

Rummel, R. J. (1992). Megamurders. *Society* (September/October), 47–52.

Siegel, J. S. (1993). *A generation of change*. New York: Russell Sage.

World Bank. (1992). *World development report*. New York: Oxford University Press.

Notes

1. Thanatology is the study of death and dying, after Thanatos, the mythological Greek god of death, twin of Hypnus, the god of sleep.
2. This passage is from the chapter, "The Funeral," in Herman Melville's masterpiece, *Moby Dick*.

DIMENSIONS OF DEATH

Contents

DEATH IS A WORD THAT HAS MULTIPLE MEANINGS. Some of these meanings describe various "dimensions" of death. (It almost sounds as though Death were a reified corpse being measured for a coffin.)

In contemporary discussions, these dimensions include the distinction between death and dying, the important distinction between "my death" and "your death" (i.e., all other deaths), the pivotal role played by the denial of death, the ways in which some deaths are more "appropriate" than others, and the twentieth-century pornography of death. Part I teaches us that no single-sentence definition of death is likely to encompass the diverse meanings and multiple dimensions contained in that complicated concept.

The selection by Robert Kastenbaum reports the result of a study in which respondents were asked to describe what sort of person death would be, were death a person. What emerges are several different personifications of death, personifications that can be found in Western art and literature over the past several hundred years. Kastenbaum discusses the relevance of The Gay Deceiver personification (the devil in modern dress?) to the current AIDS epidemic. Readers are urged to think about the ways in which the personifications of death by American college students described in this article are similar to and different from those by the Hungarian children described in the selection by Nagy.

Avery Weisman is a distinguished Harvard psychiatrist. He presents his analysis of what constitutes a befitting and appropriate death and how the answer to the question varies from one individual to another. While he does not explicitly discuss Elisabeth Kübler-Ross's stage theory, it is clear that he would not agree with her stages of death or with the view that her fifth stage, acceptance, is the universal best way to die. Weisman argues that an appropriate and befitting death for each person is the death that he or she would choose if such a choice were possible.

Gorer, an anthropologist, explores the concepts of pornography and obscenity in different cultural contexts. He then applies these concepts first in an analysis of sexuality during the Victorian era and then to death during the twentieth century. His thesis is that there has been a shift over the past century: Sexuality has become more freely discussed and death has become less openly discussed and, in a sense, more pornographic. This argument seems to be a more accurate description of American and British society up through the mid-1960s, when this essay was written; however, given the number of books, TV specials, films, and college courses on death and dying that we have seen in recent decades, it is less obvious that Gorer's article accurately describes American society of the 1990s. Yet, if we take a closer look, we may find that with all of this open discussion of death there are many contexts in which a large number of people feel uncomfortable discussing death-related issues. The reader is urged to explore some of the contexts in which discussion of death creates discomfort or is considered to be an inappropriate topic for polite conversation.

The article by Kearl explores the theme of death as reflected in several aspects of contemporary American popular culture, particularly television, the cinema, and popular music. He discusses the frequency with which Americans are exposed to homicides on television, the race or gender bias with respect to who the homicide victims are, and the way in which commercial considerations shape the kinds of deaths that get emphasized on television. Extensive reference is made to "pornographic death"; we leave it to the reader to decide whether the pornographic death as described by Kearl is the same as the pornography of death as described by Gorer.

The selection by Becker presents his unusual thesis that much of what we do in our entire lifetime represents an effort to deny death. Where Freud sees the sex drive at the core of much that we do in life, Becker sees the fear of death as at the core. This selection also outlines Becker's interpretation of our need for heroic figures. He argues that we have created heroes in part due to our fear of death. The hero is one who has the courage to face death without cowardice. This selection also deals with the distinction between healthy-minded arguments about the fear of death (that the fear of death is the product of socialization) and morbidly-minded arguments (that death anxiety is natural and will occur quite independent of socialization). In this nature-nurture debate Becker comes down on the side of the biological, innate view—perhaps too simplistically.

1 The Personification of Death ❦

Robert Kastenbaum

ROBERT KASTENBAUM, a psychologist, is professor of gerontology at Arizona State University. He is editor of *Omega: Journal of Death and Dying* and of *The International Journal of Aging and Human Development*. He is also a past president of the American Association of Suicidology. He is the author of numerous books, including *Death, Society, and Human Experience* and *The Psychology of Death*, the book from which this selection is drawn. In this article Kastenbaum discusses four very different personifications of death: The Macabre, The Gentle Comforter, The Gay Deceiver, and the Automaton. He also explores the link between The Gay Deceiver personification and the current AIDS epidemic.

THE TENDENCY TO VISUALIZE DEATH AS A PERSON has been demonstrated throughout history. *Personifications* had appeared in art, literature, drama, and mythology long before Death starred as a sardonic chess player in Ingmar Bergman's masterful film *The Seventh Seal*. Awareness of this tradition stimulated the pioneering efforts of McClelland (1963) and Greenberger (1965) to explore death personifications as a distinctive source of information in personality theory and research. Nagy (1959) also found spontaneous personifications in her studies with children. We will concentrate here on studies of death personification in adults.

My early research on death personification was summarized in the original *Psychology of Death* (Kastenbaum & Aisenberg, 1972). In the first study, a set of open-ended questions was posed to 240 adults; another sample of 421 responded to a multiple-choice version. Most of the respondents in both samples were college students.

The open-ended version included the following questions:

If death were a person, what sort of a person would Death be? Think of this question until an image of death-as-a-human being forms in your mind. Then describe Death physically, what Death would look like. . . . Now, what would Death be like? What kind of personality would Death have?

The age and sex imagined for Death was obtained by follow-up questions, if not clear from the first response. Additionally, respondents were asked to indicate their sources for their images of death and the degree of difficulty the task had held.

The multiple-choice version was established after analyzing data from the open-ended version.

1. In stories, plays and movies, death is sometimes treated as though a human being. If you were writing a story in which one character would represent Death, would you represent Death as (a) a young man, (b) an old man, (c) a young woman, (d) an old woman? If other, please specify.

2. Would Death be (a) a cold, remote sort of person, (b) a gentle, well-meaning sort of person, (c) a grim, terrifying sort of person?

Four clear types of personification emerged from these studies. These were labeled The Macabre, The Gentle Comforter, The Gay Deceiver, and The Automaton.

The Macabre was characterized as a powerful, overwhelming, and repulsive figure. The image often was of an emaciated or decaying human, or of a monster with only faint resemblance to human form. The image of a "death-like death" was also given by some respondents. For example, death would be portrayed as an animated corpse or as an assailant who was himself disintegrating or being consumed. Macabre personifications also tended to be emotionally close to their creators. One young man, for example, reported that "a shivering and nausea overwhelms me" when he thinks about the image he has produced. A young woman pictured death as a "gigantic being of superhuman strength. A body to which one would relinquish all hopes of resistance. He would be cold and dark, in such a way that one glance would reveal his mission. He would be always dressed in black and would wear a hat which he wore tightly over his head . . . self-confident with an abundance of ego. He would naturally be callous and would enjoy his occupation. He would get a greater thrill when the person whom he was claiming was enjoying life to a great degree." The Macabre personification often was presented in the form of a hideous old man.

The Gentle Comforter is embued with the theme of soothing welcome. It could be seen as an adult of any age. When presented as an old man, Father Time received much credit as a source. The Gentle Comforter was an image that came readily to many respondents. The idea of a powerful force quietly employed in a kindly way is perhaps at the core of this personification. The respondents often felt they were emotionally close to their Gentle Comforter image, but not in a threatened manner. One woman's response well typifies this type of personification:

A fairly old man with long white hair and a long beard. A man who would resemble a biblical figure with a long robe which is clean but shabby. He would have very strong features and despite his age would appear to have strength. His eyes would be very penetrating and his hands would be large. Death would be calm, soothing, and comforting. His voice would be of an alluring nature and, although kind, would hold the tone of the mysterious. Therefore, in general, he would be kind and understanding and yet be very firm and sure of his actions and attitudes.

The Gay Deceiver was pictured as an attractive and sensuous person of either sex, often elegant and worldly. Poised and sophisticated, The Gay Deceiver entices its victim, a knowing companion one might seek out for amusement, adventure, or excitement. Those who depict this type of personification often state explicitly that The Gay Deceiver tempts and lures us on, and "Then you would learn who he really is, and it would be too late." That "who he really is" might be a modern dress version of the devil is a possibility, and there are occasional direct references (e.g., "He is a little on the slim side though looks fairly powerful. He has a very dark goatee coming to a point. . . . wearing a dark suit. . . . I see death right now almost in the same way as the devil"). Another respondent imagined death in the following way:

Death is either a man and/or a woman. This death person is young to middle-aged and very good looking. The man is about 35 or 40 with dark hair, graying at the sides. The woman is tall, beautiful with dark hair and about 30. . . . Both have very subtle and interesting personalities. They're suave, charming, but deceitful, cruel, and cold. . . . Both are really sharp. You like them and they lead you on.

The Gay Deceiver seems to embody characteristics of both an ego ideal (for some people), and a con man. Perhaps on one level, The Gay Deceiver is a character who has stepped out of a morality play—one of the temptations from *Everyman*, or Sportin' Life in *Porgy and Bess*. The explosive rise in use of illicit drugs in recent years (mostly since this study was done) also suggests a connection between the Gay Deceiver and the pusher.

The AIDS epidemic may be an even more potent intensifier of the Gay Deceiver image. "Come with me—what a time we will have!" is not only The Gay Deceiver's lure, but also resonates with the facts of AIDS transmission through sexual intercourse as well as drug injections with contaminated needles. The biological fact is that heterosexual as well as homosexual intercourse can transmit the AIDS virus. The sociohistorical fact, however, is that the first wave of AIDS in the United States was associated with flagrantly promiscuous homosexual activity in several major cities. Among our various personifications of death, The Gay Deceiver is the image most suited to the AIDS epidemic, at least in its early phase.

Perhaps on another level, however, The Gay Deceiver represents the respondents' own efforts to divert themselves from the prospect of death. In effect, one declares: "By immersing myself in all the pleasures that life has to offer, I will have neither the time nor the inclination to admit dark thoughts. The very fact that I revel in sophisticated enjoyments suggests that death cannot really be catastrophic—Am I kidding myself? Of course! But that's the solution I prefer."

The Automaton may be in a class by itself: the image of death as an objective, unfeeling instrument in human guise. The Automaton looks like a normal person but lacks human qualities. Unlike the other personifications, he (usually a male) does not establish a human relationship of any kind. He advances with neither diabolical pleasure nor gentle compassion, but as an automatic—soulless—apparatus. One example from respondents follows:

> *He is sort of a blank in human form. I don't know what he looks like. . . . Probably he is not very short or very tall or very good-looking or very ugly. He is just somebody you would never notice because he just goes his own way. He looks angry or sullen, but he really doesn't feel anything. I guess he is more like a machine than anything else. You would probably never have anything in common with a guy like that. Death, we will not call him Mr., is not the frightening person one would imagine, but he is not a jolly sort of person either. Physically he is above average height with dark hair and clear brown eyes. . . . dressed in a dark suit with a conservative tie. His walk is almost military, as if he were a man who is formal in most of his dealings. . . . Psychologically, he has no feeling of emotion about his job—either positive or negative. He simply does his job. He doesn't think about what he is doing, and there is no way to reason with him. There is no way to stop him or change his mind. When you look into his eyes you do not see a person. You see only death.*

A special problem is posed by The Automaton: What are the victims to do with their own feelings? The macabre personifications might terrify, but terror is at least a human condition: One can respond to the terrifying with terror. Even such grotesque personages as the vampire and the werewolf have the reputation of establishing some kind of relationship with their victims. By contrast, one can express nothing to a "blank in human form."

Perhaps The Automaton is a creature of our own times, representing the indifferent, machined termination of a failed apparatus (the human body) rather than a death that holds a spiritual meaning of some kind.

This pair of studies also found that death was most often represented as a man, and as a person of middle or advanced adult years. The Gentle Comforter type of image was the most frequently given—suggesting that "death anxiety" may be alleviated rather than intensified through this fantasy modality for most people. For what it might be worth, funeral directors and students of mortuary sciences were the subsamples with by far the highest percentage of "no personifications," encountering some type of inner resistance to a task most others did not find very difficult. Among less frequent types of personification, the depiction of Death as a shapeless void was noted.

The most systematic follow-up to these studies has been done by Richard Lonetto and his colleagues (Lonetto, 1982). Building a link with more traditional studies, this research team found that women who depicted Death as female had the highest levels of self-reported death anxiety. Men who saw Death as a male were particularly concerned with the sight of a dead body, with the prospect of another world war, and with the shortness of life. Several other findings also contributed to sketching the relationship between the "sex of Death" and the respondent's level and type of death concerns. The Lonetto series confirmed the existence of the types of personification found in our studies, but also found some differences and examined the components in more detail. Although The Macabre image remained less frequent than the others, The Gay Deceiver type of imagery proved the commonest. Does this perhaps reflect some changes in our views of life and death during the decade between the two sets of studies? Or is it perhaps a generational shift—young adults tending to see Death as a tempter when a previous cohort was more likely to call on The Gentle Comforter imagery? Other explanations are also possible, however, so this difference serves only to suggest that there *might* be systematic changes in death fantasies over relatively short periods. In the Lonetto studies, The Gay Deceiver image "was related to the cognitive-affective component of death anxiety; specifically, to fear of dying, appearing nervous when people discuss death, the frequency of death-related thoughts, and being troubled by thoughts of life after death" (Lonetto & Templer, 1986, p. 75).

References

Greenberger, E. (1965). Fantasies of women confronting death. *Journal of Consulting Psychology*, *29*, 252–260.

Kastenbaum, R., & Aisenberg, R. (1972). *The psychology of death*. New York: Springer.

Lonetto, R. (1982). Personifications of death and death anxiety. *Journal of Personality Assessment*, *46*, 404–408.

Lonetto, R., & Templer, D. I. (1986). *Death anxiety*. New York: Hemisphere Publishing.

McClelland, D. (1963). The harlequin complex. In R. White (ed.), *The study of lives* (pp. 94–119). New York: Atherton Press.

Nagy, M. H. (1959). The child's theories concerning death. In H. Feifel (ed.), *The meaning of death* (pp. 79–98). New York: McGraw-Hill.

❧ 2 A Befitting and Appropriate Death

Avery D. Weisman

AVERY WEISMAN is professor of psychiatry emeritus, Harvard Medical School; and senior psychiatrist, Massachusetts General Hospital. He is one of the most thoughtful writers in the field of thanatology today. One of his most felicitous contributions to the field of thanatology is the concept of an "appropriate death"—a consummatory end each person would seek were he or she able to do so. The selection presented here is from his most recent book, *The Vulnerable Self*. It updates his treatment of the same issue in his earlier book, *On Dying and Denying*. In this selection he describes a "befitting and appropriate death" as the death one would choose, if one had the choice. He argues that an appropriate death is not only befitting, it also has several other characteristics described in this selection.

A FAUSTIAN BARGAIN WITH DEATH SEEMS OUT OF THE QUESTION. Negotiation with mortality must include accommodation to the various declines and deprivations of life which are unfailingly negative. The only way to bring all these negatives together into a more acceptable whole, with a positive sign, would be to make a bad bargain into a good death. A good death, in a preliminary, not a final, version, accepts with renunciation and regret, like an unwelcome invitation to a party one does not wish to attend, yet is forced to by outside pressure. The major task in a befitting death is to combine the inclination to die with the drive to survive.

The meaning of "befitting" is defined as realization of the best one could be, which fits with a sense of harmony, responsibility, and compatibility in transactions with the world. A befitting and appropriate life is what, at best, is sought and expected from psychotherapy. In adapting this concept to negotiation with mortality, I doubt if we could do much better than to imagine a similar goal.

If it were possible to picture actually sitting down with death, as novelists and playwrights have occasionally imagined, I doubt if a satisfactory solution would be an unqualified and unlimited survival. This is not because death needs human sacrifice, or that prolonged existence might produce a population explosion. Rather, the fact or possibility of unrestricted and unconditional survival might be more threatening than death. Legends about hellfire and damnation, along with myths of eternal and unrelieved anguish, such as the myth of Sisyphus, presuppose no release from loneliness and suffering. Immortality of this variety would be like an interminably debilitating disease, or a torture that stops short of killing outright. No repose, no respite. There are plenty of very sick patients who want to die, but cannot, and would find death wholly acceptable. Some sick patients want desperately to recover and get on with life, but cannot. Death is anything but acceptable, and far from appropriate. Whether a patient can actually will death, yielding passively, is still moot. But there are surely people, sick or disabled, who are predilected to death, finding it right and proper to die, and sometimes do. Largely, however, in our heterogeneous culture, people clutch at life on almost any terms, so intensely that the very desire to die without an exceedingly unambiguous reason is scorned. With all of the current discussion and dispute about "physician-assisted suicide" in cases of terminal illness, both the medical profession and others are dreadfully afraid of making death too easy and too attractive for some.

Negotiating with mortality implies dealing with death and its outcomes, and these include good deaths, bad deaths, equivocal deaths, and befitting deaths. There are people, sometimes patients, who live too long, while others die far too prematurely. When the right time to die occurs is an ultimate question on a par with the best way to live.

There is no better way to describe an appropriate death, along with a befitting demise, than a death we might choose, had we a choice. Hospice care for incurable disease can have no better objective. Aside from eliminating more obvious negatives contained in suffering, whether from pain, desertion, invalidism, incontinence, poverty, and abandonment of those we love, a good death has significance and status, in retaining much of what made living valuable. It might even have morale. A good death, having so much of a good life, is one we could live with. An appropriate death is not only befitting, but has at least four outstanding characteristics: awareness, acceptance, propriety, and timeliness.

My examples are drawn from the predicament of a cancer patient for whom no further treatment is available, and yet has positive expectations of the future, despite death in the offing.

Awareness of impending death comes at about the same time as learning that nothing more can be done, except for good medical, nursing, and considerate care by others. There are some doctors, friends, and families who insist that telling patients about their illness, especially if no treatment is feasible, will cause hopelessness, and despair, and serve no useful purpose. As if hope were contingent upon illusion. Others claim that a well-informed patient is a better patient, able to participate in decisions affecting the outcome, and post-therapeutic management. As if coping with the prospect of death depended on knowing and being able to act upon potential consequences of that knowledge. Experience with patients who opt for hospice care indicates that awareness does not harm patients, and that denial of an incipient demise is apt to be foolhardy, since most patients know from various clues what their situation is. Moreover, coping with the problems standing in the way of a better death does not seem consistent or compatible with denial of the outcome.

Acceptance of death is very inconstant: it may depend on the person speaking with a patient, and with whom a patient is ready to speak. Sometimes, patients with full knowledge and, seemingly, acceptance of the outlook, will shade the truth from family and friends, to spare them pain and embarrassment, possibly also to forestall being categorized as someone unacceptable. On the other hand, some patients simulate a philosophic acceptance when they are actually frozen with terror. But one strategy for coping turns necessity into choice. "I choose to stop all transfusions, and chemotherapy that just makes me sick!" For the very aged, death may finally be acceptable as the natural finish of the trajectory, despite no gold at the end of the rainbow. Here, as elsewhere, social support consists of normalization and acceptability, two qualities that assuredly apply to death and dying.

Propriety seems harder to define than awareness and acceptance, but that is because propriety refers to the non-medical features of illness that distinguish a good death from something more objectionable. But propriety is *not* propitious or ideal, nor does it depend on the outside judgment of someone in authority. The essentials of propriety are based on what a patient *decides* is right and proper, and what seems befitting according to the pertinent community's expectations and standards needed to preserve esteem and respect.

The first essential includes such matters as place of death, home or hospital, number and kind of visitors, degree of sharing decisions, protection of individuality and decorum, and so forth. Much of personal propriety for some patients is having a say and a choice in what happens to significant survivors, such as children.

The second essential does not necessarily mean a standard funeral service, nor a glowing eulogy within convention and under the canopy of professed religion. But it might be whatever social and community standards do to guarantee respect and regard for the deceased and his survivors. An elderly, unmarried, former teacher was besieged by calls from former students who wanted to visit her in a public hospital's geriatric division. They did not know or seemingly care that this very private and cultured woman was confined to a cot in the middle of a large ward, where privacy was out of the question and individuality something nonexistent. There were disturbed, confused, and moribund patients all around her, and she received little but routine care. As a result, despite telephone calls about visiting, she refused, asking, instead, to be sent notes and post-cards with good wishes. She clearly wanted to be remembered as she once was, not as she now was forced to become. Obviously, her death, under these circumstances, could not be one of propriety.

"Living your own life" is a defiant motto, voiced mostly by the young during a period when they are forced to comply with parental standards and codes, before they have had much chance to lead any independent life. "Dying your own death" is a somber parallel of the same thought, which is not heard as frequently. It defies what those in authority think is best. Dying your own death, however, reflects token autonomy or propriety. Many dying patients, for example, choose where and even how death will occur, together with specific funeral plans. When this happens, one can hardly doubt that the finality of the dying process requires abundant courage, moral and physical, if morale is to be maintained.

Timeliness is the fourth characteristic of the befitting, appropriate demise. It is the question, perhaps ultimate, of when is the best time to die. The question has had numerous and humorous rejoinders. But serious answers have not been much more appropriate. However, there are some patients, not at all suicidal or depressed, who decide forthrightly that, were they to live longer, nothing more could be expected. Consequently, the time is *now*; they are ripe to die, say, following a relatively benign operation or an illness that ordinarily responds to medical treatment.

In our society, however, almost any death is considered premature ("He had so much to live for!"), except, of course, for those richly deserving to die, or who linger too long for the best plans of potential survivors. Very aged and infirm patients who somehow continue to live before dying fail to die timely deaths. Instead, they have hyper-mature deaths, the kind that Glaser and Strauss described so well.

Theoretically, if we are to believe the conventional statements about premature deaths, that they occur too soon, and that some others take too long, there should be numerous deaths that occur at the right moment, when the expectation ratio is one. This might be the opportune occasion, indicating that further existence would be meaningless, and that death now would be particularly significant.

3 The Pornography of Death

Geoffrey Gorer

GEOFFREY GORER was a noted English anthropologist who wrote about Africa, Bali and Angkor, Himalayan villages, and the American people. His first book was entitled *The Revolutionary Ideas of the Marquis de Sade*. This selection, which is taken from his book, *Death, Grief, and Mourning*, has become a classic of its kind. In it, Gorer proposes and brilliantly advances the dramatic thesis that death is treated in our society as obscene and pornographic; that while sex was the pornography of the Victorians, death is the pornography of our times.

Birth, and copulation, and death. That's all the facts when you come to brass tacks; Birth, and copulation, and death.

T. S. ELIOT, *Sweeney Agonistes* (1932)

PORNOGRAPHY IS, NO DOUBT, THE OPPOSITE FACE, the shadow, of prudery, whereas obscenity is an aspect of seemliness. No society has been recorded which has not its rules of seemliness, of words or actions which arouse discomfort and embarrassment in some contexts, though they are essential in others. The people before whom one must maintain a watchful seemliness vary from society to society: all people of the opposite sex, or all juniors, or all elders, or one's parents-in-law, or one's social superiors or inferiors, or one's grandchildren have been selected in different societies as groups in whose presence the employment of certain words or the performance of certain actions would be considered offensive; and then these words or actions become charged with affect. There is a tendency for these words and actions to be related to sex and excretion, but this is neither necessary nor universal; according to Malinowski, the Trobrianders surround eating with as much shame as excretion; and in other societies personal names or aspects of ritual come under the same taboos.

Rules of seemliness are apparently universal; and the nonobservance of these rules, or anecdotes which involve the breaking of the rules, provoke that peculiar type of laughter which seems identical the world over; however little one may know about a strange society, however little one may know about the functions of laughter in that society (and these can be very various) one can immediately tell when people are laughing at an obscene joke. The topper of the joke may be "And then he ate the whole meal in front of them!" or "She used her husband's name in the presence of his mother!" but the laughter is the same; the taboos of seemliness have been broken and the result is hilarious. Typically, such laughter is confined to one-sex groups and is more general with the young, just entering into the complexities of adult life.

Obscenity then is a universal, an aspect of man and woman living in society; everywhere and at all times there are words and actions which, when misplaced, can produce shock, social embarrassment, and laughter. Pornography on the other hand, the description of tabooed activities to produce hallucination or delusion, seems to be a very much rarer phenomenon. It probably can only arise in literate societies, and we certainly have no records of it for nonliterate ones; for whereas the enjoyment of obscenity is predominantly social, the enjoyment of pornography is predominantly private. The fantasies from which pornography derives could of course be generated in any society; but it seems doubtful whether they would ever be communicated without the intermediary of literacy.

The one possible exception to this generalization is the use of plastic arts without any letterpress. I have never felt quite certain that the three-dimensional *poses plastiques* on so many Hindu temples (notably the "Black Pagoda" at Konarak) have really the highfalutin worship of the life force or glorification of the creative aspect of sex which their apologists claim for them; many of them seem to me very like "feelthy" pictures, despite the skill with which they are executed. There are too the erotic woodcuts of Japan; but quite a lot of evidence suggests that these are thought of as laughter provoking (i.e., obscene) by the Japanese themselves. We have no knowledge of the functions of the Peruvian pottery.

As far as my knowledge goes, the only Asian society which had a long-standing tradition of pornographic literature is China; and, it would appear, social life under the Manchus was surrounded by much the same haze of prudery as distinguished the nineteenth century in much of Europe and the Americas, even though the emphasis fell rather differently; women's deformed feet seem to have been the greatest focus of peeking and sniggering, rather than their ankles or the cleft between their breasts; but by and large life in Manchu China seems to have been nearly as full of "unmentionables" as life in Victoria's heyday.

Pornography would appear to be a concomitant of prudery, and usually the periods of the greatest production of pornography have also been the periods of the most rampant prudery. In contrast to obscenity, which is chiefly defined by situation, prudery is defined by subject; some aspect of human experience is treated as inherently shameful or abhorrent, so that it can never be discussed or referred to openly, and experience of it tends to be clandestine and accompanied by feelings of guilt and unworthiness. The unmentionable aspect of experience then tends to become a subject for much private fantasy, more or less realistic, fantasy charged with pleasurable guilt or guilty pleasure; and those whose power of fantasy is weak, or whose demand is insatiable, constitute a market for the printed fantasies of the pornographer.

Traditionally, and in the lexicographic meaning of the term, pornography has been concerned with sexuality. For the greater part of the last two hundred years copulation and (at least in the mid-Victorian decades) birth were the "umentionables" of the triad of basic human experiences which "are all the facts when you come to brass tacks," around which so much private fantasy and semiclandestine pornography were erected. During most of this period death was no mystery, except in the sense that death is always a mystery. Children were encouraged to think about death, their own deaths and the edifying or cautionary deathbeds of others. It can have been a rare individual who, in the nineteenth century with its high mortality, had not witnessed at least one actual dying, as well as paying their respect to "beautiful corpses"; funerals were the occasion of the greatest display for working class, middle class, and aristocrat. The cemetery was the center of every old-established village, and they were prominent in most towns. It was fairly late in the nineteenth century when the execution of criminals ceased to be a public holiday as well as a public warning.

In the twentieth century, however, there seems to have been an unremarked shift in prudery; whereas copulation has become more and more "mentionable," particularly in the Anglo-Saxon societies, death has become more and more "unmentionable" *as a natural process*. I cannot recollect a novel or play of the last twenty years or so which has a "deathbed scene" in it, describing in any detail the death "from natural causes" of a major character; this topic was a set piece for most of the eminent Victorian and Edwardian writers, evoking their finest prose and their most elaborate technical effects to produce the greatest amount of pathos or edification.

One of the reasons, I imagine, for this plethora of deathbed scenes—apart from their intrinsic emotional and religious content—was that it was one of the relatively few experiences that an author could be fairly sure would have been shared by the vast majority of his readers. Questioning my old acquaintances, I cannot find one over the age of sixty who did not witness the agony of at least one near relative; I do not think I know a single person under the age of thirty who has had a similar experience. Of course my acquaintance is neither very extensive nor particularly representative; but in this instance I do think it is typical of the change of attitude and "exposure."

The natural processes of corruption and decay have become disgusting, as disgusting as the natural processes of birth and copulation were a century ago; preoccupation about such processes is (or was) morbid and unhealthy, to be discouraged in all and punished in the young. Our great-grandparents were told that babies were found under gooseberry bushes or cabbages; our children are likely to be told that those who have passed on (fie! on the gross Anglo-Saxon monosyllable) are changed into flowers, or lie at rest in lovely gardens. The ugly facts are relentlessly hidden; the art of the embalmers is an art of complete denial.

It seems possible to trace a connection between the shift of taboos and the shift in religious beliefs. In the nineteenth century most of the inhabitants of Protestant countries seem to have subscribed to the Pauline beliefs in the sinfulness of the body and the certainty of the afterlife. "So also is the resurrection of the dead. It is sown in corruption; it is raised in incorruption: it is sown in dishonour; it is raised in glory." It was possible to insist on the corruption of the dead body, and the dishonour of its begetting, while there was a living belief in the incorruption and the glory of the immortal part. But in England, at any rate, belief in the future life as taught in Christian doctrine is very uncommon today even in the minority who make church going or prayer a consistent part of their lives; and without some such belief natural death and physical decomposition have become too horrible to contemplate or to discuss. It seems symptomatic that the contemporary sect of Christian Science should deny the fact of physical death, even to the extent (so it is said) of refusing to allow the word to be printed in the *Christian Science Monitor*.

During the last half century public health measures and improved preventive medicine have made natural death among the younger members of the population much more uncommon than it had been in earlier periods, so that a death in the family, save in the fullness of time, became a relatively uncommon incident in home life; and, simultaneously, violent death increased in a manner unparalleled in human history. Wars and revolutions, concentration camps, and gang feuds were the most publicized of the causes for these violent deaths; but the diffusion of the automobile, with its constant and unnoticed toll of fatal accidents, may well have been most influential in bringing the possibility of violent death into the expectations of law-abiding people in time of peace. While natural death became more and more smothered in prudery, violent death has played an evergrowing part in the fantasies offered to mass audiences—detective stories, thrillers, Westerns, war stories, spy stories, science fiction, and eventually horror comics.

There seem to be a number of parallels between the fantasies which titillate our curiosity about the mystery of sex, and those which titillate our curiosity about the mystery of death. In both types of fantasy, the emotions which are typically concomitant of the acts—love or grief—are paid little or no attention, while the sensations are enhanced as much as a customary poverty of language permits. If marital intercourse be considered the natural expression of sex for most of humanity most of the time, then "natural sex" plays as little role as "natural death" (the ham-fisted attempts of D. H. Lawrence and Jules Romains to describe "natural sex" realistically but high-mindedly prove the rule). Neither type of fantasy can have any real development, for once the protagonist has done something, he or she must proceed to do something else, with or to somebody else, more refined, more complicated, or more sensational than what had occurred before. This somebody else is not a person; it is either a set of genitals, with or without secondary sexual characteristics, or a body, perhaps capable of suffering pain as well as death. Since most languages are relatively poor in words or constructions to express intense pleasure or intense pain, the written portions of both types of fantasy abound in onomatopoeic conglomerations of letters meant to evoke the sighs, gasps, groans, screams and rattles concomitant to the described actions. Both types of fantasy rely heavily on adjective and simile. Both types of fantasy are completely unrealistic, since they ignore all physical, social or legal limitations, and both types have complete hallucination of the reader or viewer as their object.

There seems little question that the instinct of those censorious busybodies preoccupied with other people's morals was correct when they linked the pornography of death with the pornography of sex. This, however, seems to be the only thing which has been correct in their deductions or attempted actions. There is no valid evidence to suggest that either type of pornography is an incitement to action; rather are they substitute gratifications. The belief that such hallucinatory works would incite their readers to copy the actions depicted would seem to be indirect homage to the late Oscar Wilde, who described such a process in *The Picture of Dorian Gray*. I know of no authenticated parallels in real life, though investigators and magistrates with bees in their bonnets can usually persuade juvenile delinquents to admit to exposure to whatever medium of mass communication they are choosing to make a scapegoat.

Despite some gifted precursors, such as Andréa de Nerciat or Edgar Allan Poe, most works in both pornographics are aesthetically objectionable; but it is questionable whether, from the purely aesthetic point of view, there is much more to be said for the greater part of the more anodyne fare provided by contemporary mass media communication. Psychological Utopians tend to condemn substitute gratifications as such, at least where copulation is involved; they have so far been chary in dealing with death.

Nevertheless, people have to come to terms with the basic facts of birth, copulation, and death, and somehow accept their implications; if social prudery prevents this being done in an open and dignified fashion, then it will be done surreptitiously. If we dislike the modern pornography of death, then we must give back to death—natural death—its parade and publicity, readmit grief and mourning. If we make death unmentionable in polite society—"not before the children"—we almost ensure the continuation of the "horror comic." No censorship has ever been really effective.

4 Death in Popular Culture ❧

Michael C. Kearl

MICHAEL C. KEARL is professor of sociology at Trinity University in San Antonio, Texas. He is the author of *Endings*, the book from which this selection is drawn. Kearl explores the theme of death as expressed in three major facets of contemporary American popular culture: television, the cinema, and popular music. He discusses the extent to which television and cinema have been bringing increasingly graphic depictions of death to their audiences. He explores some of the reasons for this trend and some of its consequences.

DEATH AND TELEVISION

By the age of sixteen, according to the National Institute of Mental Health, the typical American has witnessed some eighteen thousand homicides on television. These killings come in various guises, energizing the plots of conflicts between cowboys and Indians, cops and robbers, earthlings and aliens, as well as between the living and the dead. These homicides are packaged either individually, such as when the good guy outdraws and kills the outlaw, or collectively, as when an entire populated planet is destroyed by Darth Vader. Even the advertisements carry thanatological messages: there's Charlie Tuna, who desires to be hooked and cannibalized by Starkist purchasers (slightly reminiscent of a Tennessee Williams play). The trade journal *Adweek* noted that "for some arcane reason, if you're in the business of creating TV commercials, funerals are funny. So is the reading of last wills and testaments" (1984). What are the consequences of young receptive minds absorbing so many lessons in death? One fifteen-year-old youth, accused of murdering an eighty-three-year-old woman in her Miami Beach home, held the defense that he had become intoxicated with violence from watching violent television. Though the jury was not convinced, the case marked an interesting precedent and further legitimized the belief that we are all possibly subconsciously susceptible to media influences.

In considering the symbolic messages implicit within such presentations,

George Gerbner claims that death "is just another invented characterization, a negative resource, a sign of fatal flaw or ineptitude, a punishment for sins or mark of tragedy" (1980, p. 66). In addition, the medium's death lessons are unwittingly "calculated to cultivate a sense of insecurity, anxiety, fear of the 'mean world' out there, and dependence on some strong protector" (p. 66). So who is most likely to kill, and who is most likely to die? In Gerbner's sample of television programs between 1969 and 1978, women and minorities were most vulnerable. . . .

In addition to the action programs, sit-coms, and soap operas, death is a frequent theme of the feature-magazine-format shows, the disease-of-the-month telethons, comedy (NBC's *Saturday Night Live* comes to mind), and children's cartoons (Gerbner [1980, p. 67] reported an average of five violent incidents per hour during prime time and eighteen per hour in weekend daytime children's programming). When television handles the actual deaths of public figures, Michael Arlen notes that "for the most part, . . . what it commonly does is to attend briskly and meticulously to the *famousness* of the departed, and to leave the death, and everything that humanly has to do with death, at arm's length" (1975, p. 76).

The greatest density of televised death stories is to be found on the evening news. Death is news, and it attracts viewers just as it sells newspapers. The day of the space shuttle *Challenger* explosion, the regular network evening newscasts scored a combined rating of 40 in twelve major markets, compared to a 30 rating the preceding week (*New York Times* 1986). As the medium evolved, it discovered the difference, say, between reporting one hundred air-crash fatalities and actually recording a single disaster. Editorial taste dictated whether the camera's lens was focused on the covered corpses being carried from the scene of the accident or on the human fragments intertwined in the wreckage. But technological innovation and growing public callousness toward televised death was to inflate the visual requirements. The synchronization of the Vietnam War with the development and dispersal of color television and satellite relays produced a new death experience: live war deaths during the supper hour. Certainly, the ability to capture death on a visual medium is a major accomplishment of technology, timing, and skill. The crash of the *Hindenburg* remains, after half a century, a clear and terrifying experience, with most Americans having witnessed the famous newsreel footage of the crash and heard the terror in the voice of the commentator on the spot.

Since the mid-1970s, Americans have witnessed a local newscaster committing suicide during the evening news, Los Angeles police killing members of the Symbionese Liberation Army during a 1975 shootout (carried live and commercial-free on California television stations), and the presence of television cameras perhaps inciting South African blacks to even further violence against the apartheid regime. So necessary has the staple of death become on the evening news that people object if certain deaths are not adequately covered. In 1985, Puerto Ricans complained that the American news media gave limited coverage to the mud slide that had killed five hundred of their people, "as if it had taken place in a far-off country" (Campbell 1985).

The medium is not incapable of showing real death and real grief. In 1976, WGBH of Boston aired a documentary entitled *Dying*. Said producer-director Michael Roemer, "You can't learn to die as though it were a skill. People die in the way they have lived. Death becomes the expression of everything you are, and you can bring it only what you have brought to your life" (*Time* 1976). The show began with an interview of a young widow whose husband, age twenty-nine, had been diagnosed as having lymphosarcoma. She said of the day of his death: "in a strange way it was a good day. We were able to share things. I read to Mark. I gave him his last bath. Then early in the evening he kissed me and said, 'Let's call it quits, Pooh.' And he died about half an hour later." The program also revealed the wrenching aspects of death, such as for a woman in her early thirties who, feeling frustrated and angered by her husband's mortal illness, could only make him feel guilty for dying and leaving her with two sons to raise. Such shows, however, are rare. The emotions and fears they evoke are too great, their exhibition too "real" for the comfort of their escapist viewers, to garner the viewer ratings required to subsidize their production.

DEATH IN CINEMA

According to Geoffrey Gorer (1965), the American appetite for violence and perverse forms of death has produced an ethos of "pornographic death." The motif is pornographic as it involves the culture's twentieth-century prudery toward and denial of natural death. As sex becomes pornographic when divorced from its natural human emotion, which is affection, so death becomes pornographic when abstracted from its natural human emotion, which is grief (May 1973, p. 105). Perhaps nowhere is this more evident than in the cinematic medium, wherein, over time, such deaths have become increasingly vivid.

There are a number of ways to approach the evolution of pornographic death in cinema. In part, it is a function of the medium itself, which focuses on observable action and not on the subjective perspectives of individuals, which is one of the hallmarks of literature. The medium, exhibited to be larger than life and designed to be publicly viewed, must be attention-getting to hold the interest of large numbers of people, and it is death, not grief, that commands attention. To continue holding interest, cinema must constantly outdo itself, whether by producing increasingly absorbing plots (seasoned with shock or surprise), showing increasing amounts of action sequences, employing increasingly spectacular special effects, or featuring dying film stars. Features achieving commercially successful chemistries of these elements spawn genres of sequels and imitations.

Another strategy, however, is to focus on the sociocultural factors shaping the public's receptivity to particular pornographic themes. A movie becomes successful at a particular point in time not only because of its technical or artistic merits but also because of its social context. Accordingly, one sociological enterprise has been to correlate cinematic themes with their sociohistorical settings. It was no coincidence, for instance, that the horror movie became a successful genre during the 1920s and early 1930s. Exploring the contests between good and evil as well as the conflict between our animal impulses and higher human traits, this cinematic motif first succeeded in the era of the *Scopes* monkey trial, a period of intellectual self-doubt and disillusionment following the atrocities of the "war to end all wars" and the time when Victorian mores were being eroded by an ethos of materialism and hedonism. In the context of prohibition, *Dr. Jekyll and Mr. Hyde* premiered, reaffirming the evil of drugs and reminding us of the beast that lurks within. In 1932, during the depths of the Depression, both *Dracula* (an immortal creature who must subsist on the blood of the living) and *Frankenstein* (a monster comprised of parts of dead bodies) were released, providing cathartic relief in ways reminiscent of Greek tragedy. The following year, perhaps to the delight of the economically oppressed, *King Kong* attacked the symbols of the establishment in New York. When society had to cope with all of the real death of World War II, these images of terror were to be employed for humor, as in *Abbott and Costello Meet Frankenstein* (PBS 1983). Following World War II, the uncertainties and fears of the nuclear legacy were symbolized by new monsters, unintended mutations produced by clumsy attempts to technologically harness this new force of death.

Another cinematic motif was the western, which used death to differentiate the good from the bad. During the 1930s and 1940s, the heroes—Roy Rogers, Gene Autry, and Red Ryder—avenged the deaths of innocents with more death. There was not much blood in these black-and-white episodes and always time for the outlaw to acknowledge his guilt before expiring (Rodabough 1980). By the late 1960s and early 1970s, however, in the context of the Vietnam War, the bloody protest movements, and the assassinations of John and Robert Kennedy and Martin Luther King, the pornographic obsession was to be fed by the gory "spaghetti westerns." Here the cowboy, now the symbol of true individualism, took it upon himself to execute evil, this time graphically and in "living" color.

Several death leitmotifs received extensive elaboration during the 1970s. One involved the theme of man controlling death: there was *Logan's Run*, in which, because of population pressures, individuals had only thirty years of life before being ritually destroyed. *Zardoz* dealt with the clash of two cultures, one a technological commune in which there was no aging process and no death, and the other a dying world populated with brutal inhabitants. The

Vietnam War spawned its own celluloid explorations of war and death (*The Deer Hunter, Apocalypse Now*), as did urban violence. In March 1979, a gang film called *The Warriors* was released by Paramount with the following ad: "These are the Armies of the Night. They are 100,000 strong. They outnumber the cops five to one. They could run New York City. Tonight they're all out to get the warriors." The film's first link to actual killing came in a Palm Springs drive-in in a racial incident involving a white group, the Family, and a black one, the Blue Coats. The following night in Oxnard, California, a scuffle broke out in the lobby following the first showing of *The Warriors*, leaving a white youth stabbed to death by a black youth. In Boston, there was a nonracial event in which a member of the Dorchester gang yelled, "I want you!"—a line from the script—and a youth died of stab wounds six hours later. Then there was *Cruising*, a film focusing on a killer preying on New York homosexuals, yielding gay protests from coast to coast, fearing copycat violence. United Artists, the movie's distributor, said that theater owners could deduct extra security costs from receipts.

One additional death motif of cinema during the 1970s involved attacks on humanity by the natural order. Why during this era should people be attacked by rats, frogs, bees, sharks, meteors, earthquakes, and tidal waves? There was a dramatic increase in the number of such deaths during this decade, but that probably had little effect on the cinematic expositions of the theme. Instead, perhaps people had grown tired of man-made death and had become desensitized to its terror. Further, having become fully urbanized, nature had become an unknown, its forces of destruction no longer respected when compared to our own potential for evil. In a sense, then, the motif represented a rediscovery of the natural order, bolstered by the culture's growing environmental awareness and reappreciation of ecological interdependencies.

During the decade that followed, cinema returned death to human control in an era marked by international terrorism and increasing militarization. By the mid-1980s, it was military violence that gained immense popularity, epitomized by *Rambo* and its sequels and imitations. In the original, not counting the groups of individuals who were slaughtered in more than seventy explosions, there were forty-four specific killings—one every 2.1 minutes (Powell 1985). War became romanticized, and the message was that it takes violence to resolve complex problems. In addition, the fears of random, meaningless deaths were to be dramatized in the *Halloween* and *Mad Max* series of films. It has been hypothesized that these movies, attracting two disenfranchised groups (specifically, the young and those of working-class backgrounds), provided an outlet for class antagonisms, and their ambiguous endings dramatize the loss of faith in the "just world" assumption disseminated by the upper classes (Hensley and LaBeff 1986).

With the advent of video cassettes, the ability to view uncensored death in the privacy of one's home further dramatizes Gorer's notion of pornographic death. As opposed to the obscene, which produces social embarrassment and is enjoyed socially, pornography produces fantasy and is enjoyed privately. During 1985, *Faces of Death* appeared in American video rental outlets. Here actual death was displayed, with images of suicides, executions, and autopsies. The popularity of this film among teenagers—whose suicide rate was skyrocketing—prompted editorial reflection. One movie reviewer said he couldn't tell what was acting and what was real.

DEATH AND MUSIC

Except for simple conversation, perhaps the oldest vehicle by which to express death fears and transcendent hopes, to share stories of death and how others have met it, is music. American folk music, for example, features numerous songs of death spawned by war and violence (e.g., "Mountain Meadows Massacre"), work and class oppression ("John Henry"), disease ("The TB Is Whipping Me," "Meningitis Blues"), and fatal accidents ("The Wreck of the Old 97"). Music not only reflects a culture's death ethos but possibly shapes it as well. The 1933 song "Gloomy Sunday," written by Rezso Seress and lyricist Laszlo Javor, was banned from the airwaves of Budapest because of the seventeen suicides inspired by the piece. This publicity led to its import to the United States, where "The Famous Hungarian Suicide Song" ("Angels have no thought of ever returning you. . . . Would they be angry if I thought of joining you?") received three recorded versions (from bandleaders Paul Whiteman, Hal Kemp, and Harry King).

To explore some of the relationships between death and music, let us here focus on the postwar music identified with American adolescents: rock and roll.

While academicians argued about the culture's death denials, the music of the postwar baby-boomers became imbued with death, not only being a frequent theme of its songs but also the premature fate of its performers (around whom dead-rock-star cults were to emerge). According to folk-pop singer-songwriter Don McLean ("American Pie," 1972), Buddy Holly's 1959 death in an aircrash was "the day the music died." Well, yes and no. Though the death of Holly, one of the forces behind the new rock-and-roll music of the late 1950s, was a blow to the music industry, it did not end rock and roll. If anything, it sanctified the movement and gave it its dark side. An intimacy with death was to be created that eventually was reflected even in the names of its groups: the Grateful Dead, the Zombies, the Dead Kennedys, Sharon Tate's Baby, the Clash, D-Day, the Explosives, Megadeath, and Terminal Mind.

In the early years of rock, the death of a loved one was often romanticized in song (in a sense, it was rock's Victorian era): in Mark Dinning's "Teen Angel," she ran back to the stalled car to get his high school ring but was killed by the oncoming train; in "Last Kiss," "she's gone to heaven so I've got to be good, so I can see my baby when I leave this world." Denisoff (1972, p. 172) refers to these as "coffin songs," often featuring a Romeo and Juliet motif. What could be a more effective rebuff to adults' claim that it is only puppy love?

Thanks to the mass media of the 1960s, this was to be the best informed of young generations, and the youth of America were to become increasingly politicized against the situation in Vietnam. They were frustrated by their inability to vote and yet their duty to fight in an unpopular war. This led to the rise of protest music, stimulated by the 1965 release of Barry Maguire's "Eve of Destruction." Strangely, in the following year, the number one single in the United States was a song dedicated to the warriors, Barry Sadler's "The Ballad of the Green Berets." The late 1960s continued the morbid themes of the previous years. With dead soldiers being returned in body bags by the thousands and with the assassinations of Bobby Kennedy and Martin Luther King, the world seemed to be falling apart. Nothing of the establishment (which was taken to be those over age thirty) was to be believed, and in such a context the rumor of the death of Beatle Paul McCartney swept coast to coast.

Death was not only a frequent theme of the music of the time, but it also was to become the fate of many of its performers. Death came prematurely not only to Buddy Holly (age twenty-two at the time of his fatal crash) but to Elvis Presley (drug-related coronary, age forty-two), Jim Morrison (heart attack, twenty-seven), Jimi Hendrix (drug-related, twenty-seven), Janis Joplin (substance abuse, twenty-seven), Otis Redding (thirty-six), Keith Relf (of the Yardbirds, electrocution from guitar, thirty-three), Jim Croce (plane crash, thirty), Ronnie Van Zant (Lynyrd Skynyrd, plane crash), Keith Moon (the Who, drugs), Brian Jones (Rolling Stones, drug-related drowning), Lowell George (Little Feat, drugs), Sid Vicious (Sex Pistols, suicide), Pig Pen (Grateful Dead), Cass Elliot (Mamas and Papas, age thirty), Minnie Ripperton (cancer), Duane Allman (motorcycle accident), John Lennon (murdered, age forty), Bill Haley, and Karen Carpenter. Of those musicians appearing in the film of the 1968 Monterey Pops Concert, ten were dead by 1981. During the late 1970s and early 1980s, the posthumous releases by these dead stars often outsold the recordings of the living.

Not only was death a theme of rock-and-roll songs and the fate of some performers, but the audience became involved as well. Mass murderer Charles Manson supposedly believed that the Beatles were sending him messages through the lyrics of songs from their "white album," particularly "Helter Skelter." At Altamont Speedway near San Francisco, it proved unfortunate to mix the Rolling Stones with the Hell's Angels motorcycle gang, which had been hired to provide security. When a fan attempted to gain access to the stage, he was beaten and stabbed to death by the Angels, all in view of the movie cameras that were filming the concert movie *Gimme Shelter*. In Cincinnati, Ohio, the crush of a crowd at a Who concert left six trampled to death. In Pueblo,

Mexico, during a 1983 performance of the Puerto Rican group Menudo, thousands of fans stampeded toward the only open exit after a concert, crushing three to death and injuring eighty others.

References

Adweek (Southwest ed.). 1984. "What's New Portfolio." November 26, p. 37.

Arlen, Michael. 1975. "The Air, the Cold, Bright Charms of Immortality." *New Yorker*. January 27, pp. 73–78.

Campbell, Colin. 1985. "News Coverage of Mud Slide in Puerto Rico Is Criticized as Inadequate." *New York Times*. October 15, p. 9.

Denisoff, R. Serge. 1972. *Sing a Song of Social Significance*. Bowling Green, Ohio: Bowling Green University Popular Press.

Gerbner, George. 1980. "Death in Prime Time: Notes on the Symbolic Functions of Dying in the Mass Media." *Annals* 447:64–70.

Gorer, Geoffrey. 1965. *Death, Grief, and Mourning*. New York: Doubleday Anchor Books.

Hensley, John, and Emily LaBeff. 1986. "A Sociological Analysis of Motion Picture Violence as Class-Related Fantasy Aggression." Paper presented at the Southwest Social Science Association Meetings, San Antonio.

May, William. 1973. "The Sacral Power of Death in Contemporary Experience." In Arien Mack, ed., *Death in American Experience*. New York: Schocken Books, pp. 97–122.

New York Times. 1986. "For Shuttle Coverage, a Huge Audience." January 30, p. 23.

Powell, Stewart. 1985. "What Entertainers Are Doing to Your Kids." *U.S. News & World Report*. October 28, pp. 46–49.

PBS (Public Broadcasting System). 1983. "The Horror of It All." February 23.

Rodabough, Tillman. 1980. "The Cycle of American Perspectives toward Death." *Journal of the American Studies Association of Texas* 11:22–27.

Time. 1976. "Death Watch." May 3, p. 69.

5 The Terror of Death

Ernest Becker

ERNEST BECKER won the Pulitzer Prize for general nonfiction for *The Denial of Death*. After receiving a Ph.D. in cultural anthropology from Syracuse University, Dr. Becker taught at the University of California at Berkeley, San Francisco State College, and Simon Fraser University in Canada. He was the author of *The Birth and Death of Meaning*, *Revolution in Psychiatry*, *The Structure of Evil*, *Angel in Armor*, and *Escape from Evil*.

Becker's main theme in *The Denial of Death* is that our entire lives are organized around our fear and denial of death. The selection included here is from the chapter entitled "The Terror of Death"; it presents a discussion of this deep-seated fear especially in relation to its opposite, heroism.

It is not for us to confess that in our civilized attitude towards death we are once more living psychologically beyond our means, and must reform and give truth its due. Would it not be better to give death the place in actuality and in our thoughts which properly belongs to it, and to yield a little more prominence to that unconscious attitude towards death which we have hitherto so carefully suppressed? This hardly seems indeed a greater achievement, but rather a backward step . . . but it has the merit of taking somewhat more into account the true state of affairs. . . .

SIGMUND FREUD[1]

THE FIRST THING WE HAVE TO DO WITH HEROISM is to lay bare its underside, show what gives human heroics its specific nature and impetus. Here we introduce directly one of the great rediscoveries of modern thought: That of all things that move man, one of the principal ones is his terror of death. After Darwin the problem of death as an evolutionary one came to the fore, and many thinkers immediately saw that it was a major psychological problem for man.[2] They also very quickly saw what real heroism was about, as Shaler wrote just at the turn of the century:[3] heroism is first and foremost a reflex of the terror of death. We admire most the courage to face death; we give such valor our highest and most constant adoration; it moves us deeply in our hearts because we have doubts about how brave we ourselves would be. When we see a man bravely facing his own extinction we rehearse the greatest victory we can imagine. And so the hero has been the center of human honor and acclaim since probably the beginning of specifically human evolution. But even before that our primate ancestors deferred to others who were extrapowerful and courageous and ignored those who were cowardly. Man has elevated animal courage into a cult.

Anthropological and historical research also began, in the nineteenth century, to put together a picture of the heroic since primitive and ancient times. The hero was the man who could go into the spirit world, the world of the dead, and return alive. He had his descendants in the mystery cults of the Eastern Mediterranean, which were cults of death and resurrection. The divine hero of each of these cults was one who had come back from the dead. And as we know today from the research into ancient myths and rituals, Christianity itself was a competitor with the mystery cults and won out—among other reasons—because it, too, featured a healer with supernatural powers who had risen from the dead. The great triumph of Easter is the joyful shout "Christ has risen!", an echo of the same joy that the devotees of the mystery cults enacted at their ceremonies of the victory over death. These cults, as G. Stanley Hall so aptly put it, were an attempt to attain "an immunity bath" from the greatest evil: death and the dread of it.[4] All historical religions addressed themselves to this same problem of how to bear the end of life. Religions like Hinduism and Buddhism performed the ingenious trick of pretending not to want to be reborn, which is a sort of negative magic: claiming not to want what you really want most.[5] When philosophy took over from religion it also took over religion's central problem, and death became the real "muse of philosophy" from its beginnings in Greece right through Heidegger and modern existentialism.[6]

We already have volumes of work and thought on the subject, from religion and philosophy and—since Darwin—from science itself. The problem is how to make sense out of it; the accumulation of research and opinion on the fear of death is already too large to be dealt with and summarized in any simple way. The revival of interest in death, in the last few decades, has alone already piled up a formidable literature, and this literature does not point in any single direction.

THE "HEALTHY-MINDED" ARGUMENT

There are "healthy-minded" persons who maintain that fear of death is not a natural thing for man, that we are not born with it. An increasing number of careful studies on how the actual fear of death develops in the child[7] agree fairly well that the child has no knowledge of death until about the age of three to five. How could he? It is too abstract an idea, too removed from his experience.

He lives in a world that is full of living, acting things, responding to him, amusing him, feeding him. He doesn't know what it means for life to disappear forever, nor theorize where it would go. Only gradually does he recognize that there is a thing called death that takes some people away forever; very reluctantly he comes to admit that it sooner or later takes everyone away, but this gradual realization of the inevitability of death can take up until the ninth or tenth year.

If the child has no knowledge of an abstract idea like absolute negation, he does have his own anxieties. He is absolutely dependent on the mother, experiences loneliness when she is absent, frustration when he is deprived of gratification, irritation at hunger and discomfort, and so on. If he were abandoned to himself his world would drop away, and his organism must sense this at some level; we call this the anxiety of object-loss. Isn't this anxiety, then, a natural organismic fear of annihilation? Again, there are many who look at this as a very relative matter. They believe that if the mother has done her job in a warm and dependable way, the child's natural anxieties and guilts will develop in a moderate way, and he will be able to place them firmly under the control of his developing personality.[8] The child who has good maternal experiences will develop a sense of basic security and will not be subject to morbid fears of losing support, of being annihilated, or the like.[9] As he grows up to understand death rationally by the age of nine or ten, he will accept it as part of his world view, but the idea will not poison his self-confident attitude toward life. The psychiatrist Rheingold says categorically that annihilation anxiety is not part of the child's natural experience but is engendered in him by bad experiences with a depriving mother.[10] This theory puts the whole burden of anxiety onto the child's nurture and not his nature. Another psychiatrist, in a less extreme vein, sees the fear of death as greatly heightened by the child's experiences with his parents, by their hostile denial of his life impulses, and more generally, by the antagonism of society to human freedom and self-expansiveness.[11]

As we will see later on, this view is very popular today in the widespread movement toward unrepressed living, the urge to a new freedom for natural biological urges, a new attitude of pride and joy in the body, the abandonment of shame, guilt, and self-hatred. From this point of view, fear of death is something that society creates and at the same time uses against the person to keep him in submission; the psychiatrist Moloney talked about it as a "culture mechanism," and Marcuse as an "ideology."[12] Norman O. Brown, in a vastly influential book that we shall discuss at some length, went so far as to say that there could be a birth and development of the child in a "second innocence" that would be free of the fear of death because it would not deny natural vitality and would leave the child fully open to physical living.[13]

It is easy to see that, from this point of view, those who have bad early experiences will be most morbidly fixated on the anxiety of death; and if by chance they grow up to be philosophers they will probably make the idea a central dictum of their thoughts—as did Schopenhauer, who both hated his mother and went on to pronounce death the "muse of philosophy." If you have a "sour" character structure or especially tragic experiences, then you are bound to be pessimistic. One psychologist remarked to me that the whole idea of the fear of death was an import by existentialists and Protestant theologians who had been scarred by their European experiences or who carried around the extra weight of a Calvinist and Lutheran heritage of life-denial. Even the distinguished psychologist Gardner Murphy seems to lean to this school and urges us to study *the person* who exhibits the fear of death, who places anxiety in the center of his thought; and Murphy asks why the living of life in love and joy cannot also be regarded as real and basic.[14]

THE "MORBIDLY-MINDED" ARGUMENT

The "healthy-minded" argument just discussed is one side of the picture of the accumulated research and opinion on the problem of the fear of death, but there is another side. A large body of people would agree with these observations on early experience and would admit that experiences may heighten natural anxieties and later fears, but these people would also claim very strongly that nevertheless the fear of death is natural and is present in everyone, that it is the basic fear that influences all others, a fear from which no one is immune, no matter how disguised it may be. William James spoke very early for this school, and with his usual colorful realism he called death "the worm at the core" of man's pretensions to happiness.[15] No less a student of human nature than Max Scheler thought that all men must have some kind of certain intuition of this "worm at the core," whether they admitted it or not.[16] Countless other authorities—some of whom we shall parade in the following pages—belong to this school: students of the stature of Freud, many of his close circle, and serious researchers who are not psychoanalysts. What are we to make of a dispute in which there are two distinct camps, both studded with distinguished authorities? Jacques Choron goes so far as to say that it is questionable whether it will ever be possible to decide whether the fear of death is or is not the basic anxiety.[17] In matters like this, then, the most that one can do is to take sides, to give an opinion based on the authorities that seem to him most compelling, and to present some of the compelling arguments.

I frankly side with this second school—in fact, this whole book is a network of arguments based on the universality of the fear of death, or "terror" as I prefer to call it, in order to convey how all-consuming it is when we look it full in the face. The first document that I want to present and linger on is a paper written by the noted psychoanalyst Gregory Zilboorg; it is an especially penetrating essay that—for succinctness and scope—has not been much improved upon, even though it appeared several decades ago.[18] Zilboorg says that most people think death fear is absent because it rarely shows its true face; but he argues that underneath all appearances fear of death is universally present:

> *For behind the sense of insecurity in the face of danger, behind the sense of discouragement and depression, there always lurks the basic fear of death, a fear which undergoes most complex elaborations and manifests itself in many indirect ways. . . . No one is free of the fear of death. . . . The anxiety neuroses, the various phobic states, even a considerable number of depressive suicidal states and many schizophrenias amply demonstrate the ever-present fear of death which becomes woven into the major conflicts of the given psychopathological conditions. . . . We may take for granted that the fear of death is always present in our mental functioning.*[19]

Hadn't James said the same thing earlier, in his own way?

> *Let sanguine healthy-mindedness do its best with its strange power of living in the moment and ignoring and forgetting, still the evil background is really there to be thought of, and the skull will grin in at the banquet.*[20]

The difference in these two statements is not so much in the imagery and style as in the fact that Zilboorg's comes almost a half-century later and is based on that much more real clinical work, not only on philosophical speculation or personal intuition. But it also continues the straight line of development from James and the post-Darwinians who saw the fear of death as a biological and evolutionary problem. Here I think he is on very sound ground, and I especially like the way he puts the case. Zilboorg points out that this fear is actually an expression of the instinct of self-preservation which functions as a constant drive to maintain life and to master the dangers that threaten life:

> *Such constant expenditure of psychological energy on the business of preserving life would be impossible if the fear of death were not as constant. The very term "self-preservation" implies an effort against some force of disintegration; the affective aspect of this is fear, fear of death.*[21]

In other words, the fear of death must be present behind all our normal functioning, in order for the organism to be armed toward self-preservation. But the fear of death cannot be present constantly in one's mental functioning, else the organism could not function. Zilboorg continues:

> *If this fear were as constantly conscious, we should be unable to function normally. It must be properly repressed to keep us living with any modicum of comfort. We know very well that to repress means more than to put away and to forget that which was put away and the place where we put it. It means also to maintain a constant psychological effort to keep the lid on and inwardly never relax our watchfulness.*[22]

And so we can understand what seems like an impossible paradox: the ever-present fear of death in the normal biological functioning of our instinct of self-preservation, as well as our utter obliviousness to this fear in our conscious life.

> *Therefore in normal times we move about actually without ever believing in our own death, as if we fully believed in our own corporeal immortality. We are intent on mastering death. . . . A man will say, of course, that he knows he will die some day, but he does not really care. He is having a good time with living, and he does not think about death and does not care to bother about it—but this is a purely intellectual, verbal admission. The affect of fear is repressed.*[23]

The argument from biology and evolution is basic and has to be taken seriously; I don't see how it can be left out of any discussion. Animals in order to survive have had to be protected by fear-responses, in relation not only to other animals but to nature itself. They had to see the real relationship of their limited powers to the dangerous world in which they were immersed. Reality and fear go together naturally. As the human infant is in an even more exposed and helpless situation, it is foolish to assume that the fear response of animals would have disappeared in such a weak and highly sensitive species. It is more reasonable to think that it was instead heightened, as some of the early Darwinians thought: early men who were most afraid were those who were realistic about their situation in nature, and they passed on to their offspring a realism that had a high survival value.[24] The result was the emergence of man as we know him: a hyperanxious animal who constantly invents reasons for anxiety even where there are none.

The argument from psychoanalysis is less speculative and has to be taken even more seriously. It showed us something about the child's inner world that we had never realized: namely, that it was more filled with terror, the more the child was different from other animals. We could say that fear is programmed into the lower animals by ready-made instincts; but an animal who has no instincts has no programmed fears. Man's fears are fashioned out of the ways in which he perceives the world. Now, what is unique about the child's perception of the world? For one thing, the extreme confusion of cause-and-effect relationships; for another, extreme unreality about the limits of his own powers. The child lives in a situation of utter dependence; and when his needs are met it must seem to him that he has magical powers, real omnipotence. If he experiences pain, hunger, or discomfort, all he has to do is to scream and he is relieved and lulled by gentle, loving sounds. He is a magician and a telepath who has only to mumble and to imagine and the world turns to his desires.

But now the penalty for such perceptions. In a magical world where things cause other things to happen just by a mere thought or a look of displeasure, anything can happen to anyone. When the child experiences inevitable and real frustrations from his parents, he directs hate and destructive feelings toward them; and he has no way of knowing that malevolent feelings cannot be ful-filled by the same magic as were his other wishes. Psychoanalysts believe that this confusion is a main cause of guilt and helplessness in the child. In his very fine essay Wahl summed up his paradox:

> . . . *the socialization processes for all children are painful and frustrating, and hence no child escapes forming hostile death wishes toward his socializers. Therefore, none escape the fear of personal death in either direct or symbolic form. Repression is usu-ally . . . immediate and effective. . . .*[25]

The child is too weak to take responsibility for all this destructive feeling, and he can't control the magical execution of his desires. This is what we mean by an immature ego: the child doesn't have the sure ability to organize his per-ceptions and his relationship to the world; he can't control his own activity; and he doesn't have sure command over the acts of others. He thus has no real con-trol over the magical cause-and-effect that he senses, either inside himself or outside in nature and in others: his destructive wishes could explode, his par-ents' wishes likewise. The forces of nature are confused, externally and inter-nally; and for a weak ego this fact makes for quantities of exaggerated potential power and added terror. The result is that the child—at least some of the time—lives with an inner sense of chaos that other animals are immune to.[26]

Ironically, even when the child makes out real cause-and-effect relation-ships they become a burden to him because he overgeneralizes them. One such generalization is what the psychoanalysts call the "talion principle." The child crushes insects, sees the cat eat a mouse and make it vanish, joins with the fam-ily to make a pet rabbit disappear into their interiors, and so on. He comes to know something about the power relations of the world but can't give them relative value: the parents could eat him and make him vanish, and he could likewise eat them; when the father gets a fierce glow in his eyes as he clubs a rat, the watching child might also expect to be clubbed—especially if he has been thinking bad magical thoughts.

I don't want to seem to make an exact picture of processes that are still un-clear to us or to make out that all children live in the same world and have the same problems; also, I wouldn't want to make the child's world seem more lu-rid than it really is most of the time; but I think it is important to show the pain-ful contradictions that must be present in it at least some of the time and to show how fantastic a world it surely is for the first few years of the child's life. Perhaps then we could understand better why Zilboorg said that the fear of death "undergoes most complex elaborations and manifests itself in many in-direct ways." Or, as Wahl so perfectly put it, death is a *complex symbol* and not any particular, sharply defined thing to a child:

> . . . *the child's concept of death is not a single thing, but it is rather a composite of mu-tually contradictory paradoxes . . . death itself is not only a state, but a complex sym-*

bol, the significance of which will vary from one person to another and from one culture to another.[27]

We could understand, too, why children have their recurrent nightmares, their universal phobias of insects and mean dogs. In their tortured interiors radiate complex symbols of many inadmissible realities—terror of the world, the horror of one's own wishes, the fear of vengeance by the parents, the disappearance of things, one's lack of control over anything, really. It is too much for any animal to take, but the child has to take it, and he wakes up screaming with almost punctual regularity during the period when his weak ego is in the process of consolidating things.

The "disappearance" of the fear of death

Yet, the nightmares become more and more widely spaced, and some children have more than others: we are back again to the beginning of our discussion, to those who do not believe that the fear of death is normal, who think that it is a neurotic exaggeration that draws on bad early experiences. Otherwise, they say, how do we explain that so many people—the vast majority—seem to survive the flurry of childhood nightmares and go on to live a healthy, more-or-less optimistic life, untroubled by death? As Montaigne said, the peasant has a profound indifference and a patience toward death and the sinister side of life; and if we say that this is because of his stupidity, then "let's all learn from stupidity."[28] Today, when we know more than Montaigne, we would say "let's all learn from repression"—but the moral would have just as much weight: repression takes care of the complex symbol of death for most people.

But its disappearance doesn't mean that the fear was never there. The argument of those who believe in the universality of the innate terror of death rests its case mostly on what we know about how effective repression is. The argument can probably never be cleanly decided: if you claim that a concept is not present because it is repressed, you can't lose; it is not a fair game, intellectually, because you always hold the trump card. This type of argument makes psychoanalysis seem unscientific to many people, the fact that its proponents can claim that someone denies one of their concepts because he represses his consciousness of its truth.

But repression is not a magical word for winning arguments; it is a real phenomenon, and we have been able to study in many of its workings. This study gives it legitimacy as a scientific concept and makes it a more-or-less dependable ally in our argument. For one thing, there is a growing body of research trying to get at the consciousness of death denied by repression that uses psychological tests such as measuring galvanic skin responses; it strongly suggests that underneath the most bland exterior lurks the universal anxiety, the "worm at the core."[29]

For another thing, there is nothing like shocks in the real world to jar loose repressions. Recently psychiatrists reported an increase in anxiety neuroses in children as a result of the earth tremors in Southern California. For these children the discovery that life really includes cataclysmic danger was too much for their still-imperfect denial systems—hence open outbursts of anxiety. With adults we see this manifestation of anxiety in the face of impending catastrophe where it takes the form of panic. Recently several people suffered broken limbs and other injuries after forcing open their airplane's safety door during take-off and jumping from the wing to the ground; the incident was triggered by the backfire of an engine. Obviously underneath these harmless noises other things are rumbling in the creature.

But even more important is how repression works: it is not simply a negative force opposing life energies; it lives on life energies and uses them creatively. I mean that fears are naturally absorbed by expansive organismic striving. Nature seems to have built into organisms an innate healthy-mindedness; it expresses itself in self-delight in the pleasure of unfolding one's capacities into the world, in the incorporation of things in that world, and in feeding on its limitless experiences. This is a lot of very positive experience, and when a powerful organism moves with it, it gives contentment. As Santayana once put it: a lion must feel more secure that God is on his side than a gazelle. On the most elemental level the organism works actively against its own fragility by seeking to expand and perpetuate itself in living experience; instead of shrinking, it moves toward more life. Also, it does one thing at a time, avoiding needless distractions from all-absorbing activity; in this way, it would seem, fear of death can be carefully ignored or actually absorbed in the life-expanding processes. Occasionally we seem to see such a vital organism on the human level: I am thinking of the portrait of *Zorba the Greek* drawn by Nikos Kazantzakis. Zorba was an ideal of the nonchalant victory of all-absorbing daily passion over timidity and death, and he purged others in his life-affirming flame. But Kazantzakis himself was no Zorba—which is partly why the character of Zorba rang a bit false—nor are most other men. Still, everyone enjoys a working amount of basic narcissism, even though it is not a lion's. The child who is well nourished and loved develops, as we said, a sense of magical omnipotence, a sense of his own indestructibility, a feeling of proven power and secure support. He can imagine himself, deep down, to be eternal. We might say that his repression of the idea of his own death is made easy for him because he is fortified against it in his very narcissistic vitality. This type of character probably helped Freud to say that the unconscious does not know death. Anyway, we know that basic narcissism is increased when one's childhood experiences have been securely life-supporting and warmly enhancing to the sense of self, to the feeling of being really special, truly Number One in creation. The result is that some people have more of what the psychoanalyst Leon J. Saul has aptly called "Inner Sustainment."[30] It is a sense of bodily confidence in the face of experience that sees the person more easily through severe life crises and even sharp personality changes; it almost seems to take the place of the directive instincts of lower animals. One can't help thinking of Freud again, who had more inner sustainment than most men, thanks to his mother and a favorable early environment; he knew the confidence and courage that it gave to a man, and he himself faced up to life and to a fatal cancer with a Stoic heroism. Again we have evidence that the complex symbol of fear of death would be very variable in its intensity; it would be, as Wahl concluded, "profoundly dependent upon the nature and the vicissitudes of the developmental process."[31]

But I want to be careful not to make too much of natural vitality and inner sustainment. As we will see in Chapter Six, even the unusually favored Freud suffered his whole life from phobias and from death-anxiety; and he came to fully perceive the world under the aspect of natural terror. I don't believe that the complex symbol of death is ever absent, no matter how much vitality and inner sustainment a person has. Even more, if we say that these powers make repression easy and natural, we are only saying the half of it. Actually, they get their very power from repression. Psychiatrists argue that the fear of death varies in intensity depending on the developmental process, and I think that one important reason for this variability is that the fear is transmuted in that process. If the child has had a very favorable upbringing, it only serves all the better to hide the fear of death. After all, repression is made possible by the natural identification of the child with the powers of his parents. If he has been well cared for, identification comes easily and solidly, and his parents' powerful triumph over death automatically becomes his. What is more natural to banish one's fears than to live on delegated powers? And what does the whole growing-up period signify, if not the giving over of one's life-project? I am going to be talking about these things all the way through this book and do not want to develop them in this introductory discussion. What we will see is that man cuts out for himself a manageable world: he throws himself into action uncritically, unthinkingly. He accepts the cultural programming that turns his nose where he is supposed to look; he doesn't bite the world off in one piece as a giant would, but in small manageable pieces, as a beaver does. He uses all kinds of techniques, which we call the "character defenses": he learns not to expose himself, not to stand out; he learns to embed himself in other-power, both of concrete persons and of things and cultural commands; the result is that he comes to exist in the imagined infallibility of the world around him. He doesn't have to have fears when his feet are solidly mired and his life mapped out in a ready-made maze. All he has to do is to plunge ahead in a compulsive style of drivenness in the "ways of the world" that the child learns and in which he lives later as a kind of grim equanimity—the "strange power of living in the moment and ignoring and forgetting"—as James put it. This is the deeper reason that Montaigne's peasant isn't troubled until the very end, when the Angel of Death, who has always been sitting on his shoulder, extends his wing. Or at least until he is prematurely startled into dumb awareness, like the "Husbands" in John Cassavetes' fine film. At times like this, when the awareness dawns that has always been blotted out by frenetic, ready-made activity, we see the transmutation of repression redistilled, so to speak, and the fear of death emerges in pure essence. This is why people have psychotic breaks when repression no longer works, when the forward momentum of activity is no longer possible. Besides, the peasant mentality is far less romantic than Montaigne would have us believe. The peasant's equanimity is usually immersed in a style of life that has elements of real madness, and so it protects him: an undercurrent of constant hate and bitterness expressed in feuding, bullying, bickering and family quarrels, the petty mentality, the self-deprecation, the superstition, the obsessive control of daily life by a strict authoritarianism, and so on. As the title of a recent essay by Joseph Lopreato has it: "How would you like to be a peasant?"

We will also touch upon another large dimension in which the complex symbol of death is transmuted and transcended by man—belief in immortality, the extension of one's being into eternity. Right now we can conclude that there are many ways that repression works to calm the anxious human animal, so that he need not be anxious at all.

I think we have reconciled our two divergent positions on the fear of death. The "environmental" and "innate" positions are both part of the same picture; they merge naturally into one another; it all depends from which angle you approach the picture: from the side of the disguises and transmutations of the fear of death or from the side of its apparent absence. I admit with a sense of scientific uneasiness that whatever angle you use, you don't get at the actual fear of death; and so I reluctantly agree with Choron that the argument can probably never be cleanly "won." Nevertheless something very important emerges: there are different images of man that he can draw and choose from.

On the one hand, we see a human animal who is partly dead to the world, who is most "dignified" when he shows a certain obliviousness to his fate, when he allows himself to be driven through life; who is most "free" when he lives in secure dependency on powers around him, when he is least in possession of himself. On the other hand, we get an image of a human animal who is overly sensitive to the world, who cannot shut it out, who is thrown back on his own meagre powers, and who seems least free to move and act, least in possession of himself, and most undignified. Whichever image we choose to identify with depends in large part upon ourselves. Let us then explore and develop these images further to see what they reveal to us.

Notes

1. S. Freud, "Thoughts for the Times on War and Death," 1915, *Collected Papers*, Vol. 4 (New York: Basic Books, 1959), pp. 316–317.
2. Cf., for example, A. L. Cochrane, "Elie Metschnikoff and His Theory of an '*In-*

stinct de la Mort,'" *International Journal of Psychoanalysis* 1934, 15:265–270; G. Stanley Hall, "Thanatophobia and Immortality," *American Journal of Psychology*, 1915, 26:550–613.

3. N. S. Shaler, *The Individual: A Study of Life and Death* (New York: Appleton, 1900).

4. Hall, "Thanatophobia," p. 562.

5. Cf. Alan Harrington, *The Immortalist* (New York: Random House, 1969), p. 82.

6. See Jacques Choron's excellent study: *Death and Western Thought* (New York: Collier Books, 1963).

7. See H. Feifel, ed., *The Meaning of Death* (New York: McGraw-Hill, 1959), Chapter 6; G. Rochlin, *Griefs and Discontents* (Boston: Little, Brown, 1967), p. 67.

8. J. Bowlby, *Maternal Care and Mental Health* (Geneva: World Health Organization, 1952), p. 11.

9. Cf. Walter Tietz, "School Phobia and the Fear of Death," *Mental Hygiene*, 1970, 54:565–568.

10. J. C. Rheingold, *The Mother, Anxiety and Death: The Catastrophic Death Complex* (Boston: Little, Brown, 1967).

11. A. J. Levin, "The Fiction of the Death Instinct," *Psychiatric Quarterly*, 1951, 25:257–281.

12. J. C. Moloney, *The Magic Cloak: A Contribution to the Psychology of Authoritarianism* (Wakefield, Mass.: Montrose Press, 1949), p. 217; H. Marcuse, "The Ideology of Death," in Feifel, *Meaning of Death*, Chapter 5.

13. LAD, p. 270.

14. G. Murphy, "Discussion," in Feifel, *The Meaning of Death*, p. 320.

15. William James, *Varieties of Religious Experience: A Study in Human Nature*, 1902 (New York: Mentor Edition, 1958), p. 121.

16. Choron, *Death*, p. 17.

17. *Ibid.*, p. 272.

18. G. Zilboorg, "Fear of Death," *Psychoanalytic Quarterly*, 1943, 12:465–475. See Eissler's nice technical distinction between the anxiety of death and the terror of it, in his book of essays loaded with subtle discussion: K. R. Eissler, *The Psychiatrist and the Dying Patient* (New York: International Universities Press, 1955), p. 277.

19. Zilboorg, "Fear of Death," pp. 465–467.

20. James, *Varieties*, p. 121.

21. Zilboorg, "Fear of Death," p. 467. Or, we might more precisely say, with Eissler, fear of annihilation, which is extended by the ego into the consciousness of death. See *The Psychiatrist and the Dying Patient*, p. 267.

22. *Ibid.*

23. *Ibid.*, pp. 468–471 *passim*.

24. Cf. Shaler, *The Individual*.

25. C. W. Wahl, "The Fear of Death," in Feifel, pp. 24–25.

26. Cf. Moloney, *The Magic Cloak*, p. 117.

27. Wahl, "Fear of Death," pp. 25–26.

28. In Choron, *Death*, p. 100.

29. Cf., for example, I. E. Alexander *et al.*, "Is Death a Matter of Indifference?" *Journal of Psychology*, 1957, 43:277–283; I. M. Greenberg and I. E. Alexander, "Some Correlates of Thoughts and Feelings Concerning Death," *Hillside Hospital Journal*, 1962, No. 2:120–126; S. I. Golding *et al.*, "Anxiety and Two Cognitive Forms of Resistance of the Idea of Death," *Psychological Reports*, 1966, 18: 359–364.

30. L. J. Saul, "Inner Sustainment," *Psychoanalytic Quarterly*, 1970, 39:215–222.

31. Wahl, "Fear of Death," p. 26.

PART TWO

HISTORICAL AND CROSS-CULTURAL PERSPECTIVES

Contents

ALTHOUGH IT MAY BE BANAL to say that death is as old as humankind, it is nonetheless interesting to note that reflecting on the topic of death is a development that distinguishes human beings from every other creature. Currently there are many obvious changes in the thanatological wind. These changes include the increase in general longevity, the secularization of death, debates over assisted suicide and health care rationing, and a general concern with reconceptualizing the psychological dimensions of death in light of changes in our knowledge of the human condition.

To understand the contemporary American discussions and disputations about death, we need to know something about the ways in which human beings come to grips with this topic in other cultures and at other times in history. Such a review will also help us put the contemporary AIDS epidemic and our response to it in better perspective.

The article by Ariès uses sculpture, paintings, and other such cultural artifacts to trace the evolution of thinking about the nature of death in the Western world, beginning with a seventh-century tomb panel depicting the resurrection of the dead at the end of the world but lacking any notion of a link between salvation and individual responsibility. By the twelfth century, due to the emergence of individualism, we see evidence in other artistic creations depicting a Last Judgment at which souls are individually judged and separated. By the thirteenth century, the emphasis is very much on judgment at the time of death (as opposed to the Second Coming). By the fifteenth and sixteenth century, the emphasis is no longer on judging the good and evil deeds done throughout one's life; rather, it is on dying well—that is, on one's conduct in connection with the final temptations linked to a life review during the final minutes or hours of life.

The selection by Renouard explores the profound social consequences of the fourteenth-century Black Plague on the subsequent history of Europe. It illustrates the way in which a megadeath (in this case, an epidemic) can radically alter the course of history. The case of the Black Death should be considered as an introduction to the two articles dealing with the current AIDS epidemic.

The article by Farmer and Kleinman contrasts the experience of dying of AIDS in the United States with such an experience in Haiti. The authors explore the ways in which family and community responses to those with AIDS reflect differences in cultural values. In the American context, the response reflects a reliance on technological answers to medical problems. In Haiti, there is much less emphasis on individual accountability, and as a result there is less of a tendency to blame the victim. The Haitian cultural emphasis on the primacy of familial relationships contributes to more acceptance of those with AIDS.

The article by Gladwell takes a look at contemporary policies designed to deal with the AIDS epidemic. Of late, considerable attention has been given to the call for safe sex. He points out that this educational effort is unlikely to be effective among those most at risk for AIDS. He argues that to deal with AIDS effectively, we must start by making basic health care much more available to the highest risk groups, particularly the inner-city poor. This article illustrates the problems that arise when middle-class policy makers formulate social policies directed largely at the poor that do not take into consideration class differences in values and behavioral patterns.

The article by Metcalf contrasts American mortuary practices with those among the Berawan, a tribe in Borneo. Some aspects of the four-stage funeral rites will strike many readers as strange. The practice of collecting the secretions of a decomposing corpse, mixing this fluid with rice, and then eating it will be considered disgusting by most Americans. Also of note is the discussion of how members of this tribe respond to what they consider the shocking way in which Americans deal with their dead, particularly efforts to delay the decomposition of the corpse through embalming. Metcalf explains how American rituals and practices are viewed as equally strange and shocking to the Berawan as their rites are to Americans.

The selection by Green presents an historical analysis of certain contemporary Mexican death rituals. We will see how the origins of these practices can be traced to related pre-Columbian Aztec practices and medieval Spanish practices. In some instances, the very same practice is found both among the pre-Columbian Aztecs and in medieval Spain.

6 Western Attitudes toward Death ❧

Philippe Ariès

PHILIPPE ARIÈS was a French civil servant—a botanist—who became famous for his books on social history. Among his works are *Centuries of Childhood: A Social History of Family Life*, *The Hour of Our Death*, and *Western Attitudes toward Death: From the Middle Ages to the Present*, the book from which the present excerpt is drawn. In this selection, the focus is on changes in Western conceptions of death between the early and late Middle Ages. In the seventh century, salvation was seen as an event that would take place for all Christians at the end of the world. With the emergence of individualism in the twelfth century, we begin to see a change: Salvation became viewed as something that might or might not happen, depending on the balance between good and evil as reflected in one's deeds throughout life. By the fifteenth century, yet another conception of death emerged; according to this new conception, one's salvation was determined by choices made between the powers of good and evil during the process of dying.

THE PORTRAYAL OF THE LAST JUDGMENT

In about 680 Bishop Agilbert was buried in the funeral chapel which he had had constructed adjacent to the monastery of Jouarre (Seine-et-Marne), to which he had retired and where he died. His tomb is still standing. What do we find there? On a small panel in the Christ in Majesty surrounded by the four Evangelists. This is the image inspired by the Apocalypse, of Christ returning at the end of the world. On the large panel adjoining it we find the resurrection of the dead on the last day. The elect, their arms upraised, acclaim the returning Christ, who holds in his hands a scroll, no doubt the Book of Life. No judgment or condemnation is in evidence. This image is in keeping with the general eschatology of the early centuries of Christendom. The dead who belonged to the Church and who had entrusted their bodies to its care (that is to say to the care of the saints), went to sleep like the seven sleepers of Ephesus . . . and were at rest . . . until the day of the Second Coming, of the great return, when they would awaken in the heavenly Jerusalem, in other words in Paradise. There was no place for individual responsibility, for a counting of good and bad deeds. The wicked, that is to say those who were not members of the Church, would doubtlessly not live after their death; they would not awaken and would be abandoned to a state of nonexistence. An entire quasi-biological population, the saintly population, thus would be granted a glorious afterlife following a long, expectant sleep.

But in the twelfth century the scene changed. In the sculptured tympana of the romanesque churches of Beaulieu or Conques the apocalyptic vision of the Majesty of Christ still predominates. But beneath the portrayal of Christ appears a new iconography, inspired this time by the book of Matthew: the resurrection of the dead, the separation of the just and the damned, the Last Judgment (at Conques, Christ's halo bears the word *Judex*), and the weighing of souls by the archangel Michael.

In the thirteenth century the apocalyptic inspiration and the evocation of the Second Coming were almost blotted out. The idea of the judgment won out and the scene became a court of justice. Christ is shown seated upon the judgment throne surrounded by his court (the apostles). Two acts had become increasingly important: the weighing of souls and the intercession of the Virgin and St. John, who kneel, their hands clasped, on either side of Christ the Judge. Each man is to be judged according to the balance sheet of his life. Good and bad deeds are scrupulously separated and placed on the appropriate side of the scales. Moreover, these deeds have been inscribed in a book. In the magnificent strains of the *Dies irae* the Franciscan authors of the thirteenth century portrayed the book being brought before the judge on the last day, a book in which everything is inscribed and on the basis of which everyone will be judged. . . .

This book, the *liber vitae*, must first have been conceived of as a cosmic book, the formidable census of the universe. But at the end of the Middle Ages it became an individual account book. At Albi, in the vast fresco of the Last Judgment dating from the end of the fifteenth or the beginning of the sixteenth century, the risen wear this book about their necks, like a passport, or rather like a bank book to be presented at the gates of eternity. A very curious change has occurred. This "balance" or balance sheet is closed not at the moment of death but on the *dies illa*, the last day of the world, at the end of time. Here we can see the deep-rooted refusal to link the end of physical being with physical decay. Men of the period believed in an existence after death which did not necessarily continue for infinite eternity, but which provided an extension between death and the end of the world.

Thus, the idea of the Last Judgment is linked with that of the individual biography, but this biography ends on the last day, and not at the hour of death.

IN THE BEDCHAMBER OF THE DYING

The second phenomenon consisted of suppressing the eschatological time between death and the end of the world, and of no longer situating the judgment in space at the Second Coming, but in the bedchamber, around the deathbed.

This new iconography is to be found in the woodcuts, spread by the new technique of printing, in books which are treatises on the proper manner of dying: the *ars moriendi* of the fifteenth and sixteenth centuries. . . .

The dying man is lying in bed surrounded by his friends and relations. He is in the process of carrying out the rituals which are now familiar to us. But something is happening which disturbs the simplicity of the ceremony and which those present do not see. It is a spectacle reserved for the dying man alone and one which he contemplates with a bit of anxiety and a great deal of indifference. Supernatural beings have invaded his chamber and cluster about the bed of the recumbent figure, the "*gisant.*" On one side are the Trinity, the Virgin, and the celestial court; on the other, Satan and a monstrous army of demons. Thus the great gathering which in the twelfth and thirteenth centuries had taken place on the last day, in the fifteenth century had moved to the sickroom.

How are we to interpret this scene?

Is it still really a judgment? Properly speaking, no. The scales in which good and evil are weighed no longer play a part. The book is still present, and all too frequently the demon has grabbed it with a triumphant gesture, because the account book and the person's life story are in his favor. But God no longer appears with the attributes of a judge. In the two possible interpretations, interpretations which probably can be superimposed, God is rather the arbiter or the observer.

The first interpretation is that of a cosmic struggle between the forces of good and evil who are fighting for possession of the dying man, and the dying man himself watches this battle as an impartial witness, though he is the prize.

This interpretation is suggested by the graphic composition of this scene in the woodcuts of the *artes moriendi*. But if one reads carefully the inscriptions that accompany these woodcuts one will see that they deal with a different matter, which is the second interpretation. God and his court are there to observe how the dying man conducts himself during this trial—a trial he must endure before he breathes his last and which will determine his fate in eternity. This test consists of a final temptation. The dying man will see his entire life as it is contained in the book, and he will be tempted either by despair over his sins, by the "vainglory" of his good deeds, or by the passionate love for things and persons. His attitude during this fleeting moment will erase at once all the sins of his life if he wards off temptation or, on the contrary, will cancel out all his good deeds if he gives way. The final test has replaced the Last Judgment.

Here we must make two important observations.

The first concerns the juxtaposition of the traditional portrayal of death in bed and that of the individual judgment of each life. Death in bed, as we have seen, was a calming rite which solemnized the necessary passing, the "*trépas*," and leveled the differences between individuals. No one worried about the fate of one particular dying man. Death would come to him as it did to all men, or rather to all Christians at peace with the Church. It was an essentially collective rite.

On the other hand, the judgment—even though it took place in a great cosmic activity at the end of the world—was peculiar to each individual, and no one knew his fate until the judge had weighed the souls, heard the pleas of intercessors, and made his decision.

Thus the iconography of the *artes moriendi* joins in a single scene the security of a collective rite and the anxiety of a personal interrogation.

My second observation concerns the increasingly close relationship established between death and the biography of each individual life. It took time for this relationship to gain ascendency. In the fourteenth and fifteenth centuries it became firmly fixed, no doubt under the influence of the mendicant orders. From then on it was thought that each person's entire life flashed before his eyes at the moment of death. It was also believed that his attitude at that moment would give his biography its final meaning, its conclusion.

Thus we understand how the ritual solemnity of the deathbed, which persisted into the nineteenth century, by the end of the Middle Ages had assumed among the educated classes a dramatic character, an emotional burden which it had previously lacked.

We must, however, note that this evolution strengthened the role played by the dying man himself in the ceremonies surrounding his own death. He was still at the center of activity, presiding over the event as in the past, and determining the ritual as he saw fit.

These ideas were bound to change in the seventeenth and eighteenth centuries. Under the influence of the Counter Reformation, spiritual writers struggled against the popular belief that it was not necessary to take such pains to live virtuously, since a good death redeemed everything. However, they continued to acknowledge that there was a moral importance in the way the dying man behaved and in the circumstances surrounding his death. It was not until the twentieth century that this deeply rooted belief was cast off, at least in industrialized societies.

7 The Black Death as a Major Event in World History ❧

Yves Renouard

YVES RENOUARD was a professor first at the University of Bordeaux and subsequently at the Sorbonne. He specialized in the social history of the later Middle Ages. In this article, he presents a social history of the Black Death epidemic that lasted from 1348 to 1350. The labor shortage in rural areas and the lack of labor on the feudal estates contributed to a breakdown of the feudal order and the shift to a wage-based capitalistic economy and to increased class conflict. It also had a major impact on the Church, due, in part, to the rise of religious movements such as the Flagellants (committed to mortification) and also to the loss of a high proportion of the educated clergy. This, in turn, led to the ordination of many who were illiterate and in other ways unfit.

THE BLACK DEATH OF 1348, because of its universal nature, the demographic collapse it caused throughout the Western and Mediterranean world, and its profound effect on all facets of life, was probably the most important event of fourteenth-century history. . . .

Epidemics were frequent in the Middle Ages. Efforts to combat them effectively were hindered by lack of hygiene and the inadequacies of medical science. On the average, one could expect a serious or even disastrous epidemic every quarter-century.

Many epidemics first appeared in the great urban centers of the Near and Middle East, where a number of diseases are still endemic. Caravans and ships then spread them abroad. We do not know exactly where or how, in 1347, the Black Death began. The first manifestation of the plague appeared in the great Genoese colony of Kaffa in the Crimea, on the shores of the Black Sea. Janibeg, the Mongol khan of the Kipchaks, besieged this port, which was easily supplied by sea. When an epidemic of the plague broke out in his army, he used catapults to hurl the dead into the town. He did this not only to rid himself of the bodies, but also in the hope that the plague would spread among the besieged, weakening their resistance. Here, with this simple operation, we already have chemical warfare.

From Yves Renouard, "La Peste Noire de 1348–50," *La Revue de Paris*, LVII (March, 1950), pp. 107–119. Translated by William M. Bowsky.

Actually, Janibeg's scheme failed; he was unable to take Kaffa. The defenders greatly limited the spread of the contagion by immediately throwing into the sea the corpses with which they were bombarded, and they were able to resist. But it was enough that some fell ill and that after the siege certain of these returned to the west for the "Black Death" to spread rapidly.

The disease only later received the name Black Death from the dark-colored blemishes that developed on the limbs of the sick. Without doubt it was the bubonic plague, characterized by the swelling of tumors, or buboes, on the arms and groin, a gangrenous inflammation of the throat and lungs, violent chest pains, vomiting and spitting blood, and the stench of the victim's body.

It was spread by objects touched by the sick as well as by direct contact. The suddenness and rapidity of the disease were such that a subject could pass from perfect health to death in one day. Generally the illness lasted only from three to five days, during the course of which the patient was overcome by fever and tortured by an intense thirst. . . .

In the space of two and a half years the Black Death traversed the whole of Europe. It was not that men failed to try to halt its advance or at least protect themselves from it. All the physicians of the time were concerned with the plague. A highly esteemed Italian doctor, Gentile da Foligno, renowned for his teaching at Padua, wrote *Consilia contra pestilentiam* [Treatises against the pestilence]; but he died in June 1348, a victim of his devotion to the sick, who had pressed around him. At Montpellier, where the university was famous for the skill of its medical faculty, all the doctors died of the plague. When the plague neared Paris, King Philip VI sought advice from the Paris Faculty of Medicine. It produced a *Compendium de epidemia per collegium Facultatis medicorum Parisius ordinatum* [Compendium concerning the epidemic composed by the College of the Paris Faculty of Medicine] which remains outstanding. But it was a descriptive rather than a therapeutic work.

Nevertheless, the plague continued its inexorable progress toward the north. Before it reached the gates of Reims, Pierre de Damouzy, a doctor from Champagne, composed an interesting treatise on its prevention. He began by explaining that the fact that the plague struck some and spared others was due to the influence of the stars. But he went on to give some practical advice on how to avoid infection. He repeated Rhazes' old prescription: to protect himself from the plague a person should stay at home with doors and windows shut; if he absolutely has to go out, he should carry camphor, amber, or some other disinfectant. Further, Damouzy recommended bleeding, purging, and a lightened diet; he absolutely forbade bathing and lovemaking. Although many of his prescriptions seemed sensible and judicious, the plague continued to spread.

The spread of the Black Death marked the complete failure of contemporary medicine. It also showed the futility of conceiving of charity and religion as a prophylaxis. Some religious orders were tirelessly devoted to the care of plague victims, but they saved only a very small number of the sick, and many religious brotherhoods lost their entire memberships. Ecclesiastical authorities instituted suitable prayers; Pope Clement VI established a special office to win God's mercy. This was largely in vain, just as it was in vain for popular piety to turn to Saint Sebastian, Saint Anthony, and Saint Adrian, holy protectors who were reputed to fight epidemics.

The blind barbarity that turned the wrath of the credulous masses against the Jews had no more success. The Jews were accused of spreading the epidemic by poisoning wells. They were persecuted everywhere, but it was particularly in Spain that terror of the plague stirred up the flames of anti-Semitism. At Avignon, the Pope protected the Jews from all violence.

The only preventive measure that had any efficacy was, by definition, the tactic of cowards. Those who were able to flee to a healthy part of the countryside, far from population centers, before they were infected succeeded in escaping the plague. But this was a rich man's defense, available especially to kings, princes, and lords. After having shown a great deal of courage Pope Clement VI finally withdrew to Villeneuve-les-Avignon. Many rich bourgeois also had recourse to this defense, witness the eight young women and two young men of the *Decameron*, who sought amusement and health in a villa in the Tuscan hills.

Thus, despite practical and scholarly cures, despite prayer and popular wrath, men all over Europe continued to die. The number of dead was such that contemporaries viewed the epidemic as an unprecedented disaster.

Boccaccio estimates that more than a hundred thousand died in Florence; a chronicler of Rouen gives the same number for that city, and Gilles li Muisit notes twenty-five thousand for Tournai. Froissart devoted only one sentence of his long work to the plague, but it has become famous: "In this time a disease which is called an epidemic raged generally throughout the world, and a good third of the world died of it." Simon de Couvin of Montpellier estimates that the plague carried off half the population.

These figures are clearly exaggerated; those given for towns even exceed the total number of their inhabitants. Moreover, if a third or half of the total population had perished, Europe would have become a kind of wasteland. But events after 1350 testify that a dense population still existed.

The plague did not strike all regions, all human groupings, and all social categories with the same intensity. As was to be expected, population centers were particularly hard hit. The towns, where hygiene was deplorable, suffered much more than the countryside. And in the towns social groups that lived crowded together, such as members of the working class and friars of the mendicant orders, suffered most. . . .

No weddings took place during the pestilence, but once it seemed over there were unusually many. The parish register of Givry mentions no weddings in 1348, but 86 in 1349, of which 42 took place between January 14 and February 24. And this was among a population reduced to a few hundred inhabitants. Evidently, surviving widowers, whatever their age, remarried with a young man's haste. Guillaume de Nangis's continuator notes this in his chronicle: "At the end of this epidemic, pestilence, and mortality, men and women married each other." It was necessary to restore the hearths in villages where perhaps only one still remained. But however fecund these new unions were, only in time could they remedy the severe demographic setback that the plague had caused throughout the world. For at least a generation Europe was again in that state of underpopulation from which it had wrested itself since the twelfth century.

This swift and unequal demographic collapse following immediately upon the psychological and mental shock caused by the epidemic (during which each person felt himself menaced and lived through frightful hours) had the greatest consequence in all areas.

Frightened by the approach of the plague, which they saw as God's instrument of vengeance for the punishment of their sins, certain men sought to appease divine wrath by penances as exceptional as the plague itself. Thus a preventive movement of mortification and mysticism began in Germany. Men and women assembled and left their homes in bands of several hundred under the leadership of one or more chiefs, whom they called masters in imitation of the mendicant orders. In each locality that they traversed they stopped and publicly whipped themselves with cruel violence while singing laments:

> Let us strike our "flesh" [carrion] sharply while remembering the Lord's great passion and his piteous death.

In imitating Christ's passion, these Flagellants sought to obtain God's pardon through the intercession of the Virgin. This mixture of mortification and piety, which well expressed the collective panic of the population, disquieted the authorities. But the mental contagion spread almost as quickly as the contagion it wished to destroy. Before the movement finally ended, the Flagellants had spread to Bohemia and Hungary in the east and to Picardie and Champagne in the west.

The collective mental shock, which reached its high point with the Flagellants, did not spare many of their contemporaries. Fear of the plague and the spectacle of disease and corpses aroused in most persons ideas of penitence and the constant thought of death. The passion of Christ, which the Flagellants wanted to suffer in their own bodies, became a theme of habitual meditation. It is reproduced in scenes that decorate religious edifices and private oratories. Also, the cult of the Five Wounds of Christ became prevalent. The frescoes of the Camposanto of Pisa show how strongly the epidemic turned men's imaginations to the mystery of death. . . . Macabre themes multiplied in the figurative arts.

Only heroes and heroines of romances such as Fiammetta, Pampinea, and their friends had the will and the ability to forget so many scenes of horror while residing in the beautiful gardens to which they had fled, amid dancing, feasting, siestas, and stories that aroused laughter and exalted the joy of living. Some contemporaries reacted against the destroying menace, by which they felt immeasurably burdened, by giving themselves over to sensual pleasures, free of care and with feverish violence. They abandoned themselves to debauchery, gluttonously satisfying all their appetites. During the same period that the mystical crisis we mentioned occurred, a wave of immorality shook the entire West. "After the great pestilence of the past year, each person lived according to his own caprice . . . ," notes the Sienese Agnolo di Tura.

In the countryside as in the towns, the plague carried off proportionally more peasants and workers than lords and bourgeois. Suddenly the supply of labor had dwindled.

On certain English manors all the tenants died. At the beginning of the epidemic, this rural mortality caused the halt of all work in the countryside. In certain areas, such as northern Italy, by the testimony of John of Parma, the harvest of 1348 remained in the fields. The relative abundance of products in relation to the suddenly decimated population and people's concern simply with living, no longer worrying about gain or the future, caused an initial price drop. But things changed quickly. The peak of the plague passed, and survivors abandoned poor or badly situated land in order to settle on the best land, to which lords attracted them by giving them the concessions they craved: enfranchisement if they were serfs, better conditions of tenure and high wages (wages at least 50 to 100 percent higher than before the plague).

The agrarian structure of the West was considerably disrupted. The system of the seigneurial reserve, which was already declining, disappeared completely in many regions. This was because the peasants tended to cultivate only their own tenures, whose produce they kept for themselves. The lords, both lay and ecclesiastical, suffered an unbelievable diminution in revenue from ground rents. Rents dropped by half, sometimes by three-quarters, because of the immense amount of land that was abandoned and because conditions had become very favorable for tenants on the lands that remained in cultivation. Offerings to churches decreased in the same proportion. The old class of landed proprietors, the nobility and the clergy, had its principal source of power severely shaken; castles, churches, rural monasteries, and even hospitals fell into ruin.

The scarcity of agrarian products and of fish caused their prices to soar; this had grave consequences for the urban population.

In the towns the heavy mortality led to a scarcity of artisanal and industrial labor even greater than the shortage of labor in the countryside. It also caused severe disorganization of local and long-distance commerce, since not only was the local clientele reduced, but nearly all foreign markets were affected as well. The workers, less numerous and no longer able to subsist because of the rise in food prices, demanded wage increases. The richest artisans profited from the situation by attracting all available laborers into their shops or under their control, thus ruining their competitors. Lesser officials made the same demands as the workers, for the same reasons. In 1349 the trumpeters of the commune of Florence explained to the authorities that they were no longer able to live on their wages. That same year the wax-warmers of the pontifical chancery and other employees of the palace service "no longer wished to work if their salary was not increased."

The scarcity of labor permitted survivors to obtain wage increases that were proportionally perhaps a bit greater than the increases in food prices. Thus the miserable level of their lives was slightly improved. The increase in urban wages varied from 50 to 150 percent, according to the town and the trade.

The ordinances enacted by the authorities in 1351 (especially by the kings of France and England) to hinder workers from quitting their employers and demanding wages higher than those of 1347 remained inoperative. The enactment of such ordinances was demanded primarily by landed proprietors and frightened consumers. Despite the adoption of regulations, those badly adapted to the new circumstances were crushed by the inexorable play of fundamental economic laws.

The crisis caused by the Black Death entailed a definite rise in the price of manufactured goods and the stagnation of commerce. The stagnation of commerce was caused by the sudden loss of some of its clientele. The English merchant companies, which leased their right to export wool from the king, were ruined in a few months. The king, who wished to use these companies also for borrowing money, was forced to revise his entire economic policy and to receive foreign merchants favorably.

The states of Europe suffered the consequences of these economic disturbances. The numerical decline in population and the ruin of taxpayers caused a drop in revenue which left the principal political nations of the West powerless for a time, just at the moment when their fiscal development allowed them to conceive of great enterprises.

The king of France, the king of England, the pope, and the Italian republics had to renounce temporarily their extensive political and military activities. The plague had made the raising of armies difficult, not only by terrifying the population from which the soldiers must come, but also by causing a decline in the revenue needed to pay them. After the initial success of the Dauphin Humbert's crusade, a truce was concluded between Christians and Saracens in 1348. It was broken only eleven years later after Peter I of Lusignan gained the throne of Cyprus. The threat of war between the two coalitions formed by Venice and Genoa in 1345 did not materialize until 1351, when hostilities began. Finally, after the [French] defeat at Crécy and the loss of Calais the Franco-English conflict was abated by a truce signed in 1347, which was renewed till 1355. Even the civil war in Flanders, caused by the fall of Artevelde in 1346, stopped when the plague entered that country.

Political circumstances do not perhaps alone explain the general abatement of conflicts.

The reduction in revenues which struck the princes caused them to dispute more harshly the revenues they shared. For several decades the English king had been enduring, with difficulty, the intensification of the papal hold on the English clergy. It was significant that after the outbreaks of the plague in 1351 and 1353, Edward III enacted the celebrated statutes against papal conferment of English ecclesiastical benefices and against abuses of the pontifical fisc. The impoverished English clergy was no longer able to pay taxes to both the king and the pope.

In the countryside, a great many ruined nobles took up brigandage, even before the great mercenary companies were formed in France.

The social consequences of the plague were particularly significant in the towns, where men lived more closely together than in the countryside and dealt more constantly with one another. By causing a large number of the bourgeois to perish, the plague allowed the survivors to gain possession of the property of the dead. The Black Death thus created enormous fortunes. The workers and artisans, however, who escaped death inherited only the worn-out clothing of their deceased relatives. While the plague made the rich richer, it left the poor as before; the total wretchedness of the poor continued while the affluence of the rich reached unprecedented levels of opulence. In the urban microcosm the contrast between wealth and poverty became greater than ever before. Patrician ostentation and sumptuousness burst forth even in Florence, where business men were experiencing terrible financial troubles, which since 1342 had caused the successive collapse of all the greatest commercial companies. A great many citizens, after having seen their whole family die, bequeathed all their property to charitable institutions. Thus, the Company of San Michele, to which all the great merchants contributed, increased its patrimony by 350,000 florins. It should have distributed this money to the poor, but taking into consideration that the plague had killed a great many of these, it decided to use part of this sum to construct a tabernacle to shelter the miraculous Madonna, the company's emblem. Andrea Orcagna was charged with constructing and decorating the splendid tabernacle. This example shows clearly the collective wealth and egoism of the surviving patricians in an impoverished town.

It is understandable that such a mentality offended the common people, the shop workers. Their wretchedness and the memory of the plague only made their feverish souls more responsive to the communistic preaching of the apostles of poverty, the Fraticelli and the Spirituals (who were attached to the great Franciscan order).

The aggravation of social contrasts in the town, like the severe disequilibrium of the landed nobility, was a result of the plague. These effects of the plague intensified the hostility between the ruined nobility and peasantry (who refused to give up any of their newly won advantages) in the countryside, and between the rich bourgeoisie and the miserable proletariat in the cities. It was in this climate of class hatred brought on by the plague that there broke out, in the second half of the century, for different reasons, a series of violent social conflicts which had no equivalent in the preceding period. The rural insurrections included the Jacquerie (1358) and the Tuchins (1381–1382) in France and the Laborers (1381) in England. The insurrections of the urban proletariat included the Ciompi in Florence (1378), the Weavers in Gand (1379), the Harelle in Rouen (1380), and the Maillotins in Paris (1382).

Finally, the Black Death had a profound effect even on intellectual and spiritual matters. In striking the clergy severely, it brutally deprived the population of a large proportion of its spiritual guides; in depopulating especially the urban monasteries of the mendicant orders, it suddenly removed the intellectual elite among the clergy.

The vacancies so abruptly caused by the plague had to be filled. Everywhere new priests were quickly ordained and new monks tonsured. These were for the most part fairly young or fairly old people, neither group having any priestly experience or the moral and intellectual preparation needed to exercise the office worthily. Most of the new religious, as was true of certain of the surviving priests, were attracted to the priesthood only by benefices. They sought the most profitable ones, striving to accumulate several, and they worried little about the care of souls. During a crisis period when the population had the greatest need of its spiritual guides, worldliness, immorality, and ignorance suddenly developed among the clergy. Abandoned to themselves, often demoralized and panic-stricken, the people lived slack moral lives and their religion became little more than a collection of superstitions. Traditional practices, belief in liturgical prayers, the habit of common prayer, and in some places even the divine service disappeared. The pious turned to a more personal religion, while the more material satisfied themselves with superstition. Everywhere the emotional triumphed over the rational. Thus the stage was set for the criticisms of reformers, who, from the end of the century on, preached an inner religion based upon the Bible. These reformers had great sport deriding and making a scandal of the unworthiness of too many clerics.

The plague, which greatly aggravated the long-standing ill of unfit clerics, also hindered remedying it. The Order of Friars Preachers [the Dominicans] devoted itself to preaching and teaching, and constituted the intellectual elite among the clergy. The Black Death, as we have seen, depopulated the monasteries of the Order. Faced with either closing some monasteries and concentrating the survivors in others, or with replacing the deceased friars as quickly as possible to keep all the monasteries open, the superiors general chose the second solution. Now quantity was preferred to quality. A run to the monasteries began; the practice of offering ten- to fourteen-year-old children to the Friars and Preachers as oblates became general.

Such recruits often lacked zeal or aptitude. Ignorance crept into Saint Thomas's order; the novices' studies were often insufficient, and the general meeting of 1376 emphasized that many young friars could neither read nor write. This grave intellectual decline did not allow the Dominican Order to rectify the new tendencies resulting from the deplorable recruitment of the clergy, itself also an effect of the shock of the Black Death.

The Black Death of 1348 caused general disorder throughout Europe. It is not astonishing that so violent an epidemic had such severe and lasting consequences. Actually the entire epidemic lasted at least a generation, and it was even longer before its demographic effects were wiped out. Both in violence and extent this was one of the most severe epidemics that mankind has undergone. Above all, the epidemic of 1348–1350 did not completely disappear. After the first great spate of killing, there followed during the next half-century sporadic outbreaks of the plague, which seems to have survived in a latent state almost everywhere. For example, there was the plague of 1361 in Aquitaine, the plague of 1362 in England (known as the second plague), the plague of 1363 in Florence and in southern France, the plagues of 1369 and 1375 in England, and those of 1371, 1374, 1390, and 1400 in Florence. These outbreaks once again showed the ineffectiveness of contemporary medicine and preventive measures. Throughout Europe they prolonged for several decades the effect of the 1348 epidemic.

Thus the Black Death of 1348, by the very violence of the blow it dealt mankind and by the magnitude of its consequences (reinforced by later outbreaks), clearly qualifies as a major historical event. It ended the prosperity which had prevailed in the West during the end of the thirteenth century and the first part of the fourteenth. It brought great misery everywhere and for a time impeded the course of political and military events. It promoted some profound social changes: the ruin of the nobility and the clergy, the rise of the bourgeoisie, the appearance of social strife between bourgeoisie and proletariat in the towns and between nobility and peasantry in the countryside. It also considerably hastened intellectual and moral change: the development of a lay spirit and the birth of national cultures. Finally, it caused, in an overexcited and restless population, the most frenzied and superstitious forms of religious life, which the decimated and substandard clergy could not correct. This is why certain historians, declaring how this universal event indeed ended a period, by oversimplification have wanted to see in the Black Death of 1348 the veritable terminus which separates medieval from modern civilization.

8 AIDS as Human Suffering

Paul Farmer and Arthur Kleinman

PAUL FARMER is MacArthur Fellow in Social Medicine at Harvard University. ARTHUR KLEINMAN is a professor of anthropology and psychiatry at Harvard University. This article contrasts the experience of dying of AIDS in the United States for an American named Robert, who has access to much modern medical technology, with that of Anita, a poor young woman in Haiti with no such access to medical resources. While the experience of dying was in many respects very oppressive for Anita due to the nature of the disease and her grinding poverty, she did not experience the revulsion from health-care professionals or from the community that is so common for AIDS patients in the United States. The authors argue that the way in which these two people are treated and the way in which these two very different communities are responding to the AIDS epidemic reflect profound differences in cultural values.

This plague has attracted the inevitable swarm of AIDS researchers, officials, businessmen, and journalists, and they are the ones who have monopolized the media. We people with AIDS, who devote each waking moment to our own survival, have been unable to prevent those loquacious experts from stealing our thunder and robbing us of the only thing we have left: our illness.
EMMANUEL DREUILHE[1]

The age-old, seemingly inexorable, process whereby diseases acquire meanings (by coming to stand for people's deepest fears) and inflict stigma is always worth challenging, and it does seem to have a more limited credibility in the modern world; the process itself is being questioned now. With this illness, one that elicits so much guilt and shame, the efforts to detach it from loaded meanings and misleading metaphors seem particularly liberating, even consoling.
SUSAN SONTAG[2]

From "AIDS as Human Suffering," reprinted by permission of *Daedalus*, Journal of the American Academy of Arts and Sciences, from the issue entitled "Living with AIDS," Spring 1989, Vol. 118, No. 2.

THAT THE DOMINANT DISCOURSE ON AIDS at the close of the twentieth century is in the rational-technical language of disease control was certainly to be expected and even necessary. We anticipate hearing a great deal about the molecular biology of the virus, the clinical epidemiology of the disease's course, and the pharmacological engineering of effective treatments. Other of contemporary society's key idioms for describing life's troubles also express our reaction to AIDS: the political-economic talk of public-policy experts, the social-welfare jargon of the politicians and bureaucrats, and the latest psychological terminology of mental-health professionals. Beneath the action-oriented verbs and reassuringly new nouns of these experts' distancing terminology, the more earthy, emotional rumblings of the frightened, the accusatory, the hate-filled, and the confused members of the public are reminders that our response to AIDS emerges from deep and dividing forces in our experience and our culture.

AIDS AND HUMAN MEANINGS

Listen to the words of persons with AIDS and others affected by our society's reaction to the new syndrome:

- "I'm 42 years old. I have AIDS. I have no job. I do get $300 a month from social security and the state. I will soon receive $64 a month in food stamps. I am severely depressed. I cannot live on $300 a month. After $120 a month for rent and $120 a month for therapy, I am left with $60 for food and vitamins and other doctors and maybe acupuncture treatments and my share of utilities and oil and wood for heat. I'm sure I've forgotten several expenses like a movie once in a while and a newspaper and a book."[3]

- "I don't know what my life expectancy is going to be, but I certainly know the quality is improved. I know that not accepting the shame or the guilt or the stigma that people would throw on me has certainly extended my life expectancy. I know that being very up-front with my friends, and my family and co-workers, reduced a tremendous amount of stress, and I would encourage people to be very open with friends, and if they can't handle it, then that's their problem and they're going to have to cope with it."

- "Here we are at an international AIDS conference. Yesterday a woman came up to me and said, 'May I have two minutes of your time?' She said, 'I'm asking doctors how they feel about treating AIDS patients.' And I said, 'Well, actually I'm not a doctor. I'm an AIDS patient,' and as she was shaking hands, her hand whipped away, she took two steps backward, and the look of horror on her face was absolutely diabolical."

- "My wife and I have lived here [in the United States] for fifteen years, and we speak English well, and I do O.K. driving. But the hardest time I've had in all my life, harder than Haiti, was when people would refuse to get in my cab when they discovered I was from Haiti [and therefore, in their minds, a potential carrier of HIV]. It got so we would pretend to be from somewhere else, which is the worst thing you can do, I think."

All illnesses are metaphors. They absorb and radiate the personalities and social conditions of those who experience symptoms and treatments. Only a few illnesses, however, carry such cultural salience that they become icons of the times. Like tuberculosis in *fin de siècle* Europe, like cancer in the first half of the American century, and like leprosy from Leviticus to the present, AIDS speaks of the menace and losses of the times. It marks the sick person, encasing the afflicted in an exoskeleton of peculiarly powerful meanings: the terror of a lingering and untimely death, the panic of contagion, the guilt of "self-earned" illness. There is the ironic meaning of a new incurable infection at a time when other infectious diseases seem to have been conquered—at least in the technologically advanced West—by a succession of magic bullets. There is the moral meaning of shame and humiliation imposed by the very commercialized culture that has made money from the images of sexuality and drugs: now these same images have been transformed, rationally but still hypocritically (since money is still to be made from the meanings), from desires into risks.

AIDS has offered a new idiom for old gripes. We have used it to blame others: gay men, drug addicts, inner-city ethnics, Haitians, Africans. And we in the United States have, in turn, been accused of spreading and even creating the virus that causes AIDS. The steady progression of persons with AIDS toward the grave, so often via the poor house, has assaulted the comforting idea that risk can be managed. The world turns out to be less controllable and more dangerous, life more fragile than our insurance and welfare models pretend. We have relegated the threat of having to endure irremediable pain and early death—indeed, the very image of suffering as the paramount reality of daily existence—to past periods in history and to other, poorer societies. Optimism has its place in the scale of American virtues; stoicism and resignation in the face of unremitting hardship—unnecessary character traits in a land of plenty—do not. Suffering had almost vanished from public and private images of our society.

Throughout history and across cultures, life-threatening disorders have provoked questions of control (What do we do?) and bafflement (Why me?). When bubonic plague depopulated fourteenth-century Europe by perhaps as many as half to three-fourths of the population, the black death was construed as a religious problem and a challenge to the moral authority as much or even more than as a public-health problem. Religious transcendence was its metaphor as much as medical crisis.[4] In the late twentieth century, it is not surprising that great advances in scientific knowledge and technological intervention have created our chief responses to questions of control and bafflement. To be sure, the international community of researchers has learned an astonishing amount about the human immunodeficiency virus (HIV) in a very short time. We have the technological expertise to prolong the lives of many people with AIDS and to ameliorate some of the horrendous bodily effects of the virus. Yet bafflement is not driven away by the advance of scientific knowledge, for it points to another aspect of the experience of persons with AIDS that has not received the attention it warrants. It points to a concern that in other periods and in other cultures is at the very center of the societal reaction to dread disease, a concern that resonates with that which is most at stake in the human experience of AIDS even if it receives little attention in academic journals—namely, suffering.

A mortal disease forces questions of dread, of death, and of ultimate meaning to arise. Suffering is a culturally and personally distinctive form of affliction of the human spirit. If pain is distress of the body, suffering is distress of the person and of his or her family and friends. The affliction and death of persons with AIDS create master symbols of suffering; the ethical and emotional responses to AIDS are collective representations of how societies deal with suffering. The stories of sickness of people with AIDS are texts of suffering that we can scan for evidence of how cultures and communities and individuals elaborate the unique textures of personal experience out of the impersonal cellular invasion of viral RNA. Furthermore, these illness narratives point toward issues in the AIDS epidemic every bit as salient as control of the spread of infection and treatment of its biological effects.

Viewed from the perspective of suffering, AIDS must rank with smallpox, plague, and leprosy in its capacity to menace and hurt, to burden and spoil human experience, and to elicit questions about the nature of life and its significance. Suffering extends from those afflicted with AIDS to their families and intimates, to the practitioners and institutions who care for them, and to their neighborhoods and the rest of society, who feel threatened by perceived sources of the epidemic and who are thus affected profoundly yet differently by its consequences. Moreover, because this condition is a pandemic affecting populations throughout the world, the experience of AIDS is refracted through greatly varying cultural lenses and social conditions, so that the human consequences of the disease are as distinctive as are these cultures themselves. To get at the culturally distinctive human consequences of such a pandemic, we shall examine the experience of persons with AIDS in the United States and in Haiti.

Our objective is to make the language of suffering more central to the academic and public-health discourse on AIDS. To discuss AIDS as suffering, we must make meanings and experience as salient to the problem of AIDS as are microbes and behavior; we need to make demoralization and threat and hope as legitimate to the public discourse on AIDS as are sexual practices, intravenous drug use, and HIV testing. If we minimize the significance of AIDS as human tragedy, we dehumanize people with AIDS as well as those engaged in the public-health and clinical response to the epidemic. Ultimately, we dehumanize us all.

ROBERT AND THE DIAGNOSTIC DILEMMA

It was in a large teaching hospital in Boston that we first met Robert, a forty-four-year-old man with AIDS.[5] Robert was not from Boston, but from Chicago, where he had already weathered several of the infections known to strike people with compromised immune function. His most recent battle had been with an organism similar to that which causes tuberculosis but is usually harmless to those with intact immune systems. The infection and the many drugs used to treat it had left him debilitated and depressed, and he had come east to visit his sister and regain his strength. On his way home, he was prevented from boarding his plane "for medical reasons." Beset with fever, cough, and severe shortness of breath, Robert went that night to the teaching hospital's emergency ward. Aware of his condition and its prognosis, Robert hoped that the staff there would help him to "get into shape" for the flight back to Chicago.

The physicians in the emergency ward saw their task as straightforward: to identify the cause of Robert's symptoms and, if possible, to treat it. In contemporary medical practice, identifying the cause of respiratory distress in a patient with AIDS entails following what is often called an algorithm. An algorithm, in the culture of biomedicine, is a series of sequential choices, often represented diagrammatically, which helps physicians to make diagnoses and select treatments. In most settings, the algorithms discussed and those actually used are quite different. But in Robert's case, step one, a chest X-ray, suggested the opportunistic lung parasite *Pneumocystis* as a cause for his respiratory distress; step two, examination of his sputum, confirmed it. He was then transferred to a ward in order to begin treatment of his lung infection. Robert was given the drug of choice, but did not improve. His fever, in fact, rose and he seemed more ill than ever. His physicians pondered the algorithm and waited.

After a few days of decline, Robert was found to have trismus: his jaw was locked shut. Because he had previously had oral candidiasis ("thrush"), his trismus and neck pain were thought to suggest the spread of the fungal infection back down the throat and pharynx and into the esophagus—a far more serious process than thrush, which is usually controlled by antifungal agents. Because Robert was unable to open his mouth, the algorithm for documenting esophagitis could not be followed. And so a "GI consult"—Robert has already had several—was called. It was hoped that the gastroenterologists, specialists at passing tubes into both ends of the gastrointestinal tract, would be better able to evaluate the nature of Robert's trismus. Robert had jumped ahead to the point in the algorithm that called for "invasive studies." The trouble is that on the night of his admission he had already declined a similar procedure.

Robert's jaw remained shut. Although he was already emaciated from two years of battle, he refused a feeding tube. Patient refusal is never part of an algorithm, and so the team turned to a new kind of logic: Is Robert mentally competent to make such a decision? Is he suffering from AIDS dementia? He was, in the words of one of those treating him, "not with the program." Another member of the team suggested that Robert had "reached the end of the algorithm," but the others disagreed. More diagnostic studies were suggested: in addition to esophagoscopy with biopsy and culture, a CT scan of the neck and head, repeated blood cultures, even a neurological consult. When these studies were mentioned to the patient, his silent stare seemed to fill with anger and despair. Doctors glanced uncomfortably at each other over their pale blue masks. Their suspicions were soon confirmed. In a shaky but decipherable hand, Robert wrote a note: "I just want to be kept clean."

Robert got a good deal more than he asked for, including the feeding tube, the endoscopy, and the CT scan of the neck. He died within hours of the last of these procedures. His physicians felt that they could not have withheld care without having some idea of what was going on.

In the discourse of contemporary biomedicine, Robert's doctors had been confronted with "a diagnostic dilemma." They had not cast the scenario described above as a moral dilemma but had discussed it in rounds as "a compliance problem." This way of talking about the case brings into relief a number of issues in the contemporary United States—not just in the culture of biomedicine but in the larger culture as well. In anthropology, one of the preferred means of examining culturally salient issues is through ethnology: in this case, we shall compare Robert's death in Boston to death from AIDS in a radically different place.

ANITA AND A DECENT DEATH

The setting is now a small Haitian village. Consisting of fewer than a thousand persons, Do Kay is composed substantially of peasant farmers who were displaced some thirty years ago by Haiti's largest dam. Before 1956, the village of Kay was situated in a broad and fertile valley near the banks of a large river. When the valley was flooded to build a hydroelectric dam, the majority of villages were forced up into the hills on either side of the new reservoir. Kay became divided into "Do" (those who settled on the stony backs of the hills) and

"Ba" (those who remained down near the new waterline). By all the standard measures, Kay is now very poor; its older inhabitants often blame their poverty on the massive buttress dam a few miles away and note bitterly that it has brought them neither electricity nor water.

When the first author of this paper began working in Kay, in May of 1983, the word *sida*, meaning AIDS, was just beginning to make its way into the rural Haitian lexicon. Interest in the illness was almost universal less than three years later. It was about then that Anita's intractable cough was attributed to tuberculosis. We first met her as a patient in a study on the determinants of the course and outcome of that disease in rural Haiti.

Questions about her illness often evoked long responses. She resisted our attempts to focus discussions. "Let me tell you the story from the beginning," she once said; "otherwise you will understand nothing at all."

Anita was a native of Kay in the true sense of the word. Her mother was born down in the valley and inherited with her brothers a choice bit of farmland that promised to keep them all prosperous and well fed. Anita's father was from a neighboring settlement. The dam altered their fortunes overnight, it seemed, and it was a dispirited woman who later gave birth, up on Do Kay, to Anita. As a little girl, Anita recalls, she was frightened by the arguments her parents would have in the dry seasons. When her mother began coughing, the family sold their livestock in order to buy "a consultation" with a distinguished doctor in the capital. Tuberculosis, he told them, and the family felt there was little they could do other than take irregular trips to Port-au-Prince and make equally irregular attempts to placate the gods who might protect the woman. Anita dropped out of school to help take care of her mother, who died shortly after the girl's thirteenth birthday.

It was very nearly the *coup de grâce* for her father, who became depressed and abusive. Anita, the oldest of five children, bore the brunt of his spleen. "One day, I'd just had it with his yelling. I took what money I could find, about $2, and left for the city. I didn't know where to go." Anita had the good fortune to find a family in need of a maid. The two women in the household had jobs in a U.S.-owned assembly plant; the husband of one ran a snack concession out of the house. Anita received a meal a day, a bit of dry floor to sleep on, and $10 per month for what sounded like incessant labor. She was not unhappy with the arrangement, which lasted until both women were fired for participating in "political meetings." Unable to make ends meet, the family made plans to emigrate to the bigger job market in the United States.

Anita wandered about for two days until she happened upon a kinswoman selling gum and candies near a downtown theater. She was, Anita related, "a sort of aunt." Anita could come and stay with her, the aunt said, as long as she could help pay the rent. And so Anita moved into Cité Simone, the sprawling slum on the northern fringes of the capital.

It was through the offices of her aunt that she met Vincent, one of the few men in the neighborhood with anything resembling a job: "He unloaded the whites' luggage at the airport." Vincent made a living from tourists' tips. In 1982, the year before Haiti became associated, in the North American press, with AIDS, the city of Port-au-Prince counted tourism as its chief industry. In the setting of an unemployment rate of greater than 60 percent, Vincent could command considerable respect. He turned his attention to Anita. "What could I do, really? He had a good job. My aunt thought I should go with him." Anita was not yet fifteen when she entered her first and only sexual union. Her lover set her up in a shack in the same neighborhood. Anita cooked and washed and waited for him.

When Vincent fell ill, Anita again became a nurse. It began insidiously, she recalls: night sweats, loss of appetite, swollen lymph nodes. Then came months of unpredictable and debilitating diarrhea. "We tried everything— doctors, charlatans, herbal remedies, injections, prayers." After a year of decline, she took Vincent to his hometown in the south of Haiti. There it was revealed that Vincent's illness was the result of malign magic: "It was one of the men at the airport who did this to him. The man wanted Vincent's job. He sent an AIDS death to him."

The voodoo priest who heard their story and deciphered the signs was straightforward. He told Anita and Vincent's family that the sick man's chances were slim, even with the appropriate interventions. There were, however, steps to be taken. He outlined them, and the family followed them, but still Vincent succumbed. "When he died, I felt spent. I couldn't get out of bed. I thought that his family would try to help me to get better, but they didn't. I knew I needed to go home."

She made it as far as Croix-des-Bouquets, a large market town at least two hours from Kay. There she collapsed, feverish and coughing, and was taken in by a woman who lived near the market. She stayed for a month, unable to walk, until her father came to take her back home. Five years had elapsed since she'd last seen him. Anita's father was by then a friendly but broken-down man with a leaking roof over his one-room, dirt-floor hut. It was no place for a sick woman, the villagers said, and Anita's godmother, honoring twenty-year-old vows, made room in her overcrowded but dry house.

Anita was diagnosed as having tuberculosis, and she responded to antituberculosis therapy. But six months after the initiation of treatment, she declined rapidly. Convinced that she was indeed taking her medications, we were concerned about AIDS, especially on hearing of the death of her lover. Anita's father was poised to sell his last bit of land in order to "buy more nourishing food for the child." It was imperative that the underlying cause of Anita's poor response to treatment be found. A laboratory test confirmed our suspicions.

Anita's father and godmother alone were apprised of the test results. When asked what she knew about AIDS, the godmother responded, "AIDS is an infectious disease that has no cure. You can get it from the blood of an infected person." For this reason, she said, she had nothing to fear in caring for Anita. Further, she was adamant that Anita not be told of her diagnosis—"That will only make her suffer more"—and skeptical about the value of the AIDS clinic in Port-au-Prince. "Why should we take her there?" asked Anita's godmother wearily. "She will not recover from this disease. She will have to endure the heat and humiliation of the clinic. She will not find a cool place to lie down. What she might find is a pill or an injection to make her feel more comfortable for a short time. I can do better than that."

And that is what Anita's godmother proceeded to do. She attempted to sit Anita up every day and encouraged her to drink a broth promised to "make her better." The godmother kept her as clean as possible, consecrating the family's two sheets to her goddaughter. She gave Anita her pillow and stuffed a sack with rags for herself. The only thing she requested from us at the clinic was "a beautiful soft wool blanket that will not irritate the child's skin."

In one of several thoughtful interviews accorded us, Anita's godmother insisted that "for some people, a decent death is as important as a decent life. . . . The child has had a hard life; her life has always been difficult. It's important that she be washed of bitterness and regret before she dies." Anita was herself very philosophic in her last months. She seemed to know of her diagnosis. Although she never mentioned the word *sida*, she did speak of the resignation appropriate to "diseases from which you cannot escape." She stated, too, that she was "dying from the sickness that took Vincent," although she denied that she had been the victim of witchcraft—"I simply caught it from him."

Anita did not ask to be taken to a hospital, nor did her slow decline occasion any request for further diagnostic tests. What she most wanted was a radio—"for the news and the music"—and a lambswool blanket. She especially enjoyed the opportunity to "recount my life," and we were able to listen to her narrative until hours before her death.

AIDS IN CULTURAL CONTEXT

We asserted at the outset that the way in which a person, a family, or a community responds to AIDS may reveal a great deal about core cultural values. Robert's story underlines our reliance on technological answers to moral and medical questions. "Americans love machines more than life itself," asserts author Philip Slater in a compelling analysis of middle-class North American culture. "Any challenge to the technological-over-social priority threatens to expose the fact that Americans have lost their manhood and their capacity to control their environment."[6] One of the less noticed but perhaps one of the farthest-reaching consequences of the AIDS epidemic has been the weakening of North America's traditional confidence in the ability of its experts to solve every kind of problem. In the words of one person with the disorder, "The terror of AIDS lies in the collapse of our faith in technology."[7]

This core cultural value is nowhere more evident than in contemporary tertiary medicine, which remains the locus of care for the vast majority of AIDS patients. Despite the uniformity of treatment outcome, despite the lack of proven efficacy of many diagnostic and therapeutic procedures, despite their high costs, it has been difficult for practitioners to limit their recourse to these interventions. "When you're at Disney World," remarked one of Robert's physicians ironically, "you take all the rides."

Robert's illness raises issues that turn about questions of autonomy and accountability. The concept of autonomous individuals who are solely responsible for their fate, including their illness, is a powerful cultural premise in North American society. On the positive side, this concept supports concern for individual rights and respect for individual differences and achievement. A more ominous aspect of this core cultural orientation is that it often justifies blaming the victims. The poor are viewed as unable to pull themselves up by their own bootstraps. Individual effects of powerful social forces beyond personal control are discounted. Alcoholics, those dependent on drugs, smokers who have developed emphysema, obese victims of heart attacks, chronic pain patients, even some sufferers from cancer—those who bottle up anger or who eat high-fat, low-fiber diets—all are seen as personally accountable for their disorders. Illness is said to be the outcome of their free choice of high-risk behavior.

This has been especially true in the AIDS epidemic, which has reified an invidious distinction between "innocent victims"—infants and hemophiliacs—and, by implication, "the guilty"—persons with AIDS who are homosexuals or intravenous drug users. Robert's lonely and medicalized death is what so many North Americans fear: "He was terrified. He knew what AIDS meant. He knew what happens. Your friends desert you, your lover kicks you out into the street. You get fired, you get evicted from your apartment. You're a leper. You die alone."[8] The conflation of correlation and responsibility has the effect of making sufferers feel guilt and shame. The validity of their experience is contested. Suffering, once delegitimated, is complicated and even distorted; our response to the sufferer, blocked.

In contrast, in Haiti and in many African and Asian societies, where individual rights are often underemphasized and also frequently unprotected, and where the idea of personal accountability is less powerful than is the idea of the primacy of social relationships, blaming the victim is also a less frequent response to AIDS. It is not that patterns of blame have not been discerned in rural Haiti: wherever AIDS strikes, it seems, accusation is never far behind. But in at least one Haitian village, what we have observed is not at all the American-style hysteria that initially, at least, spoiled our response to the disease. The reluctance of health-care professionals to care for patients, the angry parents who refuse to send their children to schools with children who have AIDS—these are not features of the rural Haitian response to AIDS. Noticeably absent is the revulsion with which AIDS patients have been faced in the United States, in both clinical settings and in their communities. This striking difference cannot be ascribed to Haitian ignorance of modes of transmission. On the contrary, the Haitians we have interviewed have ideas of etiology and epidemiology that reflect the incursion of the "North American ideology" of AIDS—that the disease is caused by a virus and is somehow related to homosexuality and contaminated blood. These are subsumed, however, in properly Haitian beliefs about illness causation. Long before the advent of AIDS to Do Kay, we might have asked the following question: some fatal diseases are known to be caused by "microbes" but may also be "sent" by someone; is *sida* such a disease?

It is, certain Haitians have told us, so accusations of witchcraft should not have come as a surprise. Although some would cast their analyses in terms of the familiar antinomy of voodoo and Christianity, our informants—who are from Do Kay or surrounding villages—speak in less Manichaean terms. A series of oppositions, rather than one, seems to guide much of our conversation about AIDS and other disorders: an illness might be caused by a microbe or by maleficence or by both. An illness might be treated by doctors or voodoo priests or "leaf doctors" or by prayer or any combination of these. The extent to which Anita believed in each of these modalities remains unclear; she had recourse to all of them. . . .

Suffering amplified by social death

In several memoirs published in North America, persons with AIDS have complained of the immediate social death their diagnosis has engendered. "For some of my friends and even family, I was dead as soon as they heard I had AIDS," a community activist informed us. "That was over two years ago." Even asymptomatic but seropositive individuals, whose life expectancy is often better than that of persons with most cancers and many common cardiovascular disorders, have experienced this reaction. Many North Americans with AIDS have made it clear that they do not wish to be referred to as victims: "As a person with AIDS," writes Navarre, "I can attest to the sense of diminishment at seeing and hearing myself referred to as an AIDS victim, an AIDS sufferer, an AIDS case—as anything but what I am, a person with AIDS. I am a person with a condition. I am not that condition."[9]

It is nonetheless necessary to plan humane care for persons with a chronic and deadly disease—"without needlessly assaulting my denial," as a young man recently put it. The very notion of hospice care will need rethinking if its intended clients are a group of young and previously vigorous persons. Similarly, our cross-cultural research has shown us that preferred means of coping with a fatal disease are shaped by biography and culture. There are no set "stages" that someone with AIDS will go through, and there can be no standard professional response. For a field best by recent attacks for its lack of humanism, biomedicine will need all the support it can get from other helping professions and from concerned communities and patient advocacy groups in order to effectively address the stigma, spoiling of identity, shame, humiliation, and outright rejection that has all too often been the ordeal of people with AIDS. These problems will require major changes in the education of health-care providers at all levels but also in the moral education of all of us.

Notes

We thank Carla Fujimoto, Haun Saussy, and Barbara de Zalduondo for their thoughtful comments on this essay.

1. Emmanuel Dreuilhe, *Mortal Embrace: Living with AIDS* (New York: Hill and Wang, 1988), 20.

2. Susan Sontag, "AIDS and Its Metaphors," *New York Review of Books* 35 (16) (27 October 1988): 88–99.

3. The first three of the four quotations cited here are the voices of persons with AIDS who attended the Third International Conference on AIDS, held in Washington, D.C. in June 1987. Their comments are published passim in 4 (1) (Winter/Spring 1988) of *New England Journal of Public Policy*. All subsequent unreferenced quotations are from tape-recorded interviews accorded the first author.

4. R. S. Gottfried, *The Black Death: Natural and Human Disaster in Medieval Europe* (New York: Free Press, 1983).

5. All informants' names are pseudonyms, as are "Do Kay" and "Ba Kay." Other geographical designations are as cited.

6. Philip Slater, *The Pursuit of Loneliness: American Culture at the Breaking Point* (Boston: Beacon Press, 1970), 49, 51.

7. Dreuilhe, 20.

8. George Whitmore, *Someone Was Here: Profiles in the AIDS Epidemic* (New York: New American Library, 1988), 26.

9. Max Navarre, "Fighting the Victim Label," in *AIDS: Cultural Analysis/Cultural Activism* (Cambridge: MIT Press, 1988), 143.

₰ 9 Strategies for Bringing the AIDS Epidemic under Control

Malcolm Gladwell

MALCOLM GLADWELL is the New York bureau chief for *The Washington Post*. In this essay, he is critical of the current war against AIDS in the United States. He presents a detailed analysis of why the condom approach is doomed to failure. In actual practice, this approach will be least effective with those who need the protection the most: low-income, single women under age 24, to say nothing of the teenage inner-city drug dealers. He makes a strong case for a greater concentration of funds in high-risk neighborhoods. He wants to see more spending on basic health care, including more aggressive efforts to control other sexually transmitted diseases in such areas—diseases that make a person much more susceptible to HIV.

AMONG THE MANY POSTERS that make up the Centers for Disease Control's public campaign against HIV, there is one with a group of young faces—white, black and brown—above the bold-lettered caption: "How much do your children know about AIDS?" The advertisement carries a familiar message, a call to greater education and awareness. But beyond that four-letter mention of AIDS there is nothing else to connect it to the real world of the epidemic. There is no one blistered or dying in the picture. The children scarcely seem old enough to understand what AIDS is, let alone engage in any of the behavior that would put them at risk for acquiring the virus. Even the fine print at the bottom of the page says only that "your children need an understanding of what it takes to be healthy." It is a message stripped of context: an appeal to the virtues of awareness that could just as easily have asked about tooth decay or taking candy from strangers or looking both ways before crossing the street.

Just over a decade after it began, the war against AIDS has become indistinguishable from the war against everything else. It has incorporated the language and psychology of contemporary self-help movements. It preaches the value of education, personal responsibility and self-discipline, as if unsafe sex were like smoking or overeating. It has created a class of advocates and scientists who line up alongside the cancer people and the heart disease people for their share of research dollars. To listen to the pleas for AIDS research money on Capitol Hill is to hear an almost perfect echo of previous appeals for the War on Cancer: if enough scientists are given enough money and pull enough all-nighters, we can lick this thing.

Nowhere in all of this is any consideration of HIV itself and the unique conditions that surround its spread in the United States. While no one involved with AIDS would ever deny that it dwarfs previous epidemics in the degree of its challenge and complexity, somehow when designing a program to stop it, we have assumed it can be fought with the same tools that we use on cigarettes and drunk driving. With the number of new HIV infections in the United States hovering stubbornly above 40,000 a year and the disease continuing to make inroads in our most vulnerable neighborhoods, it is time to question this assumption. Does AIDS haunt us because we haven't educated enough people and done enough research? Or is the problem that education and research alone are not the best way to fight this disease?

There is, to begin with, our troubling preoccupation with the condom. Because of its simplicity and its obvious ideological appeal, the condom has become the cornerstone of our AIDS prevention efforts. There remains precious little evidence, however, that the call for safe sex is actually working. Take, for example, condom use among sexually active urban adolescents, a group clearly at risk for HIV. According to a recent study by the Urban Institute, about 56.7 percent of urban males between 15 and 19 years old said they used a condom the last time they had sex, which is about double the percentage of a decade ago. Sound impressive? It shouldn't.

Of those males who had one sexual partner a year—a group whose risk of exposure to HIV is probably minimal—63 percent used a condom. The rate dropped to 56 percent for those who had two partners a year and 45 percent for those who had three. For the core risk group of highly sexually active teens with more than four partners a year—probably the only teen subset with an appreciable risk of acquiring HIV—37 percent used a condom. This is not a trend unique to teenagers. A national sex survey published earlier this year showed the same pattern among adult men; the more someone is at risk, the less likely he is to use a condom.

There is another, less obvious problem. When condoms are used, they aren't used very well, particularly by those who need protection the most. This fact has been obscured by the repeated and misleading use of the statistic that condoms are 97 percent to 98 percent effective as a barrier against pregnancy and sexually transmitted disease. The number, however, only refers to those occasions when the condom is used perfectly, every time. And who uses it perfectly, every time? Well, no one.

This is a common phenomenon with all types of contraception: "typical" effectiveness rates depend on the user. In the hands of an older, middle-class, married woman, for example, a diaphragm has an annual failure rate of 9 percent. For single, lower-income women under 20, by contrast—women who are much more likely to have sex while drunk or to use the device improperly—the annual failure rate approaches 40 percent.

The same is true of condoms. The only Americans who as a group use the method with anything approaching optimal effectiveness are (once again) married, middle-class, heterosexual couples over 30, for whom condoms have an annual success rate of 93.6 percent. That's another impressive statistic. But who cares? As a class, these people have a better chance of being hit by a meteorite than acquiring HIV through sex. Low-income, single women under 24 and their partners, by contrast, a group at great risk for the virus, use condoms so intermittently and, when they do, with such lack of competence that for them the annual failure rate is about three times higher.

Keep in mind that these numbers are for pregnancy where the vast number of mistakes don't result in any harm. They are even more worrisome for the use of condoms as prevention against sexually transmitted diseases, where every mistake has the potential to result in infection. Michael Rosenberg, a researcher at the University of North Carolina, recently estimated from available clinical evidence how much condoms in typical use among high-risk groups lowered the risk of acquiring HIV. His conclusion: about 30 percent.

This is safe sex?

There should be nothing surprising about the failure of the safe sex message among those who need it the most. To ask someone to use a condom is to ask him to perform a complicated risk-benefit analysis, to weigh the statistical likelihood of becoming infected against the inconvenience of wearing a condom. This is the kind of calculation that Americans, as part of the general infatuation with preaching individual responsibility for health, are increasingly asked to make about their diet, about smoking, about wearing a seat belt.

But not everyone is very good at this. The teenage inner-city drug dealer, half of whose peers are dead or in prison, probably doesn't worry about saturated fats. To a drunken 17-year-old, wearing a seat belt does not seem like a necessary concession to mortality. When it comes to personal risk reduction, there is a growing divide along the lines of income and education. There is a class of Americans who eat well, see their doctors regularly and attend aerobics classes. And there's a class for whom these things make little or no sense.

Somehow we have expected AIDS to be different. Condoms have been promoted as the principal agent of prevention on the blithe assumption that those who live in poverty, whose self-esteem and personal prospects are dismal, who lack the skills to communicate, who do drugs and take other risks in their daily lives will strap one on as readily as suburban couples. They haven't done it in the past. And, after a decade of tireless condom promotion, there is no evidence that they are doing it in any great numbers now.

This is not to say that we shouldn't try to convince those most hostile to condoms to take precautions. A few aggressive campaigns using sexually explicit and culturally relevant techniques have scored modest successes in reaching those most at risk. But it is one thing to expand the acceptability of condoms as part of a broader anti-AIDS campaign. It is quite another to construct an entire prevention effort in denial of everything we know about human behavior.

No less hopeful—and naive—is the expectation that science can bring an end to the AIDS epidemic. Scientists have done precisely what they are supposed to do: namely attack the problem from every conceivable angle. But they cannot be asked to play the central role in the attack on HIV, nor should they be elevated to the status of saviors of the sick. AIDS research simply is not, in and of itself, a strategy for fighting the epidemic. A strategy is a series of concrete steps with a clear goal and a predictable result. Research is a fishing expedition. There is a difference.

It is worth remembering, in this context, that the War on Cancer, while it resulted in a wonderful array of scientific breakthroughs, did not cure cancer. There is no guarantee that the war on AIDS—which has made spectacular contributions to our understanding of retroviruses and the human immune system—will cure AIDS either. Perhaps more important, there is no guarantee that even if some miraculous breakthrough were discovered, it would translate into lives saved. There are plenty of instances where researchers have answered a fundamental question about a disease only to have indifference, prejudice and stupidity get in the way of any good being done.

Imagine, for a moment, that we manage to overcome all of the considerable scientific obstacles that stand in the way of developing an AIDS vaccine. Where would it get us? This is a country that until recently could not muster the political will to vaccinate its children against measles. This is also a country that has not managed to teach birth control to teenagers, despite the existence of effective contraceptives. Indeed, this is a country that cannot even decide how sex should be discussed in the schools. How on earth could a mass immunization of teens against HIV be carried out?

"How many parents would object to having their children immunized?" asked June Osborne, chairwoman of the National Commission on AIDS, in a speech at the International AIDS Conference in Amsterdam last year. "And out of those how many would refuse out of conviction? Out of ignorance? Out of outrage at the imputation that they and theirs were even part of this epidemic risk?"

Then, Osborne pointed out, there are the limitations of the vaccine itself. Even the best vaccines against relatively simple viruses like yellow fever or measles are only 98 percent effective. HIV, obviously, is a much more formidable opponent than either of these. Many scientists say that the best we can hope for is that the first generation of AIDS vaccine will work in about 70 percent to 75 percent of those inoculated. Moreover, it wouldn't be an all-purpose vaccine. Because HIV is constantly mutating, there are few scientists who believe that it could be defeated with a one-time inoculation, like measles. Rather, it will likely have to be attacked the way influenza is attacked: by making specific vaccines against specific strains and then reimmunizing people whenever new strains emerge. What all of this means is that coming up with a vaccine isn't going to wipe out AIDS. In all likelihood it will do no more than confer temporary protection against some strains of the virus on the part of the population that agrees to be vaccinated.

It is even possible that having a vaccine would be worse than having none at all. In the spring of 1984, when Robert Gallo of the National Institutes of Health made it known that he had developed a blood test to detect HIV, then Secretary of Health and Human Services Margaret Heckler foolishly announced that she felt a vaccine would be ready for clinical testing in two years. According to Osborne, the next day Los Angeles bathhouses that had been empty for months had four-hour waiting lines. This, keep in mind, was on the basis of speculation that a vaccine might be available at some point in the future. If there actually were a vaccine—even a flawed one—one can only imagine how much more dramatic the recalculation of the risks and benefits of unsafe sexual behavior would be. As should be obvious from the condom research, the young, sexually active and less-educated are already in denial over HIV. What better invitation for further denial than a good—but imperfect—vaccine?

This, of course, wouldn't matter for those who are actually protected. But those lives saved might well be offset by an increase in infection among the unprotected 30 percent who, under the assumption that they too were protected, would feel it was safe to abandon whatever safe sexual practices they once followed.

Again there should be nothing surprising about this. Risk homeostasis—the idea that a reduction in risk in one area often triggers a compensatory (and in some cases greater) increase in risky behavior in another—is a well-described concept in the social sciences. In his classic work *Traffic Safety and the Driver*, Leonard Evans recounts that pedestrians are twice as likely to be struck by cars when they cross at marked crosswalks than when they cross at random. Why? Because the extra caution shown by cars approaching crosswalks is more than offset by the assumption of pedestrians that because there are lines on the road they no longer need to look both ways.

This is not to say that we should not have crosswalks or, for that matter, vaccines. It is to say that a technical advance does not necessarily constitute a solution to a problem. It is to say that spending billions of dollars on AIDS research, like exhorting Americans to practice safe sex, is simply not good enough.

In the end, the problem with AIDS is its singularity. It is too complicated biologically to be tackled by science as easily as, say, leukemia and too complicated behaviorally to be addressed as simply as, say, drunk driving. The epidemic in the United States is not the same as the epidemic in Africa—where it is much more of a heterosexual woman's disease—or the epidemic in Thailand, which appears to be driven by a new and highly virulent strain of HIV known as Type A. Indeed, the AIDS crisis of today hardly resembles the crisis in this country ten years ago. Epidemics are living, moving forces, their appearance as dependent on time and circumstance as their underlying biology. They are, to use a word that has fallen out of fashion in discussion of disease, fundamentally social phenomena.

Consider, for example, the mathematical shorthand used by epidemiologists to express the status of any outbreak of infectious disease. It is the ratio of those who have just been infected by a given agent to those who are no longer infectious: the ratio, in other words, between those newly claimed by a virus and those cured of or killed by it. If that ratio is greater than one—if a disease is infecting more people than it is losing—the epidemic grows. If the ratio is less than one, if more people die or are cured than are newly infected, the epidemic is doomed. No disease—not cholera, not the black plague, not AIDS—can survive if it kills its victims faster than they manage to infect others.

In the early 1980s, as HIV surged through the gay communities of San Francisco and New York, the ratio was at three and four and five. Today, it is at one. About 40,000 new people are infected with HIV each year, and about that many die of the disease in the same period, which is why the total population of infected Americans has remained fairly steady over the past few years at 1 million.

What this means is that the American AIDS epidemic is at a critical juncture. Any change for the worse could push it back into its old expansionist mode. This is not an idle fear. There is now in the Northeast, for example, a resurgence of the heroin use among young adults. Because of the purity of heroin supply at the moment, the drug is generally being sniffed. But if these new users start injecting the drug and sharing needles, then a new cycle of infection could begin.

Another potential threat comes from the growth of infection among the young. The stable epidemic ratio of HIV in the United States is actually a combination of two separate phenomena: gay males, for whom the ratio is now much less than one, and young adults, for whom the ratio is much greater than one. In other words, just as the epidemic is contracting among those who have responded to safe sex messages, it is expanding among those least responsive to the call for behavioral changes.

On the other hand, the epidemiological status of HIV presents a tremendous opportunity. Making inroads against HIV need not require some scientific breakthrough or a revolution in the behavior of every sexually active American. It need only involve finding some way to take a bite out of the 40,000 new infections every year, pushing the ratio below one, and letting the same relentless mathematics that created the epidemic work to destroy it.

Donald Des Jarlais, an AIDS expert at Beth Israel Medical Center in New York and perhaps the chief proponent of this kind of social strategy, says that a reasonable goal would be to halve the current yearly total of 40,000 new infections. "If we could do that," he says flatly, "the epidemic would die out."

This, of course, is easier said than done. But it is not impossible, and certainly easier than fighting AIDS by throwing money at scientists and condoms at schoolchildren. To begin with, there is no great mystery about who those 40,000 people are, or where they can be found. For all its much ballyhooed biological mystery, HIV is strikingly predictable in its manifestations. The epidemic, according to a recent report by the National Research Council, is "settling into spatially and socially isolated groups and possibly becoming endemic in them." To find those at risk for AIDS, the report went on, one need only look at where other bacterial and sexually transmitted diseases are epidemic: "zones of urban poverty, poor health, drug addiction and social disintegration." In New York City that translates into no more than six to ten neighborhoods in Greenwich Village, the Upper West Side, Harlem, Washington Heights and the Bronx. Nationwide, those with the greatest probability of being among HIV's yearly victims probably live in no more than several hundred clearly identifiable neighborhoods.

What we should be doing in those neighborhoods are the simple things that reduce people's risk of acquiring HIV. The first is basic health care. HIV, it should be remembered, is not a terribly infectious agent. The rough estimate used by epidemiologists to describe the risk of contracting HIV from unprotected vaginal sex once with a carrier is between 1 in 500 and 1 in 1,000, which makes it substantially less infectious than, say, hepatitis.

People tend to become infected with HIV because they have other sexually transmitted diseases that vastly increase their susceptibility to the virus. Syphilis, herpes and chancroid—the so-called ulcerative STDs—all cause genital lesions that bring to the surface of the skin precisely those cells that HIV likes to infect the most. They give the virus a gateway to the bloodstream. (To a lesser extent gonorrhea and chlamydia also increase the odds of infection.)

Every group hit by the epidemic now—or hit by AIDS in the past—has suffered from a corresponding epidemic of ulcerative sexually transmitted disease. It was true of gay men in San Francisco and New York in the late 1970s. It is true today in Africa, where, according to a paper presented at the Amsterdam conference, more than 75 percent of heterosexual male HIV infections in sub-Saharan Africa and between 20 percent and 40 percent of female infections resulted from the presence of some other sexually transmitted disease.

It is also the case that STDs are epidemic today in American inner cities. Between 1984 and 1990, the time the AIDS virus began to move from white gay communities into disadvantaged neighborhoods, the number of cases of syphilis for black males almost tripled. The number of new cases among black women in that same period almost quadrupled. The number of reported cases of chancroid, once almost unknown in the United States, has increased seven-fold over the past decade. An estimated 4 million Americans suffer from chlamydia; each year there are between 200,000 and 500,000 new cases of genital herpes. These are rates paralleled only by Third World countries.

That this has been allowed to happen during a period when the United States has been under siege by the AIDS virus is little short of criminal. Every one of these diseases is treatable—and in many cases curable—with drugs that are available and relatively inexpensive. Yet in the country's poorest neighborhoods, where these diseases are concentrated, the public health infrastructure that once existed to detect and treat STDs has deteriorated. The government today spends 23 percent less (in constant dollars) on controlling STDs than it did in 1950. In some cities, as many as 25 percent of all those people seeking treatment at publicly funded STD clinics are turned away each day for lack of resources.

Reversing this slide has to be a priority of any revitalized AIDS prevention strategy. According to the Coalition on STDs, a group of public health organizations, this would probably require adding about $110 million to the Centers for Disease Control's current STD budget of $90 million. Considering that the direct and indirect costs of HIV and AIDS in the United States last year amounted to $64 billion, that seems like a small price to pay.

Any targeted AIDS prevention campaign also has to focus on drug use. This is not just a matter of ending needle-sharing among heroin addicts. The problem is with the kind of behavior that all drug use creates. One study published this year, for example, looked at 500 adults in their 20s drawn from drug-infested, inner-city neighborhoods in New York, San Francisco and Miami. The men and women were all what might be considered at risk for HIV. They were poor and largely minority. Many were on public assistance. A sizable percentage had spent time in jail. Condom use was less than ideal. But of the 500, half were crack users and the other half never smoked it—and that made all the difference.

Among the women, for example, the crack users had six times as many sexual partners as the non-crack users. They were five times as likely to have had sex with a drug injector, three times more likely to have had an ulcerative STD and a third less likely to use a condom when they had sex with someone other than their regular partner. To fight crack use in the inner city, in other words, is to fight AIDS. To put a crack addict in drug treatment is to strike at the very heart of the behavior that results in HIV infection.

This much seems obvious, and one would think it would already be incorporated into national and local AIDS prevention programs. It is not. In New York City, funds for drug treatment have just been cut. And nationally, an estimated 2 million to 3 million Americans in need of drug treatment cannot get it, with the problem most acute among those who fall into the socioeconomic and geographic categories at risk for HIV.

Finally, any focused attack on the spread of HIV should involve behavioral modification. Think, for example, what could be done with New York City's intravenous drug users, 50 percent of whom are now HIV infected. Because of that extraordinarily high rate of infection, this group is the principal point of entry of HIV into the younger heterosexual population. Intravenous heroin users, however, are an easily identifiable group. Few are younger than 30 or 35. One AIDS prevention strategy, according to Des Jarlais, may consist of no more than this: telling teenagers and young adults in Harlem, Washington Heights and the Bronx not to have sex with people more than a few years older than themselves, thereby cutting the connection between heroin users and their habitual partners and the next generation. It may not be as effective as telling them to wear a condom. But then again, this is advice they may actually follow.

These strategies all rely on simple things: getting people to educate others in their own community, opening STD clinics in poor neighborhoods with enough doctors to handle demand, coming up with the money to open new drug treatment facilities. None requires a medical breakthrough. What they require instead is that we abandon our insistence that AIDS is a disease like any other. This, of course, is asking a lot. Dressing AIDS up like cancer or heart disease has made it much more politically appealing to a country that might otherwise have forgotten or ignored it. Many AIDS activists, combating the discrimination that accompanies their battle, continue to have good reason to insist that we "Fight AIDS, not people with AIDS," even though that only diverts attention from the fact that HIV is very much a disease of specific people in specific circumstances.

The challenge of the fight against AIDS over the next few years will be to convince Americans to continue to wage war against a disease that will probably never affect them and will only destroy those groups and people that they care least about. Had we the courage to make this argument earlier—to focus on basic health care and drug treatment rather than T.V. commercials for condoms and international conferences for research—there might be more people alive today.

10 Death Be Not Strange

Peter A. Metcalf

PETER METCALF is professor of anthropology at the University of Virginia. Among his books are *Celebrations of Death: The Anthropology of Mortuary Ritual* and *Where are You Spirits*. In this article, Metcalf contrasts the funeral rites of a remote tribe in Borneo with those in the United States. He makes an effort to explain why practices that seem strange to Americans make sense to the Berawan tribe in Borneo. He also explains why certain American practices would be as offensive to the Berawans as some of their practices would be to many Americans.

THE POPULAR VIEW OF ANTHROPOLOGY is that it is concerned with faraway places, strange peoples, and odd customs. This notion was neatly captured by a nineteenth-century wit who described the field as "the pursuit of the exotic by the eccentric." In recent decades many anthropologists have tried to shake this image. They see the exotic as dangerously close to the sensational and, therefore, a threat to the respectability of a serious academic discipline. They argue that anthropology has solid theoretical bases, and that some anthropologists routinely work in cities right here in America. And they are right. Nevertheless, anthropologists are as much involved with the exotic as ever, and I think that this concern actually works to scholarship's advantage.

This continuing involvement is a result of the characteristic *modus operandi* of anthropologists. First, we seek out the exotic, in the sense of something originating in another country or something "strikingly or excitingly different," as my *Webster's* puts it. Second, we try to fit this alien item—culture trait, custom, piece of behavior—into its social and cultural context, thereby reducing it to a logical, sensible, even necessary element. Having done that, we feel that we can understand why people do or say or think something instead of being divorced from them by what they say, think, or do.

Sir James Frazer, whose classic study of primitive religions, *The Golden Bough*, was first published in 1890, provides an excellent example of the eccentric in pursuit of the exotic. For him, the process of reducing the mysterious to the commonplace was the very hallmark of scientific progress. Like many anthropologists of his time, Frazer assumed that some societies were superior and others inferior, and that anthropology's main task was to describe how the latter had evolved into the former. To Frazer, Europe's technological achievements were proof of social, intellectual, and moral superiority. The dominance of the West represented the triumph of science, which in Frazer's evolutionary schema, superseded even the most rational of world religions. Science's clear light was to shine far and wide, driving superstition, the supernatural, and even God himself back into shadows and dimly lit corners.

But Frazer might have found a second aspect of the anthropological *modus operandi* less to his taste. In the course of making sense of someone else's behavior or ideas, we frequently begin to observe our own customs from a new angle. Indeed, this reflexive objectivity is often acclaimed as one of the great advantages of our methods and cited as a major justification for the long, expensive physical and psychic journeys that we make, seeking out societies far removed from our own cultural traditions. Less often remarked upon, however, is that the exotic possesses its own reflexive quality. As we learn to think of other peoples' ways as natural, we simultaneously begin to see our own as strange. In this sense, anthropologists import the exotic, and that, I suppose, puts us on the side of the angels.

An incident that occurred about four years ago during my fieldwork in north-central Borneo brought home to me the depth and subtlety of anthropologists' involvement with the exotic. I was working with the Berawan, a small tribe comprising four communities, each made up of several hundred people living in a massive wooden longhouse. The four longhouses stand beside the great rivers that are the only routes into the interior of Borneo. Berawan communities live on fish and on rice planted in clearings cut anew in the rain forest each year. In the late nineteenth century, which was a stormy period of tribal warfare, each longhouse was a fortress as well as a home, and the Berawan look back with pride on the military traditions of that era.

Among the things that interested me about the Berawan were their funeral rites, which involve what anthropologists call "secondary burial," although the Berawan do not usually bury the dead at all. Full rites consist of four stages: the first and third involve ritual preparation of the corpse; the second and fourth make up steps in storage of the remains. The first stage, lasting two to ten days, consists of rites performed immediately after death. During the second stage, the bereaved family stores the corpse in the longhouse or on a simple platform in the graveyard. This storage lasts at least eight months and sometimes for several years if the close kin cannot immediately afford to complete the expensive final stages. Third, if the corpse has been in the graveyard, the family brings it back to the longhouse, where it is kept for six to ten days, while the family lavishly entertains guests who have been summoned from far and wide. Finally, the remains are removed to a final resting place, an impressively proportioned mausoleum.

Within this four-part plan, details of the corpse's treatment vary considerably. During the first storage stage, the family may place the corpse in large earthenware jars or in massive coffins hewn from a single tree trunk. For secondary storage, the family may use valuable glazed jars or the coffin left over from the first stage. During the third-stage rites, the family may take out the bones of the deceased and clean them. As the corpse decomposes, its secretions may be collected in a special vessel. Some neighbors of the Berawan reportedly consume liquids of decomposition mixed with rice—a variety of endo-cannibalism.

For anthropologists, this intimate interaction with the corpse is certainly exotic. For Americans not professionally trained in the niceties of cultural relativism, Berawan burial is no doubt disgusting: keeping corpses around the house, shuttling them between the graveyard and the longhouse, storing them above ground instead of burying them, manipulating the bones, and, to Western eyes, paying macabre attention to the process of decay itself. My Berawan informants were aware that some phases of their ritual bothered Europeans. They soon learned, moreover, that I had a lot of questions about their funerals. One of the pleasures of working in Borneo is that people soon begin to cross-examine their interviewer. They are as curious about the stranger as he or she is about them. So before long, they began to quiz me about the death ways of my country.

On one memorable occasion, during a lull in ritual activity, I responded to one of these questions by outlining American embalming practices—the treatment of the corpse with preservative fluids and its display in an open coffin. I was well into my story, concentrating on finding the right words to describe this unfamiliar topic, when I became aware that a sudden silence had fallen over my audience. They asked a number of hesitant questions just to be sure that they had understood me correctly and drew away from me in disgust when they found that they had. So shocked were they that I had to backtrack rapidly and change my story. The topic was never broached again.

At the time, I did not understand why American embalming practices had so unnerved the Berawan. Now, having thought about the meaning of Berawan death rituals, I think that I do understand.

The death rituals of central Borneo early attracted the interest of explorers and ethnologists. In 1907, Robert Hertz, a young student of French sociologist Émile Durkheim, wrote an essay about these rites that has become a classic. Never having set foot in Borneo, Hertz relied on the accounts of travelers. Had he not been killed during the First World War, he might well have undertaken firsthand research himself. Nevertheless, his analysis is still routinely cited in discussions and comparisons of funeral customs. Yet, oddly, Hertz's central thesis has received very little attention. Hertz hypothesized that peoples who practice secondary burial have certain beliefs about the afterlife, namely, that the fate of the body provides a model for the fate of the soul.

Since Hertz did not know of the Berawan, they provided me with an appropriate test case for his hypothesis. I collected data on everything related to Berawan death rites: the people involved, mourning practices, related rituals, myths and beliefs, and so on. I also pressed my informants for interpretations of rituals. All the material I accumulated revealed a consistent set of ideas very similar to those described by Hertz. The Berawan believe that after death the soul is divorced from the body and cannot reanimate the already decaying corpse. However, the soul cannot enter the land of the dead because it is not yet a perfect spirit. To become one of the truly dead, it must undergo a metamorphosis. As the body rots away to leave dry bones, so the soul is transformed slowly into spirit form. As the corpse is formless and repulsive until putrefaction is completed, so the soul is homeless. It lurks miserably on the fringes of human habitation and, in its discomfort, may affect the living with illness. The third stage of the mortuary sequence, which Hertz called the "great feast," marks the end of this miserable period. The soul finally passes to the land of the dead, and the mortal remains of the deceased join those of its ancestors in the tomb.

But before this happy conclusion is reached, the hovering soul is feared because it may cause more death. Even more dread surrounds the body itself, caused not by the process of rotting, for that releases the soul of the deceased from the bonds of the flesh, but by the possibility that some malignant spirit of nonhuman origin will succeed in reanimating the corpse. Should this occur, the result will be a monster of nightmarish mien, invulnerable to the weapons of men, since it is already dead.

I once witnessed an incident that dramatically demonstrated how real is the Berawan fear of reanimated corpses. Toward sunset, a group of mourners and guests were chatting casually beside a coffin that was being displayed on the longhouse veranda in preparation for primary storage. Suddenly there was a tapping sound, apparently from inside the coffin. The noise could have come from the house timbers, contracting in the cool of the evening, but the people present saw a different explanation. After a moment of shock, the women fled, carrying their children. Some panic-stricken men grabbed up what weapons were handy, while others tied up the coffin lid with yet more bands of rattan. Calm was not restored until later in the evening when a shaman investigated and declared that nothing was amiss.

We can now see why American mortuary practices so shock the Berawan. By delaying the decomposition of corpses, we commit a most unnatural act. First, we seem to be trying to trap our nearest and dearest in the unhappiest condition possible, neither alive nor in the radiant land of the dead. Second, and even more perverse and terrifying, we keep an army of undecomposed corpses, each and every one subject to reanimation by a host of evil spirits. For the Berawan, America is a land carpeted with potential zombies.

After a couple of years of fieldwork, and an application of the ideas of Hertz and others, I can offer a relatively full account of Berawan death ways: what they express about Berawan notions of life and death; how they are manipulated by influential men in their struggles for power; how they relate to their sense of identity, art forms, and oral history. Meanwhile, I have also explored the literature on American death ways—and have found it wanting. For the most part, it is restricted to consideration of psychological variables—how people react to death, either the possibility of their own or that of close relatives and friends. None of these studies begins to explain why American funerals are the way they are; why they differ from British funerals, for instance.

Jessica Mitford, author of *The American Way of Death*, tried to explain the form that American funerals take by arguing that they are a product of the death industry's political power. But Mitford's theory does not explain the tacit support that Americans give to this institution, why successive immigrant groups have adopted it, or why reform movements have failed.

I have tried to relate American practices to popular ideas about the nature of a fulfilling life and a proper death. Despite these intellectual efforts, I am left with a prickly sense of estrangement. For, in fact, I had spared my Berawan friends the more gruesome details of embalming: replacement of the blood with perfumed formaldehyde and other chemicals; removal of the soft organs of the chest and abdomen via a long hollow needle attached to a vacuum pump; injection of inert materials. I did not mention the American undertaker's elaborate restorative techniques: the stitching up of mutilated corpses, plumping out of emaciated corpses with extra injections of waxes, or careful cosmetic care of hands and face. Nor did I tell the Berawan about the padded coffins, grave clothes ranging in style from business suits to negligees, and other funeral paraphernalia. Had I explained all this, their shock might have been transformed into curiosity, and they might have reversed our roles of social scientist and informant.

In the meantime, something of their reaction has rubbed off on me. I have reduced the celebrated mortuary rites of remote and mysterious Borneo to a kind of workaday straightforwardness, only to be struck by the exotic character of an institution in our very midst.

🪱 11 The Days of the Dead in Oaxaca, Mexico: An Historical Inquiry

Judith Strupp Green

In this article, Judith Strupp Green describes the Days of the Dead in
Mexico as occasions for elaborate celebration and extensive rituals. Many of
these rituals and much of the iconography can be traced far back in history,
either to medieval Europe or to the pre-Columbian Aztecs. She presents evidence that many present-day customs in Oaxaca, Mexico, arise directly from
these historical traditions. Some of the European folk customs discussed turn
out to have pre-Christian origins.

Días de Todos Muertos, or Days of the Dead, is the collective name by
which the Catholic holy days of All Saints' on November first and All Souls' on
November second are known in Mexico. The unique flavor of the celebration
of these universal Catholic festivals in some traditional Indian communities
and in Indian sections of larger cities has long been recognized. The Island of
Janitzio in Michoacán and Zapotec villages in the Valley of Oaxaca are two
such areas.

Among those raised in the Western heritage of death-avoidance, the observation of the Days of the Dead in traditional parts of Mexico often elicits a reaction of mild shock and even repulsion. Death iconography mingled with
gustatory delights (sugar skulls, coffin candies), toys for children (skeleton
puppets), and politics (the calaveras news-sheet) and the ordinary pursuits of
the living grates against contemporary North American and European attitudes towards death. Certain customs carried out in graveyards on these days
or nights, such as gambling or playing board games on the tombstones, or eating a picnic lunch there, have the same effect. Although these customs are actually peripheral rather than central to the ritual itself, they are consonant with
the ancient indigenous beliefs about the dead.

Below the surface of cursory examination, the Days of the Dead are revealed as a result of the amalgamation of pre-Spanish Indian ritual and belief and the imposed ritual and dogma of the Spanish Catholic Church. This study attempts to illuminate some elements of the historical and cultural backdrop to the contemporary celebration of the Dias de Todos Muertos in a traditional area—the Valley of Oaxaca. . . .

Collectively, the Days of the Dead are one of the most important festivals in Oaxaca and certainly one of the most expensive for each family. About a month before the Days of the Dead the women of the family begin to buy and store up material for the altar and the dishes and *ollas* for the preparation and serving of foods, according to Sra. Ramirez. She indicated that the purchase of all new dishes was mandatory, to please the spirits, no matter how poor any family might be.

On the thirty-first of October, Allhallows Eve, the family stays up all night. Food for the altar and for guests is prepared—including chiles, black and red *moles*, and tamales. Greatest importance is given to the preparation of tamales. When the laborious work of making them is over and they are thrown into the *ollas* to steam, boys set off firecrackers in celebration.

The altar in the home is also arrayed on that night. Either a special table is set up or the family altar, if it is large enough, is used. Sra. Ramirez stated that formerly, while living in a more spacious house, they put up both an altar for the child dead as well as that for adults. It had everything that the adult altar had in miniature, including tiny candleholders, small fruits and vegetables, and toys. Only "adult" foods, tobacco and alcohol, were omitted. An altar fitting this description was later seen at Santa Lucia del Valle. As well as being considered an altar to the child dead, it was designated as the special altar of the living child of the household.

The children's spirits arrive at 4:00 a.m. on November first, according to Sra. Ramirez. They are called *angelitos*. One tiny candle is lit at this time for each child. At 8:00 a.m. the same morning the child spirits are said to leave, and the little candles are snuffed and removed from the main altar. A mass is said in the local church on the morning of the first.

The adult spirits arrive on the afternoon of the same day, at 3:00 p.m., at which time a candle of standard size is lit for each. At 8:00 p.m. that evening the family says the rosary. No one would eat anything laid out on the altar for fear of antagonizing the spirits of the dead. Sr. Ramirez expressed the belief that the angry ghosts would tie their feet up in the night if they ate from the altar. Leaving nothing (or inferior gifts) on the altar causes the spirits to be sad and/or angry, depending on the folktale quoted. Usually however, the dead are believed to take revenge for poor treatment on this day.

The next morning, November second, is All Souls' Day; three masses are said and at 8:00 a.m. the adult spirits leave. Responses for the dead go on all day in various cemeteries in the Valley. Priests or prayer leaders bless and sprinkle the graves with holy water and say prayers for the dead. This goes on for many days after the Days of the Dead have passed, in order to reach all the cemeteries.

The evening of the second, about sundown, people in villages where the responses will be said decorate the graves in the cemetery with flowers, candles, and incense. Children's graves receive the most elaborate treatment, including tiny candles, *ollas* and miniature gourds, toys and cardboard or plaster figures, representing the dead or the afterlife.

It is this afternoon and evening, too, when relatives and friends come to visit, pray at the altar, and offer a gift to the souls. The gift is referred to as a *muerto*, and consists mainly of foods selected from those on the altar and prepared specially for the day. Guests, in return, receive food from their hosts. Hot beaten chocolate and bread of the dead were given to a Zapotec woman guest, during our visit to a home in Teotitlan on the second. She was a *comadre* (ritual co-godparent) to the family. Formerly, stated the mother of Sra. Ramirez, groups of men came to the houses in costumes and masks and sang special hymns of praise, *alabanzas*, for the dead and received gifts of fruits and altar goods. Until about two years ago they came, unmasked, to pray and sing and ask "Hay muertos?" (are there any *muertos* or gifts?), but the custom has apparently died out in the barrio. In the 1930's Parsons mentions masked men on domiciliary begging trips on the Days of the Dead at Santo Domingo Alvarrados and San Baltazar, Zapotec towns in the Valley (Parsons 1936: 282–283).

At Xochimilco Barrio the Days of the Dead are officially over on November third. The altars are not dismantled there until the fourth of November, however. Food on the altars can be eaten as soon as the spirits leave on the morning of the second, and it is used as the source of supply for the *muertos* gifts.

Informants at Santiago Ixtaltepec and Teotitlan offered different time-tables for the coming and going of the spirits, though all agreed that the child ghosts came on the first and the adults arrived on the first and left on the second.

RITUAL OBJECTS ASSOCIATED WITH THE DAYS OF THE DEAD

Aside from altar decorations, other material associated with the Days of the Dead are the gifts or *muertos*, brought to relatives and *compadres*. A *muerto* consists of items from the altar, as well as foodstuffs specially prepared for the holy days. An earthenware jar of black *mole*, or a cup of chocolate, fruits, flowers, nuts, tortillas wrapped in napkins and carried in a basket, along with a candle are typical.

Other special foods for the Days of the Dead are tamales and a sweet food made of squash, *conserva de calabaza*. The bread of the dead, *pan de los muertos*, is apparently indispensable for the celebration of these days in the Valley. Special loaves are prepared by bakers from the villages. Even the local commercial bakery in Oaxaca City brings in young men from Santo Domingo Comaltepec, "the village of the master bakers," for the occasion, solely to bake massive quantities of these loaves. The Indian bakers in the small barrios use old-fashioned brick beehive ovens to make three classes of bread of the dead, classed according to the amount of egg and types of spices used. There are minor differences in the shape and decoration of the loaves within the Valley—the baker from a Oaxaca barrio, who was originally from Ixtlan de Juarez, and those from Sto. Domingo Comaltepec fashioned them in an oval shape with a small knob at one end. On this knob was pressed a painted face or winged angel molded of white dough. In Tlacolula the larger loaves were sprinkled with hearts and crosses made of beaten egg white and colored sugar. A baker from Etla fashioned ghostly, human-looking figures with orange bean eyes.

No food is offered on the graves, although people sometimes eat their lunch in the cemetery while visiting graves, or bring bread of the dead and other food as an offering to those saying the responses, as at Santiago Ixtaltepec. Each loaf of bread represents a soul, according to informants.

Other representational artifacts include symbols of funerary equipment such as tombs, coffins, and pallbearers. Symbols of the afterlife include angels, devils, lyres, the soul in purgatory consumed in flames and the disembodied heart. These artifacts are made in sugar, clay, plaster, papier-mâché and cardboard. They may be static figures or puppets. Many depict skeletal figures engaged in everyday, or comical activities—such as laughing skeletal puppets, plaster skeletons dressed as bishops, women with babies, priests, scholars, etc. The sugar ones are edible, and those made in Etla and brought to Oaxaca from that town, which is known for its fine candies, are filled with anise flavored liqueur. Tiny pottery fruits and miniature dishes are set out on children's graves. In areas other than Oaxaca (i.e., Michoacán, Edo de Mexico, Guanajuato) more emphasis is concentrated on molded animal figures, especially in sugar.

Grave decorations consist of flowers, candles or vigil lights, and, on occasion, representational figurines, especially cardboard tombs (*tumbitas*) or paper skulls. Occasionally those visiting the graves would set out an incense burner before the cross or headstone. These examples are drawn from the graves seen at the San Felipe del Agua cemetery and that at Santiago Ixtaltepec, both small traditional ones. The larger cemetery at San Antonio Castillo de Velasco was only embellished with flower decorations, as was the main cemetery at Oaxaca City.

Another artifact connected with the cemetery ritual, at least at San Felipe, is the board game played by children on the unadorned gravestones. *El Ancla* and *La Oca* are both games played at other times of the year but, according to informants, are traditional for the Days of the Dead. Grown men played ordinary dice in the Santiago Ixtaltepec cemetery on the night the graves were blessed.

The *calaveras*, satirical verses written to lampoon local politicians and prominent persons, are printed on newssheets decorated with drawings of skeletons and distributed during the Days of the Dead. The church bells are tolled in distinctive ways. Parsons reports that at Mitla the bells ring double quick at noon on Oct. 31, as they do for children's funerals. At noon on Nov. 2 they tolled as at an adult's funeral (1936: 281–282).

OFFICIAL CATHOLIC POSITION AND CUSTOMS SANCTIONED BY THE CHURCH

The Days of the Dead are official holy days in the Catholic Calendar. November first was established in 834 A.D. as All Saints' Day by Pope Gregory IV as a day to honor all the saints, including the unrecognized as well as the canonized saints who had attained the Beatific Vision (New Catholic Encyc. 1967: Vol. 1, 318–319). It coincided with the ancient festival to Samhain, Celtic Lord of the Dead, at which human and animal sacrifices were made.

The day following All Saints' is All Souls' Day, established in the Roman Calendar by the fourteenth century, following its institution as a day of observance in the Cluniac monasteries by Odilo, Abbot of Cluny, France, in the ninth century. It was founded to honor all the faithful departed, and on it the Office of the Dead and three Requiem Masses are said by the clergy to assist the souls from purgatory to heaven.

The custom of having a procession from the church to the cemetery, visiting the graves of deceased relatives and friends, the blessing of the graves by a priest, and decorating the graves with flowers and candles is almost universal in Catholic countries (New Catholic Encyc. 1967: Vol. 1, 319) and looked upon with favor by the Church (Weiser 1952: 308–311).

The color of vestments and altar drapings on the Day of All Souls is black, according to Catholic liturgy. In some churches in New Spain, it was the custom of the clergy to erect a temporary catafalque in the church to remind the congregation of the purpose of the day, like the one that Pfefferkorn saw on All Souls' in a church in Sonora in the eighteenth century (Pfefferkorn 1949: 270). They also exhibited the relics of saints, often bones or skulls, on that day, as Felipe el Hermoso saw in the Cologne cathedral on November 1, 1501 (Lalaing in García Marcadal 1952–1962: Vol. 1, 543). In Yucatan in the 1850's John Lloyd Stephens found that the skulls of former local residents were exposed on All Souls' Day on a catafalque at the church. He said this practice was general "all over the country." Each skull was identified by name on a strip of paper spanning the forehead (Stephens 1856: Vol. 1, 420).

The Catholic Church promised heavenly rewards for those who died in the Faith and in the state of grace, pending a period of time in purgatorial flames for those who had not expiated their sins on earth, and eternal suffering in hell for those who did not die in the state of grace. The idea of purgatory was a concept that came into prominence in the High Middle Ages, for previously "the poets and theologians had been satisfied to leave the riddle of the soul's fate between death and final judgment unanswered" (Gatch 1969: 111). While theologically the idea of purgatory was accepted, the ordinary people evidently clung to some pre-Christian customs like feeding the dead which was carried over through early Christian and early Medieval times.

FOLK CUSTOMS IN MEDIEVAL TIMES

The pre-Christian practice of feeding the dead hinges on the belief that, for some time at least, the dead person continues to have needs like those of the living. The belief was apparently quite tenacious in Europe. In the fifteenth century the custom of laying out a banquet for dead family members on All Souls' Day was prevalent enough to receive an official ban by the Church in the fifteenth century. Hoyos Sainz, the Spanish folklorist, states that formerly in the Cantabrian zone of Spain, food was put into the tombs of the dead at burial, and on the night of All Saints an array of food was set in the windows as an offering for the dead (Hoyos Sainz 1945: 30–53). These practices are unknown today.

A common custom involving food with All Souls' Day was that of "souling," as it was called in Medieval England. Black-garbed friars walked through the streets ringing a bell and calling on the living to remember the dead in their prayers, while the soulers, often young men, sang verses called souling songs and begged alms and soul-cakes—square buns topped with currants.

Spain was a country so enamored of death during the reign of the Hapsburgs (1516–1700) that one scholar was provoked to say, "The Hapsburg attitude toward death was . . . in accordance with the ethical temper of their subjects, if the evidence of our series of texts is valid. The Death tradition had invaded all walks of Spanish society" (Whyte 1931: 127). Charles V retired to a monastery and ordered his own funeral to be celebrated before his death. Philip II habitually dressed in black, as did his followers; he built the remarkable Escorial which has been described as a vast mausoleum. The Dance of Death composed in Spain ca. 1450 was performed during the fifteenth and sixteenth centuries as an allegorical and devotional dance (Whyte 1931: 20, 43). Religious poems and plays about death such as "La Farsa de la Muerte," "Las Cortes de la Muerte" and "La Vida y la Muerte" were evidently popular (Whyte 1931: 75, 100, 117).

Spanish devotion to the dead was so great as to amount to a death cult, according to the versions of it given by seventeenth and eighteenth century travelers to Spain. A Jourvin who journeyed to Spain in 1672 remarks that prayers were solicited for the dead continuously in all the churches, on the public plazas, and at all crossroads. At 9:00 p.m. the church bell rang to remind people to pray for the souls in purgatory, and men wandered the streets begging alms for the souls (Jourvin in García Mercadal 1952: Vol. 2, 750). Pfefferkorn attests to the same practice, carried out by Spanish religious brotherhoods in Sonora, Mexico, in 1756–1767 (Pfefferkorn 1949: 271–272).

During the Days of the Dead devotion was intensified. Juan F. Peyron, a traveler in Spain in 1772–1773, remarks that "The love of the souls is universal in Spain; they even know the precise day when a soul ought to leave purgatory and often announce at the door of the church that 'today the soul is taken out'" (Peyron in Mercadal 1952: Vol. 3, 880). The same author reports that on the night before the "Día de los Muertos," nearly all the Spanish towns and cities had a public auction to which people were expected to donate livestock and poultry or foodstuffs to be sold for the benefit of the souls. Dances and hunts were given to raise money to have masses said for the souls as well. On the day of All Saints the people carried lighted candles to the tombs of their relatives because they believed that in the evening before All Souls' the dead held a procession, and those for whom no one had taken a candle for the grave, attended ashamedly with their arms crossed. Some people even adorned their beds that night and left them empty, so that the wandering souls could rest (Peyron in Mercadal 1952: Vol. 3, 880–881).

Hoyos Sainz, the Spanish folklorist, states that in this century the custom of giving bread of the souls (*pan de animas* and *pan de muertos*) to beggars on the Days of the Dead was still practiced in Leon, Salamanca, and Segovia (Hoyos Sainz 1945: 30–53). The Catholic Church was able to stamp out the practice of feeding the dead in Spain, possibly encouraging the giving of food and alms to the poor or to the Church to benefit the souls (i.e., the public auction). Although it was practiced in earlier times, the Catholic Church would not have introduced or encouraged this pre-Christian rite. The ritual they brought to the New World is generally considered to be a reduced and expurgated one. As Foster states, ". . . in missionizing America the Church had the opportunity to throw off these popular observances, to define Catholicism in terms of rites and observances central to dogma, to produce a theologically ideal religion" (Foster 1960: 15). The fact that they did not always take this opportunity in America, especially when the popular custom worked to the benefit of the Church—such as the giving of bread of the dead and begging alms for the souls—is apparent from the older and contemporary accounts of the Days of the Dead ritual in Mexico. Also they were faced with the New World indigenous tradition of honoring and sustaining souls by feeding them—the same custom that existed in rural Europe.

ICONOGRAPHY OF THE DEAD AND OF DEATH IN MEDIEVAL EUROPE

The obsessive concern with death and the dead found in Spain has its roots in the dominance of death themes in literature and art in most of Europe in the late Middle Ages. This trend has precedents in the thirteenth and fourteenth centuries with the theme of the *Three Living and Three Dead* and the *Art of Dying Well* and finally culminated in the *Dance of Death*. Macabre paintings inspired by these themes appear in and on Medieval European structures. One exception is Spain, which had its own *Danza de la Muerte*, but no painted representations of it have been found. The morbid spirit lasted longer in Spain than in the rest of Europe, through the Hapsburg reign. Trapier (1956: 31) feels that death themes in the forms of skulls or skeletons are more frequent in the funerary art of the seventeenth century than during the previous century, not to mention the influence of the lugubrious works of Valdés Leal.

Kurtz poses his belief that the instigation and promotion of the death theme should be attributed to the Medieval clergy who, concerned about the general decay of morals at the time, and the loss of value put on life because of devastating outbreaks of the Black Death, felt people needed the grim reminder that the sinner's life was short and that he had to repent in time to save himself (Kurtz 1934: 281). The Dominicans, so dominant in the missionization of Mexico, were cited as particularly instrumental in this movement (Whyte 1931: 13).

Vivid visual images were used to convey the idea of Death and the dead. Men dressed in painted skeleton suits acted in the *autos*, as they no doubt did for the Dance of the Dead. Cheap, popular woodcuts and the ubiquitous paintings and murals of death themes depicted the dead as near-skeletons, that is, as partly desiccated corpses. These were not always gruesome. The famous woodcuts of Holbein on death, which were available by 1555 in Spain, showed "death [as] an abstract, personified concept that enters into the daily life of the people of the world and mingles with them like another human being" (Kurtz 1934: 194). The dead in his graphics appear in contemporary clothing and indulge in practical jokes on the living. This familiar, tongue-in-cheek characterization of death was to reappear in the nineteenth century graphics of Mexican artists José Guadalupe Posada, Manuel Manilla and Santiago Hernández, as the famous skeletons known as *calaveras*.

In addition to graphics, the death motif appeared on sepulchral monuments, catafalques, architectural ornaments and jewelry, both religious and secular. These reminders of death are called *memento mori*. "What may be termed the memento mori age included the fifteenth, sixteenth, and seventeenth centuries, and the popularity of memento mori devices certainly culminated in the "Dance of Death" designs of the sixteenth century . . . memento mori devices occurred everywhere, on paintings, and prints, on sepulchral monuments, as architectural ornaments, on all kinds of jewelry (especially on memorial finger rings), in books of emblems, in books of hours and other kinds of devotional books, on devotional objects (such as rosary beads in the form of death's heads) and on medals" (Weber 1922: 135–136). The catafalque for Carlos V in Mexico was covered with skeletons called "muertes" (Cervantes Salazar 1963: 188–200). The catafalque designed for Carlos II in Coatepec, Puebla, in 1700 was similarly adorned.

Actual skulls and skeletons were not uncommon sights to the Medieval and Renaissance man. Charnel houses were integral parts of the popular cemeteries, where the bones of earlier deceased were heaped up after being exhumed to make room for others who wished to be buried there. Public executions and exposure of the victims' bodies or heads for extended periods was common practice. Parts of the bodies of saints, including hair, nails, but particularly the skull and various bones, were venerated as relics and regularly exposed in the churches (Huizinga 1924: 150).

AZTEC RITUAL FOR THE DEAD

Much more is known of pre-Columbian Aztec ritual, iconography, and eschatology than any other Mesoamerican group, thanks to the work of Sahagún and later investigators like Caso, Seler, Fernández, Angel María Garibay and León-Portilla. There may have been significant differences between their ritual and outlook and that of the pre-Columbian Zapotecs who occupied the Valley of Oaxaca. Aztec customs and beliefs as well as place names and vocabulary were known to have influenced the Zapotecs, however, after their invasion by the Aztec peoples in the fifteenth century, and previously through trade contacts (Parsons 1936: 2).

The Aztecs believed in an afterlife, though not an infinite one. The attainment of this afterlife did not hinge on the morality of one's behavior in life, except in the way that it might influence the manner of death. The way in which one died was considered a calling by a god. Those who went to the dwelling place of the sun (*Tonatiuhilhuicac*) were those who died in battle or on the sacrificial stone, and the women who died with a "prisoner in the womb" (in childbirth). Even this fate lasted only four years when they turned into various types of birds of rich plumage and color and would sip the honey of all the flowers of heaven and earth, according to Sahagún (1952: Bk. 3, 34–48).

Tlalocán, the earthly paradise, was the destined home of those chosen by Tlaloc, the god of rain. They died by drowning, lightning, dropsy or gout, which was considered the summons of the god. There is some evidence that after four years they were considered to be reborn on earth (León-Portilla 1963: 125–127). Those who died a natural death had a less pleasant fate. They had to make an arduous journey to Mictlan, the underworld, accompanied only by the little dog cremated with them, and face a series of tests, among them: trekking through eight deserts and eight hills, facing wild animals and obsidian-bladed winds. After four years they came to the ninth hill called Chiconamictlan and passed into nothingness (Sahagún 1952: Bk. 3, 39–42).

Both Parsons and Leslie, in their studies of the Zapotecs of Mitla, confirm that the villagers retain some of the fatalistic view towards death and the afterlife that was prevalent at the time of the Conquest. Despite over 400 years of missionary effort, heaven and hell in the Christian sense of reward for good or punishment for evil in this life was not accepted. *Gabihl*, the "hell" of the Zapotecs, "designated a realm of the dead coexistent with this world in which the souls lived much as they lived during this lifetime . . . Similarly, townspeople did not conceive of heaven as a dwelling place of the souls. It was for them a vague, far away place where God and some saints lived" (Leslie 1960: 49–50). Nor was the idea of purgatory internalized. "The soul of a person who died abruptly became an *alma en pena*, an afflicted soul that could not complete its transition to the other world. This idea did not, however, conform to the Catholic conception of purgatory. The soul experiencing the *pena*, pain, consequent to sudden death was not atoning for sin; it was simply harassed by the compulsion to complete the expectations and obligations that death had interrupted" (Leslie 1960: 48–49).

In pre-Hispanic times the Aztecs cremated those who died naturally. The remaining bones and ashes were placed in a jar or bowl, and upon them a green stone or lump of obsidian was laid to serve as the dead man's heart in the other world. The ash-filled bowl was buried in the home or in the tribal temple, and offerings were laid on that spot (Sahagún Bk. 3: 43).

Although Sahagún does not specify that these first offerings were burned, or of what they consisted, Torquemada states that for a chief the gifts were slaves, quail, rabbits, birds, butterflies, incense, food, wine, flowers, and canes of tobacco. At the end of a year slaves were no longer offered, but other gifts of food, flowers and incense were, accompanied with music, feasting and dancing (Torquemada 1943: Bk. 13, 521–523). Eighty days after death, says Sahagún in recounting ritual for those who died naturally, gifts and belongings were burned, and again in one year, and on the second, third and fourth anniversaries of death. After the fourth year all offerings stopped as the dead had reached their end.

The dead who went to one of the heavens, however, were honored at fixed festivals. Those who had been taken by Tlaloc to Tlalocan were feted at the feast of Tepeihuitl in the thirteenth month. Images were made of amaranth dough in the shape of clouds and human figures, which Torquemada likened to dolls, and were offered to the gods along with tamales and other food. Later they were eaten by the people (Sahagún 1951: Bk. 2, 121–123). In addition the people drank wine and uttered canticles of praise in honor of these dead holy ones.

On Quecholli in the fourteenth month, they observed a feast which honored the dead warriors by placing small arrows and torches on their graves and performing nighttime rites. The women who died in childbirth, the Cihuapipiltin, were also honored on the third movable feast in the third sign in the first house. Offerings were made to them, and these women, now goddesses, were thought to visit the earth on that day (Sahagún 1951: Bk. 2, 36).

Dr. Jacinto de la Serna noted in his *Tratado de las Idolatrías, Supersticiones,*

Dioses, Ritos, Hechicerías y Otras Costumbres Gentílicas de las Razas Aborigenes de México, first published in 1546, that the Indians adulterated Church custom by making offerings to the dead in their homes and burning candles to them there all night before All Souls'. In the churches that were not attended that night by priests they did the same, offering the dead good food and drink and later eating it themselves. On the day of All Souls' when the mass is said, he complains, the Indians had no more candles, since they had burned them the night before (de la Serna 1953: 69). He named as idolatrous their customs of offering food and drink to the dead, placing provisions in the shroud for the journey to the other life, and dressing them in new and fine clothing. When a baby died, its mother put a small cane, filled with her milk, on its breast for sustenance (de la Serna 1953: 68).

Burgoa in his seventeenth century account of Zapotec life laments the fact that the Indians continued to hold "superstitious banquets" for dead relatives and friends, sacrificing turkeys and preparing strong drink for the guests and singers (Burgoa 1934: Vol. 1, 22).

AZTEC ICONOGRAPHY OF THE DEAD AND OF DEATH

The actual remains of the dead were a familiar sight to the Aztecs, despite the cremation custom, for human sacrifices accompanied almost every festival. At the dedication of the Great Temple at Tenochtitlan about 20,000 captives were sacrificed. The skulls were sometimes spitted on racks known as *tzompantli*, and the skins of victims were worn by the priests for certain observances.

The custom of venerating parts of the bodies of the dead, especially those dead considered to have gone to paradise, was prevalent and undoubtedly aided the clergy in spreading belief in the efficacy of saintly relics after the conquest. Trophy heads of important war victims, dried and preserved, were kept, and there is evidence of a jawbone cult in Tlatelolco (Ruz 1968: 201). The arms, hands, and middle finger of women who died in childbirth were much sought after by young warriors as a source of supernatural power. So great was their value, that the family of the dead woman had to guard her grave for some time after death.

Although death motifs may have reached their apogee in Aztec art, symbols of death in the forms of skull and skeleton, corpse, or the perhaps characteristically Mesoamerican representation of a human that is vertically divided into skeleton and living person, appear from pre-Classic times through the Classic and post-Classic in all the important civilizations of Mesoamerica. The death's-head was the symbol of a particular month in one of the Aztec calendars, which was derived in turn from the Maya.

Although the fragile materials such as wood and cloth are gone, the death themes have been found in painting, sculpture, architectural ornament, pottery figurines, and jewelry.

Obviously the symbol of death to the Aztecs was not an admonition to reform since the forces controlling an individual's destiny were superhuman and his fate was established irrevocably at birth. Westheim feels that the Aztec *calavera* (skull) was an allusion to immortality and a sign of coming resurrection (1953: 54). But if life after death was a mere four years, and that fraught with danger and trial for the ordinary man, it is doubtful if it could mean that to the Aztec individual. Perhaps it was a device used by the religious hierarchy to keep the idea of the necessity of death—human sacrifice—before the people, since it was the only means by which the Aztecs believed they could avoid the destruction of their world by the gods (León-Portilla 1963: 36–37).

SUMMARY

The outward form of ritual prescribed by the Catholic Church for the Days of the Dead are: the obligatory mass on All Saints' Day, the celebration of three masses on All Souls' Day (a custom established by the Spanish Dominicans in the fifteenth century), and the recitation of the Office of the Dead. Common customs established by the Church in Europe such as the parish procession to the cemetery, the blessing of the graves, and the decoration by the people of relatives' tombstones with flowers and candles were no doubt introduced by the friars into Mexico, recognizing that placing offerings at the place of burial was already an Aztec custom.

Certain aspects of the Spanish death cult reached the New World, such as the custom of forming religious brotherhoods whose members solicited alms for the dead, ringing bells in special ways for the dead, and possibly erecting catafalques and exposing human skulls in the churches. The custom of begging for the souls in Spain obviously relates to the singing and soliciting alms at homes in Oaxaca on All Saints'. The meaning this ritual had to the Zapotec Indians as opposed to the meaning it had to the Spanish settlers may be quite different, however.

Related to this is the old Spanish tradition of giving visitors bread of the souls or bread of the dead. Noting that bread is listed among the death-offerings that the Indians brought to the church, in the sixteenth century by Motolinía (1951: 144–145), and in the early seventeenth century by Thomas Gage (Thompson 1958: 238–239), it is very possible that bread of the dead as part of the Days of the Dead ritual was introduced early in the Colonial period. Although the Aztecs did make figures of amaranth to offer to the dead and this custom may have been influential in the custom's acceptance, the purely Spanish technology of the bread-making and identical term used in Spain for it suggests that it was an Hispanic introduction.

The iconography of death for the Days of the Dead shows Spanish elements in the catafalque, coffin, and symbols of the afterlife such as the lyre, angels, valentine-type hearts, devils and souls in purgatory. Black and purple, used on these days for decoration, are the colors used in the Catholic liturgy for death and penance. To my knowledge the desiccated corpse or skin-and-bones figure does not appear in the Mesoamerican death iconography, but the skeleton itself, of course, does.

Many of the elements of ritual and iconography in the Oaxacan version of the Days of the Dead are syncretic. That is, they are the result of a process of integration of both Spanish and Indian traits during the missionization period and later. The Mesoamerican Indians honored and made offerings to their dead. The Spanish did too, but when they attempted to impose Catholic ritual on the Indians, they found that their converts sometimes changed the form to better fit with their own pre-Hispanic ritual and belief. When they accepted the form, they imbued it with a meaning more consistent with their own body of beliefs. Some of the acceptance or rejection patterns depended on the Spanish friars' tolerance, of course. The feeding of the dead, deplored by de la Serna and Burgoa, apparently was tolerated in the New World as it was in Spain as a superstition rather than idolatry or heresy. The Indians' all-night vigil awaiting the visit of the dead fall into the same category.

Symbols of death in the form of sugar skulls and animals have been documented only to the 1840's when Madam Calderón de la Barca reported the rows of sugar skulls and animals in the zócalo in Mexico City before All Saints' (1966: 541–542).

These ephemeral objects, along with the cardboard catafalques, seem to be replacements for the real skulls, sacrificial animals and catafalques once part of the Days of the Dead observance. The transference of death themes to toys and candies for children is entirely consonant with ancient and modern Indian beliefs regarding childhood participation in religious ritual. And there is no need to hide the facts of death from the Indian child. It is an event with which he is intimately familiar, not only because of the depressingly high mortality rate, but because death, like birth, takes place in the home and with the family.

References

Burgoa, F. *Geográfica descripción de la parte septentrional del polo artico de la América, y nueva iglesia de las indías occidentales.* Mexico: Talleres Gráficos de la Nación, 1934.

Calderón de la Barca, F. In H. T. Fisher and M. H. Fisher (Eds.), *Life in Mexico. The letters of Fanny Calderón de la Barca.* Garden City, New York: Doubleday, 1966.

Catholic University of America. *The new Catholic encyclopedia.* New York: McGraw-Hill, 1967.

Cervantes de Salazar, F. *México en 1554, y túmulo imperial.* Mexico: Editorial Porrua, S. A., 1963.

de la Serna, J. *Tratado de las idolatrías, supersticiones, dioses, ritos, hechicerías y otras costumbres gentílicas de las razas aborigenes de México.* Mexico, 1953.

Foster, G. M. *Culture and conquest: America's Spanish heritage.* New York: Viking Fund Publications in Anthropology, No. 27, 1960.

García Mercadal, J. *Viajes de extranjeros por España y Portugal.* Madrid: Aguilar, 1952–1962. 3 vols.

Gatch, M. M. *Death: Meaning and mortality in Christian thought and contemporary culture.* New York: Seabury Press, 1969.

Green, J. S. *Laughing souls: The days of the dead in Oaxaca, Mexico.* San Diego: San Diego Museum of Man, 1969, Popular Series, No. 1.

Hoyos Sainz, Luis. Folklore español del culto a los muertos. *Revista de Dialectología y Tradiciones Populares,* 1945, *1.* (Madrid)

Huizinga, J. *The waning of the Middle Ages.* London: E. Arnold, 1924.

Kurtz, Leonard P. The dance of death and the macabre spirit in European literature. (Ph.D. dissertation, Columbia University, New York), 1934.

León-Portilla, M. *Aztec thought and culture: A study of the ancient Nahuatl.* Norman, Oklahoma: University of Oklahoma Press, 1963.

Leslie, C. M. *Now we are civilized.* Detroit: Wayne State University Press, 1960.

Motolinía, T. *History of the Indians of New Spain.* Translated and annotated by F. B. Steck. Washington, D.C.: Academy of American Franciscan History, 1951.

Parsons, E. C. *Mitla, town of the souls, and other Zapotec-speaking pueblos of Oaxaca, Mexico.* Chicago: University of Chicago Press, 1936.

Pfefferkorn, I. *Sonora, a description of the province.* Translated and annotated by T. Treutlein. Albuquerque: University of New Mexico Press, 1949.

Ruz Lhuillier, A. *Costumbres funerarias de los antiguos mayas.* Mexico: UNAM, 1968.

Sahagún, B. *General history of the things of New Spain; Florentine codex.* Translated and annotated by A. J. O. Anderson and C. E. Dibble. Santa Fe: School of American Research, 1950.

Stephens, J. L. *Incidents of travel in Yucatan.* New York: Harper and Brothers, 1856. 2 vols.

Thompson, J. E. S. (Ed.) *Thomas Gage's travels in the New World.* Norman, Oklahoma: University of Oklahoma Press, 1958.

Torquemada, J. *Los veinte i un libros rituales i Monarchia Indiana.* Mexico: Chaves Hayhoe, 1943.

Trapier, E. D. G. *Valdés Leal, baroque concept of death and suffering in his paintings.* New York: Hispanic Society of America, 1956.

Weber, F. P. *Aspects of death and correlated aspects of life in art, epigram, and poetry.* (4th ed. rev.) London: Lewis, 1922.

Weiser, F. X. *Handbook of Christian feasts and customs.* New York: Harcourt, Brace, and World, 1952.

Westheim, P. *La calavera.* Traducción de Mariana Frenk. Mexico: Antigua Librería Robredo, 1953.

Whyte, F. *The dance of death in Spain and Catalonia.* Baltimore: Waverly Press, 1931.

DYING IN VARIOUS SETTINGS

Contents

PART III CONTAINS FIVE PAPERS. The first three deal with dying in a hospital setting, the fourth deals with dying in a nursing home, and the fifth deals with dying at home with the support of a hospice organization. These are the settings in which most Americans die today. The article by Friedland gives a brief history of the current AIDS epidemic in the United States from the perspective of a health-care provider who works with HIV patients. This article also includes a discussion of how AIDS differs from other life-threatening diseases such as cancer. It may be equally appropriate to read this article in connection with the two others on AIDS included in Part II.

The Glaser and Strauss article deals with the ways in which the hospital staff and the patient both contribute to the pretense that the patient is not dying—part of a more general understanding of the control of information about a patient's true condition. Sudnow deals with differences in the quality of treatment given to different individuals based on characteristics such as age and appearance (well-groomed versus disheveled), as well as moral categories (such as prostitute). The focus of these articles is on the social organization of work within hospitals by those who attend to the dying and the dead.

While the Gubrium book deals with dying in nursing homes from the perspective of three categories of actors (top staff, the floor staff, and the clients), the selection included here deals with only one of those worlds: dying as witnessed and experienced by the clients.

The focus of the Gentile and Fello article is on dying at home with hospice care. This article reflects that emphasis in the American hospice movement, but it is also important to discuss the special nature of hospice inpatient facilities as well. The hospice is generally presented as the humanistic alternative to impersonal high-tech dying in a hospital. While there is a great deal of truth to this conception, it is important to give some thought to those situations and those categories of patients for whom dying in a hospital setting is preferable to the hospice alternative. It may also be of value to think about those aspects of hospice care that can be (and in some cases have been) introduced into nursing home and hospital settings, as well as the structural factors that make it difficult to introduce other aspects of the hospice model.

12 Clinical Care in the AIDS Epidemic ∿

Gerald H. Friedland

GERALD FRIEDLAND is codirector of the AIDS Center at Montefiore Medical Center and professor of medicine at the Albert Einstein College of Medicine in the Bronx, New York. This article is written from the perspective of health-care providers, particularly professionals dealing with AIDS patients. It provides a brief history of the evolution of the AIDS epidemic and a discussion of the various stages in the disease process. Of particular interest is the discussion of the ways in which AIDS may be different from many other fearful diseases.

The word plague had just been uttered for the first time. Everybody knows that pestilences have a way of recurring in the world; yet somehow we find it hard to believe in ones that crash down on our heads from a blue sky. There have been as many plagues as wars in history; yet always plagues and wars take people equally by surprise. . . . Our townsfolk were not more to blame than others; they forgot to be modest, that was all, and thought that everything was still possible for them; which presumed that pestilences were impossible. . . . They fancied themselves free, and no one will ever be free so long as there are pestilences.

ALBERT CAMUS[1]

THE LAST THING I HAD TIME FOR on that busy autumn morning in 1983 was a telephone call about an AIDS patient in distress. Clinical teaching rounds with interns and residents were about to begin, and I was scheduled to lecture later that morning.

"The parents of your patient Jose Quintero told me to call you," a nurse exclaimed anxiously.

I had seen Jose the evening before and knew he was soon to die. Years of cocaine abuse and careless sex had brought him to the edge. AIDS had been

From "Clinical Care in the AIDS Epidemic," reprinted by permission of *Daedalus*, Journal of the American Academy of Arts and Sciences, from the issue entitled "Living with AIDS," Spring 1989, Vol. 118, No. 2.

particularly cruel to him—multiple hospitalizations for pneumocystis pneumonia, fevers, pain, emaciation, and now swelling of his small body and another episode of pneumonia. He was an impossibly angry man, demanding of everyone with such urgency and insistence that both his family and the doctors and nurses caring for him often found it hard to be compassionate. But he elicited a grudging respect as well. Although his anger was diffuse and unfocused, nothing made him more angry than this illness. He accepted neither his disease nor its resultant disabilities. When he was no longer able to drive his taxi, he had his father drive it for him while he sat in the front seat going through the motions of his business. Rarely keeping routine clinic appointments, instead he usually showed up only when he was sick and always expected immediate care. Each diagnostic test and therapeutic maneuver offered to him he met first with sneering refusal, yet eventually he would reluctantly agree to it. I knew he was grateful for our efforts, but he hated his dependency and loss of control. Never ceasing to fight with us and his disease, Jose lived longer than we had expected. I used to quip that he was so angry he scared his dwindling immune system into working overtime to keep him alive. Earlier in the week, after we discussed his illness and prognosis, he and his family decided that if he required intubation—being placed on a respirator—he would refuse and take his chances. He knew his death was imminent, and he was not going to be dependent on a machine to keep him alive.

"He's asking for you, and I think you should come as quickly as you can," the nurse on the phone insisted.

I momentarily worried about not meeting my organized schedule for the day but went off to Jose's room. There he sat, still alive, upright in a chair beside his bed, bloated and breathing fitfully, an oxygen mask over his mouth and an intravenous line in one arm. His parents were hovering nearby, and the young nurse who had called me was sitting at his side. He grasped her hand tightly, holding onto her as his life ebbed. She had cared for him the previous day, and moved by his courage and recognizing his final stage of illness, had chosen to stay through the night with him. As I stepped into the room, he lifted his swollen eyelids, stared directly into my eyes, and slowly nodded.

In the spring of 1981, I returned to live and work as a physician in New York City after a thirteen-year absence. I came to Montefiore Medical Center/North Central Bronx Hospital and Albert Einstein College of Medicine in the Bronx, a borough of New York City, to help supervise the training of medical students and young physicians in internal medicine and to teach infectious diseases. This was the specialty in which I had been trained and which I had practiced for over a decade in the United States, Africa, and the Middle East.

In August of 1981, I saw the first three patients with *Pneumocystis carinii* pneumonia. They were desperately ill young men, and two of them were on respirators. A similar bizarre illness had been reported among gay men in California and New York City earlier in the summer, but these three men were not gay. Instead, all had histories of intravenous drug use. I recalled that a young woman with the same mysterious illness had been cared for during the previous spring at Montefiore, and we later learned that her infant had also been hospitalized with an unusual and unknown immunodeficiency. I can remember a mixture of feelings at the time—dispassionate clinical interest in what appeared to be a most unusual and challenging cluster of cases, personal distress at the terror and pain of those young men whose lungs could no longer bear the assault of infection and whose lives were hanging in the balance on those mechanical respirators, a clear and deep sense of disbelief, foreboding, and dread—that something not only different and unusual but also cruel and malevolent was occurring, and that this was just the beginning.

During the first year of what we now know to be the AIDS epidemic, an additional fourteen patients were diagnosed with the still unnamed syndrome at my institution. During the second year, the number doubled.

I remember a disturbing recurring dream in those early years. I was walking along Jerome Avenue in the Bronx at midday. I felt the vibration of the overhead subway trains, but there was no sound. Buses maneuvered through the lines of double-parked cars and greengrocer stands pushed onto the sidewalk with bins of tropical fruit, but there was no color. Everything looked right and as it should have been, but there were no people; the silent, secret epidemic had carried them away. I've long since stopped having this dream, but flashes of its images sometimes break into my consciousness.

Since the early 1980s remarkable biologic, epidemiologic, and clinical progress has been made in the AIDS epidemic. The human immunodeficiency virus (HIV) causing AIDS and other related illness has been discovered, characterized, and examined.[2] Its routes of transmission have been carefully documented, and the ways in which it is not transmitted have been established as well.[3] Surveillance methodologies have been elaborated so that the numerical and geographic extent of infection and disease have been tracked,[4] and a fuller appreciation of the spectrum of illness induced by HIV has evolved.[5] Clinical diagnosis and treatment of both HIV infection and the myriad of complicating secondary infections and malignancies have progressed both in specific instances and on a broad and advancing front.[6] Some relevant and innovative systems of care for HIV-infected persons and those with AIDS have been developed,[7] and finally, local as well as larger national and international societies in which HIV infection occurs have slowly responded in policy and allocation of resources.[8]

As this exceptional progress has taken place and even accelerated, the number of new cases of AIDS has multiplied. By September 1988, seven years after those initial three cases were diagnosed, over 800 men, women, and children have been diagnosed with AIDS at the hospitals in which I work. During this time 16,663 cases have been diagnosed in New York City,[9] 72,645 in the United

States,[10] and more than 250,000 cases in the entire world.[11] These, of course, represent the tip of the iceberg of HIV infection, now estimated to be between 5 million and 10 million worldwide.[12] At my institution and elsewhere, most patients diagnosed with AIDS during the past seven years have now died or are in the terminal stages of their illness. Their median life expectancy from time of diagnosis of AIDS to death has been less than a year.[13] Some have survived substantially longer, and others have succumbed quickly. I've learned to believe that the angry patients are likely to live longer—that fighting with their disease and care providers, as Jose did, is better than passivity and acceptance. But ultimately for all, the outcome is the same—a cruel, progressive, lingering demise. Epidemiologic studies have demonstrated that almost half those infected with HIV will develop AIDS within ten years,[14] and the proportion rises with each year, so that at the very least the majority, if not all, will develop AIDS. Thus, the full force of the HIV epidemic has not yet been experienced; the worst is yet to come. Indeed, the simple, irrefutable fact is that we are at the beginning of the epidemic. Although of great consequence world-wide, this fact is of special significance in areas of high prevalence like central Africa and New York City. Only a few years ago, new cases appeared at my institution in the Bronx at the rate of 1 or 2 per month. Now approximately 5 new cases are seen each week and added to our patient roster. On any day of the week, 50 to 60 patients with AIDS are hospitalized in our wards. In New York City in June 1988, 1,498 acute-care beds were in use citywide for AIDS patients, representing 6 percent of all medical-surgical beds in the city.[15] The need for acute-care beds for AIDS patients will increase to 2,700 by 1991, or 11 percent of the total hospital beds in New York City.[16] Some projections forecast that up to one-third of all beds in New York City will be occupied by AIDS cases by 1991.[17] Projections based on New York City AIDS cases already reported indicate that in 1991 between 7,876 and 11,232 new cases will be diagnosed—possibly more cases in one year than in the first seven years of the epidemic.[18] During this year, there may be 10,000 persons alive with AIDS, and perhaps 100,000 living persons will have AIDS-related illness.

The statistics of epidemiology are human beings with the tears removed. They capture the number of sufferers but not the quality or the weight of the suffering that is being endured, for the fundamental reality of AIDS is that it slowly, prematurely, and with great cruelty robs young men and women of their function, their plans and dreams, and ultimately, their lives. Further, the numbers do not capture the profound effect of the epidemic on health-care workers, who by the nature of their work have been placed in the path of the epidemic.

In my professional routine and that of my colleagues, what was initially an exotic curiosity has now become our daily fare. Among health-care workers, including myself, the initial interest and even clinical excitement about a new disease has long since given way under the weight of the steady, unrelenting procession of new patients. Challenging but disturbing personal and professional ethical issues have surfaced, including the appropriateness of treatment in the terminal stages of illness, the limits of confidentiality of medical information, and even the refusal of some health-care workers to care for patients. A paradoxical comfort and familiarity have set in because the diagnosis and treatment have become so common. A kind of routinization of available technical care has developed, but the systems to provide necessary comprehensive care are not adequately developed or they are faltering. At the beginning I could individualize each AIDS patient's care, but as the numbers have increased, knowing each patient with AIDS personally has become impossible. Gratifyingly, others have joined the ranks and teams of health-care workers now struggle with the myriad complex clinical and social issues that invariably characterize each case. But whatever is put into place is soon obsolete or inadequate. A self-selected core of physicians, nurses, social workers, community volunteers, and others have been drawn to AIDS as a primary professional activity, and many more when called have simply tried as best they could to do their jobs. Increasingly, there is the danger of resignation, futility, and burnout among those on the front lines.

There is a growing sense of anxiety about the future. Yet in the midst of it all and despite personal experience, uniform predictions for increasing numbers of cases, and calls for national and international mobilization,[19] personal, institutional, and societal disbelief persists and the fantasy of a quick and easy solution remains. Planning and provision of resources, particularly human resources, lag behind the pace of new cases. AIDS is now with us for the duration of human history, but this new and now permanent reality in our lives resists acceptance. "How many years do you think it will take to find a cure?" I'm asked repeatedly, rather than "How will we learn to live and manage with AIDS and HIV infection in our midst now and in the future?" Whether society, the health-care system, and health-care workers will effectively adjust to this new reality is unclear. For clinicians, fear of personal jeopardy, related to the risk of HIV transmission, the daily inescapable confrontation with death and dying, and the weariness engendered by overwork, hovers just below the surface. The fear breaks into full view periodically and unquestionably influences caregivers' daily function. Many, particularly those in training, rethink future professional plans. As I watch the caseload increase and the pressures on young doctors, nurses, and social workers mount, I wonder who will care for the huge number of AIDS patients in the future.

To understand the full complexity of medical-care issues confronting the clinician and health-care system, one must understand the clinical course of HIV infection and relate various stages to the array of health-care needs at each point. A familiar epidemiologic concept describes HIV infection or any infectious disease as a pyramid or an iceberg. The visible, symptomatic disease, in this case AIDS, represents only the tip above the surface. The bulk of infection lies below the surface, invisible but potentially of grave danger. Successive layers of increasingly healthy but infected individuals descend from the surface in an ever-widening base. To this epidemiologic image might be added a contiguous iceberg or a pyramid representing the need for clinical care and services. In this image the form is inverted, with the tip of need below the surface and the resource need widening as the illness grows more severe. Thus, although they may represent only a small fraction of people infected, the sickest patients require the greatest number of resources. As infection progresses over time, initially healthy infected individuals become sicker and resource needs increase. The hundreds of thousands of healthy infected individuals at the base of the pyramid now require minimal resources, but as they ascend to the iceberg tip, their care needs will widen beyond our resources.

It is essential to view HIV infection as a chronic viral illness progressing inexorably over time. Within weeks of acquiring HIV infection, a patient may develop a self-limited viral-like illness termed the acute retroviral syndrome.[20] Mostly unrecognized, it may require few resources. Infection then progresses to an asymptomatic stage with or without swollen lymph glands, which may persist for years, perhaps even decades. Technical medical care is usually not necessary, but if blood testing for HIV infection is performed, or if an individual perceives him- or herself to be at risk, severe psychologic symptoms may occur, including anxiety, depression, guilt, and fear of abandonment. In addition, loss of job or other forms of discrimination may occur. Minor medical problems are invariably interpreted as HIV related, and physician or clinic visits may result. Health-care providers must be available to assess clinical status, to counsel and educate about HIV transmission, and to effectively treat psychosocial problems and offer preventive medical services. Community-based organizations, if available, may be of great value here in providing support services.

Later, perhaps five or six years after the acquisition of HIV infection, clinical symptoms may appear. These may be vague and insidious or abrupt in onset, consisting of fevers, malaise, fatigue, weight loss, diarrhea, and skin and mucous-membrane infection. In addition to increased psychologic stress, technical medical needs begin to appear. Physician visits and occasional hospitalizations become necessary. Diagnosis and treatment of both HIV and complicating secondary infections begin. The need for outpatient and inpatient care is accompanied by diminishing independence and sometimes full disability with loss of employment or ability to perform usual functions. Entitlements and arrangements for income, health care, and housing are often necessary.

The next stage in this continuum of infection is the onset of AIDS or more severe symptomatic HIV infection. This is associated with increasing hospitalization need and progressive debilitation. These have averaged 56 days per year per patient at our institution, or 25 percent of an individual's remaining life.[21] Neurologic dysfunction may occur in one-third of the patients and will progress to dementia in many. The array of complex, often invasive technical services for the treatment of infections, cancers, and neurologic complications widens. Home health services, including nursing care, homemaker services, and infusion of medications, may be necessary; and loss of job and housing often results in need for scarce long-term care facilities, and finally, if available, for hospice care. The ability to pay for health-care services or for supporting daily needs such as food and housing melts away as health and energy fail. Usually public facilities and resources, already strained and inadequate, are required.

Certainly in my work over the past twenty years, I've learned that there are other fearful diseases, but AIDS is clearly different and more difficult. Why are the care needs of patients and demands on health-care workers so extraordinary? The reasons are varied. Foremost among these is unquestionably *the nature of the disease itself.* AIDS is an excruciatingly cruel and relentless disease that is invariably fatal. Its repetitive onslaughts and the wasting, disfigurement, neurologic dysfunction, and disability it produces are disturbing. Gaunt, slow in movement, some breathless, others bedridden, AIDS patients increasingly populate the hospital landscape. I find myself looking at healthy young men and women who are well and functioning even after the initial AIDS diagnosis, and like a witness to an all too familiar drama, I see them in my mind's eye months or several years later wasted and suffering, shadows of their present selves.

Second, *the afflicted are mostly young*—men and women in the third and fourth decades of life—a time of productivity and achievement or at least vigor. Although familiar in developing countries, in our society, death on this scale in this age group, except during a war, is something we are not accustomed to. The recurrent scenes of still young parents caring for their sick and debilitated young-adult or infant children and then burying them when they die is not one that fits our worldview. Death belongs to the old, not the young. AIDS causes an inversion of the expected life cycle. For health-care workers, particularly young doctors and nurses, this is especially difficult. Caring for dying young men and women of a similar age makes identification unavoidable and confrontation with their own mortality and vulnerability inescapable.

Third, all this is not a collection of isolated events but *an epidemic* of death and dying among the young. In areas like New York City, the numbers alone are both numbing and overwhelming. The experience is not one of an occasional dying young man with leukemia or a young woman mangled in an automobile accident. It is dozens and dozens of young men and women, in an increasing torrent over a very short period of time.

Fourth, there is a continuing *fear of transmission* among most members of our society, among health-care workers in particular. Although the risk to health-care workers is reassuringly low,[22] it is not zero. Measures exist to reduce the risk further, but there is no doubt that inadvertent, accidental injury may occur and cause infection. Made more frightening by being placed in daily contact with suffering people with HIV infection, this fear is constant among health-care workers, but mostly hidden.[23] It is essential to be sensitive to and understanding of health-care workers' fears and not to harshly condemn them. "To assume that health-care professionals need only a statistical appreciation of risk to assume the mantle of professional virtue in caring for AIDS patients is to deny their humanity."[24]

"I see something in the back of my throat and I'm sure it's thrush. I must have AIDS." A young intern accosted me in panic earlier this year. I examined him and explored his history. I was convinced it was a minor sore throat and not thrush, a throat infection characteristic of HIV, and that he was not at risk for and had not acquired AIDS, but it was impossible to dispel his panic. It was only after his HIV antibody test turned out to be negative two weeks later that he was able to resume functioning normally.

Another young doctor appeared unexpectedly at my office early one morning: "I slashed my hand last night with a needle while I was doing a spinal tap on a woman with a history of IV drug use. I can't think straight. I couldn't sleep all night. What should I do? What should I tell my wife?" Although his test eventually turned out negative as well, it took months before he could definitely be told that he was not infected with HIV. He continued to work, but like so many others at risk, lived in fear until his final negative test result came back.

Paradoxically, I still see young doctors preferring to deny that they may be at risk and not wearing gloves as they draw blood from patients with AIDS. The flip side of their fear of infection is to deny it completely and thereby put themselves at greater risk. After seven years of working with AIDS patients, knowing well the minimal statistical risks, I must admit that I remain frightened. When I notice a blemish on my skin, I can't help wondering if it could be Kaposi's sarcoma. I still interpret minor illness in myself as the beginning of the "expected" HIV infection although rationally I know better. The essential position for me and for other health-care workers is to recognize the fear but to act on the reassuring fact that the incidence of transmission is low. It is necessary to be sensitive and understanding of these fears among health-care workers, but we must be clear about our expectations in the AIDS epidemic. Although doctors have fled plagues in the past,[25] we cannot condone such behavior.

The risk of HIV acquisition is substantially less than for other infectious diseases such as tuberculosis, yellow fever, cholera, and plague. Further, we have the advantage of understanding routes of transmission, virology, and disease etiology. To deny or compromise the treatment of any patient on the ground that a medical risk is posed to the provider is to break the fundamental trust between patient and caregiver and between caregiver and society. Nevertheless, some have chosen not to give care. The difficulty is that the refusal is often subtle. It is passive and not overt and hard to identify. Mostly among some surgeons and others who perform "invasive" procedures, it takes the form of avoidance rather than refusal: "I don't think surgery—or a bronchoscopy—is necessary in this patient. Let's try antibiotics first and not operate."

Frustrating and difficult to combat, this behavior, in my experience, has been the exception and not the rule among most other health-care workers. Whereas for some health-care workers special risks may exist, these have not been documented and are not unique. Blood-bank and laboratory workers, obstetricians and midwives, interns and nurses are also exposed and for the most part have quietly and without complaint (although not without fear) done their jobs. In fact, although we concentrate on concern about health-care workers' refusal to care for AIDS patients, the predominant response is a remarkable story of personal and professional behavior of the highest standards. Tens of thousands of health-care workers—mostly young, vulnerable, and at the start of their careers—have faced the panic and their own personal discomfort and fears head on and have exemplified the very best in human and professional behavior. In many ways these are the unsung heroes and heroines of the AIDS epidemic.

AIDS is different from other diseases for a fifth reason. AIDS is deeply *rooted in our views of the social worth of individuals and the acceptability of behavior.* From the outset AIDS has been associated with illicit intimacy—it is a "dirty disease." For many, it remains a disease of homosexuals and intravenous drug users and is thereby bound to intimate behavior not felt to be acceptable. There is a related intolerance or at best unfamiliarity and lack of understanding of differences in race, ethnicity, and social class that characterizes the present demography of AIDS. This view has been enhanced inadvertently by the designation of persons with AIDS into "risk groups." Although useful for epidemiologic surveillance purposes, this designation creates the illusion that nonmembership in an arbitrarily defined and seemingly homogenous group conveys protection. HIV transmission is the result of specific behaviors, not group identity. There is further belief that most of the infected have brought their illness on themselves and are therefore unworthy of compassion. It's a "blame the victim" mentality. Finally, there is a temptation to behave differently toward certain individuals with HIV infection than toward others. Infants, hemophiliacs, and transfusion recipients are characterized as "innocent victims" or "blameless," thereby implying that others infected with HIV are "guilty" and "blamable."

It is assumed that all those infected through drug use or sexual activity acquired infection willfully and knowingly. However, HIV was widely disseminated among homosexual men and intravenous drug users in the early 1980s before its existence was known. In addition, since those at risk are concerned about their health and future, many have reduced their risk of acquiring HIV. Motivated by fear of HIV acquisition, substantial reduction in risk behavior has been reported not only among homosexual men but also among intravenous drug users in recent years.[26] But even if this was not the case (and for the individual patient, it may not be) the issue of blame is irrelevant. So much of the illness we treat has its roots in behavior, and the behaviors that result in transmission of HIV are ubiquitous—sex and drug use. Sexually transmitted diseases have always been surrounded by disapproval and stigma, and intravenous drug use and its associated medical illnesses have received even greater reproach. Illicit intravenous drug use is criminal and results in serious health risks but in many respects is not dissimilar from alcohol abuse, cigarette smoking, and the abuse of diazepam (Valium) or other drugs we prescribe and administer.

Only a theoretical and abstract perspective makes blaming the victim easy. It is more difficult when one personally witnesses the suffering endured by AIDS patients and their loved ones and appreciates their courage in the face of this final adversity.

Most of the patients with AIDS treated at my institution have been intravenous drug users. They have the reputation of being difficult, frustrating patients. Engaged in an illegal activity, secretive in their behavior, and rarely having an established, ongoing relationship with a health-care provider, many intravenous drug users elicit disapproval from health-care workers and, in turn, are distrustful and expect judgmental treatment. I have found that when treated with attention to their medical needs in a straightforward, clinical manner, most intravenous drug users can be disarmingly open about their life-style and no more or less difficult than other patients. The essential point is that each person, intravenous drug user or otherwise, is unique and does not comfortably conform to a stereotype.

Instead of blaming the victim, it would be more constructive to examine the societal conditions that promote unhealthy risk-taking behavior and ask who is responsible for them. This is particularly true for intravenous drug use. It is not a matter of chance that rates of intravenous drug use are highest among poor minorities in the inner city. Illicit intravenous drug use is grounded in and the product of hopelessness. It is engrafted on unemployment, poverty, racism, and depression. Without doubt, it is perpetuated by greed and corruption at many levels in our society. It should be seen as a personal and societal symptom of deeper unaddressed ills. The final common pathway may lead to the intravenous drug user on the streets of the South Bronx and Harlem, but the genesis of drug use can be traced back through many levels of our society. Although certainly responsible for his or her own actions, the drug user is also the victim of powerful, disturbing, unconscionable social forces and conditions. In a sense, drug abuse heralds many of the unaddressed problems of this society, which have now come to haunt us in the form of the AIDS epidemic.

Intravenous drug use should be viewed as a medical and societal illness. It has remained refractory to efforts to eliminate it, which have largely been punitive and directed by law-enforcement agencies. Instead of insisting on cure or complete abstinence, we should seek reduction in the amount and frequency of drug use and advocate safer drug-use practices. A medical model of treatment should be our goal for all drug users. It remains a disturbing paradox that in the face of the AIDS epidemic we are able to provide specific treatment for no more than 10 percent of those actively using illicit drugs and we have been unwilling to mount programs that may make drug use safer.

Instead of blaming the victim, we would serve society better by talking openly about all risky behaviors, advocating broader and targeted education about the risks of unhealthy behavior, and providing treatment for those in need.

Finally, AIDS is different because *it forces us, particularly those of us who are physicians, to confront our own vulnerability and inability to substantially alter the power and force of natural events.* Trained during the decades since World War II and in the era of antibiotics and other interventions, most physicians believe that they can cure most diseases. Certainly they were taught to believe this in the field of infectious diseases, my own specialty. The administration of an appropriately chosen antibiotic could remarkably reverse the course of a virulent illness. A decade earlier while working in Africa, I learned that even with potent antibiotics, the social and environmental conditions that breed infection conspire to produce it again—that antibiotics are potent and magical but limited. We are now learning that lesson in this society as well. Most serious illness in our society is the result of chronic and not acute disease and is not amenable to seemingly magical technical interventions. Nevertheless, we still *believe* that the goal of our endeavors should be to cure and that anything less is failure. AIDS assaults this belief and this unrealistic goal and creates the uncomfortable feeling of inadequacy and failure in physicians. Although the goal of curing is of course paramount, the parallel ethic of prolonging life, improving the quality of life, and alleviating suffering is more realistic and appropriate. With these as goals, we can feel somewhat successful in treating most AIDS patients and people infected with HIV.

Notes

I am indebted to countless patients and their families and loved ones, who at a time of great adversity have brought me closest to what is essential: courage, humility, and doing what needs to be done. I am grateful to my colleagues at Montefiore Medical Center for their dedication, competence, support, and generosity of spirit and to Ms. Lucy Carrion for her expert secretarial assistance.

1. From Albert Camus, *The Plague*, trans. Stuart Gilbert (New York: Alfred A. Knopf, 1983).

2. F. Barre-Sinoussi, J. C. Chermann, F. Rey, et al., "Isolation of a T-Lymphotropic Retrovirus from a Patient at Risk for the Acquired Immunodeficiency Syndrome (AIDS)," *Science* 220 (4599) (1983):868–71; and R. Gallo, S. Z. Salahuddin, and M.

Popovic, "Frequent Detection and Isolation of Cytopathic Retroviruses (HTLVIII) from Patients with AIDS and at Risk for AIDS," *Science* 224 (April 1984):500–503.

3. G. H. Friedland and R. S. Klein, "Transmission of the Human Immunodeficiency Virus," *New England Journal of Medicine* 317 (October 1987):1125–35.

4. Centers for Disease Control, "Human Immunodeficiency Virus Infection in the Untied States: A Review of Current Knowledge," *Morbidity and Mortality Weekly Report* 36 (1987):5–6.

5. Centers for Disease Control, "Classification System for Human T-Lymphotropic-Associated Virus Infections," *Morbidity and Mortality Weekly Report* 35 (1986):334–39.

6. A. Glatt, K. Chirgwin, and S. Landesman, "Treatment of Infections Associated with Human Immunodeficiency Virus," *New England Journal of Medicine* 318 (June 1988):1439–48; and S. Broder and A. Fauci, "Progress in Drug Therapies for HIV Infection," *Public Health Reports* 225 (May–June 1988):224–28.

7. Institute of Medicine and National Academy of Sciences, *Confronting AIDS, Directions for Public Health, Health Care and Research* (Washington, D.C.: National Academy Press, 1986); and Institute of Medicine and National Academy of Sciences, *Confronting AIDS, Update 1988* (Washington, D.C.: National Academy Press, 1988).

8. *Assuring Care of New York City AIDS Population* (New York: Mayor's Task Force on AIDS, September 1988); *New York City Strategic Plan for AIDS* (New York: Interagency Task Force on AIDS, May 1988); *Report of the Presidential Commission on the Human Immunodeficiency Virus Epidemic* (Washington, D.C., June 1988); and P. Piot, F. Plummer, and F. Mhala, "AIDS: An International Perspective," *Science* 239 (February 1988):573–79.

9. AIDS Surveillance Unit, *AIDS Surveillance Update* (New York: New York City Department of Health, 28 September 1988).

10. AIDS Program, *AIDS Weekly Surveillance Report* (Atlanta, Ga.: Centers for Disease Control, September 1988).

11. J. M. Mann, J. Chin, P. Piot, and T. Quinn, "The International Epidemiology of AIDS," *Scientific American* 259 (4) (October 1988):82–89.

12. Ibid.

13. B. R. Saltzman, G. H. Friedland, R. S. Klein, J. Vileno, K. Freeman, and L. K. Schrager, "Factors that Predict Survival of AIDS Patients, Experience at a Single New York City Medical Center," Fourth International Conference on AIDS, Stockholm, June 1988.

14. N. A. Hessol, G. W. Rutherford, A. R. Lifson, P. M. O'Malley, L. S. Doll, W. W. Darrow, H. W. Jaffe, and D. Werdegar, "The Natural History of HIV Infection in a Cohort of Homosexual Men: A Decade of Followup," Fourth International Conference on AIDS, Stockholm, June 1988.

15. *New York City Strategic Plan for AIDS.*

16. *Assuring Care of New York City AIDS Population.*

17. M. Alderman, E. Drucker, A. Rosenfield, and C. Healton, "Predicting the Future of the AIDS Epidemic and Its Consequences for the Health Care System of New York City," *Bulletin of the New York Academy of Medicine* 14 (March 1988): 175–83.

18. *New York City Strategic Plan for AIDS.*

19. *Confronting AIDS, Directions for Public Health, Health Care and Research*; *Confronting AIDS, Update 1988*; *Report of the Presidential Commission on the Human Immunodeficiency Virus Epidemic*; and Mann, Chin, Piot and Quinn.

20. "Classification System for Human T-Lymphotropic-Associated Virus Infections."

21. Alderman, Drucker, Rosenfield, and Healton.

22. Friedland and Klein; and "Recommendations for Prevention of HIV Transmission in Health-Care Settings," *Morbidity and Mortality Weekly Report* 36 (2S) (1987):35–18S.

23. R. N. Link, A. R. Feingold, M. H. Charap, K. Freeman, and S. P. Shelov, "Concerns of Medical and Pediatric House Officers About Acquiring AIDS from their Patients," *American Journal of Public Health* 78 (April 1988):455–59.

24. *Update 1988*.

25. A. Zuger and S. H. Miles, "Physicians, AIDS, and Occupational Risk: Historic Traditions and Ethical Obligations," *Journal of the American Medical Association* 258 (October 1987):14; and J. K. Kim, and J. R. Perfect, "To Help the Sick: A Historical and Ethical Essay Concerning the Refusal to Care for Patients with AIDS," *American Journal of Medicine* 84 (January 1988):135–38.

26. P. S. Selwyn, C. Feiner, C. Cox, S. Lipshultz, and R. Cohen, "Knowledge About AIDS and High Risk Behavior Among IV Drug Users in New York," *AIDS* 1 (October 1987):247–54.

13 The Ritual Drama of Mutual Pretense

Barney G. Glaser and Anselm L. Strauss

BARNEY GLASER and ANSELM STRAUSS are sociologists in the symbolic interactionist tradition. Among their books are *Time for Dying* and *Awareness of Dying*, the book from which this selection is taken. This book is based on ethnographic research conducted in several hospitals in the San Francisco Bay Area, focusing on the social organization of care for the dying. The mutual pretense awareness context described in this article is one of four awareness contexts discussed in the book, the other three being closed awareness, suspicion awareness, and open awareness. The mutual pretense awareness context is one in which the patient and the caregiver (or family member) both know that the patient is dying, but both interact as if they are unaware of this. The authors explore how mutual pretense is initiated, why it is initiated, and some of the consequences.

WHEN PATIENT AND STAFF BOTH KNOW that the patient is dying but pretend otherwise—when both agree to act as if he were going to live—then a context of mutual pretense exists. Either party can initiate his share of the context; it ends when one side cannot, or will not, sustain the pretense any longer.

The mutual-pretense awareness context is perhaps less visible, even to its participants . . . because the interaction involved tends to be more subtle. On some hospital services, however, it is the predominant context. One nurse who worked on an intensive care unit remarked about an unusual patient who had announced he was going to die: "I haven't had to cope with this very often. I may know they are going to die, and the patient knows it, but (usually) he's just not going to let you know that he knows."

Once we visited a small Catholic hospital where medical and nursing care for the many dying patients was efficiently organized. The staff members were supported in their difficult work by a powerful philosophy—that they were doing everything possible for the patient's comfort—but generally did not talk with patients about death. This setting brought about frequent mutual pretense. This awareness context is also predominant in such settings as county hospitals, where elderly patients of low socioeconomic status are sent to die; patient and staff are well aware of imminent death but each tends to go silently about his own business.[1] Yet, as we shall see, sometimes the mutual pretense context is neither silent nor unnegotiated.

The same kind of ritual pretense is enacted in many situations apart from illness. A charming example occurs when a child announces that he is now a storekeeper, and that his mother should buy something at his store. To carry out his fiction, delicately cooperative action is required. The mother must play seriously, and when the episode has run its natural course, the child will often close it himself with a rounding-off gesture, or it may be concluded by an intruding outside event or by the mother. Quick analysis of this little game of pretense suggests that either player can begin; that the other must then play properly; that realistic (nonfictional) action will destroy the illusion and end the game; that the specific action of the game must develop during interaction; and that eventually the make-believe ends or is ended. Little familial games or dramas of this kind tend to be continual, though each episode may be brief.

For contrast, here is another example that pertains to both children and adults. At the circus, when a clown appears, all but the youngest children know that the clown is not real. But both he and his audience must participate, if only symbolically, in the pretense that he is a clown. The onlookers need do no more than appreciate the clown's act, but if they remove themselves too far, by examining the clown's technique too closely, let's say, then the illusion will be shattered. The clown must also do his best to sustain the illusion by clever acting, by not playing too far "out of character." Ordinarily nobody addresses him as if he were other than the character he is pretending to be. That is, everybody takes him seriously, at face value. And unless particular members return to see the circus again, the clown's performance occurs only once, beginning and ending according to a prearranged schedule.

Our two simple examples of pretense suggest some important features of the particular awareness context to which we shall devote this [discussion]. The make-believe in which patient and hospital staff engage resembles the child's game much more than the clown's act. It has no institutionalized beginning and ending comparable to the entry and departure of the clown; either the patient or the staff must signal the beginning of their joint pretense. Both parties must act properly if the pretense is to be maintained, because, as in the child's game, the illusion created is fragile, and easily shattered by incongruous "realistic" acts. But if either party slips slightly, the other may pretend to ignore the slip.[2] Each episode between the patient and a staff member tends to be brief, but the mutual pretense is done with terrible seriousness, for the stakes are very high.[3]

INITIATING THE PRETENSE

This particular awareness context cannot exist, of course, unless both the patient and staff are aware that he is dying. Therefore all the structural conditions which contribute to the existence of open awareness (and which are absent in closed and suspicion awareness) contribute also to the existence of mutual pretense. In addition, at least one interactant must indicate a desire to pretend that the patient is not dying and the other must agree to the pretense, acting accordingly.

A prime structural condition in the existence and maintenance of mutual pretense is that unless the patient initiates conversation about his impending death, no staff member is required to talk about it with him. As typical Americans, they are unlikely to initiate such conversation; and as professionals they have no rules commanding them to talk about death with the patient, unless he desires it. In turn, he may wish to initiate such conversation, but surely neither hospital rules nor common convention urges it upon him. Consequently, unless either the aware patient or the staff members break the silence by words or gestures, a mutual pretense rather than an open awareness context will exist; as, for example, when the physician does not care to talk about death, and the patient does not press the issue though he clearly does recognize his terminality.

The patient, of course, is more likely than the staff members to refer openly to his death, thereby inviting them, explicitly or implicitly, to respond in kind. If they seem unwilling, he may decide they do not wish to confront openly the fact of his death, and then he may, out of tact or genuine empathy for their embarrassment or distress, keep his silence. He may misinterpret their responses, of course, but . . . he probably has correctly read their reluctance to refer openly to his impending death.

Staff members, in turn, may give him opportunities to speak of his death, if they deem it wise, without their directly or obviously referring to the topic. But if he does not care to act or talk as if he were dying, then they will support his pretense. In doing so, they have, in effect, accepted a complementary assignment of status—they will act with pretense toward his pretense. (If they have misinterpreted his reluctance to act openly, then they have assigned, rather than accepted, a complementary status.)

Two related professional rationales permit them to engage in the pretense. One is that if the patient wishes to pretend, it may well be best for his health, and if and when the pretense finally fails him, all concerned can act more realistically. A secondary rationale is that perhaps they can give him better medical and nursing care if they do not have to face him so openly. In addition, as noted earlier, they can rely on common tact to justify their part in the pretense. Ordinarily, Americans believe that any individual may live—and die—as he chooses, so long as he does not interfere with others' activities, or, in this case, so long as proper care can be given him.

To illustrate the way these silent bargains are initiated and maintained, we quote from an interview with a special nurse. She had been assigned to a patient before he became terminal, and she was more apt than most personnel to encourage his talking openly, because as a graduate student in a nursing class that emphasized psychological care, she had more time to spend with her patient than a regular floor nurse. Here is the exchange between interviewer and nurse:

INTERVIEWER: Did he talk about his cancer or his dying?

NURSE: Well, no he never talked about it. I never heard him use the word cancer . . .

INTERVIEWER: Did he indicate that he knew he was dying?

NURSE: Well, I got that impression, yes . . . It wasn't really openly, but I think the day that his roommate said he should get up and start walking, I felt that he was a little bit antagonistic. He said what his condition was, that he felt very, very ill that moment.

INTERVIEWER: He never talked about leaving the hospital?

NURSE: Never.

INTERVIEWER: Did he talk about his future at all?

NURSE: Not a thing. I never heard a word . . .

INTERVIEWER: You said yesterday that he was more or less isolated, because the nurses felt that he was hostile. But they have dealt with patients like this many many times. You said they stayed away from him?

NURSE: Well, I think at the very end. You see, this is what I meant by isolation . . . we don't communicate with them. I didn't, except when I did things for him. I think you expect somebody to respond to, and if they're very ill we don't . . . I talked it over with my instructor, mentioning things that I could probably have done; for instance, this isolation, I should have communicated with him . . .

INTERVIEWER: You think that since you knew he was going to die, and you half suspected that he knew it too, or more than half; do you think that this understanding grew between you in any way?

NURSE: I believe so . . . I think it's kind of hard to say but when I came in the room, even when he was very ill, he'd rather look at me and try to give me a smile, and gave me the impression that he accepted . . . I think this is one reason why I feel I should have communicated with him . . . and this is why I feel he was rather isolated . . .

From the nurse's account, it is difficult to tell whether the patient wished to talk openly about his death, but was rebuffed; or whether he initiated the pretense and the nurse accepted his decision. But it is remarkable how a patient can flash cues to the staff about his own dread knowledge, inviting the staff to talk about his destiny, while the nurses and physicians decide that it is better not to talk too openly with him about his condition lest he "go to pieces." The patient, as remarked earlier, picks up these signals of unwillingness, and the mutual pretense context has been initiated. A specific and obvious instance is this: an elderly patient, who had lived a full and satisfying life, wished to round it off by talking about his impending death. The nurses retreated before this prospect, as did his wife, reproving him, saying he should not think or talk about morbid matters. A hospital chaplain finally intervened, first by listening to the patient himself, then by inducing the nurses and the wife to do likewise, or at least to acknowledge more openly that the man was dying. He was not successful with all the nurses.

The staff members are more likely to sanction a patient's pretense than his family's. The implicit rule is that though the patient need not be forced to speak of his dying, or to act as if he were dying, his kin should face facts. After all, they will have to live with the facts after his death. Besides, staff members usually find it less difficult to talk about dying with the family. Family members are not inevitably drawn into open discussion, but the likelihood is high, particularly since they themselves are likely to initiate discussion or at least to make gestures of awareness.

Sometimes, however, pretense protects the family member temporarily against too much grief, and the staff members against too immediate a scene. This may occur when a relative has just learned about the impending death and the nurse controls the ensuing scene by initiating temporary pretense. The reverse situation also occurs: a newly arrived nurse discovers the patient's terminality, and the relative smooths over the nurse's distress by temporary pretense.

THE PRETENSE INTERACTION

An intern whom we observed during our fieldwork suspected that the patient he was examining had cancer, but he could not discover where it was located. The patient previously had been told that she probably had cancer, and she was now at this teaching hospital for that reason. The intern's examination went on for some time. Yet neither he nor she spoke about what he was searching for, nor in any way suggested that she might be dying. We mention this episode to contrast it with the more extended interactions with which this [selection] is concerned. These have an episodic quality—personnel enter and leave the patient's room, or he occasionally emerges and encounters them—but their extended duration means that special effort is required to prevent their breaking down, and that the interactants must work hard to construct and maintain their mutual pretense. By contrast, in a formally staged play, although the actors have to construct and maintain a performance, making it credible to their audience, they are not required to write the script themselves. The situation that involves a terminal patient is much more like a masquerade party, where one masked actor plays carefully to another as long as they are together, and the total drama actually emerges from their joint creative effort.

A masquerade, however, has more extensive resources to sustain it than those the hospital situation provides. Masqueraders wear masks, hiding their facial expressions; even if they "break up" with silent laughter (as a staff member may "break down" with sympathy), this fact is concealed. Also, according to the rules ordinarily governing masquerades, each actor chooses his own status, his "character," and this makes his role in the constructed drama somewhat easier to play. He may even have played similar parts before. But terminal patients usually have had no previous experience with their pretended status, and not all personnel have had much experience. In a masquerade, when the drama fails it can be broken off, each actor moving along to another partner; but in the hospital the pretenders (especially the patient) have few comparable opportunities.

Both situations share one feature—the extensive use of props for sustaining the crucial illusion. In the masquerade, the props include not only masks but clothes and other costuming, as well as the setting where the masquerade takes place. In the hospital interaction, props also abound. Patients dress for the part of not-dying patient, including careful attention to grooming, and to hair and makeup by female patients. The terminal patient may also fix up his room so that it looks and feels "just like home," an activity that supports his enactment of normalcy. Nurses may respond to these props with explicit appreciation—"how lovely your hair looks this morning"—even help to establish them, as by doing the patient's hair. We remember one elaborate pretense ritual involving a husband and wife who had won the nurses' sympathy. The husband simply would not recognize that his already comatose wife was approaching death, so each morning the nurses carefully prepared her for his visit, dressing her for the occasion and making certain that she looked as beautiful as possible.

The staff, of course, has its own props to support its ritual prediction that the patient is going to get well: thermometers, baths, fresh sheets, and meals on time! Each party utilizes these props as he sees fit, thereby helping to create the pretense anew. But when a patient wishes to demonstrate that he is finished with life, he may drive the nurses wild by refusing to cooperate in the daily routines of hospital life—that is, he refuses to allow the nurses to use their props. Conversely, when the personnel wish to indicate how things are with him, they may begin to omit some of those routines.

During the pretense episodes, both sides play according to the rules implicit in the interaction. Although neither the staff nor patient may recognize these rules as such, certain tactics are fashioned around them, and the action is partly constrained by them. One rule is that dangerous topics should generally be avoided. The most obviously dangerous topic is the patient's death; another is events that will happen afterwards. Of course, both parties to the pretense are supposed to follow the avoidance rule.

There is, however, a qualifying rule: Talk about dangerous topics is permissible as long as neither party breaks down. Thus, a patient refers to the distant future, as if it were his to talk about. He talks about his plans for his family, as if he would be there to share their consummation. He and the nurses discuss today's events—such as his treatments—as if they had implications for a real future, when he will have recovered from his illness. And some of his brave or foolhardy activities may signify a brave show of pretense, as when he bathes himself or insists on tottering to the toilet by himself. The staff in turn permits his activity. (Two days before he returned to the hospital to die, one patient insisted that his wife allow him to travel downtown to keep a speaking engagement, and to the last he kept up a lively conversation with a close friend about a book they were planning to write together.)

A third rule, complementing the first two, is that each actor should focus determinedly on appropriately safe topics. It is customary to talk about the daily routines—eating (the food was especially good or bad), and sleeping (whether one slept well or poorly last night). Complaints and their management help pass the time. So do minor personal confidences, and chatter about events on the ward. Talk about physical symptoms is safe enough if confined to the symptoms themselves, with no implied references to death. A terminal patient and a staff member may safely talk, and at length, about his disease so long as they skirt its fatal significance. And there are many genuinely safe topics having to do with movies and movie stars, politics, fashions—with everything, in short, that signifies that life is going on "as usual."

A fourth interactional rule is that when something happens, or is said, that tends to expose the fiction that both parties are attempting to sustain, then each must pretend that nothing has gone awry. Just as each has carefully avoided calling attention to the true situation, each now must avert his gaze from the unfortunate intrusion. Thus, a nurse may take special pains to announce herself before entering a patient's room so as not to surprise him at his crying. If she finds him crying she may ignore it or convert it into an innocuous event with a skillful comment or gesture—much like the tactful gentleman who, having stumbled upon a woman in his bathtub, is said to have casually closed the bathroom door, murmuring, "Pardon me, sir." The mutuality of the pretense is illustrated by the way a patient who cannot control a sudden expression of great pain will verbally discount its significance, while the nurse in turn goes along with his pretense. Or she may brush aside or totally ignore a major error in his portrayal, as when he refers spontaneously to his death. If he is tempted to admit impulsively his terminality, she may, again, ignore his impulsive remarks or obviously misinterpret them. Thus, pretense is piled upon pretense to conceal or minimize interactional slips.

Clearly then, each party to the ritual pretense shares responsibility for maintaining it. The major responsibility may be transferred back and forth, but each party must support the other's temporary dominance in his own action. This is true even when conversation is absolutely minimal, as in some hospitals where patients take no particular pains to signal awareness of their terminality, and the staff makes no special gestures to convey its own awareness. The pretense interaction in this case is greatly simplified, but it is still discernible. Whenever a staff member is so indelicate, or so straightforward, as to act openly as if a terminal patient were dying, or if the patient does so himself, then the pretense vanishes. If neither wishes to destroy the fiction, however, then each must strive to keep the situation "normal."[4]

THE TRANSITION TO OPEN AWARENESS

A mutual pretense context that is not sustained can only change to an open awareness context. (Either party, however, may again initiate the pretense context and sometimes get cooperation from the other.) The change can be sudden, when either patient or staff distinctly conveys that he has permanently abandoned the pretense. Or the change to the open context can be gradual: nurses, and relatives, too, are familiar with patients who admit to terminality more openly on some days than they do on other days, when pretense is dominant, until finally pretense vanishes altogether. Sometimes the physician skillfully paces his interaction with a patient, leading the patient finally to refer openly to his terminality and to leave behind the earlier phase of pretense.

Pretense generally collapses when certain conditions make its maintenance increasingly difficult. These conditions have been foreshadowed in our previous discussion. Thus, when the patient cannot keep from expressing his increasing pain, or his suffering grows to the point that he is kept under heavy sedation, then the enactment of pretense becomes more difficult, especially for him.

Again, neither patient nor staff may be able to avoid bringing impending death into the open if radical physical deterioration sets in, the staff because it has a tough job to do, and the patient for other reasons, including fright and panic. Sometimes a patient breaks his pretense for psychological reasons, as when he discovers that he cannot face death alone, or when a chaplain convinces him that it is better to bring things out into the open than to remain silent. (Sometimes, however, a patient may find such a sympathetic listener in the chaplain that he can continue his pretense with other personnel.) Sometimes he breaks the pretense when it no longer makes sense in light of obvious physical deterioration.

Here is a poignant episode during which a patient dying with great pain and obvious bodily deterioration finally abandoned her pretense with a nurse:

> *There was a long silence. Then the patient asked, "After I get home from the nursing home will you visit me?" I asked if she wanted me to. "Yes, Mary, you know we could go on long drives together . . ." She had a faraway look in her eyes as if daydreaming about all the places she would visit and all the things we could do together. This continued for some time. Then I asked, "Do you think you will be able to drive your car again?" She looked at me, "Mary, I know I am daydreaming; I know I am going to die." Then she cried, and said, "This is terrible, I never thought I would be this way."*

In short, when a patient finds it increasingly difficult to hang onto a semblance of his former healthy self and begins to become a person who is visibly dying, both he and the staff are increasingly prone to say so openly, whether by word or gesture. Sometimes, however, a race occurs between a patient's persistent pretense and his becoming comatose or his actual death—a few more days of sentience or life, and either he or the staff would have dropped the pretense.

Yet a contest may ensue when only one side wishes to keep up the pretense. When a patient openly displays his awareness but shows it unacceptably, as by apathetically "giving up," the staff or family may try to reinstate the pretense. Usually the patient then insists on open recognition of his own impending death, but sometimes he is persuaded to return to the pretense. For instance, one patient finally wished to talk openly about death, but her husband argued against its probability, although he knew better; so after several attempts to talk openly, the patient obligingly gave up the contest. The reverse situation may also occur: the nurses begin to give the patient every opportunity to die with a maximum of comfort—as by cutting down on normal routines—thus signaling that he should no longer pretend, but the patient insists on putting up a brave show and so the nurses capitulate.

We would complicate our analysis unduly if we did more than suggest that, under such conditions, the pretense ritual sometimes resembles Ptolemy's cumbersomely patched astronomical system, with interactants pretending to pretend to pretend! We shall only add that when nurses attempt to change the pretense context into an open context, they generally do this "on their own" and not because of any calculated ward standards or specific orders from an attending physician. And the tactics they use to get the patient to refer openly to his terminality are less tried and true than the more customary tactics for forcing him to pretend.

CONSEQUENCES OF MUTUAL PRETENSE

For the patient, the pretense context can yield a measure of dignity and considerable privacy, though it may deny him the closer relationships with staff members and family members that sometimes occur when he allows them to participate in his open acceptance of death. And if they initiate and he accepts the pretense, he may have nobody with whom to talk although he might profit greatly from talk. (One terminal patient told a close friend, who told us, that when her family and husband insisted on pretending that she would recover, she suffered from the isolation, feeling as if she were trapped in cotton batting.) For the family—especially more distant kin—the pretense context can minimize embarrassment and other interactional strains; but for closer kin, franker concourse may have many advantages. . . . Oscillation between contexts of open awareness and mutual pretense can also cause interactional strains. We once observed a man persuading his mother to abandon her apathy—she had permanently closed her eyes, to the staff's great distress—and "try hard to live." She agreed finally to resume the pretense, but later relapsed into apathy. The series of episodes caused some anguish to both family and patient, as well as to the nurses. When the patient initiates the mutual pretense, staff members are likely to feel relieved. Yet the consequent stress of either maintaining the pretense or changing it to open awareness sometimes may be considerable. Again, both the relief and the stress affect nurses more than medical personnel, principally because the latter spend less time with patients.

But whether staff or patient initiates the ritual of pretense, maintaining it creates a characteristic ward mood of cautious serenity. A nurse once told us of a cancer hospital where each patient understood that everyone there had cancer, including himself, but the rules of tact, buttressed by staff silence, were so strong that few patients talked openly about anyone's condition. The consequent atmosphere was probably less serene than when only a few patients are engaged in mutual pretense, but even one such patient can affect the organizational mood, especially if the personnel become "involved" with him.

A persistent context of mutual pretense profoundly affects the more permanent aspects of hospital organization as well. (This often occurs at county and city hospitals.) Imagine what a hospital service would be like if all terminal patients were unacquainted with their terminality, or if all were perfectly open about their awareness—whether they accepted or rebelled against their fate.[5] When closed awareness generally prevails the personnel must guard against disclosure, but they need not organize themselves as a team to handle continued pretense and its sometimes stressful breakdown. Also, a chief organizational consequence of the mutual pretense context is that it eliminates any possibility that staff members might "work with" patients psychologically, on a self-conscious professional basis. This consequence was strikingly evident at the small Catholic hospital referred to a few pages ago. It is also entirely possible that a ward mood of tension can be set when (as a former patient once told us) a number of elderly dying patients continually communicate to each other their willingness to die, but the staff members persistently insist on the pretense that the patients are going to recover. On the other hand, the prevailing ward mood accompanying mutual pretense tends to be more serene—or at least less obviously tense—than when open suspicion awareness is dominant.

Notes

1. Robert Kastenbaum has reported that at Cushing Hospital, "a Public Medical Institution for the care and custody of the elderly" in Framingham, Massachusetts, "patient and staff members frequently have an implicit mutual understanding with regard to death . . . institutional dynamics tend to operate against making death 'visible' and a subject of open communication. . . . Elderly patients often behave as though they appreciated the unspoken feelings of the staff members and were attempting to make their demise as acceptable and unthreatening as possible." This observation is noted in Robert Kastenbaum, "The Interpersonal Context of Death in a Geriatric Institution," abstract of paper presented at the Seventeenth Annual Scientific Meeting, Gerontological Society (Minneapolis: October 29–31, 1964).

2. I. Bensman and I. Garver, "Crime and Punishment in the Factory," in A. Gouldner and H. Gouldner (eds.), *Modern Society* (New York: Harcourt, Brace and World, 1963), pp. 593–96.

3. A German communist, Alexander Weissberg, accused of spying during the great period of Soviet spy trials, has written a fascinating account of how he and many other accused persons collaborated with the Soviet government in an elaborate pretense, carried on for the benefit of the outside world. The stakes were high for the accused (their lives) as well as for the Soviet. Weissberg's narrative also illustrated how uninitiated interactants must be coached into their roles and how they must be cued into the existence of the pretense context where they do not recognize it. See Alexander Weissberg, *The Accused* (New York: Simon and Schuster, 1951).

4. A close reading of John Gunther's poignant account of his young son's last months shows that the boy maintained a sustained and delicately balanced mutual pretense with his parents, physicians and nurses. John Gunther, *Death Be Not Proud* (New York: Harper and Bros., 1949). Also see Bensman and Garver, *op. cit.*

5. For a description of a research hospital where open awareness prevails, with far-reaching effects on hospital social structure, see Renée Fox, *Experiment Perilous* (New York: Free Press of Glencoe, 1959).

14 Death, Uses of a Corpse, and Social Worth ❧

David Sudnow

DAVID SUDNOW has served on the faculty at the University of California at Irvine and at Brooklyn College. He has written a number of books, including *Ways of the Hand*, *Pilgrim in the Microworld*, and *Passing On*, the book from which our selection is taken. *Passing On* presents an ethnographic study of the social organization of "death work" in an urban general hospital for the indigent. This selection describes the rather startling treatment accorded both the living and the dead as they pass through the hospital's emergency room.

IN COUNTY'S EMERGENCY WARD, the most frequent variety of death is what is known as the "DOA" [dead on arrival] type. Approximately forty such cases are processed through this division of the hospital each month. The designation "DOA" is somewhat ambiguous insofar as many persons are not physiologically dead upon arrival, but are nonetheless classified as having been such. A person who is initially classified as "DOA" by the ambulance driver might retain such a classification even though he might die some hours after his arrival at the hospital.

When an ambulance driver suspects that the person he is carrying is dead, he signals the Emergency Ward with a special siren alarm as he approaches the entrance driveway. As he wheels his stretcher past the clerk's desk, he restates his suspicion with the remark "possible," a shorthand reference for "Possible DOA." The use of the term *possible* is required by law which insists, primarily for insurance purposes, that any diagnosis unless made by a certified physician be so qualified. The clerk records the arrival in a logbook and pages a physician, informing him, in code, of the arrival. Often a page is not needed as physicians on duty hear the siren alarm and expecting the arrival wait at the entranceway. The "person" is rapidly wheeled to the far end of the ward corridor and into the nearest available foyer or room, supposedly out of sight of other patients and possible onlookers from the waiting room. The physician

From David Sudnow, *Passing On: The Social Organization of Dying*, © 1967, pp. 100–107. Reprinted by permission of Prentice Hall, Englewood Cliffs, New Jersey.

arrives, makes his examination and pronounces the patient dead or alive. A nurse then places a phone call to the coroner's office, which is legally responsible for the removal and investigation of all DOA cases.

Neither the hospital nor the physician has medical responsibility in such cases. In many instances of clear death, ambulance drivers use the hospital as a depository for disposing of a body, which has the advantages of being both closer and less bureaucratically complicated a place than the downtown coroner's office. The hospital stands as a temporary holding station, rendering the community service of legitimate and free pronouncements of death for any comers. In circumstances of near-death, it functions more traditionally as a medical institution, mobilizing lifesaving procedures for those for whom they are still of potential value, at least as judged by the ER's [emergency room] staff of residents and interns. The boundaries between near-death and sure-death are not, however, altogether clearly defined.

In nearly all DOA cases, the pronouncing physician, commonly that physician who is the first to answer the clerk's page or spot the incoming ambulance, shows, in his general demeanor and approach to the task, little more than passing interest in the event's possible occurrence and the patient's biographical and medical circumstance. He responds to the clerk's call, conducts his examination, and leaves the room once he has made the necessary official gesture to an attending nurse (the term "kaput," murmured in differing degrees of audibility depending upon the hour and his state of awakeness, is a frequently employed announcement). It happened on numerous occasions, especially during the midnight-to-eight shift, that a physician was interrupted during a coffee break to pronounce a DOA and returned to his colleagues in the canteen with, as an account of his absence, some version of "Oh, it was nothing but a DOA."

It is interesting to note that while the special siren alarm is intended to mobilize quick response on the part of the ER staff, it occasionally operates in the opposite fashion. Some ER staff came to regard the fact of a DOA as decided in advance, and exhibited a degree of nonchalance in answering the siren or page, taking it that the "possible DOA" most likely is "D," and in so doing gave authorization to the ambulance driver to make such assessments. Given that time lapse which sometimes occurs between that point at which the doctor knows of the arrival and the time he gets to the patient's side, it is not inconceivable that in several instances patients who might have been revived died during this interim. This is particularly likely as apparently a matter of moments may differentiate the revivable state from the irreversible one.

Two persons in "similar" physical condition may be differentially designated as dead or not. For example, a young child was brought into the ER with no registering heartbeat, respiration, or pulse and was, through a rather dramatic stimulation procedure involving the coordinated work of a large team of doctors and nurses, revived for a period of eleven hours. On the same evening, shortly after the child's arrival, an elderly person who presented the same physical signs, with what a doctor later stated, in conversation, to be no discernible differences from the child in skin color, warmth, etc., "arrived" in the ER and was almost immediately pronounced dead, with no attempts at stimulation instituted. A nurse remarked later in the evening: "They (the doctors) would never have done that to the old lady (attempt heart stimulation) even though I've seen it work on them too." During the period when emergency resuscitation equipment was being readied for the child, an intern instituted mouth-to-mouth resuscitation. This same intern was shortly relieved by oxygen machinery and when the woman "arrived," he was the one who pronounced her dead. He reported shortly afterwards that he could never bring himself to put his mouth to "an old lady's like that."

It is therefore important to note that the category "DOA" is not totally homogeneous with respect to actual physiological condition. The same is generally true of all deaths, death involving, as it does, some decisional considerations, at least in its earlier stages.

There is currently a movement in progress in some medical and lay circles to undercut the traditional distinction between "biological" and "clinical" death, and procedures are being developed and their use encouraged for treating any "clinically dead" person as potentially reviveable.[1] This movement, unlike late nineteenth-century arguments for life after death, is legitimate by modern medical thinking and technology. Should such a movement gain widespread momentum, it would foreseeably have considerable consequence for certain aspects of hospital social structure, requiring, perhaps, that much more continuous and intensive care be given "dying" and "dead" patients than is presently accorded them, at least at County. At Cohen Hospital, where the care of the "tentatively dead" is always very intensive, such developments would more likely be encouraged than at County.

Currently, at County, there seems to be a rather strong relationship between the age, social backgrounds, and perceived moral character of patients and the amount of effort which is made to attempt revival when "clinical death signs" are detected, as well as the amount of effort given to forestalling their appearance in the first place. As one compares practices at different hospitals, the general relationship seems to hold, although at the private, wealthier institutions, like Cohen, the overall amount of attention given to "initially dead" patients is greater. At County, efforts at revival are admittedly superficial, with the exception of the very young and occasionally wealthier patient, who by some accident, ends up at County's ER. No instances have been witnessed, at County, where external heart massage was given a patient whose heart was stethoscopically inaudible, if that patient was over forty years of age. On the other hand, at Cohen Hospital heart massage is a normal routine at that point, and more drastic measures, such as injection of adrenalin directly into the heart, are not uncommon. While these practices are undertaken for many patients at Cohen if "tentative death" is discovered early, as it generally is because of the attention "dying" patients are given, at County they are reserved for a very special class of cases.

Generally, the older the patient the more likely is his tentative death taken to constitute pronounceable death. Before a twenty-year-old who arrives in the ER with a presumption of death, attached in the form of the ambulance driver's assessment, will be pronounced dead by a physician, very long listening to his heartbeat will occur, occasionally efforts at stimulation will be made, oxygen administered, and oftentimes stimulative medication given. Less time will elapse between initial detection of an inaudible heartbeat and nonpalpable pulse and the pronouncement of death if the person is forty years old, and still less if he is seventy. As well as can be detected, there appeared to be no obvious difference between men and women in this regard, nor between white and Negro "patients." Very old patients who are considered to be dead, on the basis of the ambulance driver's assessment, were seen to be put in an empty room to "wait" several moments before a physician arrived. When a young person is brought in as a "possible," the ambulance driver tries to convey some more alarming sense to the arrival by turning the siren up very loud and continuing it after he has already stopped, so that by the time he has actually entered the wing, personnel, expecting "something special," act quickly and accordingly. When it is a younger person that the driver is delivering, his general manner is more frantic. The speed with which he wheels his stretcher in, and the degree of excitement in his voice as he describes his charge to the desk clerk, are generally more heightened than with the elderly "DOA." One can observe a direct relationship between the loudness and length of the siren alarm and the considered "social value" of the person being transported.

The older the person, the less thorough is the examination he is given; frequently, elderly people are pronounced dead on the basis of only a stethoscopic examination of the heart. The younger the person, the more likely will an examination preceding an announcement of death entail an inspection of the eyes, attempt to find a pulse and touching of the body for coldness. When a younger person is brought to the hospital and while announced by the driver as a "possible" is nonetheless observed to be breathing slightly, or have an audible heart beat, there is a fast mobilization of effort to stimulate increased breathing and a more rapid heartbeat. If an older person is brought in in a similar condition there will be a rapid mobilization of similar efforts; however, the time which will elapse between that point at which breathing noticeably ceases and the heart audibly stops beating, and when the pronouncement of death is made, will differ according to his age.

One's location in the age structure of the society is not the only factor which will influence the degree of care he gets when his death is considered to have possibly occurred. At County Hospital a notable additional set of considerations can be generally termed as the patient's presumed "moral character." The detection of alcohol on the breath of a "DOA" is nearly always noticed by the examining physician, who announces to his fellow workers that the person is a drunk, and seems to constitute a feature he regards as warranting less than strenuous effort to attempt revival. The alcoholic patient is treated by hospital physicians, not only when the status of his body as alive or dead is at stake, but throughout the whole course of medical treatment, as one for whom the concern to treat can properly operate somewhat weakly. There is a high proportion of alcoholic patients at County, and their treatment very often involves an earlier admission of "terminality" and a consequently more marked suspension of curative treatment than is observed in the treatment of nonalcoholic patients. In one case, the decision whether or not to administer additional needed blood to an alcoholic man who was bleeding severely from a stomach ulcer was decided negatively, and that decision was announced as based on the fact of his alcoholism. The intern in charge of treating the patient was asked by a nurse, "Should we order more blood for this afternoon?" The doctor answered, "I can't see any sense in pumping it into him because even if we can stop the bleeding, he'll turn around and start drinking again and next week he'll be back needing more blood." In the DOA circumstance, alcoholic patients have been known to be pronounced dead on the basis of a stethoscopic examination of the heart alone, even though that person was of such an age that were he not an alcoholic he would have likely received much more intensive consideration before being so designated. Among other categories of persons whose deaths will be more quickly adjudged, and whose "dying" more readily noticed and used as a rationale for palliative care, are the suicide, the dope addict, the known prostitute, the assailant in a crime of violence, the vagrant, the known wife-beater, and other persons whose moral characters are considered reproachable.

Within a limited temporal perspective at least, but one which is not necessarily to be regarded as trivial, the likelihood of "dying" and even of being "dead" can thus be said to be partially a function of one's place in the social structure, and not simply in the sense that the wealthier get better care, or at least not in the usual sense of the fact.[2] If one anticipates having a critical heart attack, he best keep himself well-dressed and his breath clean if there is a likelihood he will be brought into the County Emergency Unit as a "possible."

There are a series of practical consequences of publicly announcing that a patient is dead in the hospital setting. His body may be properly stripped of clothing and jewelry, wrapped up for discharge, the family notified of the death, and the coroner informed in the case of DOA deaths. In the Emergency Unit there are a special set of procedures which are partially definitive of death. DOA cases are very interestingly "used" in many American hospitals. The inflow of dead bodies, or what can properly be taken to be dead bodies, is regarded as a collection of "guinea pigs," in the sense that a set of procedures can be performed upon those bodies for the sake of teaching and research.

In any "teaching hospital" (in the case of County, I use this term in a weak sense, a hospital which employs interns and residents; in other settings a "teaching hospital" may mean systematic, institutionalized instruction), the environment of medical events is regarded not merely as a collection of treatable cases, but as a collection of experience-relevant information. It is a continually enforced way of looking at the cases one treats under the auspices of a concern for experience with "such cases." This concern can legitimately warrant the institution of a variety of procedures, tests, and inquiries which lie outside and may even, on occasion, conflict with the strict interests of treatment; they fall within the interests of learning "medicine," gaining experience with such cases and acquiring technical skills. A principle for organizing medical care activities in the teaching hospital, and perhaps more so in a county hospital where patients' social value is often not highly regarded, is the relevance of any particular activity to the acquisition of skills of general import. Physicians feel that among the greatest values of such institutions is the ease with which they can selectively organize medical attention so as to maximize the benefits to knowledge and technical proficiency which working with a given case expectably affords. The notion of the "interesting case" is, at County, not simply a casual notion, but an enforced principle for the allocation of attention. The private physician is in a more committed relation to each and every one of his patients, and while he may regard this or that case as more or less interesting, he ideally cannot legitimate the interestingness of his patients' conditions as bases for devoting varying amounts of attention to them. His reward for treating the uninteresting case is, of course, the fee, and physicians are known to give more attention to the patients who will be paying more.

At County Hospital, a case's degree of interest is a crucial fact, and one which is invoked to legitimate the way a physician does and should allocate his attention. In surgery I found many examples. If on a given morning in one operating room a "rare" procedure was scheduled, and in another a "usual" procedure planned, there would be no special difficulty in getting personnel to witness and partake in the "rare" procedure, whereas work in the "usual" case was considered as merely work, regardless of such considerations as the relative fatality rate of each procedure or the patient's physical condition. It is not uncommon to find interns at County interchange among themselves in scrubbing for an appendectomy, each taking turns going next door to watch the skin graft or chest surgery. At Cohen,[3] such house staff interchanging was not permissible. Interns and residents were assigned to a particular surgical suite and required to stay throughout the course of the procedure. On the medical wards, on the basis of general observation, it seems that one could obtain a high order correlation between the amount of time doctors spent discussing and examining patients and the degree of unusualness of their medical problems.

I introduce this general feature to point to the predominant orientation, at County, to such matters as "getting practice," and the general organizational principle which provides for the propriety of using cases as the basis for this practice. Not only are live patients objects of practice, so are dead ones.

There is a rule, in the Emergency Unit, that with every DOA a doctor should attempt to insert an "endotracheal" tube. This should be done only after the patient is pronounced dead. The reason for this practice (and it is a rule on which new interns are instructed as part of their training in doing emergency medicine) is that such a tube is extremely difficult to insert, requiring great yet careful force and, insofar as it causes great pain, cannot be "practiced" on live patients. The body must be positioned with the neck held at an angle so that this large tube will go down the proper channel. In some circumstances when it is necessary to establish a rapid "airway" (an open breathing canal), the endotracheal tube can apparently be an effective substitute for the tracheotomy incision. The DOA's body, in its transit from the scene of the death to the morgue, constitutes an ideal experimental opportunity. The procedure is not done on all deceased patients, the reason apparently being that it is part of the training one receives on the Emergency Unit, and to be learned there. Nor is it done on all DOA cases, for some doctors, it seems, are uncomfortable in handling a dead body whose charge as a live one they never had, and handling it in the way such a procedure requires. It is important to note that when it is done, it is done most frequently and most intensively with those persons lowly situated in the social structure. No instances were observed where a young child was used as an object for such practice, nor where a well-dressed, middle-aged, middle-class adult was similarly used.

On one occasion a woman, who had seemingly ingested a fatal amount of Clorox, was brought to the Emergency Unit and after her death several physicians took turns trying to insert an endotracheal tube, after which one of them suggested that the stomach be pumped to examine its contents to try to see what effects the Clorox had on the gastric secretions. A lavage was set up and the stomach contents removed. A chief resident left the room and gathered together a group of interns with the explanation that they should look at this woman because of the apparent results of such ingestion. In effect, the doctors conducted their own autopsy investigation without making any incisions.

On several similar occasions, physicians explained that with these cases they didn't really feel like they were prying in handling the body, but that they often did in the case of an ordinary or "natural death" of a morally proper person. Suicidal victims are frequently the object of curiosity, and while among the nursing staff there is a high degree of distaste in working with such patients and their bodies, doctors do not express such a high degree of distaste. There was a woman who came into the Emergency Unit with a self-inflicted gunshot wound, which ran from her sternum downward and backward, passing out through a kidney. She had apparently bent over the rifle and pulled the trigger. Upon her "arrival" in the Emergency Unit she was quite alive and talkative, and while in great pain and very fearful, was able to conduct something of a conversation. She was told that she would need immediate surgery, and was taken off to the OR. She was followed by a group of physicians, all of whom were interested in seeing what damage the path of the bullet had done. One doctor said aloud, quite near her stretcher, "I can't get my heart into saving her, so we might as well have some fun out of it." During the operation, the doctors regarded her body much as they would during an autopsy. After the critical damage was repaired and they had reason to feel the woman would survive, they engaged in numerous surgical side ventures, exploring muscular tissue in areas of the back through which the bullet had passed but where no damage requiring special repair had to be done, with the exception of tying off bleeders and suturing. One of the operating surgeons performed a side operation, incising an area of skin surrounding the entry wound on the chest, to examine, he announced to his colleagues, the structure of the tissue through which the bullet passed. He explicitly announced his project to be motivated by curiosity. One of the physicians spoke of the procedure as an "autopsy on a live patient," about which there was a little laughter.

In another case, a man was wounded in the forehead by a bullet, and after the damage was repaired in the wound, which resembled a natural frontal lobotomy, an exploration was made of an area adjacent to the path of the bullet, on the forehead proper below the hairline. During this exploration the operating surgeon asked a nurse to ask Dr. X to come in. When Dr. X arrived, the two of them, under the gaze of a large group of interns and nurses, made a further incision, which an intern described to me as unnecessary in the treatment of the man, and which left a noticeable scar down the side of the temple. The purpose of this venture was to explore the structure of that part of the face. This area of the skull, that below the hairline, cannot be examined during an autopsy because of a contract between local morticians and the Department of Pathology, designed to leave those areas of the body which will be viewed, free of surgical incisions. The doctors justified the additional incision by pointing out that since he would have a "nice scar as it was, a little bit more wouldn't be so serious."

During autopsies themselves, bodies are routinely used to gain experience in surgical techniques, and many incisions and explorations are conducted that are not essential to the key task of uncovering the cause of the death. On frequent occasions, specialists-in-training came to autopsies having no interest in the patient's death. They would await the completion of the legal part of the procedure, at which point the body is turned over to them for practice. Mock surgical procedures are staged on the body, oftentimes with two coworkers simulating actual conditions, tying off blood vessels which obviously need not be tied or suturing internally.

When a patient died in the Emergency Unit, whether or not he had been brought in under the designation "DOA," there occasionally occurred various mock surgical procedures on his body. In one case a woman was treated for a chicken bone lodged in her throat. Rapidly after her arrival via ambulance a tracheotomy incision was made in the attempt to establish an unobstructed source of air, but the procedure was not successful and she died as the incision was being made. Several interns were called upon to practice their stitching by closing the wound as they would on a live patient. There was a low peak in the activity of the ward, and a chief surgical resident used the occasion to supervisorily teach them various techniques for closing such an incision. In another case the body of a man who died after being crushed by an automobile was employed for instruction and practice in the use of various fracture-setting techniques. In still another instance several interns and residents attempted to suture a dead man's dangling finger in place on his mangled hand.

Notes

1. There is a large popular and scientific literature developing on efforts to "treat the dead," the import of which is to undercut traditional notions of the nonreversibility of death. Some of this discussion goes so far as to propose the preservation of corpses in a state of nondeterioration until such time as medical science will be able to do complete renovative work. See particularly R. Ettinger, *The Prospect of Immortality* (Garden City: Doubleday & Company, Inc., 1964). The Soviet literature on resuscitation is most extensive. Soviet physicians have given far more attention to this problem than any others in the world. For an extensive review of the technical literature, as well as a discussion of biomedical principles, with particular emphasis on cardiac arrest, see V. A. Negovskii, *Resuscitation and Artificial Hypothermia* (New York: Consultants Bureau Enterprises, Inc., 1962). See also, L. Fridland, *The Achievement of Soviet Medicine* (New York: Twayne Publishers, Inc., 1961), especially Chapter Two, "Death Deceived," pp. 56–57. For an account of the famous saving of the Soviet physicist Landau's life, see A. Dorozynski, *The Man They Wouldn't Let Die* (New York: The Macmillan Company, 1956).

    For recent popular articles on "bringing back the dead" and treating death as a reversible process, see "The Reversal of Death," *The Saturday Review*, August 4, 1962; "A New Fight Against Sudden Death," *Look*, December 1, 1964.

    Soviet efforts and conceptions of death as reversible might be seen to have their ideological basis in principles of dialectics:

    For everyday purposes we know and can say, e.g., whether an animal is alive or not. But, upon closer inquiry, we find that this is, in many cases, a very complex question, as the jurists know very well. They have cudgelled their brains in vain to discover a rational limit beyond which the killing of a child in its mother's womb is murder. It is just as impossible to determine absolutely the moment of death, for physiology provides that death is not an instantaneous, momentary phenomenon, but a very protracted process. In like manner, every organized being is every moment the same and not the same.

    From F. Engels, *Socialism: Utopian and Scientific* (New York: International Publishers Co., 1935), p. 47.

    For a discussion of primitive conceptions of death with particular attention to the passage between life and death, see I. A. Lopatin, *The Cult of the Dead Among the Natives of the Amur Basin* (The Hague: Mouton and Company, 1960), pp. 26–27 and 39–41.

2. The "DOA" deaths of famous persons are reportedly attended with considerably prolonged and intensive resuscitation efforts. In Kennedy's death, for example, it was reported:

Medically, it was apparent the President was not alive when he was brought in. There was no spontaneous respiration. He had dilated, fixed pupils. It was obviously a lethal head wound.

Technically, however, by using vigorous resuscitation, intraveneous tubes and all the usual supportive measures, we were able to raise the semblance of a heartbeat.

The New York Times, November 23, 1963, p. 2.

3. Editor's Note: A private hospital in the same city.

15 Dying at Murray Manor ❧

Jaber F. Gubrium

JABER GUBRIUM is professor of sociology at the University of Florida. He is
editor of the *Journal of Aging Studies* and the author of numerous books,
including *Living and Dying at Murray Manor*. That ethnographic book examines the social organization of care in a nursing home he calls Murray Manor.
This selection is taken from the chapter that deals with dying and death.

The clientele at Murray Manor are divided between residents who are
capable of relatively independent living and patients who require more
intensive nursing care and are typically showing more obvious signs of
dying. Gubrium describes the lengths to which the residents go to distinguish themselves from the patients, and he discusses the social organization
of dying from the perspective of three categories of actors: the top staff
(administrators), the floor staff (nurses and aides on the ward), and the clientele (the residents and patients). The focus of the selection presented here is
on the clientele's view of experiencing and witnessing death.

UNLIKE PATIENTS' CONCERN with watching automobiles or top staff's attempt
to write total care plans, dying and death are commonly recognized occasions
considered characteristic of the Manor's setting by all its participants. However, all do not consider them in the same way. Although all may be able to talk
"casually" about them together and separately, not all talk is tacitly grounded
in the same assumptions. Three worlds of dying and death exist in the home,
adhered to separately by top staff, floor staff, and clientele. When the participants of one world deal with the participants of another, they may make trouble for each other.

EXPERIENCING VERSUS WITNESSING

When dying or death occurs at the Manor, it is clientele who physically *experience* them. Every day, patients and residents live with the knowledge that
dying and death are imminent events for them. Not only do they experience
dying and death themselves, but each one is also a *witness* to the experiences of

others. If he is not seriously experiencing or witnessing, he still sees what he easily might become by observing those around him who are dying or dead.

Patients and residents differ somewhat as far as the continuity of their experiences with dying is concerned. When elders are admitted to the Manor as patients or become patients after entering as residents, staff considers them to be showing "obvious" signs of potentially dying. Both staff and clientele believe all residents and patients to be terminal in that they are aged, reside in the home, and are not fully expected to return to society "out there." Patients, however, are more likely than residents to show either certain "pointable" signs of dying (e.g., being completely bedridden, moaning, being emaciated, visibly decaying, or being virtually unintelligible) or to be defined by staff and clientele as soon to acquire these signs. Residents experience only periodic episodes of dying. Some have occasional epileptic seizures. Others have mild heart attacks or chest pains. Most take medications for nondisabling but chronic illnesses.

Patients and residents all define their futures in terms of death. In that respect, they all believe they are dying. Only the actual time of death is unknown. Take the following typical comments about their futures:

Gus Marsh [resident]: My future, hell! What future is there for me? Blink! I'm the last of my family. No one's got a future here.

Homer Wilson [resident]: At eighty-six? All I can think about is that God will call me someday. They'll take me out and bury me. I don't think about nothin'. I take it day by day. I don't plan on anything, because generally when you plan on somethin', it never turns out that way anyway. So I don't try to think or make any plans whatsoever. I take it day by day and leave the rest in God's hands.

Pearl Smith [resident]: Well, I tell you. I take a day at a time. And you don't plan what might transpire because you just know it may all end anytime. So I might as well adjust myself and be happy and go along day by day.

Joan Borden [resident]: I don't know. Well, if it comes, it comes. If it comes tomorrow, it comes. It's coming for all of us anyway, sooner than later. No, it's no use to think about my future. It's settled! I wanna make use of my money first. I don't leave any money for anybody else. That's all I worked for—what I got.

John Varady [resident]: Lots of time, in my mind, I say it be better if I die. I got in Calvary cemetery—I got lot there and stone and everything. Lots of time I think, "Let me out, quick so I can go." What use we all here? We all going soon.

Katy Miles [resident]: I don't worry about it, if that's what you mean. I know just about what will happen, where I'll be buried, and all. So I don't worry about it. I just don't wanna be laying around here for months. That's all. Well, I've got everything taken care of so that if anything happens to me, I'll be taken care of. I don't plan much no more. I don't think I can. Not at my age. I suppose age makes a person stop planning. I don't know. My legs aren't too good either that I can run around even if I could. I think there's a lot more places that I could go to and do things, but I have arthritis.

BERNICE HOGAN [RESIDENT]:   Could we go on? There's no future. I just as soon die. I just ask God to please take me home. What should I live for? I ain't got nothing to live for. Kids don't come to see you. We're all sick here and upstairs they're worse. All we have left to look forward to is the end.

ELIZABETH TANNER [PATIENT]:   There is no future for me. That's gone. I have nowhere to turn. What would I look forward to? Just sitting here? There's no future in that. I just feel hopeless. I did make plans at first, but none now. I just let Mother Nature take its course, I guess.

BERTHA THOMAS [PATIENT]:   I have no future. Tell me, when you're eighty-five, what are you going to do? There is no life here. If I could walk better . . . if it wasn't for that, I would call one of my friends, an attorney, and say, "You tell my daughter you wanna get me out of here." No. I would welcome, and I mean *welcome* if I could go to sleep. How do you like that? I hope I die. My minister gets mad. I say, "Please, please pray that I should die. I don't wanna live." I have nothing to stay for.

LAURA KOWALSKI [PATIENT]:   No future. Not now anymore. I used to have a future before I got here. Nothing in particular but I did love my home. I used to plan a lot what I would like to do, see the grandchildren. You know, stuff like that. But not now. I don't know. I just feel that I'm stuck here and that . . . [weeps] I don't know what the future looks like. I don't know.

STELLA IMOGENE [PATIENT]:   What kind of future could I think about? I don't make no plans because I can't walk around. See, it's a handicap for me. Now, I'm a person that lives day to day . . . ever since I was ill for so long, for so many years. They say the way my heart is, I could be dead tomorrow. See, when you have heart trouble, you don't know. People fall dead on the street and you never knew they were sick. That is the way I would like to. . . .

BETTY WHITE [PATIENT]:   I don't know. I can't see no future. When I get down in the dumps, I think I'm better off than some people. At least, I can wait on myself and I still have my mind. But it's hard to think that way. Well, I don't see no future . . . just death. That's all. Well, I don't know about death. It's a puzzle. Nobody's ever come back to tell us. I think I'm ready anytime.

Patients witness continuously what they define as vivid scenes of dying. Residents, on the other hand, witness what they believe is vivid dying on four occasions. First, when one of them experiences a physical crisis, such as a seizure or heart attack, other residents consider this to be an event when "he [or she] could have died."

Second, if the crisis is disabling to the degree that the person affected is believed to need skilled nursing care, he is transferred to the third or fourth floor and becomes a patient. To residents, a crisis that is followed by a "transfer upstairs" is considered evidence of "really dying." Such transfers are felt to be not only possible personal endings but also a social demise. As is often said after a resident witnesses a transfer that has followed a disabling crisis, "Poor thing. She's going and will probably never live a normal [first-floor] life again."

Third, several services at the Manor are located in places that make it necessary for those residents desiring to use them to observe dying patients. For example, the beauty and barber shop is located on the third floor. Also, many activities planned by the top staff include both patients and residents. This too provides residents with an opportunity to witness dying.

When residents enter the premises of those known to be dying, they are visibly wary. As soon as the elevator doors open onto a floor that houses dying patients, they give the premises much more careful scrutiny than is typical in other situations at the Manor. When the floor area immediately surrounding the elevator is believed to be adequately free from signs of dying, they proceed quickly to their destinations. Rarely do they continue to look about.

Fourth, two residents have wives on the third floor. Their daily reports to other residents on the health status of their spouses contribute to the vicarious witnessing of dying by those who listen. Another kind of vicarious witnessing occurs when residents inform others on the first floor of the status of friends whom they occasionally visit on the third and fourth floors.

Residents who have friends on patient floors try to avoid visiting them there. They sometimes go so far as to fetch patient friends from patient floors. When they can't do this, their visits on patient floors are notably short, infrequent, and uncomfortable. They sit in patients' rooms or lounges with obvious apprehension. When someone who shows what they consider to be signs of dying appears before them, they grimace or turn away.

Patients and residents differ in the extent to which each is likely to experience or witness death. Both believe that patients are more likely to die than residents. References are often made to the "fact that up there [or here], you're likely to go anytime." However, because they are ambulatory, residents are somewhat more likely to witness death than patients, and especially more than bedridden ones. In addition, when one resident hears about a death in the home, all are likely to know of it in short order. Among patients, there is a less comprehensive network of social contacts along which death news can spread. Although a few ambulatory patients may be witnesses to more deaths than any resident, residents as a whole hear of deaths or observe death clues more than patients do.

Bodies may be carried out of the building in two ways. Sometimes, especially at night, they are taken through the lobby and out the front entrance. This route is more visible to residents than to patients. More often, they are taken to the basement in the elevator and placed in an ambulance or hearse that has been parked at the rear of the building on the service ramp. When a body is released via the basement, both residents and patients whose rooms face the southeast or who sit and watch in the south lounge may witness death; in this case, see a body removed. This entrance is used mostly for deliveries of various

goods, garbage pickups, and retrieval of bodies. If the first two are not occurring when vehicles park there, the third is likely to be.

Members of the floor staff do not die in the Manor. They are, however, more frequent witnesses of both dying and death than patients and residents. Not only does floor staff witness more dying and death, but it does so more in-timately than either patients or residents, for the most part. For example, as an integral part of its routine work, floor staff handles and examines such evi-dence of dying as extreme emaciation and extensive physical decay. Clientele may observe these conditions, but they don't handle or treat them.

Floor staff is also a more intimate witness of dying and death than patients and residents in that it makes frequent and periodic inspection of dying patients in the course of bed-and-body work. It is witness to histories of dying. Be-cause it observes dying and its symptoms over a period of time, floor staff is not as upset as clientele are when it encounters it. As one aide explained, "You get use to even the worst ones when you work around them a while."

In contrast to the floor staff, top staff does not witness dying and death to any great extent, nor does it extensively witness patient and resident responses to either. The witnessing of dying and death that top staff does primarily in-volves the administrator, administrative nurses, and the chaplain. Dying is witnessed indirectly by the administrative nurses in their periodic checks of routine floor work. They don't usually deal with the dying person nor with other patients' responses to dying per se. Rather, what they witness is only a by-product of their main concern with routine administrative work. What top staff sees of death is primarily an outcome of presiding over floor staff's work. A top staff nurse verifies a floor nurse's death diagnosis, calls the physician, and obtains a death pronouncement. If the administrator is in the building, he man-ages the death scene in terms of both space and timing: he sees to it that all floor personnel are properly involved and that clientele are kept distant; he may su-pervise the entire sequencing of events from death to removal of the body. The chaplain performs a variety of religious rituals depending, to some extent, upon the religious affiliation of the deceased.

Top staff's regular administrative work affects its witnessing of death and dying in two ways. First, dying is believed to be part of the routine work of floor personnel, not of top staff. Second, when top staff witnesses death, it is involved administratively, officially or unofficially. As one aide put it, "They do their bit and if the funeral men take too long to come, they leave."

DEATH WORLDS

Clientele and Death

Talk of dying is never completely separate from talk of death among patients and residents. Dying is suffering and, as they say, "Who wants to suffer!" To them, it is only "sensible" to want to be dead if one is suffering. As for the dead, they are believed to have finished with the "worry" that comes from having to "be a burden" on others. The following express their practical view of the intimate link between dying and death.

> Well, for her I was grateful [that she died]. 'Cause they said there was nothing to her. And I know she was a good person and if there was a heaven she would go there.

> Not that I like to hear of anybody dying, but as far as that [death] bothers one—no. We all have to go, and we don't know when. And she was ninety-three years old.

> As long as God leaves Mother [wife] here with me, I'll stay with Mother. When God calls her—which is a terrible thing to say—I hope it comes soon. When you know that she can't get well, it's pitiful to sit there and watch her. She's in pain most of the time . . . very severe diabetes. And I hope it's tonight. That's an awful thing to say. Awful. 'Cause I dearly love her.

> I hope that I don't live to be too old. That's all. I mean I hate to be a burden or a worry all my life to someone. I have never been before. And then you wonder and just hope that when your time comes, you go quickly. That's all.

I took part in many informal conversations about dying and death at the Manor. On occasion, I deliberately tried to steer talk toward either dying or death alone, but I was rarely successful. In a gathering one time, a participant pointedly asked me, "How can you talk about one without the other? You tell me that." In another attempt, a man flatly stated, "When you're dying, you're dead. That's all there is to it."

When someone dies at the Manor, there is no general gloom among other patients and residents. As many suggest, death is a very reasonable thing to expect "in a place like this." When anyone hears of the death of someone he did not know well, he may be curious and politely sympathetic, but he is not especially mournful or depressed.

As patients and residents gather in the lounges or other public places, they exchange opinions about dying and death whenever one of them mentions that he "just happened to look in on" or "heard about" a dying person at the Manor. Typically, the ensuing exchange involves at least two kinds of statements. First, someone says that the suffering is "terribly depressing." Occasionally, another person adds that the dying person is "taking it very hard" or "taking it very well." Second, talk of death closes the conversation. This usually takes one of two forms, depending on whether discussion has turned to their own futures or is still oriented to the dying person. When it is centered on their own futures, comments are made about the personal desirability of death should one begin "really suffering" [dying]. Everyone agrees. When it is still oriented to the dying person, it is likely to be said that "death would be a blessing for him" or "I hope she passes for her sake, the poor thing."

On occasion, a person who is quite visibly dying appears or is pushed into the company of a group of residents or "alert" patients. When this occurs, the group becomes increasingly irritated the longer the intruder remains with them. It is not uncommon for the "alerts" to look away or to show both consternation and anxiety. Their comments also make it obvious that they are persons "rudely" being subjected to the frightening symptoms of dying, "without any regard for *our* feelings."

In such "uncalled for" circumstances, talk of dying is exasperated but whispered. Anyone may lean over to another and complain, "They shouldn't bring people who are that bad in here!" "It's best to keep those poor people separated." When such an intrusion occurred in his area of the dining room, one patient, who later claimed to have lost his appetite, whispered through clenched teeth: "See that man. He must be suffering. I'd rather be dead than that way. How can anyone eat with that around?"

Patients and residents claim to "feel sorry" for the dying—to them, a proper sentiment to express—but this does not mean that they are willing to personally indulge them. They "feel sorry" at a distance. For example, residents are usually quite willing to talk about "visitation programs" to the sick, and they may complain among themselves or to the activity director about the "need" for scheduled visits. This usually is punctuated with talk of "Christian duty," "those poor people suffering alone," and "everyone wanting a visitor or a kind voice in time of need." But whenever visitation is scheduled, residents typically are reluctant to engage in it. As they say, "I just don't have time today," or "I've just been so tired lately that I better not," or "I'm expecting a visitor this afternoon." Others groan or simply "forget."

When dying patients talk of dying, they express an urgent desire for death. Some say that it is unfortunate that one has to suffer so before he "passes." Others complain that it is the waiting that is so agonizing. Three of them put it this way:

> Why do we have to suffer? That's the thing. God help us. I wish it would come soon. Let it end. When? When?

> Who likes life, anyhow? Well, it's just that I wanna pass away. That's the one. I wanna pass away. That's it. Well, what should I do? The rest of the afternoon I don't know what I'm gonna do. God help me. I wanna go. I'd like to pass away. It would be quiet and nice.

> I'm bad and they're [other dying patients] worse yet. So why a person has to live that kind of life? If you're old, you should die and be done with. They're no good to nobody. They're just like a vegetable. I hope someday I go to sleep and I don't get up. I only ask God to give me peace as soon as possible. Take me out of this world.

Clientele are rather perfunctory in referring to death. Dying patients matter of factly describe the characteristics of death as opposite to what they consider the most prominent features of dying. If dying for them means pain, death is blissful relief. If dying means being annoyed by others' complaints of the burden involved, death means quiet solitude. Residents and patients who are not dying describe the character of death in a simpler fashion than do visibly dying patients. Since dying, for them, means chronic dependence, death is simply the "end of useless living," of "being a burden."

The one exception to this occurs when patients and residents talk about a close or intimate friend who has died. Friendship makes death an interpersonal ending in addition to a public one at the Manor. When a patient's or resident's close friend dies, he usually refers to the death mournfully. The deceased is missed. Occasionally, those who survive the friendship are in despair at the loss. A resident recalls her friend in this way:

> *There's one that died from this floor. She came the same day I did. She was Miss Custer. She'd never been married. She was a schoolteacher. She was a very nice person, and real friendly. I miss her. I'm really sorry that she's gone. She was as lonesome as I was. I was alone. So we used to visit each other. Yes, I liked her very much. I felt awful bad when she died.*

And a male patient, when asked about being depressed by news of a death at the Manor, said:

> *Oh, not unless he's a personal friend. Otherwise, I don't give a damn. Of course, I feel it because I know it's a life, but it doesn't affect you that much. Now George [roommate who's his friend] . . . if there's anything wrong with George, I would feel sorry for him. I like George and I think he's a hell of a nice fella.*

16 Hospice Care for the 1990s: A Concept Coming of Age ॐ

Marian Gentile and Maryanne Fello

MARIAN GENTILE is Hospice Manager at Forbes Hospice in Pittsburgh.
MARYANNE FELLO is Director of Cancer Services at Forbes Health System,
also in Pittsburgh. Both are registered nurses who have been part of the hospice movement since 1979. Working together at Forbes, they have taken the
program from its inception to one of the largest full-service programs in the
country. This selection provides a good overview of the form that the hospice approach to care for the dying has taken in the United States during the
1990s. It also provides a brief discussion of the evolution of the modern hospice movement in England and the United States.

THE ROOTS OF HOSPICE

Even though its roots can be traced to the Middle Ages, the modern hospice
program did not take shape until the mid-1960s. At that time, the work of two
remarkable physicians, Elizabeth Kübler-Ross and Dame Cicely Saunders,
converged to bring the emotional and physical needs of the dying to the
forefront.

In 1970, Kübler-Ross' landmark book, *On Death and Dying*,[1] revolution-
ized the psychologic approaches to patients with terminal illness. After several
years of observation and actual interviews with the dying, Kübler-Ross created
a theoretic framework describing the psychologic stages of dying and pointed
out to health care workers a sobering fact: as dying patients needed *more* attention and support, they were actually receiving *less*. Indeed, Kübler-Ross
brought death and dying "out of the closet," making health care providers and
society in general more aware that death is a part of life and a legitimate part of
clinical care, and that with sensitivity and understanding it can be faced openly
and honestly.

In 1967, while Kübler-Ross was working at the University of Chicago
Hospital, a British physician, Cicely Saunders, MD, opened the doors of St

Reprinted from M. Gentile and M. Fello, "Hospice Care for the 1990s: A Concept Coming
of Age," *Journal of Home Health Care Practice*, Vol. 3, No. 1, pp. 1–15, with the permission
of Aspen Publishers, Inc., © 1990.

Christopher's Hospice in London. Trained as a nurse and social worker, she received her medical degree and set about her life's work to improve the care of the dying—and what better background? Some have called Saunders "a whole hospice team wrapped up in one person"!

Saunders' approach to the dying was first and foremost geared to achieving and maintaining comfort. Her approach to pain management has shaped the development of a pain control philosophy that has become a benchmark of hospice care.

Her model, prescribing an interdisciplinary team, communicating effectively, treating symptoms of terminal disease, including the patient *and* family,[2] has been replicated in concept over 1,400 times in the United States today.

HOSPICE IN THE UNITED STATES

In the early 1970s, as the work of Kübler-Ross and Saunders became known, individuals in the United States became eager to put their concepts into action. The United States programs, however similar in concept to the British world, were very different in design. The first US hospice, Hospice of Connecticut (New Haven) began to deliver care to the dying at home, since funding problems forced delays in the construction of a free-standing facility. After 6 years of delays an inpatient unit was christened in 1980 "but its early years as a home care program left an indelible impression on the purposes and practices of the hospice staff and administrators. It provided the country with a new and different model of care for the dying, care focused primarily on patients at home."[3]

As the hospice movement spread across the United States, programs took on various shapes and sizes. In most instances the shape of each hospice was determined by its genesis. For example, if a hospital felt that its commitment included the provision of terminal care, its hospice program would probably be a hospital-based hospice; if a group of active lay volunteers began a program, it might be a consortium model hospice. In all, there are at least six common program designs for hospice.

In an effort to more exactly define this concept, the National Hospice Organization (NHO) and the then Joint Commission on Accreditation of Hospitals (JCAH) developed standards of care to which hospice should adhere. Standards were developed in seven areas: (1) the patient and family as the unit of care, (2) interdisciplinary team services, (3) continuity of care, (4) home care services, (5) symptom control, (6) bereavement, and (7) quality assurance.

Most significant in the creation of uniformity of hospice programming was the addition of hospice to the Federal Medicare Program in 1982. Maintenance of a certification to deliver hospice care calls for rigid adherence to the standards developed. As we look toward the 1990s, many uncertainties still exist, many questions remain unanswered, such as

- What is the best model for delivery of hospice care?
- Will hospice in the United States face a dilemma as larger programs force out small, community programs?
- Will hospice care be assimilated into mainstream health care, or can it only stand alone?
- Will patients be *forced* to participate in hospice?
- What will be the impact of high technology on the dying process?

CRITERIA FOR ADMISSION

Probably the most crucial in the management of a hospice in today's society is the development of the program's admission criteria. Surely the kinds of support the hospice offers might be well received by any patient and family facing a major illness, but just when during that illness does a patient become eligible?

After years of developing a careful decision-making process, the authors' hospice has developed a fairly rigid set of three criteria for admission:

1. completion of all active, curative treatment
2. patient's awareness of diagnosis and prognosis
3. patient and family's clear understanding of the goals of hospice care.

Clearly these criteria bring to mind grey areas for questioning such as, "What if a patient is receiving palliative chemotherapy?" "What if a patient knows the diagnosis but not the prognosis?" "What if the family is divided about how the patient's illness should be treated?" And more recently, "What if the patient wants no life supports, but does want artificial hydration and nutrition?" These so-called grey areas demand that each patient's application for hospice care is reviewed in depth with the *most* important question: "Are the patient and family choosing supportive care for a terminal disease with the care delivered primarily in the home setting?"

WHO WORKS IN A HOSPICE PROGRAM?

In this age of nursing shortages across the country, the opportunity to work in a hospice setting still draws nurses. Why?

Two reasons come to mind. The first is the satisfaction of the work itself. To assist the patient and family during the dying process carries many rewards.

Becoming involved after a family has been told "there is nothing more to be done" can restore the family's faith that it will not be abandoned even though curative medical treatment has been exhausted. Helping a family know what to expect, putting effective symptom management skills into practice, and supporting with effective counseling skills makes a hero of many nurses in the eyes of grateful families.

The second draw is the role of the nurse within the hospice team itself. Medical intervention takes a back seat to nursing intervention in terminal care. This fact thrusts the nurse into a primary role for both direct care and the coordination of the care provided by other members of the team. More will be said about that role later in the discussion of the interdisciplinary team.

An early study done by Amenta[4] has proven itself true many times: nurses (and others) who are drawn to hospice tend to be religious, realistic revolutionaries and they find in a hospice program a setting that is just short of an ideal medium for fundamental, holistic, independent nursing practice.

THE INTERDISCIPLINARY TEAM

The essence of hospice care is derived from the multifaceted and comprehensive approach of the hospice interdisciplinary team, whose members look for solutions to a patient's medical, psychosocial, and spiritual problems. The diversity of talent, cultural and ethnic backgrounds, life style, and educational background creates a blend that can sort out various problems to find the approach most suitable for that individual patient and family. A well-coordinated, confident group of hospice professionals can work together with everyone having equal say in most matters only if each team member is comfortable offering information from his or her experience and knowledge as well as listening to and accepting the differing contributions of others.

"Role blurring" (overlapping of duties of various professional disciplines) is acceptable and actually encouraged to some extent within hospice programs. Every team member has an area of expertise accompanied by some primary responsibilities but each also must have some knowledge of other disciplines and be sensitive to problems and needs not directly related to the particular area of expertise. A common example of role blurring is when a hospice nurse spends time with family members advising them on how to approach the children about an impending death. There is no need (and often, no time) to wait until the counselor can be called to talk or meet with the family. A well-trained, experienced, and sensitive hospice nurse can give meaningful and accurate information in this situation. However, the lines must be drawn when the problems require more specific expertise and that team member must defer to another member of the team. Furthermore, sharp distinctions must be made in some areas because of primary responsibility and liabilities (i.e., the patient's physician has the final decision in the ordering of medications, treatments, etc.). Hospice personnel need to be cognizant of and comfortable with role blurring and to know their boundaries.

THE COMPOSITION OF THE INTERDISCIPLINARY TEAM AND THE MEMBERS' ROLES

The composition of the hospice team may vary from program to program depending on the model and whether the program is Medicare certified to provide hospice care. Typical members are discussed below.

Hospice Nurse

Often the nucleus of a hospice team, the nurse may find herself or himself in the role of coordinating the care of most patients. Because the majority of hospice patients need some assistance with symptom management along with accompanying problems related to their physical care, the discipline of nursing is drawn on heavily by hospice care. It is the hospice nurse who is available 24 hours a day as needed by patients and families; it is usually the nurse who has the most day-by-day contact with the families, who visits regularly and calls frequently to give added reassurance and guidance. Regardless of the setting, the nurses are the principal support to patients and their families.

Clinical competence coupled with sensitivity and kindness seem to be key ingredients in the practice of hospice nursing. Hospice nurses generally have a great deal of autonomy on the job which, in itself, means that they must have good decision-making skills in addition to better than average communication abilities. The ability to communicate is demonstrated most keenly when a patient and family have chosen an avenue of treatment (or more often, nontreatment) that is contrary to the physician's plan. On the other hand, the hospice nurse may need to help a patient understand why no further treatment is advocated by the patient's physicians; the nurse must then employ gentle methods of reinforcing bad news. By staying open to communication from many directions, the hospice nurse can open up meaningful and useful dialogue not only for that patient and family but also for the community at large.

Hospice Aide

Working closely with the hospice nurses, the home health aide is one of the most valuable members of the hospice team. Formally the home health aide's role is to help provide personal care and light housekeeping duties in the home.

The home health aide is encouraged to provide the care in the way that is most satisfying to the family—either by working with the family member to help provide the care or by doing the care alone to allow the family a much needed rest. (It is important for some families to feel like they have "done it all" even when it drives them to the point of exhaustion.) By working *with* the family they give the family members some assistance and help lighten the load and still allow them to feel that they really have done it all.

Light housekeeping duties can be of great importance in some households. At times the primary caregiver is somewhat incapacitated or just plain tired. Having someone clean up last night's supper dishes or launder a few loads of clothes can be supportive to a caregiver and an emotional boost as well.

Without question, however, the home health aide plays an important informal role. The aide's visits are generally longer than those of other members of the team (except the volunteer) and are geared to giving the caregiver a break. This may be the time the family relaxes just a bit more than usual and starts talking. Relationships between families and home health aides often become very intimate. Caregivers may derive their greatest support from the chance to talk over coffee with their friend, the home health aide. There is less professional distance obvious in these relationships. And, even though the relationships are encouraged, the aide must attempt to remain objective and not become enmeshed in family problems.

Counselor

The person looking most closely at families and family dynamics is the hospice counselor. The counselor's educational background is generally in the areas of psychology or social work. This specialized training is brought into practice in the usual ways of seeking out community resources, and finding help with financial, legal, and insurance issues. With hospice patients these problems take on exaggerated proportions because so much is happening at once in their lives. Sorting through these issues can bring about some peace of mind for the patient and caregivers but also permits insight into the more critical areas of the family system. Developing a relationship while working on the more tangible problems is a natural link into the more private (and thus guarded) family relationships. The crux of many of the difficulties for hospice families can be found within the family system. The counselor must employ special skills and sensitivity to help the families work through their issues. Most important, the counselor must sort through the details of the particular difficulty and offer options but allow the family to make the actual decision. This is a formidable task at times because many families have great difficulty making decisions or may be asking the counselor to rescue them. Developing skills that help people adapt to the crisis of terminal illness and all of its ramifications requires much emotional fortitude and keen perceptive talents on the part of the counselor.

Therapists

Physical therapists, occupational therapists, and speech therapists contribute in their own way to the enhancement of each day of life for a hospice patient. Physical therapists usually teach families transfer techniques, proper positioning, and maintenance exercises for the patients. Because rehabilitation is generally not feasible for the terminally ill patient, the emphasis is on maintaining strength and mobility as long as possible. In conjunction with this maintenance plan the occupational therapist evaluates the patient and the home setting for ways to continue a semblance of the patient's former activities of daily living. In both cases the emphasis is on maintaining function as long as possible and conserving energy so that remaining energy can be channeled into the patient's most important activities. Speech therapists emphasize communication and swallowing problems, both of which might be seen in the same patient (such as patients with brain tumor or amyotrophic lateral sclerosis [ALS]). Some hospice programs also include music and art therapists as part of the interdisciplinary team. Each of these therapists, using individual expertise, tries to enable patients to maximize their diminishing physical and communication abilities.

Nutritionist

Specializing in the nutritional aspects of terminal illness, the nutritionist counsels families on the special needs of these patients. The nutritionist focuses on understanding the meaning of food in each individual family system. Recognizing different ethnic and cultural views relating to food, the nutritionist attempts to help families look at these nutritional problems from their own perspective. Families for whom food was the center of life and pleasure need to continue to work on feeding and nourishing their dying family member. For them the emphasis is on getting as much nourishment as possible into every bite while knowing that the patient's food intake will probably continue to decline. At the same time the nutritionist emphasizes that what is most important at this stage of life is to eat and *enjoy*—not just to eat for the sake of eating. Families need to be told that nutritional problems are commonplace and that it is not their failing if the patient continues to lose weight and has a poor appetite. No one says that more convincingly than the hospice nutritionist.

Medical Director

A major force within the interdisciplinary team is the medical director. The medical director presents the physician's view within the hospice framework and then represents the hospice approach to the medical community whose members often are struggling with decisions related to terminal illness in other settings such as acute care. The medical director must possess expertise in clinical aspects of symptom management in order to help implement effective palliative care. The medical director plays a variety of parts. On one hand, the medical director may actually manage the care of some hospice patients or act as a consultant to the care in other cases. Acting as a teacher, the medical director works with the rest of the hospice staff and interdisciplinary team to understand the various disease processes and their clinical implications. It is the hospice medical director who can most fully see the patient in the context of prior medical history and who, because of the physician's knowledge of the natural history of the disease process, will be instrumental in helping the team plan for the patient's medical care in the days ahead. The hospice medical director must display compassion and patience to the other team members while often acting as a stabilizing force within the group framework.

Chaplain

Spiritual care is an integral component of the hospice concept. Clergy serving as hospice chaplains form the most formal aspect of a hospice pastoral care program. All members of a hospice team must be able to attend to the spiritual needs of patients and families as questions and fears arise when death becomes more imminent. But the chaplain is a resource to both the staff, as staff persons address the spiritual concerns of patients and families, and the terminally ill patients and their families who are grappling with those life and death issues.

Chaplains represent faith and a link to God and eternity. They must be careful to help patients explore spiritual dimensions in a broad sense, not within one particular denomination or religious affiliation unless requested by the patient. Many of the patients to whom hospice chaplains minister have been alienated from formal religion and now are feeling a need to reestablish themselves with their spiritual roots. Caution and sensitivity, along with a caring and loving nature, enable the chaplain to explore areas sometimes unreachable by anyone else.

The hospice chaplain represents the religious community within the context of the interdisciplinary team and, in turn, represents the hospice program in the community. Chaplains not only work directly with patients and families but also may participate in staff and volunteer training and continuing education. Hospice chaplains participate regularly in interdisciplinary team meetings where each patient's medical, social, and spiritual picture is reviewed. And the chaplain's involvement continues into the bereavement period when spiritual care may be the most important ingredient in grief support.

Volunteers

Embracing the spirit of hospice care, the volunteers donate their time to hospice programs and the terminally ill patients the programs serve. It is doubtful that any other area of health care involves volunteers to the extent that hospices do. Many hospice programs could not continue to operate without their volunteer constituency and no program could be considered a full-service hospice without a strong volunteer component.

Volunteers are in a position to provide a tremendous contribution to the hospice program and to individual patients and families. Because expectations of the volunteers are naturally high it is vital that they are carefully selected and trained. Hospice programs gear their selection and training programs to their own needs with training usually comprised of 20 to 40 hours of lectures, group discussion, outside reading, and instruction on physical care including hands-on nursing care. Then the volunteers begin assisting the hospice staff, all the while becoming entrenched in the care of terminally ill patients and their families. At the same time it is important for staff to supervise volunteers and provide them with outlets for emotional support.

Every component of a hospice program might include volunteers from in-patient care to home care and bereavement care, but they also help with office duties, speaker's bureau work, and fundraising. Some serve on hospice boards and help formulate and enact policy changes. Each area has its own needs and calls upon many different kinds of talents.

The most common area of hospice volunteering is the home care setting. Volunteers in the home act in the capacity of a friend—one who knows how to care for a sick person. Most commonly the volunteer provides respite for the caregivers by affording them an opportunity to get out of the home during the volunteer's visit. Even if the caregivers do not choose to leave the home, they have a chance to rest or do other chores without having to be concerned with the patient's care. Other home care volunteer duties include light housekeeping, laundry, grocery shopping, meal preparation, errands, even babysitting to give caregivers more time with the patient.

Volunteers give an added dimension to the families and the programs they serve. Their perspective is one of kindness and caring, along with a belief in maintaining human dignity in the dying process. They give much of themselves and reap only the gratification that comes from helping people in their darkest hour.

THE ROLE OF THE FAMILY IN HOSPICE CARE

In the early days of the hospice programming, many held the view that hospice staff was essential to do *for* the family, to be a substitute for the family in the care of the patient. Hospice, by its very nature, seemed to attract those helpers caught up with the notion of the "rescue fantasy." This, combined with an underestimation of what families are capable of doing, made for much over-functioning and early warning signs of staff burnout.

As staff members learned together about the nature of family systems and how best to be helpful, they realized that the primary role of the hospice nurse was to be an enabler. When staff members share their competence in caring with families, rather than taking over, families are able to feel as if *they* did everything they could until their loved one died. One of the highest compliments to hospice staff is the thank-you note that says, "You gave us what it took to be able to do it ourselves. . . .

PAIN MANAGEMENT

Probably the most valuable contribution to the health care system at large has been the development of the body of knowledge by hospice professionals regarding pain management. Even though only approximately 50% of hospice patients have moderate to severe pain problems, pain is often what patients and families fear most. Some of the most important pain management concepts follow.

- Chronic pain management requires regularly scheduled (not prn) delivery of appropriate analgesia *in advance of* the return of pain.
- Patients do *not* exhibit signs of drug addiction (i.e., drug-seeking behavior, ever-escalating dosages) when placed on an appropriate pain management program.
- Various routes of administration (i.e., sublingual, rectal, oral) can be equally effective to the IV route when used in equianalgesic ratios.
- Morphine and its derivatives are by far the most useful drugs in the management of intractable pain.
- Knowledge of combinations of drugs such as narcotics with nonsteroidal antiinflammatory drugs can be very effective for bone pain.
- Careful assessment of pain and all of its components is essential to developing an effective intervention.

Before dealing with some of the more complex psychosocial problems such as loss and grief, the hospice nurse must make a thorough evaluation of all symptoms, particularly pain. As Maslow[5] suggested in his theory of human motivation, basic physiologic needs must be addressed and satisfied before higher needs can be considered.

NUTRITIONAL PROBLEMS IN THE TERMINALLY ILL

Even more common than pain management, nutritional problems call for much expertise from hospice staff. The fundamental piece of information for staff to gather is the meaning of food during the patient's illness and in the life of that patient and family. It is important for the hospice staff to deal with this issue sensitively because of strong individual and cultural beliefs about the importance of food.

Nutritional deficiencies usually result from nausea, with or without subsequent vomiting; mouth soreness, which may be caused by treatment or vitamin deficiencies; or anorexia. Nausea can generally be at least partially controlled by antiemetics. As with pain management, regular and prophylactic administration of antiemetics is important. Mouth soreness can usually be remedied by healing mouthwashes, topical anesthetics, and vitamin supplements. Anorexia is more complex. Quite commonly, terminally ill cancer patients simply have no appetite. Food is unappealing and may taste different from what they recall, and early satiety is the norm. "Two bites and they can't eat another thing" is an often heard lament from many a family. Anorexia as a symptom in this situation is not easily remedied. Families should learn not to make nutrition a battleground; they should encourage the patient to eat but not force feed. The nutritional content of food is far less important at this stage in life than being able to eat and to enjoy the experience of eating. Beer and pizza may be just the thing to get a little nourishment into that disease-ravaged body. No amount of nutrition will stop the progress of the disease but attempting to maintain protein stores can help skin integrity and the patient may not weaken quite so quickly.

More critical is the issue of hydration. A person can live quite a while without food (as evidenced by hunger strikers who do not eat but ingest fluids) but a human being cannot live for any length of time without fluids. IV therapy questions are often raised by families and hospice nurses must be prepared to discuss this sensitive issue. An assessment must be made of the patient's performance status, the rapidity of dehydration, level of consciousness with accompanying thirst, and patient and family views concerning hydration and other invasive procedures.

If a patient has been ambulatory but is weakening and is dehydrated, a liter or two of fluid can certainly enhance quality of life temporarily. If, however, the patient is in an extremely debilitated state, is bedridden and is barely conscious, starting IVs could be considered invasive and will probably not add an iota of quality. In the authors' experience, slow dehydration caused by ingestion of less and less fluids and finally no fluid does not usually create much discomfort. The usual symptoms created by this slow dehydration process are slight elevation of body temperature, which can be counteracted by acetaminophen suppositories, and drying of the mucous membranes like the nose and mouth, which should be kept moistened. Rapid dehydration, on the other hand, which is usually caused by prolonged vomiting, severe diarrhea, or mechanical evacuation of stomach contents, can be significantly more uncomfortable. Without replacement IVs a person will weaken and die quickly. Some patients choose to forego IV therapy knowing full well the eventual outcome.

VISIT PATTERNS

Most hospice referrals (75%) are made at the point of a patient's discharge from an acute care facility. Many times, families are asked by the facility to give home care one more try. Often during the hospital stay the patient has been evaluated and "tuned up," providing for a stable medical condition, at least initially. The visit pattern for hospice patients starts moderately at the time of admission to the program with an increase in the frequency of visits as the patient's condition begins to change. This can be contrasted with a referral of a nonterminal patient to a home health agency where the patient's needs are the greatest initially and diminish over a period of weeks (e.g., a patient with a new colostomy). Generally, the hospice visits increase in number and duration as death approaches. It is vital to be able to increase the number of visits as the patient deteriorates, thus allowing the family to feel the ever-increasing support from the hospice staff.

PREPARATION FOR A HOME DEATH

A person dying at home surrounded by family and the familiar smells, sounds, and sights can be an exceedingly beautiful experience. Almost nothing can make family members feel any better about themselves than caring for someone they love and being able to keep the loved one at home for the duration of the illness. For some a home death is the ultimate gift. For others the very thought of someone dying at home is repugnant. A hospice nurse's greatest challenge may be discerning the choice relating to home death for each patient and family. Some families feel a home death would be wonderful but unmanageable for them, while others may see a home death in much simpler terms than are accurate and are inadequately prepared physically and emotionally. The hospice nurse needs to convey to these families the sense that (1) a home death is manageable for nearly every patient and family if they have proper support; (2) it is important to address needs as they arise, so that a crisis does not occur because of unrealistic or inadequate preparation; (3) not every patient can die at home no matter how much he or she is loved and supported. It is not an indication of failure if an institutional death is necessary or is chosen by the family.

Preparing for a home death is really not too difficult if the professional people supporting the family believe home death is acceptable and are willing to help the family through it. Most patients and families say that they fear not the death but rather the dying. They are concerned about suffering.

First and foremost it must be explained that the physical symptoms will be kept to a minimum, and that the hospice staff and the patient's physician will see to it that enough of the needed medication will be supplied to keep the symptoms at bay. Some families worry about emotional suffering, but most people worry about physical suffering.

The hospice staff must be aware that many families crumble temporarily and need extra visits, telephone calls, and pats on the back to get through that time when they believe they cannot get through it. One of these crises is generally all that is seen, and the sailing is usually much smoother after that. Families may be more intent than ever to achieve a home death because now they know they can.

It is useful to alert the patient's physician and funeral home that a home death is expected. When a patient dies at home, the physician may not always be required to come and pronounce the patient dead. In some states a nurse may do the pronouncement and in other states the family may simply notify the physician and their funeral home. The words "expected home death" can be magic if the funeral home is called and its staff decides to call the local coroner. Regulations differ from state to state and accepted practices differ from municipality to municipality, but notification of the physician and the funeral home can allay many problems and their accompanying heartache. Somehow being forced to have your loved one's body taken to a local emergency department if no physician (or nurse in some locales) is available lacks the dignity that we strive for when people die at home.

ON-CALL SYSTEM

Essential to the success of a hospice program is the development of a nurse on-call system. Terminal care problems have no respect for the usual 9-to-5 Monday through Friday work week. Families need to be assured that they are only a telephone call away from expert advice or a home visit. It is extremely comforting to a family to know that someone who understands the problems can be reached regardless of the time or the day of the week. Problems always seem worse in the middle of the night and it is important to be able to reach someone and discuss them. That, coupled with the option of a home visit if needed, is often a major reason why hospice patients can remain at home until they die.

Staffing an on-call schedule is done many different ways. Most hospices use their own staff on a rotating basis, others hire extra nurses to work on call, and some use their own staff during the week with the extra staff being on call for weekends and holidays. When hospices are using their own nurses for on call they may change the person on call every day, every few days or even weekly. Whatever works best for each individual program is the right way to manage an on-call system because being on call is, perhaps, one of the most stressful parts of hospice nursing. It is difficult to work all day or all week and then be on call that night or for the weekend. On the other hand, each nurse has a slightly different way of doing things and sometimes the nurse prefers to be the person on call for better continuity of care and follow through with his or her patients. Opinions on this aspect of hospice nursing are as diverse as the many models of hospice care.

STAFF BURNOUT

One of the common concerns of outsiders viewing a hospice team in action is the expectation of "burnout" of team members. With the experience of successive losses, there is pervasive fear that the staff will not be able to survive in this working environment for long.

With this in mind, the early hospice team developers created support systems, both formal and informal, to prevent burnout from happening. Much to the surprise of hospice managers, the issue of burnout has not been a problem. Staff members come to hospice with an expectation that they will lose every patient they meet, and so for the most part they gear their involvement accordingly. It is wonderful to watch a well-integrated team taking turns with families; moving toward and away from intimacy with patients, knowing that the hospice team as a whole provides even more than the sum of its parts.

What is apparent about burnout, however, is that staff is susceptible to common work setting problems such as patient workload demands, shrinking continuing education monies, and staff personality differences. Hospice staff members have needs similar to those of any workers in a health care setting: They need to feel support from their managers, to see that their good work is valued by the agency, and to be treated fairly with scheduling, work space, patient load, time-off requests, and compensation.

Staff members leave the hospice setting for all the normal reasons: to pursue education, to change location, to spend more time with children. And, yes, it is sometimes a healthy decision to leave hospice to seek a more varied or diverse health care experience. With each person's coping abilities differing so greatly, there is no standard 2-year or 3-year stint prescribed for hospice. More important, each individual must continually evaluate job satisfaction, self-esteem, and overall personal and career goals.

References

1. Kübler-Ross, E. *On Death and Dying*. New York, NY: Macmillan, 1970.
2. Torrens, P. R. *Hospice Programs and Public Policy*. Chicago, Ill.: American Hospital Publishing, Inc., 1985.
3. Ibid., p. 11.
4. Amenta, M. O., and Bohnet, N. L. *Nursing Care of the Terminally Ill*. Boston, Mass.: Little, Brown, 1986.
5. Maslow, A. H. *Motivation and Personality*. New York, NY: Harper & Row, 1954.

FUNERALS

Contents

THE ARTICLE BY MITFORD IS TAKEN from perhaps the most widely read book about the funeral industry written in the past thirty years. While the social movement for funeral practice reform that grew up in response to this book (and a few others) has produced some changes (particularly since the 1980s), much of what she had to say in this book is as true today as it was in 1963. It will not take much to convince many readers of the truth of what Mitford had to say, but there are many other views on this emotion-laden issue that mixes money and sentiment.

The second article is by Vanderlyn Pine, who had extensive experience as a practicing funeral director prior to his becoming an academic sociologist. In this article he describes in detail the steps in the process of planning a funeral, from the first call to the funeral home through the end of the funeral itself. What makes his description useful is the sociological interpretation of events at each stage. We see how the funeral director influences the clients' decisions without making that fact obvious. The tone of this article—descriptive, rather than that of a social critic—can be contrasted with that of the Mitford selection.

Peter Metcalf's article, "Death Be Not Strange," describes funeral rites in both Borneo and the United States (making reference to Jessica Mitford's book). While that article has been included in Part II, it would fit as well here.

17 The American Way of Death ∿

Jessica Mitford

Social critic JESSICA MITFORD has written a number of influential books
over the years, but none has been more influential than *The American Way of
Death*. This book is highly critical of the materialism of the contemporary
American funeral and of a number of practices that, in her opinion, take
unfair advantage of consumers at a time when they are very vulnerable. She
is very critical of the attempt to prettify death and the many euphemisms
used by those in the funeral industry. Many have argued that the movement
stimulated by Mitford's book was an important factor leading to the implementation of the Federal Trade Commission's 1984 "Trade Regulation Rule
on Funeral Industry Practices." The selection included here is the introductory chapter of her book.

*How long, I would ask, are we to be subjected to the tyranny of custom and
undertakers? Truly, it is all vanity and vexation of spirit—a mere mockery of
woe, costly to all, far, far beyond its value; and ruinous to many; hateful, and
an abomination to all; yet submitted to by all, because none have the moral
courage to speak against it and act in defiance of it.*

LORD ESSEX

O DEATH, WHERE IS THY STING? O grave, where is thy victory? Where, indeed. Many a badly stung survivor, faced with the aftermath of some relative's
funeral, has ruefully concluded that the victory has been won hands down by a
funeral establishment—in disastrously unequal battle.

Much has been written of late about the affluent society in which we live,
and much fun poked at some of the irrational "status symbols" set out like
golden snares to trap the unwary consumer at every turn. Until recently, little
has been said about the most irrational and weirdest of the lot, lying in ambush
for all of us at the end of the road—the modern American funeral.

If the Dismal Traders (as an eighteenth-century English writer calls them)
have traditionally been cast in a comic role in literature, a universally recog-

nized symbol of humor from Shakespeare to Dickens to Evelyn Waugh, they have successfully turned the tables in recent years to perpetrate a huge, macabre and expensive practical joke on the American public. It is not consciously conceived as a joke, of course; on the contrary, it is hedged with admirably contrived rationalizations.

Gradually, almost imperceptibly, over the years the funeral men have constructed their own grotesque cloud-cuckooland where the trappings of Gracious Living are transformed, as in a nightmare, into the trappings of Gracious Dying. The same familiar Madison Avenue language, with its peculiar adjectival range designed to anesthetize sales resistance to all sorts of products, has seeped into the funeral industry in a new and bizarre guise. The emphasis is on the same desirable qualities that we have all been schooled to look for in our daily search for excellence: comfort, durability, beauty, craftsmanship. The attuned ear will recognize too the convincing quasi-scientific language, so reassuring even if unintelligible.

So that this too, too solid flesh might not melt, we are offered "solid copper—a quality casket which offers superb value to the client seeking long-lasting protection," or "the Colonial Classic Beauty—18 gauge lead coated steel, seamless top, lap-jointed welded body construction." Some are equipped with foam rubber, some with innerspring mattresses. Elgin offers "the revolutionary 'Perfect-Posture' bed." Not every casket need have a silver lining, for one may choose between "more than 60 color matched shades, magnificent and unique masterpieces" by the Cheney casket-lining people. Shrouds no longer exist. Instead, you may patronize a grave-wear couturière who promises "handmade original fashions—styles from the best in life for the last memory—dresses, men's suits, negligees, accessories." For the final, perfect grooming: "Nature-Glo—the ultimate in cosmetic embalming." And, where have we heard that phrase "peace of mind protection" before? No matter. In funeral advertising, it is applied to the Wilbert Burial Vault, with its ⅜-inch precast asphalt inner liner plus extra-thick, reinforced concrete—all this "guaranteed by Good Housekeeping." Here again the Cadillac, status symbol par excellence, appears in all its gleaming glory, this time transformed into a pastel-colored funeral hearse.

You, the potential customer for all this luxury, are unlikely to read the lyrical descriptions quoted above, for they are culled from *Mortuary Management* and *Casket and Sunnyside*, two of the industry's eleven trade magazines. For you there are ads in your daily newspaper, generally found on the obituary page, stressing dignity, refinement, high-caliber professional service and that intangible quality, *sincerity*. The trade advertisements are, however, instructive, because they furnish an important clue to the frame of mind into which the funeral industry has hypnotized itself.

A new mythology, essential to the twentieth-century American funeral rite, has grown up—or rather has been built up step by step—to justify the peculiar customs surrounding the disposal of our dead. And, just as the witch doctor must be convinced of his own infallibility in order to maintain a hold over his clientele, so the funeral industry has had to "sell itself" on its articles of faith in the course of passing them along to the public.

The first of these is the tenet that today's funeral procedures are founded in "American tradition." The story comes to mind of a sign on the freshly sown lawn of a brand-new Midwest college: "There is a tradition on this campus that students never walk on this strip of grass. This tradition goes into effect next Tuesday." The most cursory look at American funerals of past times will establish the parallel. Simplicity to the point of starkness, the plain pine box, the laying out of the dead by friends and family who also bore the coffin to the grave—these were the hallmarks of the traditional funeral until the end of the nineteenth century.

Secondly, there is the myth that the American public is only being given what it wants—an opportunity to keep up with the Joneses to the end. "In keeping with our high standard of living, there should be an equally high standard of dying," says the past president of the Funeral Directors of San Francisco. "The cost of a funeral varies according to individual taste and the niceties of living the family has been accustomed to." Actually, choice doesn't enter the picture for the average individual, faced, generally for the first time, with the necessity of buying a product of which he is totally ignorant, at a moment when he is least in a position to quibble. In point of fact the cost of a funeral almost always varies, not "according to individual taste" but according to what the traffic will bear.

Thirdly, there is an assortment of myths based on half-digested psychiatric theories. The importance of the "memory picture" is stressed—meaning the last glimpse of the deceased in open casket, done up with the latest in embalming techniques and finished off with a dusting of makeup. A newer one, impressively authentic-sounding, is the need for "grief therapy," which is beginning to go over big in mortuary circles. A historian of American funeral directing hints at the grief-therapist idea when speaking of the new role of the undertaker—"the dramaturgic role, in which the undertaker becomes a stage manager to create an appropriate atmosphere and to move the funeral party through a drama in which social relationships are stressed and an emotional catharsis or release is provided through ceremony."

Lastly, a whole new terminology, as ornately shoddy as the satin rayon casket liner, has been invented by the funeral industry to replace the direct and serviceable vocabulary of former times. Undertaker has been supplanted by "funeral director" or "mortician." (Even the classified section of the telephone directory gives recognition to this; in its pages you will find "Undertakers— see Funeral Directors.") Coffins are "caskets"; hearses are "coaches," or "professional cars"; flowers are "floral tributes"; corpses generally are "loved ones," but mortuary etiquette dictates that a specific corpse be referred to by name only—as, "Mr. Jones"; cremated ashes are "cremains." Euphemisms such as "slumber room," "reposing room," and "calcination—the *kindlier* heat" abound in the funeral business.

If the undertaker is the stage manager of the fabulous production that is the modern American funeral, the stellar role is reserved for the occupant of the open casket. The decor, the stagehands, the supporting cast are all arranged for the most advantageous display of the deceased, without which the rest of the paraphernalia would lose its point—*Hamlet* without the Prince of Denmark. It is to this end that a fantastic array of costly merchandise and services is pyramided to dazzle the mourners and facilitate the plunder of the next of kin.

Grief therapy, anyone? But it's going to come high. According to the funeral industry's own figures, the *average* undertaker's bill in 1961 was $708 for casket and "services," to which must be added the cost of a burial vault, flowers, clothing, clergy and musician's honorarium, and cemetery charges. When these costs are added to the undertaker's bill, the total average cost for an adult's funeral is, as we shall see, closer to $1,450.

The question naturally arises, *is* this what most people want for themselves and their families? For several reasons, this has been a hard one to answer until recently. It is a subject seldom discussed. Those who have never had to arrange for a funeral frequently shy away from its implications, preferring to take comfort in the thought that sufficient unto the day is the evil thereof. Those who have acquired personal and painful knowledge of the subject would often rather forget about it. Pioneering "Funeral Societies" or "Memorial Associations," dedicated to the principle of dignified funerals at reasonable cost, have existed in a number of communities throughout the country, but their membership has been limited for the most part to the more sophisticated element in the population—university people, liberal intellectuals—and those who, like doctors and lawyers, come up against problems in arranging funerals for their clients.

Some indication of the pent-up resentment felt by vast numbers of people against the funeral interests was furnished by the astonishing response to an article by Roul Tunley, titled "Can You Afford to Die?" in *The Saturday Evening Post* of June 17, 1961. As though a dike had burst, letters poured in from every part of the country to the *Post*, to the funeral societies, to local newspapers. They came from clergymen, professional people, old-age pensioners, trade unionists. Three months after the article appeared, an estimated six thousand had taken pen in hand to comment on some phase of the high cost of dying. Many recounted their own bitter experiences at the hands of funeral directors; hundreds asked for advice on how to establish a consumer organization in communities where none exists; others sought information about pre-need plans. The membership of the funeral societies skyrocketed. The funeral industry, finding itself in the glare of public spotlight, has begun to engage in serious debate about its own future course—as well it might.

Is the funeral inflation bubble ripe for bursting? A few years ago, the United States public suddenly rebelled against the trend in the auto industry towards ever more showy cars, with their ostentatious and nonfunctional fins, and a demand was created for compact cars patterned after European models. The all-powerful auto industry, accustomed to *telling* the customer what sort of car he wanted, was suddenly forced to *listen* for a change. Overnight, the little cars became for millions a new kind of status symbol. Could it be that the same cycle is working itself out in the attitude towards the final return of dust to dust, that the American public is becoming sickened by ever more ornate and costly funerals, and that a status symbol of the future may indeed be the simplest kind of "funeral without fins"?

18 Public Behavior in the Funeral Home

Vanderlyn R. Pine

VANDERLYN PINE was a practicing funeral director for more than ten years prior to becoming a sociologist. For many years he was professor of sociology at the State University of New York at New Paltz. Today he is a national consultant on death, dying, and bereavement. Among his books are *Responding to Disaster, Acute Grief and the Funeral, Unrecognized and Unsanctioned Grief,* and *Caretaker of the Dead*, the book that the present selection is taken from. In this selection, he describes how funeral directors carry out the public aspects of their work. From a symbolic interactionist perspective, he discusses such issues as the prospective client's first call to the funeral director, the process of making the funeral arrangement, selecting the casket, visitation, and the funeral itself. A great deal of attention is given to issues linked to impression management.

THIS CHAPTER DESCRIBES, discusses, and analyzes how funeral directors carry out the public aspects of their work. It is largely through the conduct of the funeral director and the carrying out of his conception of relevant funeral activities that the bereaved develop a notion of "appropriate" funeral behavior. In this way, the funeral director helps establish the context in which funerals occur much as doctors collectively help set the boundaries of illness.[1] Therefore, we focus on the funeral director's *public* behavior in the funeral home.

THE FIRST CALL

Whenever the telephone rings in a funeral home, it represents a potential summons for the funeral director, for it may be a "call" that informs of a death. If it is an initial summons, it is referred to as the "first call." Someone has died and the funeral home must direct its activities to take care of that dead person and his bereaved survivors. All funeral directors try to treat their first calls calmly and patiently.

No matter what else is said, the Community Funeral Home directors make an effort to assure the family that "We will take care of all the necessary details and get things under control right away, and we will do everything we can to make the next few days easier." This assurance may be met with silence on the part of the calling family, or there may be questions or requests; at other times, statements may be made about funeral plans. The funeral director usually offers as the next bit of information:

> *I'm very sorry for your troubles. For the time being, you needn't worry about anything. We'll take care of all the necessary details. However, it would be a good idea if you and your family could collect your thoughts, organize your ideas, and plan to come to the funeral home to make the funeral arrangements. At that time, we can work out your wishes for the funeral.*

What the funeral director really means by this statement is that he will remove the deceased from the place of death and ready himself for the encounter with the family. This encounter is to complete making funeral arrangements, to gather the statistical information regarding the bereaved and deceased, and to provide an opportunity for the funeral director to offer to the bereaved his various services, facilities, and merchandise. It is felt that the funeral director's seeming imperturbability and professional competence is important to demonstrate at this time. By carefully weighing each word and paying close attention to what the bereaved say, the funeral directors of the Community Funeral Home generally are able to effect the impression of deep concern and knowledgeable control.

When a first call is received at the Cosmopolitan Funeral Home, it is answered by the switchboard operator, who transfers the call to one of the funeral counselors. The counselor's method of handling first calls is different from the one described above for the Community Funeral Home directors. The counselor's main concern is getting enough information so that most of the funeral arrangements can be made without waiting for the family to come into the funeral home.

Each counselor is careful to identify himself individually to affect a sense of personal service. Then, he offers some words of sympathy to foster this impression. Once these preliminaries are over, the counselor begins to ascertain every possible bit of pertinent information. By carefully measuring his words and not rushing the bereaved with questions, the counselor elicits a great deal of information in a short period of time. He fills out three sets of cards while he is talking and generally gathers all of the statistical information for the death certificate in a matter of minutes.

Both the Community Funeral Home directors and the Cosmopolitan Funeral Home counselors appear to be competent professionals carrying out an important aspect of their job when handling first calls. The difference between them is emphasis and direction. The funeral directors of the Community Funeral Home are concerned primarily with giving the appearance over the phone that they are concerned, knowledgeable, and anxious to be of assistance, but that they want to deal with the bereaved in a face-to-face personal situation at the funeral home. The Cosmopolitan Funeral Home counselors, on the other hand, use this occasion to gather information and do not waste their time with comforting efforts that have little functional value for them.

Having spoken to a number of families about such first calls, it seems that the funeral directors of both firms were successful in what they were trying to do. Some families served by the Community Funeral Home said such things as, "Once I had made the call, I felt so much at ease. They seemed to know just what they were doing," and, "You just know they care and will do the best job possible after talking with them on the phone." The remarks of the families served by the Cosmopolitan Funeral Home went typically like this: "After talking with the funeral director, I felt relieved because he obviously knew what he was talking about. He seemed to be so efficient at his work that I figured he must know what he's doing," or, "It was really a pleasure to talk with him. After dealing with those people at the hospital switchboard, I expected somebody who couldn't tell me anything. Instead I got a man who knew exactly what was going on and why."[2] . . .

MAKING ARRANGEMENTS

It is customary that following the first call and sometime before, during, or after the removal of the deceased from the place of death, the funeral director and the family sit down together and plan the funeral, that is, "they make arrangements."[3] This process is an important aspect of every funeral call, and all funeral directors take particular care in assuring that their setting is appropriate and that they are psychologically prepared for such an encounter. Sometimes the notification of the death is made by people in person at the funeral home, and while there, they make the complete plans and arrangements for the funeral. In such a case the first call actually occurs at the same time as the making of arrangements, but for present purposes we treat them as two separate events.

In the Community Funeral Home those making the arrangements for the funeral gather in the office of the funeral director. The conversation often includes a discussion of general funeral customs, the specific customs that the particular family wishes to carry out, and the schedule which will be followed for the next few days of the funeral. During this period the funeral director usually ascertains all of the necessary vital statistics for filing the death certificate and burial permit.[4] Most questions are asked in a straightforward fashion and the answers recorded on a standard form provided by the state's Department of

Health. Such additional items as the names of survivors and the deceased's educational background are gathered by the funeral director at this time. It is during this period that many families voluntarily discuss the dying period, how they learned of the deceased's death, and similar matters. Although the funeral directors do not make note of this extra information, it is offered commonly in a general conversational way by many families.[5]

Much of this statistical and obituary information is gathered at the time of the first call by the counselors for the Cosmopolitan Funeral Home. If not, it is recorded by the counselor while making arrangements. Usually, his questions review the information previously gathered, and he quickly goes over pertinent matters to be certain that the forms are correct. It is interesting that a great many families working with the counselors divulge similar extra information as those dealing with the Community Funeral Home directors. Notably, there appears to be a desire to talk about one's problems, and on numerous occasions bereaved families use the counselor as a sounding board for their thoughts about the deceased and his death. They seemed to be seeking some form of personal attention from the counselors. To some extent, they receive it, for the counselors are good listeners and most of them give the impression of being sympathetic and understanding of the problems the bereaved mention. During the course of making arrangements, therefore, the counselors for the Cosmopolitan Funeral Home seem to provide professional services, even though the way in which they foster this impression is through bureaucratically oriented and efficiently conceived procedures.

During this arrangement period, funeral directors at both firms explain as many aspects of the funeral as possible. They offer advice and suggestions when they are solicited. The following questions are typical of the advice sought and questions asked.

"Should we look at the body?"
"Should we have visiting hours?"
"Should we bring the children to the funeral?"
"What should we do when people come into the funeral home?"
"What cemetery should we buy a plot in?"
"Where should we buy flowers?"
"What should we do about the insurance policy?"
"What about social security?"
"What about joint bank accounts?"
"Should we get a lawyer?"

It was observed on many occasions that the bereaved funeral arrangers depended on the funeral director's answers to these questions for much of their subsequent behavior.[6] In most instances, the funeral directors attempted to appear knowledgeable and concerned. For example, there were no outright fabrications to increase either the family's social involvement or their financial obligation.

Of course, by refraining from such fabrications, the funeral director has a chance to demonstrate his professional skill as a nonpartisan funerary specialist. Furthermore, the funeral director, like other professionals, derives a large measure of work satisfaction from actually helping bereaved families.[7] . . .

In addition to deciding upon the type of service, and selecting the casket, an important outcome of making arrangements is designating the time, place, and date for the funeral service. For the most part this is contingent upon arrangements the family have made or will make with a clergyperson. At this point an interesting difference between the Community Funeral Home and the Cosmopolitan Funeral Home stands out.

Apparently, because of the Community Funeral Home directors' wish to please people and to gain respect, they seem to bend over backwards to make the scheduling of the funeral compatible with everyone's wishes, largely excluding the convenience or inconvenience to themselves. They schedule funerals to suit the family, the clergy, and the cemetery, and, then, they manipulate their staff and facilities to fit. This emphasizes that the Community Funeral Home directors aim their behavior at and modify it primarily for the bereaved and the public rather than themselves or other funeral directors.

Such a practice stands out as one of the unique features of funeral directing as a service occupation, especially since it disrupts their personal lives. For instance, they all mentioned how much they dislike to be called out on weekends; however, they always added the postscript, "Well, that's just the nature of things, people can't help it when they die."

The scheduling of funeral services for the Cosmopolitan Funeral Home is geared to the desires of the bereaved family to some extent. However, the concerns of the firm are more important in determining the exact time of the funeral. In one sense, this is a matter of logistics, because to handle a large number of services in a given amount of time requires precise scheduling to eliminate overlap.

The counselors handle this organizational necessity in an interesting fashion. When talking with the bereaved family they unobtrusively check the master schedule which shows the times and locations of funeral services, and then they suggest the time to the family by asking a question such as this: "Now, let's see, today is Monday. This means you would probably want the funeral Wednesday or Thursday. Possible Wednesday afternoon at 3:00 or Thursday morning at 10:00?" In most cases, the family feels that it has a choice between two times, a morning service or an afternoon service, and they seem pleased when they make their final decision, as if the time had been their idea in the first place. . . .

Making arrangements for a funeral involves more than merely scheduling the time for the actual services. One of the important results of making arrangements is the selection of the casket to be used for the service. Although the casket is a mercantile item, it has become an integral part of American funeral service, and funeral directors at both firms look upon its selection as an important element of making arrangements.

SELECTING THE CASKET

In almost all instances, the casket is selected by the next of kin of the deceased. There is a wide range of available types, styles, and prices of caskets, and both funeral homes display a fairly large selection of caskets and other funeral merchandise in their selection rooms.

The funeral directors in the Community Funeral Home believe that it is not their job to try to "sell caskets," but they do feel that it is part of their job to explain the differences between caskets for the family's information if requested. Most of the time, however, they merely enter the selection room with the family and mention that each casket is marked with a price card showing its cost. They go on to explain that any questions the family may have will be answered willingly. Generally, at this point, they allow the family to browse through the casket selection room and make their own choice.

Importantly, the caskets are purchased by the funeral director for their attractive qualities, and the differences in price stand out rather obviously even to the inexperienced eye. All of the caskets are shown in the same room and are not separated into sections by price or quality. The Community Funeral Home directors believe that the attractiveness of their selection room and the appearance of the caskets will help in the sale and "allow the family to make this decision without pressure and yet be aware of the different values that exist."

On one occasion a bereaved family commented that they were shocked that they were left to themselves in the selection room and that the funeral director did not try to force the sale of a casket. They were so surprised and put at ease by this lack of pressure to "buy an expensive casket" that "we spent more than we had planned to, and after looking everything over, we are glad that we were able to do so." Thus, it may be that presenting themselves as professionals who are not concerned with sales, the funeral directors in the Community Funeral Home are able to handle their sales more effectively; however, they never consciously spoke of "sales" in these terms.

The counselors at the Cosmopolitan Funeral Home are considerably more professional than one would expect given the size of the operation and its form of organization. Notably, the counselors are not paid commissions for caskets sales, which means that to some extent they are able to effect a detached air about the purchase. It is important that the firm keeps extensive business records which analyze the quality of sale made by each counselor over a six-month period. So, although a specific sale is relatively uninfluenced by efforts to sell expensive caskets, the records of the firm are such that the counselor admitted that in the long run they are concerned with sales, but that it really does not influence individual transactions.[8] Of course, this enables them to behave as concerned professionals, not overly interested in selling expensive merchandise.

The selection room of the Cosmopolitan Funeral Home is separated into several sections. The largest section includes a wide range of differently priced caskets, but there are small annexes in which there are extremely low-priced and extremely high-priced caskets. It was explained that those people wishing to select an especially expensive casket deserved to be treated exclusively and to be taken to a room in which only the best were shown. Conversely, anyone wanting the cheapest casket possible also deserved to be so segregated. The room is small and crowded because it is not profitable to display inexpensive merchandise to the exclusion of moderate to more expensive merchandise. Thus, the Cosmopolitan Funeral Home also uses the physical setting and appearance to help make casket sales and still appear as a professional operation.

Let us turn from the sales techniques used by funeral directors and focus on some observations regarding funeral director orientations toward merchandise, caskets, and funeral sales. First, families assumed to have limited funds generally were discouraged by the funeral directors from purchasing beyond their assumed limit of paying ability, although they were encouraged to spend up to that limit. This observation is counter to the criticisms leveled at funeral directors for overselling their merchandise. All the funeral directors claimed that there is little sense in making big sales for which they never will be paid; therefore, concerted efforts seem to be made to encourage families with "less than adequate means" to select something within (up to the limit of) their financial reach including available insurance and bank accounts. . . .

Good purchases elicit behavior from the funeral director which is similar to that of attorneys and physicians when confronted with a client or patient whose ability to pay is well above "average."[9] While the actual services rendered may be essentially similar and there is not necessarily a deliberate effort to give these "more fortunate" people more or better service, the cordiality with which service is given is the most noticeably different thing. Wealthy families with high social status generally are treated not just to the best services available by the funeral director, but also they are treated by him in a most felicitous way.[10] . . .

VISITATION

Once the arrangements are made and the body prepared, generally the next event is "visitation." Visitation is that period during which family and friends of the deceased and of the bereaved come to "pay their respects" and to offer condolences. This period is alternately called the "wake," "visiting hours," "calling hours," or "viewing." It is the time for the regathering of scattered units, whether these be familial or friendship relationships.

Visitation usually commences with the first viewing by the immediate next of kin. This is an upsetting time for most families. It is their first exposure to the deceased either since sometime before death, or just after death occurred. The fears that "Daddy won't look the same anymore," or that "Dad was such a mess," or that "Mother had lost so much weight and had gotten so wrinkled" all loom before the family prior to the first viewing. In general, the first viewing allays many of the fears of the bereaved. Due to the restorative efforts of both firms, this first exposure generally produces a positive reaction, with surprise at "how well he looks," and relief because "things aren't as bad as I expected."

This time is also a chance for the family to break down openly and to display grief reactions to each other. Such reactions, however, must be modified fairly quickly to accommodate friends and relatives who are also interested in being involved. Throughout this period of time the Community Funeral Home directors generally remain in the background ready to assist if needed and ready to answer questions. The Cosmopolitan Funeral Home personnel merely check on how things are arranged and then leave the bereaved alone when all seems satisfactory.

Normally, there is very little reaction with the exception of tearful comments such as, "You've done a magnificent job," or, "You certainly have done more than I ever expected." It is common for the funeral director to try to learn if the deceased looks the way the bereaved want him to look without asking in so many words. Most families get the message, but some, however, see his probes differently. For instance, they make statements such as: "No, everything's not the way I want it. He's dead! Isn't he?" or "I thought the casket was darker," or "I didn't realize that flowers made such a difference. It will be nice when some more get here." If this occurs, the funeral director may drop the subject or probe a bit further and ask, "Is your mother's hair the way you want it?"

The funeral director's concern with the appearance of the dead body eventually seems to get communicated to the bereaved. The awareness of such a concern is an important aspect in helping the bereaved know just what the body of the deceased actually "should" be to them. The concern with the appearance is made openly by the funeral director and draws attention to his work, his importance, and his practical value, as well as to the lifeless body of the deceased. Thus, although the funeral director's reasons for emphasizing the dead body actually may not be the same as the social-psychological value of viewing the dead, the result often is the same. His efforts enable the family to come to an acceptance of death that would not occur if the funeral director did not attend to or concern himself with such appearances.[11] . . .

THE FUNERAL

When funeral directors refer to "the funeral" they mean the actual funeral process, including the social-psychological events for acting out feelings that are basic to therapeutic intervention.[12] The funeral may occur in the funeral home, in the home of the deceased, in a church or other public building, at the cemetery, or any place the bereaved decide to carry out the commemorative service. Whatever the setting, funeral behavior is essentially the same.

On the day of the funeral, the funeral director and his assistants are prepared well in advance, and they stand ready to greet people long before they are due to arrive. Wherever the funeral takes place, it is customary for the funeral director to seat the bereaved family in the front of the room. Usually, they usher them to this position in a slow and deliberate fashion. The front location of the family is thought to be an important part of the funeral, and on the few occasions when families seated themselves elsewhere, the funeral directors made certain that they moved to the front.

The funeral director in the Community Funeral Home is easily identifiable not only because he acts as a doorman and head usher for the bereaved family, but also because he is well known to the townspeople. Many years ago, the earlier Community Funeral Home directors made certain that they would be identifiable by wearing morning dress. Today, they emphasize their identities by their actions and reputations.

At the Cosmopolitan Funeral Home, some of the funeral directors still wear striped pants and black jackets to identify themselves. Others identify themselves by their actions. One of the commonly used devices to foster the appearance of being the funeral director is to carry an arrangement card containing notations about the funerals. In almost all instances observed, the director knew all he needed without the card; thus, it had little functional value except to identify him as the director of the service.

Funeral directors in both settings work hard to make the funeral go as smoothly as possible. This includes maintaining an orderly seating arrangement and making certain that the participants in the funeral do not do something unexpected, for surprise easily upsets the event.

One of the important but too often overlooked elements of the funeral is that it allows the bereaved to behave in a death-appropriate mask. In the setting of both funeral homes, it is appropriate for men to be seen with tears in their eyes, for women to be disheveled, and otherwise obviously affected by the death.[13] Prior to and during the funeral, all such behavior is not merely allowed, but it is encouraged by the funeral director through his activities and procedures. Thus, to some extent, it is because of his behavior that the bereaved come to have a definition of the funeral as a useful social process to attend death.

. . . When a body is donated to medical science by a family, the Community Funeral Home director usually plays very little part in the definition of the funeral situation. The family may decide to go through some kind of memorial service, but seldom do they ask the funeral home to help them arrange for such a service. This makes problems not just for the funeral director, but for the community as well, for in such an instance, it is impossible for friends and acquaintances to act out many of the parts that they usually do when someone dies.[14]

For example, the obituary which announces the death almost never mentions that the body has been donated to science. Thus, although word about the death may spread, it remains little more than news floating in space with no actual connection to "acceptable" funeral behavior. At times there may be a memorial service handled by the family and a church or other organization. Because such organizations are not usually familiar with publicity about funerals or memorial services in the same way the Community Funeral Home is, very seldom are such services adequately publicized to allow attendance of all those concerned with the deceased.

Naturally, this means that the funeral is never likely to be completed in the "standard" way. Of course, it is possible to offer condolences in other settings; the point is that it is not commonly done. Even in the funeral home setting, it is difficult enough to offer useful consolation to the bereaved, and without such a setting, the problems become considerably greater. While such problems often are treated as unimportant for society, they are always important for the funeral director whose main concern is with defining and carrying out the necessary steps to complete the funeral.

The situation of the Cosmopolitan Funeral Home regarding such an event as the donation of a body to science does not have the same impact for the funeral directors. Since each of them only attends to specific aspects of the funeral, there tends to be little feeling about not completing one. The donation of a body to science merely means that the removal man does all the work. He goes to the hospital and makes the removal and takes the body to the institution to which it was donated. He is not distressed that he does not get a chance to meet the family face to face, for he never deals face to face with families. The counselor handling the family also is not distressed not only because his work is briefer than usual, but also because he is never concerned with the completion of the funeral ceremony. Thus, none of the specialists of the Cosmopolitan Funeral Home feel the impact of a donation to science in the same way that the total practitioner does in the Community Funeral Home.

It makes sense that the funeral director's public behavior inside his funeral home helps foster and encourage many aspects of the lay public's funeral behavior. This is not to say that the funeral director's motivations for doing so are necessarily in the best interests of the bereaved in every situation. Rather, it is through his dramatic presentations that he helps implement their funerary activities. Let us now turn our attention to the ways the funeral director manages the impressions of funeral performances others receive.

FUNERAL DIRECTORS AND IMPRESSION MANAGEMENT

When the funeral director is able to work on his own home ground inside his funeral home, he is under relatively little pressure and is able to practice to the full his arts of impression management.[15] Important in this regard is the fact that the funeral director no longer goes forth to meet families in their homes as he did years ago, for it is to the funeral home that they come to make funeral arrangements.

Impression management, however, involves more than the spatial location of the funeral director's workshop, just as it involves more than the hospital as the physician's workshop, or the courtroom as the attorney's workshop, or the schoolroom as the teacher's workshop. Notably, there are a number of techniques which are commonly used to carry out impression management by funeral directors. Tact is important to the funeral director. He is careful not to offend or otherwise adversely impress the family which comes to make the funeral arrangements. This means that his attitudes, actions, and behavior are carefully modulated to reflect an aura of tact and cooperativeness that might not otherwise exist. . . .

Tact is not the only attribute required of the funeral director. Loyalty to the overall funeral is another. This refers to funeral directors strictly adhering to and remaining loyal to all of the dramaturgical demands of the funeral. For funeral directors in both firms, an important aspect of maintaining the loyalty of team members is that they are not allowed to become too sympathetically attached to the bereaved. In this way, funeral directors are seldom tempted to be disloyal to the overall funeral.[16]

The funeral team also is likely to develop considerable internal solidarity and an image of the bereaved as an audience which tends somewhat to dehumanize them and allows the funeral directors to deal with them on an impersonal emotional basis.[17] In this sense, it is important that funeral directors form a complete social unit, and that the funeral team as a society has built-in sources of support which allow its members to be protected from the doubts of the bereaved audience. This sort of esprit de corps is very important to all professional groups, and it is not merely a defense mechanism. Moreover, to the extent that funeral directors conceive of their professional role as members of an important caretaking occupation, their team behavior is built around respect and appreciation for their common role.

Funeral directors also are prevented from developing strong affective ties with the bereaved because they deal with each bereaved family separately either only once, or, on rare occasions, a few times.[18] For example, a widow arranging for her husband's funeral will not arrange for her own funeral as well, although she may act as an arranger for some other family member. The number of contacts between even the Community Funeral Home director and a particular family are limited considerably; thus, the affective contacts with the bereaved have little chance to become well developed. However, even though the length of time of any funeral is quite brief and would appear to leave little room for the development of strong affective ties between the funeral director and bereaved families in either setting, the distinction between chronological time and psychological time considerably modifies the situation. Emotional movement is rapid in times of crisis and stress, and the time the funeral director spends with a bereaved family, although short in hours, may be highly privileged and meaningful in terms of impact and development.

Another important element in maintaining the stability of the overall funeral is that the funeral team has dramaturgical discipline.[19] Funeral directors must be disciplined not to break their role, and they must be consistent in their part and not give the show away by disclosing secrets that are pertinent to it. Thus, a funeral director who observes an assistant making a blunder must be careful not to shout or run wildly to the assistant's aid, thereby drawing attention to the error. He must carry out the funeral by adhering to the strictest discipline possible, and an important part of the training of future funeral directors involves imparting to them a sense of calm during the service. Thus, apprentice funeral directors are cautioned: "Never run, even when something drastic happens, such as someone fainting beside the casket, or somebody knocking over a basket of flowers." . . .

. . . An important part in the training of a funeral director is that he learns how to appear to be appropriately solemn and yet not somber or depressing to the bereaved. His facial expression must be managed so as to give the impression of care, interest, and understanding, not dismay, fear, or panic.

It is necessary for the funeral director to make prudent preparations for the funeral itself. He must prepare in advance for contingencies which could disrupt the process. For example, someone fainting during visiting hours disrupts the supposedly smooth operation of the funeral home. In both organizations, it is common for funeral directors to be prepared for such swooning people by having small kits of ammonia capsules, and they are quick to hand these out to those members of the family who are expected to be best able to "take" the stress. . . .

A technique that is commonly available to professional practitioners staging an occupational performance which allows for dramaturgical circumspection is not always available to the funeral director. Since people come to him, the funeral director is unable to select the kind of bereaved audience that will cause a minimum of trouble in terms of the kind of funeral service he wants.[20]

Clearly, it makes it difficult that the funeral director must perform before audiences that are not necessarily optimally selected. The Cosmopolitan Funeral
Home is not nearly so limited in this regard as is the Community Funeral
Home. In large urban areas it is common for people to select funeral directors
based on such things as ethnic ties, religious affiliation, and social status. Thus,
although the funeral director in the Cosmopolitan Funeral Home does not
select his bereaved families specifically, there is usually a process of self-
selectivity which often affords him a certain amount of dramaturgical circumspection regarding audience selection. . . .

Normally, it is important for an audience to have some knowledge of the
performer in advance of any staged or real-life performance. In the Community Funeral Home this is commonly the case, for it is operated by people
whose reputations are "good," practices well known, and community relationships highly developed; however, in the Cosmopolitan Funeral Home the
situation is considerably different, and only the firm possesses such attributes.
In either event, when the bereaved family enters into a relationship with the funeral director, familiarity with his (or his firm's) techniques and practices is
often such that it allows them to judge his work as he carries it out. Because of
this relationship with the bereaved, and because the funeral director is judged
by laypeople rather than other funeral directors, it is important for him to make
obvious the important aspects of the funeral performance by his front, his
manner, and his appearance.

Funeral directors are also dramaturgically circumspect and prudent in that
they adhere to a rather strict agenda; thus, funerals seldom are run in a haphazard fashion.[21] Naturally, this reduces the possibility of disruption of the overall
funeral. Paradoxically, the funeral director also must be careful to stick to his
plan with greater diligence than if he ran things with considerable leeway.[22] Funerals are scheduled for specific times with many other operations contingent
upon that time. For instance, the use of the church, arrival at the cemetery,
arrangement for vehicles, etc., are set in advance; therefore, funerals do not
get "rained out," postponed, or similarly disrupted because of a change in
plans.

Thus, no matter what conditions arise that conceivably could disrupt a funeral, "the show must go on." For instance, cemeteries which are unable to
open graves because of frozen ground during the winter notify funeral directors well in advance that the grave opening is impossible, and arrangements are
made to store the deceased in a receiving vault until the ground allows the grave
to be opened. Never does the cemetery wait until the funeral procession arrives
for the burial, for to them that would completely disrupt the performance, and
the entire funeral would be blown to pieces. Thus, the funeral team cooperates.

Most of the defensive techniques of impression management are accompanied by a tendency on the part of an audience or an outsider to act in a reciprocally protective way, thereby allowing the performers to save their own

show.[23] One of the common techniques that allows for such protection is that individuals voluntarily stay away from those regions to which they have not been invited. For instance, the bereaved would not enter into the preparation room and accidentally stumble onto an embalming, even if the funeral director did not specifically exclude them from there. Thus, tact on the part of the funeral audience as well as exclusions by the funeral performer serve to protect the performer from disruptive behavior.

The audience also may generously forgive slips, errors, or mistakes made by the performer.[24] Thus, when a funeral director inadvertently and accidentally buries the deceased with jewelry on that was supposed to be removed, the audience may forgive him, saying such things as, "Well, she would have wanted it that way anyway, so it's probably for the best;" or, "God meant for her to have those things anyway."

There seem to be a number of reasons why bereaved audiences behave in such a tactful manner. First, the bereaved may identify with the funeral director and be hesitant to expose him because of knowing how badly he would feel. Second, it may be that the bereaved do not want to have an unpleasant scene which would prove little or nothing; therefore, they just accept things as being accidental. Third, it may be that the bereaved intend to exploit the funeral director by ingratiating themselves to him, and it may be that they display good humor and tact in hopes of reducing the funeral bill or otherwise compromising the funeral director. . . .

Notes

1. For a complete treatment of the "Social Construction of Illness" see Eliot Freidson, *Profession of Medicine: A Study in the Sociology of Applied Knowledge.* New York: Dodd, Mead, and Co., 1970, pp. 203–331.

2. For a discussion about general hospital death-related behavior see Freidson, *op. cit.*, pp. 109–36; for death-related behavior and communication see Barney G. Glaser and Anselm Strauss, *Awareness of Dying.* Chicago: Aldine Publishing Company, 1965; David Sudnow, *Passing On.* Englewood Cliffs, N.J.: Prentice-Hall, Inc., 1967; and Vanderlyn R. Pine, "Institutionalized Communication About Dying and Death," *Journal of Thanatology*, forthcoming.

3. Such arrangements are historically common to funeral behavior. A possible explanation for this is offered by Parsons and involves the concept of "keeping going" even under great stress through customary ritualized behavior. For a related theoretical discussion of this concept see Talcott Parsons, *The Social System.* New York: The Free Press, 1951, p. 304.

4. The questions include the deceased's name, age, sex, marital status, date and place of birth, parents' names, social security number, veteran's status, place of burial, etc. The cause of death is entered by the attending physician, coroner, or medical examiner.

5. The situation is similar to the case of physicians learning confidential information about their patient's private life. See Parsons, *op. cit.*, p. 452.

6. This contributes, of course, to the funeral director's ability to help the family construct funerary reality and is similar to the physician's ability to do so with a patient's illness. For a discussion of this aspect of medicine, see Freidson, *op. cit.*, pp. 286–88.

7. This is a source of satisfaction for some bureaucratic officials as is pointed out by Peter M. Blau, *The Dynamics of Bureaucracy*. Chicago: University of Chicago Press, 1955, pp. 83–86.

8. For an interesting comparison about the effect of such organizational pressures in bureaucracies see Blau, *op. cit.*, pp. 36–56; and in medicine see Freidson, *op. cit.*, pp. 98–105.

9. For comparison see Freidson, *op. cit.*, pp. 30–36, 90–93, and 362; also see Erwin O. Smigel, *The Wall Street Lawyer*. Bloomington: The Indiana University Press, 1969, pp. 176–78 and 200.

10. A similar observation is made about other professionals; see Peter M. Blau and W. Richard Scott, *Formal Organizations*. San Francisco: Chandler Publishing Company, 1962, pp. 74–81.

11. Once again, the funeral director is engaged actively in the construction of funeral behavior much as the physician is with illness. For comparison see Freidson, *op. cit.*, pp. 203–331.

12. For a fuller discussion see Parsons, *op. cit.*, pp. 443–45; and L. E. Abt and S. L. Weisman (eds.), *Acting Out: Theoretical and Clinical Aspects*. New York: Grune and Stratton, 1965.

13. For comparison with the "funeral show" see Parsons' discussion of "expressive symbolism," *op. cit.*, pp. 510–13.

14. For an additional perspective on this very problem see Parsons, *op. cit.*, pp. 443–45.

15. See Erving Goffman, *The Presentation of Self in Everyday Life*. Garden City, New York: Doubleday Co., Anchor Books, 1959, pp. 208–37.

16. For a fuller discussion see Goffman, *op. cit.*, p. 214.

17. This is similar to the way in which jazz musicians deal with their audiences. See Howard S. Becker, *Outsiders*. New York: The Free Press, 1963, pp. 79–120.

18. This is very different from what happens to physicians. See Freidson, *op. cit.*, pp. 109–36.

19. For a full discussion see Goffman, *op. cit.*, pp. 216–218.

20. For a full discussion of this sort of problem see *ibid.*, p. 219.

21. For a more detailed discussion of this aspect of occupational difficulties *ibid.*, pp. 218–28.

22. In this sense, as well as for other reasons, funerals can be thought of in terms of "routine and emergency," for even though time is not usually a crucial factor, once the funeral schedule is established it becomes more important. For comparison see Hughes, *Men and Their Work*, Glencoe, Ill.: The Free Press, 1958, pp. 54–55, and *The Sociological Eye*: Book 2. Chicago: Aldine-Atherton, 1971.

23. For an expanded treatment of how the audience protects the performer see Goffman, *op. cit.*, pp. 88–101.

24. For a discussion about occupational mistakes see Hughes, *op. cit.*, pp. 88–101.

GRIEF AND BEREAVEMENT

Contents

TO BE A SURVIVOR, to have suffered a grievous loss of someone close, is a terrible plight. If grief is not an illness, its effects are often so severe that it might as well be one. Grief and mourning are powerful and stressful emotional states that can touch off conscious and unconscious psychological reactions that jeopardize the individual's life. Studies show that loss of a loved one is at the top of the list of stressful, abrasive, and disruptive life events. For a while—at least a year or so—the grieving person is an individual at risk; more apt to neglect adequate care, more apt to be sick and hospitalized, and even more likely to die or be killed.

Currently there is much-needed concern with widows and widowers, bereaved parents, and orphaned children, who have, by and large, been rather neglected. Part V deals with the psychological needs of mourners and grievers.

The essay by Lindemann is considered a classic. What he says about the distinction between normal and morbid (abnormal, pathological) acute grief remains profoundly true. Lindemann's article is credited with starting the practice of brief psychotherapy.

The essay by Lewis is a first-hand account of the experience of grief and bereavement by a distinguished English writer. It provides a vivid and powerful statement of what that experience was like for him.

One of the conditions that contributes to what Lindemann refers to as a morbid grief reaction is unresolved grief, the topic of the selection by Rando. In this essay, she describes the various forms of unresolved grief. What these forms have in common is the presence of a disturbance that has somehow inhibited the normal trajectory toward the resolution of grief. In this article, there is also a discussion of the evidence concerning the possible link between bereavement and mortality.

The selection by Kenneth Doka deals with disenfranchised grief, the grief experienced by those who are not given adequate opportunity to acknowledge and express their sadness and who receive little, if any, social support in connection with their grief experience. The existence of those who experience disenfranchised grief can be used as a window to study society's "grieving rules." Certain categories of grievers are given support (e.g., a legitimate widow), while others are denied it (e.g., an illicit lover).

19 Symptomatology and Management of Acute Grief ❧

Erich Lindemann

ERICH LINDEMANN was professor of psychiatry at Harvard Medical School. This article is arguably the most important early study of acute grief. Much of the empirical evidence on which the paper was based was the result of the author's involvement in treating the survivors of a fire in a Boston nightclub in 1942 (the Cocoanut Grove fire) in which 492 people died. The article describes the symptoms associated with what he refers to as normal reactions to acute grief. It also includes a detailed discussion of morbid (or abnormal) acute grief reactions.

INTRODUCTION

At first glance, acute grief would not seem to be a medical or psychiatric disorder in the strict sense of the word but rather a normal reaction to a distressing situation. However, the understanding of reactions to traumatic experiences whether or not they represent clear-cut neuroses has become of ever-increasing importance to the psychiatrist. Bereavement or the sudden cessation of social interaction seems to be of special interest because it is often cited among the alleged psychogenic factors in psychosomatic disorders. The enormous increase in grief reactions due to war casualties, furthermore, demands an evaluation of their probable effect on the mental and physical health of our population.

The points to be made in this paper are as follows:

1. Acute grief is a definite syndrome with psychological and somatic symptomatology.

2. This syndrome may appear immediately after a crisis; it may be delayed; it may be exaggerated or apparently absent.

3. In place of the typical syndrome there may appear distorted pictures, each of which represents one special aspect of the grief syndrome.

From *American Journal of Psychiatry*, vol. 101, pp. 141–148, 1944. Copyright © 1944, the American Psychiatric Association. Reprinted by permission.

4. By appropriate techniques these distorted pictures can be successfully transformed into a normal grief reaction with resolution.

Our observations comprise 101 patients. Included are (1) psychoneurotic patients who lost a relative during the course of treatment, (2) relatives of patients who died in the hospital, (3) bereaved disaster victims (Cocoanut Grove fire) and their close relatives, (4) relatives of members of the armed forces.

The investigation consisted of a series of psychiatric interviews. Both the timing and the content of the discussions were recorded. These records were subsequently analysed in terms of the symptoms reported and of the changes in mental status observed progressively through a series of interviews. The psychiatrist avoided all suggestions and interpretations until the picture of symptomatology and spontaneous reaction tendencies of the patients had become clear from the records. The somatic complaints offered important leads for objective study. Careful laboratory work on spirograms, g.-i. functions, and metabolic studies are in progress and will be reported separately. At present we wish to present only our psychological observations.

Symptomatology of normal grief

The picture shown by persons in acute grief is remarkably uniform. Common to all is the following syndrome: sensations of somatic distress occurring in waves lasting from twenty minutes to an hour at a time, a feeling of tightness in the throat, choking with shortness of breath, need for sighing, and an empty feeling in the abdomen, lack of muscular power, and an intense subjective distress described as tension or mental pain. The patient soon learns that these waves of discomfort can be precipitated by visits, by mentioning the deceased, and by receiving sympathy. There is a tendency to avoid the syndrome at any cost, to refuse visits lest they should precipitate the reaction, and to keep deliberately from thought all references to the deceased.

The striking features are (1) the marked tendency to sighing respiration; this respiratory disturbance was most conspicuous when the patient was made to discuss his grief. (2) The complaint about lack of strength and exhaustion is universal and is described as follows: "It is almost impossible to climb up a stairway." "Everything I lift seems so heavy." "The slightest effort makes me feel exhausted." "I can't walk to the corner without feeling exhausted." (3) Digestive symptoms are described as follows: "The food tastes like sand." "I have no appetite at all." "I stuff the food down because I have to eat." "My saliva won't flow." "My abdomen feels hollow." "Everything seems slowed up in my stomach."

The sensorium is generally somewhat altered. There is commonly a slight sense of unreality, a feeling of increased emotional distance from other people (sometimes they appear shadowy or small), and there is intense preoccupation with the image of the deceased. A patient who lost his daughter in the Cocoanut Grove disaster visualized his girl in the telephone booth calling for him and was much troubled by the loudness with which his name was called by her and was so vividly preoccupied with the scene that he became oblivious of his surroundings. A young navy pilot lost a close friend; he remained a vivid part of his imagery, not in terms of a religious survival but in terms of an imaginary companion. He ate with him and talked over problems with him, for instance, discussing with him his plan of joining the Air Corps. Up to the time of the study, six months later, he denied the fact that the boy was no longer with him. Some patients are much concerned about this aspect of their grief reaction because they feel it indicates approaching insanity.

Another strong preoccupation is with feelings of guilt. The bereaved searches the time before the death for evidence of failure to do right by the lost one. He accuses himself of negligence and exaggerates minor omissions. After the fire disaster the central topic of discussion for a young married woman was the fact that her husband died after he left her following a quarrel, and of a young man whose wife died because he fainted too soon to save her.

In addition, there is often disconcerting loss of warmth in relationship to other people, a tendency to respond with irritability and anger, a wish not to be bothered by others at a time when friends and relatives make a special effort to keep up friendly relationships.

These feelings of hostility, surprising and quite inexplicable to the patients, disturbed them and again were often taken as signs of approaching insanity. Great efforts are made to handle them, and the result is often a formalized, stiff manner of social interaction.

The activity throughout the day of the severely bereaved person shows remarkable changes. There is no retardation of action and speech; quite to the contrary, there is a push of speech, especially when talking about the deceased. There is restlessness, inability to sit still, moving about in an aimless fashion, continually searching for something to do. There is, however, at the same time, a painful lack of capacity to initiate and maintain organized patterns of activity. What is done is done with lack of zest, as though one were going through the motions. The bereaved clings to the daily routine of prescribed activities; but these activities do not proceed in the automatic, self-sustaining fashion which characterizes normal work but have to be carried on with effort, as though each fragment of the activity became a special task. The bereaved is surprised to find how large a part of his customary activity was done in some meaningful relationship to the deceased and has now lost its significance. Especially the habits of social interaction—meeting friends, making conversation, sharing enterprises with others—seem to have been lost. This loss leads to a strong dependency on anyone who will stimulate the bereaved to activity and serve as the initiating agent.

These five points—(1) somatic distress, (2) preoccupation with the image of the deceased, (3) guilt, (4) hostile reactions, and (5) loss of patterns of conduct—seem to be pathognomonic for grief. There may be added a sixth characteristic, shown by patients who border on pathological reactions, which is not so conspicuous as the others but nevertheless often striking enough to color the whole picture. This is the appearance of traits of the deceased in the behavior of the bereaved, especially symptoms shown during the last illness, or behavior which may have been shown at the time of the tragedy. A bereaved person is observed or finds himself walking in the manner of his deceased father. He looks in the mirror and believes that his face appears just like that of the deceased. He may show a change of interests in the direction of the former activities of the deceased and may start enterprises entirely different from his former pursuits. A wife who lost her husband, an insurance agent, found herself writing to many insurance companies offering her services with somewhat exaggerated schemes. It seemed a regular observation in these patients that the painful preoccupation with the image of the deceased described above was transformed into preoccupation with symptoms or personality traits of the lost person, but now displaced to their own bodies and activities by identification.

Course of normal grief reactions

The duration of a grief reaction seems to depend upon the success with which a person does the *grief work*, namely, emancipation from the bondage to the deceased, readjustment to the environment in which the deceased is missing, and the formation of new relationships. One of the big obstacles to this work seems to be the fact that many patients try to avoid the intense distress connected with the grief experience and to avoid the expression of emotion necessary for it. The men victims after the Cocoanut Grove fire appeared in the early psychiatric interviews to be in a state of tension with tightened facial musculature, unable to relax for fear they might "break down." It required considerable persuasion to yield to the grief process before they were willing to accept the discomfort of bereavement. One assumed a hostile attitude toward the psychiatrist, refusing to allow any references to the deceased and rather rudely asking him to leave. This attitude remained throughout his stay on the ward, and the prognosis for his condition is not good in the light of other observations. Hostility of this sort was encountered on only occasional visits with the other patients. They became willing to accept the grief process and to embark on a program of dealing in memory with the deceased person. As soon as this became possible there seemed to be a rapid relief of tension and the subsequent interviews were rather animated conversations in which the deceased was idealized and in which misgivings about the future adjustment were worked through.

Examples of the psychiatrist's rôle in assisting patients in their readjustment after bereavement are contained in the following case histories. The first shows a very successful readjustment.

A woman, aged 40, lost her husband in the fire. She had a history of good adjustment previously. One child, ten years old. When she heard about her husband's death she was extremely depressed, cried bitterly, did not want to live, and for three days showed a state of utter dejection.

When seen by the psychiatrist, she was glad to have assistance and described her painful preoccupation with memories of her husband and her fear that she might lose her mind. She had a vivid visual image of his presence, picturing him as going to work in the morning and herself as wondering whether he would return in the evening, whether she could stand his not returning, then, describing to herself how he does return, plays with the dog, receives his child, and gradually tried to accept the fact that he is not there any more. It was only after ten days that she succeeded in accepting his loss and then only after having described in detail the remarkable qualities of her husband, the tragedy of his having to stop his activities at the pinnacle of his success, and his deep devotion to her.

In the subsequent interviews she explained with some distress that she had become very much attached to the examiner and that she waited for the hour of his coming. This reaction she considered disloyal to her husband but at the same time she could accept the fact that it was a hopeful sign of her ability to fill the gap he had left in her life. She then showed a marked drive for activity, making plans for supporting herself and her little girl, mapping out the preliminary steps for resuming her old profession as secretary, and making efforts to secure help from the occupational therapy department in reviewing her knowledge of French.

Her convalescence, both emotional and somatic, progressed smoothly, and she made a good adjustment immediately on her return home.

A man of 52, successful in business, lost his wife, with whom he had lived in happy marriage. The information given him about his wife's death confirmed his suspicions of several days. He responded with a severe grief reaction, with which he was unable to cope. He did not want to see visitors, was ashamed of breaking down, and asked to be permitted to stay in the hospital on the psychiatric service, when his physical condition would have permitted his discharge, because he wanted further assistance. Any mention of his wife produced a severe wave of depressive reaction, but with psychiatric assistance he gradually became willing to go through this painful process, and after three days on the psychiatric service he seemed well enough to go home.

He showed a high rate of verbal activity, was restless, needed to be occupied continually, and felt that the experience had whipped him into a state of restless overactivity.

As soon as he returned home he took an active part in his business, assuming a post in which he had a great many telephone calls. He also took over the rôle of amateur psychiatrist to another bereaved person, spending time with him and comforting him for his loss. In his eagerness to start anew, he developed a plan to sell all his former holdings, including his house, his furniture, and giving away anything which could remind him of his wife. Only after considerable discussion was he able to see that this would mean avoiding immediate grief at the price of an act of poor judgment. Again he had to be encouraged to deal with his grief reactions in a more direct manner. He has made a good adjustment.

With eight to ten interviews in which the psychiatrist shares the grief work, and with a period of from four to six weeks, it was ordinarily possible to settle an uncomplicated and undistorted grief reaction. This was the case in all but one of the 13 Cocoanut Grove fire victims.

MORBID GRIEF REACTIONS

Morbid grief reactions represent distortions of normal grief. The conditions mentioned here were transformed into "normal reactions" and then found their resolution.

a. *Delay of Reaction.* The most striking and most frequent reaction of this sort is *delay* or *postponement.* If the bereavement occurs at a time when the patient is confronted with important tasks and when there is necessity for maintaining the morale of others, he may show little or no reaction for weeks or even much longer. A brief delay is described in the following example.

A girl of 17 lost both parents and her boy friend in the fire and was herself burned severely, with marked involvement of the lungs. Throughout her stay in the hospital her attitude was that of cheerful acceptance without any sign of adequate distress. When she was discharged at the end of three weeks she appeared cheerful, talked rapidly, with a considerable flow of ideas, seemed eager to return home and to assume the rôle of parent for her two younger siblings. Except for slight feelings of "lonesomeness" she complained of no distress.

This period of griefless acceptance continued for the next two months, even when the household was dispersed and her younger siblings were placed in other homes. Not until the end of the tenth week did she begin to show a true state of grief with marked feelings of depression, intestinal emptiness, tightness in her throat, frequent crying, and vivid preoccupation with her deceased parents.

That this delay may involve years became obvious first by the fact that patients in acute bereavement about a recent death may soon upon exploration be found preoccupied with grief about a person who died many years ago. In this manner a woman of 38, whose mother had died recently and who had responded to the mother's death with a surprisingly severe reaction, was found to be but mildly concerned with her mother's death but deeply engrossed with unhappy and perplexing fantasies concerning the death of her brother, who died twenty years ago under dramatic circumstances from metastasizing carcinoma after amputation of his arm had been postponed too long. The discovery that a former unresolved grief reaction may be precipitated in the course of the discussion of another recent event was soon demonstrated in psychiatric interviews by patients who showed all the traits of a true grief reaction when the topic of a former loss arose.

The precipitating factor for the delayed reaction may be a deliberate recall of circumstances surrounding the death or may be a spontaneous occurrence in the patient's life. A peculiar form of this is the circumstance that a patient develops the grief reaction at the time when he himself is as old as the person who died. For instance, a railroad worker, aged 42, appeared in the psychiatric clinic with a picture which was undoubtedly a grief reaction for which he had no explanation. It turned out that when he was 22, his mother, then 42, had committed suicide.

b. *Distorted Reactions.* The delayed reactions may occur after an interval which was not marked by any abnormal behavior or distress, but in which there developed an *alteration* in the patient's *conduct* perhaps not conspicuous or serious enough to lead him to a psychiatrist. These alterations may be considered as the surface manifestations of an unresolved grief reaction, which may respond to fairly simple and quick psychiatric management if recognized. They may be classified as follows: (1) *overactivity without a sense of loss*, rather with a sense of wellbeing and zest, the activities being of an expansive and adventurous nature and bearing semblance to the activities formerly carried out by the deceased, as described above; (2) *the acquisition of symptoms belonging to the last illness of the deceased.* This type of patient appears in medical clinics and is often labelled hypochondriasis or hysteria. To what extent actual alterations of physiological functions occur under these circumstances will have to be a field of further careful inquiry. I owe to Dr. Chester Jones a report about a patient whose electrocardiogram showed a definite change during a period of three weeks, which started two weeks after the time her father died of heart disease.

While this sort of symptom formation "by identification" may still be considered as conversion symptoms such as we know from hysteria, there is another type of disorder doubtlessly presenting (3) a recognized *medical disease*, namely, a group of psychosomatic conditions, predominantly ulcerative colitis, rheumatoid arthritis, and asthma. Extensive studies in ulcerative colitis have produced evidence that 33 out of 41 patients with ulcerative colitis developed their disease in close time relationship to the loss of an important person. Indeed, it was this observation which first gave the impetus for the present detailed study of grief. Two of the patients developed bloody diarrhea at funerals. In the others it developed within a few weeks after the loss. The course of the ulcerative colitis was strikingly benefited when this grief reaction was resolved by psychiatric technique.

At the level of social adjustment there often occurs a conspicuous (4) *alteration in relationship to friends and relatives.* The patient feels irritable, does not want to be bothered, avoids former social activities, and is afraid he might antagonize his friends by his lack of interest and his critical attitudes. Progressive social isolation follows, and the patient needs considerable encouragement in re-establishing his social relationships.

While overflowing hostility appears to be spread out over all relationships, it may also occur as (5) *furious hostility against specific persons*; the doctor or the surgeon are accused bitterly for neglect of duty and the patient may assume that foul play has led to the death. It is characteristic that while patients talk a good deal about their suspicions and their bitter feelings, they are not likely to take any action against the accused, as a truly paranoid person might do.

(6) Many bereaved persons struggled with much effort against these feelings of hostility, which to them seem absurd, representing a vicious change in their characters and to be hidden as much as possible. Some patients succeed in hiding their hostility but become wooden and formal, with affectivity and conduct *resembling schizophrenic pictures*. A typical report is this, "I go through all the motions of living. I look after my children. I do my errands. I go to social functions, but it is like being in a play; it doesn't really concern me. I can't have any warm feelings. If I were to have any feelings at all I would be angry with everybody." This patient's reaction to therapy was characterized by growing hostility against the therapist, and it required considerable skill to make her continue interviews in spite of the disconcerting hostility which she had been fighting so much. The absence of emotional display in this patient's face and actions was quite striking. Her face had a mask-like appearance, her movements were formal, stilted, robot-like, without the fine play of emotional expression.

(7) Closely related to this picture is a *lasting loss of patterns of social interaction*. The patient cannot initiate any activity, is full of eagerness to be active—restless, can't sleep—but throughout the day he will not start any activity unless "primed" by somebody else. He will be grateful at sharing activities with others but will not be able to make up his mind to do anything alone. The picture is one of lack of decision and initiative. Organized activities along social lines occur only if a friend takes the patient along and shares the activity with him. Nothing seems to promise reward; only the ordinary activities of the day are carried on, and these in a routine manner, falling apart into small steps, each of which has to be carried out with much effort and without zest.

(8) There is, in addition, a picture in which a patient is active but in which most of his activities attain a coloring which is *detrimental to his own social and economic existence*. Such patients with uncalled for generosity, give away their belongings, are easily lured into foolish economic dealings, lose their friends and professional standing by a series of "stupid acts," and find themselves finally without family, friends, social status or money. This protracted self-punitive behavior seems to take place without any awareness of excessive feelings of guilt. It is a particularly distressing grief picture because it is likely to hurt other members of the family and drag down friends and business associates.

(9) This leads finally to the picture in which the grief reaction takes the form of a straight *agitated depression* with tension, agitation, insomnia, feelings of worthlessness, bitter self-accusation, and obvious need for punishment. Such patients may be dangerously suicidal.

A young man aged 32 had received only minor burns and left the hospital apparently well on the road to recovery just before the psychiatric survey of the disaster victims took place. On the fifth day he had learned that his wife had died. He seemed somewhat relieved of his worry about her fate; impressed the surgeon as being unusually well-controlled during the following short period of his stay in the hospital.

On January 1st he was returned to the hospital by his family. Shortly after his return home he had become restless, did not want to stay at home, had taken a trip to relatives trying to find rest, had not succeeded, and had returned home in a state of marked agitation, appearing preoccupied, frightened, and unable to concentrate on any organized activity. The mental status presented a somewhat unusual picture. He was restless, could not sit still or participate in any activity on the ward. He would try to read, drop it after a few minutes, or try to play pingpong, give it up after a short time. He would try to start conversations, break them off abruptly, and then fall into repeated murmured utterances: "Nobody can help me. When is it going to happen? I am doomed, am I not?" With great effort it was possible to establish enough rapport to carry on interviews. He complained about his feeling of extreme tension, inability to breathe, generalized weakness and exhaustion, and his frantic fear that something terrible was going to happen. "I'm destined to live in insanity or I must die. I know that it is God's will. I have this awful feeling of guilt." With intense morbid guilt feelings, he reviewed incessantly the events of the fire. His wife had stayed behind. When he tried to pull her out, he had fainted and was shoved out by the crowd. She was burned while he was saved. "I should have saved her or I should have died too." He complained about being filled with an incredible violence and did not know what to do about it. The rapport established with him lasted for only brief periods of time. He then would fall back into his state of intense agitation and muttering. He slept poorly even with large sedation. In the course of four days he became somewhat more composed, had longer periods of contact with the psychiatrist, and seemed to feel that he was being understood and might be able to cope with his morbid feelings of guilt and violent impulses. On the sixth day of his hospital stay, however, after skillfully distracting the attention of his special nurse, he jumped through a closed window to a violent death.

If the patient is not conspicuously suicidal, it may nevertheless be true that he has a strong desire for painful experiences, and such patients are likely to desire shock treatment of some sort, which they picture as a cruel experience, such as electrocution might be.

A 28-year-old woman, whose 20-month-old son was accidentally smothered developed a state of severe agitated depression with self-accusation, inability to enjoy anything, hopelessness about the future, overflow of hostility against the husband and his parents, also with excessive hostility against the psychiatrist. She insisted upon electric-

shock treatment and was finally referred to another physician who treated her. She responded to the shock treatments very well and felt relieved of her sense of guilt.

It is remarkable that agitated depressions of this sort represent only a small fraction of the pictures of grief in our series.

PROGNOSTIC EVALUATION

Our observations indicate that to a certain extent the type and severity of the grief reaction can be predicted. Patients with obsessive personality make-up and with a history of former depressions are likely to develop an agitated depression. Severe reactions seem to occur in mothers who have lost young children. The intensity of interaction with the deceased before his death seems to be significant. It is important to realize that such interaction does not have to be of the affectionate type; on the contrary, the death of a person who invited much hostility, especially hostility which could not well be expressed because of his status and claim to loyalty, may be followed by a severe grief reaction in which hostile impulses are the most conspicuous feature. Not infrequently the person who passed away represented a key person in a social system, his death being followed by disintegration of this social system and by a profound alteration of the living and social conditions for the bereaved. In such cases readjustment presents a severe task quite apart from the reaction to the loss incurred. All these factors seem to be more important than a tendency to react with neurotic symptoms in previous life. In this way the most conspicuous forms of morbid identification were found in persons who had no former history of a tendency to psychoneurotic reactions.

MANAGEMENT

Proper psychiatric management of grief reactions may prevent prolonged and serious alterations in the patient's social adjustment, as well as potential medical disease. The essential task facing the psychiatrist is that of sharing the patient's grief work, namely, his efforts at extricating himself from the bondage to the deceased and at finding new patterns of rewarding interaction. It is of the greatest importance to notice that not only over-reaction but under-reaction of the bereaved must be given attention, because delayed responses may occur at unpredictable moments and the dangerous distortions of the grief reaction, not conspicuous at first, be quite destructive later and these may be prevented.

Religious agencies have led in dealing with the bereaved. They have provided comfort by giving the backing of dogma to the patient's wish for continued interaction with the deceased, have developed rituals which maintain the patient's interaction with others, and have counteracted the morbid guilt feelings of the patient by Divine Grace and by promising an opportunity for "making up" to the deceased at the time of a later reunion. While these measures have helped countless mourners, comfort alone does not provide adequate assistance in the patient's grief work. He has to accept the pain of the bereavement. He has to review his relationships with the deceased, and has to become acquainted with the alterations in his own modes of emotional reaction. His fear of insanity, his fear of accepting the surprising changes in his feelings, especially the overflow of hostility, have to be worked through. He will have to express his sorrow and sense of loss. He will have to find an acceptable formulation of his future relationship to the deceased. He will have to verbalize his feelings of guilt, and he will have to find persons around him whom he can use as "primers" for the acquisition of new patterns of conduct. All this can be done in eight to ten interviews. . . .

20 A Grief Observed

C. S. Lewis

C. S. LEWIS (1898–1963) was known to students at Cambridge University as a brilliant scholar and tutor, and to the world as an observer, author, and essayist of unusual distinction. His works include *The Screwtape Letters*, *The Allegory of Love*, *Mere Christianity*, *The Chronicles of Narnia* (an acknowledged classic of childhood fantasy), and his famous science fiction trilogy (*Out of the Silent Planet*, *Perelandra*, and *That Hideous Strength*.) He had the rare gift of translating the concepts of religion into the language and context of the everyday world.

Our selection is the first chapter of a poignant book, written under the following circumstances: In April 1956, Lewis, a confirmed bachelor, married Joy Davidman (referred to in the article as H.), an American poet with two small children. After four brief, intensely happy years, she died and Lewis found himself alone again and inconsolable. To defend himself against the loss of his belief in God, he began a journal that became an eloquent statement of rediscovered faith. He freely confesses his doubts, his rage, and his awareness of human frailty, and finally is able to find his way back to a meaningful life.

NO ONE EVER TOLD ME THAT GRIEF FELT SO LIKE FEAR. I am not afraid, but the sensation is like being afraid. The same fluttering in the stomach, the same restlessness, the yawning. I keep on swallowing.

At other times it feels like being mildly drunk, or concussed. There is a sort of invisible blanket between the world and me. I find it hard to take in what anyone says. Or perhaps, hard to want to take it in. It is so uninteresting. Yet I want the others to be about me. I dread the moments when the house is empty. If only they would talk to one another and not to me.

There are moments, most unexpectedly, when something inside me tries to assure me that I don't really mind so much, not so very much, after all. Love is not the whole of man's life. I was happy before I ever met H. I've plenty of what are called "resources." People get over these things. Come, I shan't do so badly. One is ashamed to listen to this voice but it seems for a little to be making out a good case. Then comes a sudden jab of red-hot memory and all this "common-sense" vanishes like an ant in the mouth of a furnace.

On the rebound one passes into tears and pathos. Maudlin tears. I almost prefer the moments of agony. These are at least clean and honest. But the bath of self-pity, the wallow, the loathsome sticky-sweet pleasure of indulging it—that disgusts me. And even while I'm doing it I know it leads me to misrepresent H. herself. Give that mood its head and in a few minutes I shall have substituted for the real woman a mere doll to be blubbered over. Thank God the memory of her is still too strong (will it always be too strong?) to let me get away with it.

For H. wasn't like that at all. Her mind was lithe and quick and muscular as a leopard. Passion, tenderness and pain were all equally unable to disarm it. It scented the first whiff of cant or slush; then sprang, and knocked you over before you knew what was happening. How many bubbles of mine she pricked! I soon learned not to talk rot to her unless I did it for the sheer pleasure—and there's another red-hot jab—of being exposed and laughed at. I was never less silly than as H.'s lover.

And no one ever told me about the laziness of grief. Except at my job—where the machine seems to run on much as usual—I loathe the slightest effort. Not only writing but even reading a letter is too much. Even shaving. What does it matter now whether my cheek is rough or smooth? They say an unhappy man wants distractions—some thing to take him out of himself. Only as a dog-tired man wants an extra blanket on a cold night; he'd rather lie there shivering than get up and find one. It's easy to see why the lonely become untidy; finally, dirty and disgusting.

Meanwhile, where is God? This is one of the most disquieting symptoms. When you are happy, so happy that you have no sense of needing Him, so happy that you are tempted to feel His claims upon you as an interruption, if you remember yourself and turn to Him with gratitude and praise, you will be—or so it feels—welcomed with open arms. But go to Him when your need is desperate, when all other help is vain, and what do you find? A door slammed in your face, and a sound of bolting and double bolting on the inside. After that silence. You may as well turn away. The longer you wait, the more emphatic the silence will become. There are no lights in the windows. It might be an empty house. Was it ever inhabited? It seemed so once. And that seeming was as strong as this. What can this mean? Why is He so present a commander in our time of prosperity and so very absent a help in time of trouble?

I tried to put some of these thoughts to C. this afternoon. He reminded me that the same thing seems to have happened to Christ: "Why hast thou forsaken me?" I know. Does that make it easier to understand?

Not that I am (I think) in much danger of ceasing to believe in God. The real danger is of coming to believe such dreadful things about Him. The conclusion I dread is not, "So there's no God after all," but, "So this is what God's really like. Deceive yourself no longer."

Our elders submitted and said, "They will be done." How often had bitter resentment been stifled through sheer terror and an act of love—yes, in every sense, an act—put on to hide the operation?

Of course it's easy enough to say that God seems absent at our greatest need because He *is* absent—non-existent. But then why does He seem so present when, to put it quite frankly, we don't ask for Him?

One thing, however, marriage has done for me. I can never again believe that religion is manufactured out of our unconscious, starved desires and is a substitute for sex. For those few years H. and I feasted on love; every mode of it—solemn and merry, romantic and realistic, sometimes as dramatic as a thunderstorm, sometimes as comfortable and unemphatic as putting on your soft slippers. No cranny of heart or body remained unsatisfied. If God were a substitute for love we ought to have lost all interest in Him. Who'd bother about substitutes when he has the thing itself? But that isn't what happens. We both knew we wanted something besides one another—quite a different kind of something, a quite different kind of want. You might as well say that when lovers have one another they will never want to read, or eat—or breathe.

After the death of a friend, years ago, I had for some time a most vivid feeling of certainty about his continued life; even his enhanced life. I have begged to be given even one hundredth part of the same assurance about H. There is no answer. Only the locked door, the iron curtain, the vacuum, absolute zero. "Them as asks don't get." I was a fool to ask. For now, even if that assurance came I should distrust it. I should think it a self-hypnosis induced by my own prayers.

At any rate I must keep clear of the spiritualists. I promised H. I would. She knew something of those circles.

Keeping promises to the dead, or to anyone else, is very well. But I begin to see that "respect for the wishes of the dead" is a trap. Yesterday I stopped myself only in time from saying about some trifle, "H. wouldn't have liked that." This is unfair to the others. I should soon be using "what H. would have liked" as an instrument of domestic tyranny; with her supposed likings becoming a thinner and thinner disguise for my own.

I cannot talk to the children about her. The moment I try, there appears on their faces neither grief, nor love, nor fear, nor pity, but the most fatal of all non-conductors, embarrassment. They look as if I were committing an indecency. They are longing for me to stop. I felt just the same after my own mother's death when my father mentioned her. I can't blame them. It's the way boys are.

I sometimes think that shame, mere awkward, senseless shame, does as much towards preventing good acts and straightforward happiness as any of our vices can do. And not only in boyhood.

Or are the boys right? What would H. herself think of this terrible little notebook to which I come back and back? Are these jottings morbid? I once read the sentence "I lay awake all night with toothache, thinking about toothache and about lying awake." That's true to life. Part of every misery is, so to speak, the misery's shadow or reflection: the fact that you don't merely suffer but have to keep on thinking about the fact that you suffer. I not only live each endless day in grief, but live each day thinking about living each day in grief. Do these notes merely aggravate that side of it? Merely confirm the monotonous, tread-mill march of the mind round one subject? But what am I to do? I must have some drug, and reading isn't a strong enough drug now. By writing it all down (all?—no: one thought in a hundred) I believe I get a little outside it. That's how I'd defend it to H. But ten to one she'd see a hole in the defense.

It isn't only the boys either: An odd by-product of my loss is that I'm aware of being an embarrassment to everyone I meet. At work, at the club, in the street, I see people, as they approach me, trying to make up their minds whether they'll "say something about it" or not. I hate it if they do, and if they don't. Some funk it up altogether. R. has been avoiding me for a week. I like best the well-brought-up young men, almost boys, who walk up to me as if I were a dentist, turn very red, get it over, and then edge away to the bar as quickly as they decently can. Perhaps the bereaved ought to be isolated in special settlements like lepers.

To some I'm worse than an embarrassment. I am a death's head. Whenever I meet a happily married pair I can feel them both thinking, "One or other of us must some day be as he is now."

At first I was very afraid of going to places where H. and I had been happy—our favorite pub, our favorite wood. But I decided to do it at once—like sending a pilot up again as soon as possible after he's had a crash. Unexpectedly, it makes no difference. Her absence is no more emphatic in those places than anywhere else. It's not local at all. I suppose that if one were forbidden all salt one wouldn't notice it much more in any one food than in another. Eating in general would be different, every day, at every meal. It is like that. The act of living is different all through. Her absence is like the sky, spread over everything.

But no, that is not quite accurate. There is one place where her absence comes locally home to me, and it is a place I can't avoid. I mean my own body. It had such a different importance while it was the body of H.'s lover. Now it's like an empty house. But don't let me deceive myself. This body would become important to me again, and pretty quickly, if I thought there was anything wrong with it.

Cancer, and cancer, and cancer. My mother, my father, my wife. I wonder who is next in the queue.

Yet H. herself, dying of it, and well knowing the fact, said that she had lost a great deal of her old horror at it. When the reality came, the name and the idea were in some degree disarmed. And up to a point I very nearly understood. This is important. One never meets just Cancer, or War, or Unhappiness (or Happiness). One only meets each hour or moment that comes. All manner of ups and downs. Many bad spots in our best times, many good ones in our worst. One never gets the total impact of what we call "the thing itself." But we call it wrongly. The thing itself is simply all these ups and downs: the rest is a name or an idea.

It is incredible how much happiness, even how much gaiety, we sometimes had together after all hope was gone. How long, how tranquilly, how nourishingly, we talked together that last night!

And yet, not quite together. There's a limit to the "one flesh." You can't really share someone else's weakness, or fear or pain. What you feel may be bad. It might conceivably be as bad as what the other felt, though I should distrust anyone who claimed that it was. But it would still be quite different. When I speak of fear, I mean the merely animal fear, the recoil of the organism from its destruction; the smothery feeling; the sense of being a rat in a trap. It can't be transferred. The mind can sympathize; the body, less. In one way the bodies of lovers can do it least. All their love passages have trained them to have, not identical, but complementary, correlative, even opposite, feelings about one another.

We both knew this. I had my miseries, not hers; she had hers, not mine. The end of hers would be the coming-of-age of mine. We were setting out on different roads. This cold truth, this terrible traffic-regulation ("You, Madam, to the right—you, Sir, to the left") is just the beginning of the separation which is death itself.

And this separation, I suppose, waits for all. I have been thinking of H. and myself as peculiarly unfortunate in being torn apart. But presumably all lovers are. She once said to me, "Even if we both died at exactly the same moment, as we lie here side by side, it would be just as much a separation as the one you're so afraid of." Of course she didn't *know*, any more than I do. But she was near death; near enough to make a good shot. She used to quote, "Alone into the Alone." She said it felt like that. And how immensely improbable that it should be otherwise! Time and space and body were the very things that brought us together; the telephone wires by which we communicated. Cut one off, or cut both off simultaneously. Either way, mustn't the conversation stop?

Unless you assume that some other means of communication—utterly different, yet doing the same work, would be immediately substituted. But then, what conceivable point could there be in severing the old ones? Is God a clown who whips away your bowl of soup one moment in order, next moment, to replace it with another bowl of the same soup? Even nature isn't such a clown as that. She never plays exactly the same tune twice.

It is hard to have patience with people who say, "There is no death," or, "Death doesn't matter." There is death. And whatever is matters. And whatever happens has consequences, and it and they are irrevocable and irreversible. You might as well say that birth doesn't matter. I look up at the night sky. Is anything more certain than that in all those vast times and spaces, if I were allowed to search them, I should nowhere find her face, her voice, her touch? She died. She is dead. Is the word so difficult to learn?

I have no photograph of her that's any good. I cannot even see her face distinctly in my imagination. Yet the odd face of some stranger seen in a crowd this morning may come before me in vivid perfection the moment I close my eyes tonight. No doubt, the explanation is simple enough. We have seen the faces of those we know best so variously, from so many angles, in so many lights, with so many expressions—walking, sleeping, laughing, crying, eating, talking, thinking—that all the impressions crowd into our memory together and cancel out into a mere blur. Bur her voice is still vivid. The remembered voice—that can turn me at any moment to a whimpering child.

21 Unresolved Grief

Terese Rando

TERESE RANDO is a clinical psychologist in private practice. Her books include *Treatment of Complicated Mourning* and *Grief, Dying, and Death: Clinical Interventions for Caregivers*, the work from which this selection is drawn. In this article she outlines a variety of different forms of unresolved grief, providing case-study examples to illustrate the various categories. She discusses the symptoms of unresolved grief, the reasons for unresolved grief, and the determinants of bereavement outcomes.

FORMS OF UNRESOLVED GRIEF

The following descriptions of forms of unresolved grief have been taken from the analyses of Averill (1968), Parkes and Weiss (1983), and Raphael (1983). Any of these forms may overlap. In each there are components of denial or repression of aspects of the loss or of the feelings generated, as well as an attempt to hold on to the lost relationship.

Absent grief. In this situation feelings of grief and mourning processes are totally absent. It is as if the death never occurred at all. It requires either that the mourner completely deny the death or that he remain in the stage of shock.

Inhibited grief. In this form there is a lasting inhibition of many of the manifestations of normal grief, with the appearance of other symptoms such as somatic complaints in their place. The mourner may be able to relinquish and mourn only certain aspects of the deceased and not others, for example, the positive aspects but not the negative ones.

> CASE EXAMPLE. *Ruth came to therapy because her deteriorating physical condition suggested a significant depression. She was compliant and eager to please in treatment. Investigation revealed that her estranged husband had committed suicide several years earlier. She had attended to the tasks of the funeral and then resumed her life as if nothing had occurred. There were no behavioral expressions of any grief and no inter-*

From *Grief, Dying, and Death: Clinical Interventions for Caregivers*, pp. 59–71, by T. A. Rando, 1984, Champaign, Ill.: Research Press. Copyright © 1984 by T. A. Rando. Adapted by permission.

nal processing of it. Shortly afterwards Ruth developed severe gastrointestinal difficulties and the next several years were devoted to focusing on her physical complaints.

Delayed grief. Normal or conflicted grief may be delayed for an extended period of time, up to years, especially if there are pressing responsibilities or the mourner feels he cannot deal with the process at that time. A full grief reaction may eventually be initiated by another loss or by some event related to the original loss. For instance, a pet's death can trigger a response for a loved one who died years earlier, but who had never been mourned because the griever felt he had to be strong to take care of other family members. Meanwhile, only an inhibited form of grief may be observed.

> CASE EXAMPLE. *Randi was a high-school senior when her mother died suddenly following a successful heart operation. Her father had also died unexpectedly the previous year. Randi was always the domestic one and she took over the task of managing the house and paying the bills for her two siblings and herself. She was also the "strong one" and never took time to grieve. Several years after the death of her mother Randi entered nursing school. One day she went to give a cardiac patient an injection, but instead of seeing the patient in the bed she "saw" her own mother. This initiated an acute grief reaction.*

Conflicted grief. In this grief there is frequently an exaggeration or distortion of one or more of the manifestations of normal grief, while other aspects of the grief may be suppressed at the same time. Two common patterns are extreme anger and extreme guilt. This grief reaction can be abnormally prolonged and is often associated with a previously dependent or ambivalent relationship with the deceased.

> CASE EXAMPLE. *Felicia's 10-year-old son died from acute appendicitis 8 months prior to her referral for therapy. Felicia was an overemotional woman who for years had become hysterical whenever she had to contact the pediatrician about her son. She had strong ambivalent feelings towards her son because of his father's having deserted her when she discovered she was pregnant. At the time of the appendicitis attack, the pediatrician had heard Felicia exaggerate her son's symptoms once too often and consequently responded too slowly to save the child's life. Felicia's grief continued unabated as she constantly blamed herself for not convincing the pediatrician of the gravity of the illness, and she was filled with self-reproach for the resentment she frequently had felt for her son.*

Chronic grief. In chronic grief the mourner continuously exhibits intense grief reactions that would be appropriate in the early stages of loss. Mourning fails to draw to its natural conclusion and it almost seems that the bereaved keeps the deceased alive with grief. Intense yearning, often associated with an intensely dependent relationship on the deceased fostered by the mourner's insecurity, is symptomatic of this grief. It is also evident after the loss of an irreplaceable relationship in which the bereaved had extraordinary, and possibly pathological, emotional investment.

> CASE EXAMPLE. *Bill was a shy, insecure man who was devoted to his wife and built his entire emotional world around her. She handled all the family finances, organized their social schedule, and raised the children independently. Most of his social contacts with others were through her. After she died he was both deeply depressed and isolated. He went through only the minimum attempts at communicating with others, being fearful of them. He spent most of his time alone and arranged for a housekeeper to handle the domestic duties and take responsibility for the children. Six years later he had made no changes since she died.*

Unanticipated grief. This is a form of grief reaction that only recently has been discussed in the literature (Glick et al., 1974; Parkes & Weiss, 1983). It occurs after a sudden, unanticipated loss and is so disruptive that recovery is usually complicated. In unanticipated grief, mourners are unable to grasp the full implications of the loss. Their adaptive capabilities are seriously assaulted and they suffer extreme feelings of bewilderment, anxiety, self-reproach, and depression that render them unable to function normally in any area of their lives. There is difficulty in accepting the loss, despite intellectual recognition of the death, and the death may continue to seem inexplicable. Grief symptomology persists much longer than usual.

> CASE EXAMPLE. *Jane's husband was hit by a drunk driver after he had stopped to help a motorist change a tire. Jane was completely overwhelmed when informed of the accident, and this feeling stayed with her for almost a year. She could not believe that the death had actually occurred, and she frequently had to remind herself that her husband was not going to return. Many of her grief symptoms persisted for an abnormally long period of time. Although she was able to go through the motions of putting her life back together again, Jane became chronically anxious and apprehensive, always awaiting another trauma to befall her. Jane dated, but she was never able to make a commitment to another man for fear that he would be taken from her too.*

Abbreviated grief. This reaction is often mistaken for unresolved grief. In fact, it is a short-lived but normal form of grief. It may occur because of the immediate replacement of the lost person (e.g., marrying a new spouse right after the first one dies) or an insufficient attachment to the lost person (e.g., the individual was never that attached to the person in the first place). Sometimes it occurs when a significant amount of anticipatory grief has been completed prior to a death. After the actual death occurs the individual grieves, but much of the grief work has been accomplished so that the postdeath bereavement period, while painful, may be relatively shorter.

CASE EXAMPLE. *Peter's wife succumbed to cancer after a long illness of several years. Peter had gone through a long process of anticipatory grief during the illness and consequently, after a short but intense grief reaction at the time of her death, was left with little to grieve for. He started dating within 10 weeks of his wife's death and evidenced no further symptoms of grief.*

SYMPTOMS AND BEHAVIORS OF UNRESOLVED GRIEF

The following lists adopted from Lindemann (1944), Lazare (1979), and Worden (1982) enumerate some symptoms and behaviors indicative of unresolved grief. These individual symptoms may be unremarkable during the acute stage of grief. However, they are the major signs of incomplete grief work when they are manifested *beyond* the expected time for resolution of grief. The more of these symptoms the mourner has, the stronger the diagnosis of unresolved grief.

The following manifestations of unresolved grief reaction were put forth by Lindemann (1944):

- Overactivity without a sense of loss
- Acquisition of symptoms belonging to the last illness of the deceased
- Development of a psychosomatic medical illness
- Alteration in relationships with friends and relatives
- Furious hostility against specific persons somehow connected with the death (e.g., doctor, nurse)
- Wooden and formal conduct that masks hostile feelings and resembles a schizophrenic reaction in which there is a lack of emotion
- Lasting loss of patterns of social interaction
- Acts detrimental to one's own social and economic existence (e.g., giving away belongings, making foolish economic deals)
- Agitated depression with tension, agitation, insomnia, feelings of worthlessness, bitter self-accusation, and obvious need for punishment, and even suicidal tendencies.

The following diagnostic criteria for unresolved grief were proposed by Lazare (1979). When one or more of these symptoms or behaviors transpires after a death and continues beyond 6 months to 1 year, he considers the diagnosis of unresolved grief. The greater the number of symptoms and behaviors, the greater the likelihood of unresolved grief.

- A depressive syndrome of varying degrees of severity since the time of the death, frequently a very mild, subclinical one often accompanied by persistent guilt and lowered self-esteem

- A history of delayed or prolonged grief, indicating that the person characteristically avoids or has difficulty with grief work
- Symptoms of guilt and self-reproach, panic attacks, and somatic expressions of fear such as choking sensations and shortness of breath
- Somatic symptoms representing identification with the deceased, often the symptoms of the terminal illness
- Physical distress under the upper half of the sternum, accompanied by expressions such as "There is something stuck inside" or "I feel there is a demon inside of me"
- Searching that continues over time, with a great deal of random behavior, restlessness, and moving around
- Recurrence of symptoms of depression and searching behavior on specific dates, such as anniversaries of the death, birthdays of the deceased, achieving the age of the deceased, and holidays (especially Christmas), that are more extreme than those anniversary reactions normally expected
- A feeling that the death occurred yesterday, even though the loss took place months or years ago
- Unwillingness to move the material possessions of the deceased after a reasonable amount of time has passed
- Changes in relationships following the death
- Diminished participation in religious and ritual activities that are part of the mourner's culture, including avoidance of visiting the grave or taking part in funerary rituals
- An inability to discuss the deceased without crying or having the voice crack, particularly when the death occurred over a year ago
- Themes of loss

These additional symptoms of unresolved grief were suggested by Worden (1982):

- A relatively minor event triggering major grief reactions
- False euphoria subsequent to the death
- Overidentification with the deceased leading to a compulsion to imitate the dead person, particularly if it is unconscious and the mourner lacks the competence for the same behavior
- Self-destructive impulses
- Radical changes in lifestyle

- Exclusion of friends, family members, or activities associated with the deceased
- Phobias about illness or death

These lists are not all-inclusive. Mourners can be expected to manifest widely varying symptoms of unresolved grief, and caregivers will place varying amounts of importance on the presence or absence of specific symptoms depending upon the norms they develop over time as they work with the bereaved.

Three primary variables demarcate unresolved grief: absence of a normal grief reaction, prolongation of a normal grief reaction, and distortion of a normal grief reaction (Siggins, 1966). To make a determination of unresolved grief it is necessary to know the full range of normal grief against which the behavior in question is being compared and the psychological, social, and physiological variables that would influence the individual's grief reaction. Without an understanding of and appreciation for these variables and how they affect a particular individual's grief experience, *no* judgments can be made about the person's grief response.

REASONS FOR UNRESOLVED GRIEF

Jackson (1957) feels that two conditions may provoke difficulties in accomplishing grief work and thus predispose the mourner to unresolved grief. In the first condition, the mourner is unable to tolerate the emotional distress of grief and resists dealing with the necessary tasks and feelings of grief. The second condition occurs when the mourner has an excessive need to maintain interaction with the deceased. In this case the mourner denies the loss and fails to appropriately decathect from the deceased, thereby failing in the requisite tasks of grief work. . . .

Lazare (1979) has given a number of psychological and social reasons for failure to grieve. The following factors are adapted from his work.

Psychological Factors in Unresolved Grief

Guilt. Unresolved grief may occur when mourners are afraid to grieve because reviewing their relationship with the deceased would bring up negative acts or feelings they had directed towards her, or things they had neglected to do, making them feel guilty. This concern usually develops in people with harsh superegos whose feelings towards the deceased are highly ambivalent. Guilt resulting from other factors can also block the grief process if mourners feel unable to confront the guilt. . . .

Loss of an extension of the self. Some people may be so dependent upon, or place such a high value on, the deceased that they will not grieve in order to avoid the reality of the loss. In this case, the deceased had been perceived as an extension of the bereaved and to recognize the loss and grief would constitute a severe narcissistic loss to the self. One mourner said, "Mother was my other half. I cannot be complete without her. She cannot be dead."

Reawakening of an old loss. In some cases individuals are reluctant to grieve because the current loss reawakens a more profound and painful loss that has not yet been resolved. An example of this would be the man who cannot grieve for his divorce because it resurrects the memory of the death of his mother, for whom he never appropriately grieved.

Multiple loss. Those who experience multiple losses, such as the death of an entire family or a number of sequential losses within a relatively short period of time, sometimes have difficulty grieving because the losses are too overwhelming to contemplate and deal with. Essentially they are suffering from "bereavement overload" (Kastenbaum, 1969). In the case of losing family members it is additionally complicated because those who would normally support the griever no longer exist.

Inadequate ego development. To mourn appropriately the individual needs to have achieved the state of object constancy and to have realized an adequate integration of a number of basic ego functions. Without these prerequisites, the individual responds to loss and separation with serious ego regression. Consequently, people with severe ego impairments (e.g., borderline personalities) are often unable to adequately complete the grief process because they cannot meet the necessary intrapsychic tasks. Instead, they frequently experience feelings of intense hopelessness, rage, frustration, depression, anxiety, and despair that they cannot defend against. Often psychotic behavior results when their primitive defense mechanisms fail. Such individuals are not psychologically able to successfully master the tasks of grief. For instance, one borderline patient could never complete grieving over the death of his father because he was incapable of maintaining a consistent mental image of his father from which to decathect.

Idiosyncratic resistances to mourning.

There are individuals who do not permit themselves to grieve because of specific psychological issues that interfere with the process. For example, some people will not grieve for fear of losing control or appearing weak to themselves and others. Others have expressed the concern that if they start to cry the tears will never stop. Still other grievers are afraid to give up the pain, since it binds them closely to the deceased. Any individual fear, conflict, issue, or conditioned response that interferes with the mourner's yielding to the normal process of grief will constitute a resistance to mourning and may have to be interpreted and addressed with the help of a therapist if it cannot be successfully worked through by the individual.

Social Factors in Unresolved Grief

Social negation of a loss. In this situation the loss is not socially defined as a loss, e.g., an abortion, a miscarriage, an infant given up for adoption. Although grief work is necessary, the social support for it is inadequate or nonexistent. This is what occurs in many cases involving symbolic psychosocial losses.

Socially unspeakable loss. In this case the loss is so "unspeakable" that members of the social system cannot be of any assistance to the bereaved. They tend to shy away out of ignorance of what to say to help or moral repugnance. Examples of such a loss include death by an overdose of morphine, murder, suicide, or the death of an illicit lover.

Social isolation and/or geographic distance from social support. In this instance the individual is either away from her social supports at the time of mourning or there are no existing social supports available for assistance. Geographical distance from support is becoming increasingly common as individuals are becoming more and more mobile. In addition, deaths may occur in places or at times when people may be unable to travel conveniently or quickly. The difficulties inherent in this type of situation are seen in the dilemma of the 20-year-old college student whose mother did not inform her that her father had died until after she returned from school following final examinations. By that time the family had already dealt with a great deal of their own grief and provided her with little support in her own initial stages of grief. People also fail to grieve when they have no social support in the first place. The breakdown of the nuclear family, the decline in primary group interactions with consequent depersonalization and alienation, and the diminished importance of religious institutions all account for this lack of support.

Assumption of the role of the strong one. In some situations there are certain people who are designated to be the "strong one" by those around them. They must make all the funeral arrangements, bolster the morale of others, and not show any emotion. Sometimes their very occupations or roles require this, as with priests or Army captains. Often these individuals miss the opportunity to deal with their own grief due to the roles they attempt to maintain.

Uncertainty over the loss. In cases where the loss is uncertain, such as when a boater is lost at sea or a child is kidnapped, the grievers and their social systems are often unable to commence grieving until they know the precise status of the lost person. This is why so much time, money, and effort is spent searching to recover missing bodies and confirm deaths. . . .

DETERMINANTS OF BEREAVEMENT OUTCOME

Recent findings have indicated that early intervention is successful in reducing the damaging effects of bereavement for high-risk widows and widowers, although such intervention may not benefit those in low-risk or unselected groups (Parkes, 1980; Parkes & Weiss, 1983). This means that, in order to intervene effectively, it is necessary to know which mourners are at risk. Through a series of investigations with widows and some widowers, Parkes and Weiss (1983) identified what appear to be those variables most predictive of bereavement outcome. From these they derived the three major determinants of pathological grief syndromes: bereavements that were sudden, unexpected, and untimely, leading to unanticipated grief; those associated with ambivalence towards the deceased with reactions of intense anger and/or self-reproach, resulting in conflicted grief; and those related to an abnormally dependent relationship with the deceased, generating reactions of intense yearning that became chronic grief.

In analyzing the factors that were associated with unresolved grief Parkes and Weiss identified a list of precursors. The eight variables appearing during the first 2 months after death that, combined, gave the most satisfactory prediction of bereavement outcome at 13 months (and that appeared to predict the trajectory for the future outcome) are listed in order of significance as follows:

Coders' prediction of outcome. This was an educated guess made by the coders of the Harvard Bereavement Study, from which the data for these investigations came (Glick et al., 1974).

Respondent's level of yearning (3 to 4 weeks after bereavement). Intense yearning, much greater than that typically seen, appeared to have been associated with undue dependence on the deceased. Interestingly, this further provides evidence that it is not solely those who avoid or repress grief who are most likely to become disturbed a year later.

Respondent's attitude toward own death (3 to 4 weeks after bereavement). This involved the expression, at the first interview, of the wish for one's own death. It is unclear as to why this variable had such predictive value. It arose under a variety of circumstances and did not appear associated with any particular antecedent or outcome variable. It seemed to be equally expressive of several different syndromes of pathological grief.

Duration of terminal illness. This was closely associated with the pathological syndrome of unanticipated grief.

Social class. Social class may represent a constellation of variables. For instance, low social class may indicate an environment in which there are special stresses and/or a lack of resources. Whatever social class represents, it is interesting to note that it affected the outcome of bereavement without changing the actual course of grief: respondents of lower socio-economic status grieved in much the same way as those of higher status, although the outcome appeared to be poorer. Surprisingly, poor financial status and low income did not correlate with outcome, leaving this variable requiring more analysis.

Years of marriage. The importance of a long marriage can be evaluated only in light of other evidence. While brief marriages appear to be easier to give up than longer marriages are, a long marriage cannot be assumed to be a major cause of pathological bereavement, as witnessed by the studies of older widows and widowers who appear less vulnerable to the effects of conjugal bereavement than younger ones.

Respondent's level of anger and *Respondent's level of self-reproach* (3 to 4 weeks after bereavement). Both anger and self-reproach may reflect ambivalent marriages. Since such marriages appear to result in more problematic grief, it is not surprising that these variables are associated with poorer outcome.

Several other variables appeared to be clinically important, but were not statistically significant in this study because of its design. When the design deficiencies were controlled for, it was clear that bereavement symptoms are worse for young widows and widowers than for older ones, and for widowers than widows. Other possible impediments to recovery observed during the study were a tendency to doubt one's own capacities, a lack of hope for the future, and a deathbed statement from the deceased amounting to prohibition of recovery.

PSYCHIATRIC PROBLEMS DUE TO BEREAVEMENT

Bereavement has been significantly associated with psychiatric admission (Parkes, 1965) and with first entry into psychiatric care (Stein & Susser, 1969). In 1964 Parkes found that within a 6-month period following the death of their husbands a group of London widows under 65 had tripled their psychiatric consultation rates and had received prescriptions for sedation at seven times the amount prior to the death of their husbands. Parkes and Brown (1972) found that the bereaved in their study obtained professional help more frequently and had more social difficulties in comparison to the control group. Stroebe and Stroebe (1983) noted that there is near unanimous agreement in the literature that bereavement can be a cause of mental illness. While depression is the most common disorder, other disorders such as neurotic disorders, phobias, obsessions, hypochondriasis, and conversions have been described as well (Raphael, 1983).

MORBIDITY AND MORTALITY DUE TO BEREAVEMENT

Some degree of physiological disturbance is a common component of the normal grief process. Nevertheless, it often escalates into a health risk for the bereaved. In some instances, the mourner even dies from grief-related illnesses. The following sections describe the nature and extent of the risks that bereavement poses to physical health. Despite its being discussed in this chapter, physiological symptomatology does not signify unresolved grief in and of itself; it is mentioned here to illustrate that normal physiological disturbances accompanying grief can themselves become pathological to the mourner.

Morbidity

There have been a number of investigations of the physical sequelae of a loss through death (Clayton, 1979; Glick et al., 1974; Lindemann, 1944; Maddison, 1969; Maddison & Viola, 1968; Maddison & Walker, 1967; Parkes, 1964, 1970, 1972; Parkes & Brown, 1972; Rees & Lutkins, 1967; Young, Benjamin, & Wallis, 1963; Parkes, Note 2). All of these concluded that the death of a loved one carries with it a definite physical risk for the griever much greater than that of the normal population.

Maddison (1969) summarized several studies and noted that in studying the health status of widows in Boston and Sydney 13 months after bereavement there was deterioration in 21% of Boston subjects and 32% of Sydney subjects. When matched to a control group these figures became more significant, as only 7% of the control group in Boston and 2% in Sydney reported a comparable deterioration in health. Glick et al. (1974) discovered that within 8 weeks after the death of their husbands 40% of the widows they studied had consulted their physicians because of headaches, dizziness, sleeplessness, and loss of appetite. Parkes (Note 2) reported that this same population spent considerably more time in bed than did the control group and had three times as many hospitalizations in the year following bereavement.

When comparing bereaved widows and widowers to a nonbereaved control group 13 months after the loss of their spouses, Parkes and Brown (1972) reported that bereaved subjects exceeded the control group in physical symptoms, especially in autonomic symptoms. They found that widows reported 50% more autonomic symptoms than women in the control group and widowers displayed four times as many symptoms as married men in the control group. Twelve bereaved individuals were admitted to the hospital during the year after their loss, while only four members of the comparison group had hospital admissions, and these were for conditions less serious than the bereaved group. The emotional distress of the bereaved sample was greater than the control group. Insomnia and changes in appetite and weight were also more frequent. Of the bereaved group, 28% reported an increase in smoking, 28% reported an increase in alcohol consumption, and 26% had either begun taking tranquilizers or increased their use. There had been virtually no increase in drug use in the control sample, with the exception of an unexplained increase in smoking among 20% of the married men. Other studies have suggested that bereavement is a precipitant for ulcerative colitis (Lindemann, 1944), neoplastic diseases (Klerman & Izen, 1977), thyrotoxicosis (Lidz, 1949), and asthma (McDermott & Cobb, 1939). . . .

Mortality

The combined evidence of mortality statistics suggests that there is a strong mortality risk to the bereaved. Kraus and Lilienfield (1959) found an increase in death rates of 40% for widowers in the first 6 months subsequent to the loss. In 1963, Young, Benjamin, and Wallis found almost the same 40% increase in the mortality rate of British widowers for 6 months following the death, after which it declined to expected levels. Subsequent analysis of these deaths revealed that three-quarters of the increased death rate was attributable to heart disease (Parkes, Benjamin, & Fitzgerald, 1969). Studies by Cox and Ford (1964) and Rees and Lutkins (1967) also found a significant increase in mortality for the bereaved as compared to control populations.

Stroebe et al. (1981–82) originally found that the evidence traditionally used to sustain the assumption of a "loss effect" (a predisposition to mortality due to bereavement) was insufficient, but that numerous indirect sources of evidence seemed to support it. They urged continued research on the issue, with particular attention to psychosocial processes that might cause the bereaved to either take an active self-destructive role or cease adequate health care. In a later extensive review Stroebe and Stroebe (1983) found that, compared with marriage, widowhood was associated with higher mortality for both sexes, with the excess risk being greater for men and the younger widowed. (This supports the findings of Jacobs and Ostfeld, who reviewed the literature in 1977.) Synthesizing the evidence from longitudinal studies, Stroebe and Stroebe found that for widowers there appeared to be a peak in the mortality risk during the first 6 months after the death, while for widows the period of highest risk appeared to be during the second year of bereavement.

Taken together, all these studies of morbidity and mortality corroborate clinical observations that bereavement is a state of great risk physically, as well as emotionally and socially. For this reason, the importance of adequate resolution of grief work cannot be stressed too much.

References

Averill, J. R. Grief: Its nature and significance. *Psychological Bulletin*, 1968, 70, 721–748.

Clayton, P. J. The sequelae and non-sequelae of conjugal bereavement. *Psychiatry*. 1979, 136, 1530–1534.

Cox, P., and Ford, J. R. The mortality of widows shortly after widowhood. *Lancet*, 1964, 1, 163–164.

Glick, I. O., Weiss, R. S., and Parkes, C. M. *The first year of bereavement*. New York: Wiley, 1974.

Jackson, E. N. *Understanding grief: Its roots, dynamics and treatment*. Nashville: Abington Press, 1957.

Jacobs, S., and Ostfeld, A. An epidemiological review of the mortality of bereavement. *Psychosomatic Medicine*, 1977, 39, 344–357.

Kastenbaum, R. J. Death and bereavement in later life. In A. H. Kutscher (Ed.), *Death and bereavement*. Springfield, Ill.: Charles C. Thomas, 1969.

Klerman, G. L., and Izen, J. E. The effects of bereavement and grief on physical health and general well-being. *Advances in Psychosomatic Medicine*, 1977, 9, 63–68.

Kraus, A. S., and Lilienfield, A. K. Some epidemiological aspects of the high mortality rate in the young widowed group. *Journal of Chronic Disease*. 1959, 10, 207.

Lazare, A. Unresolved grief. In A. Lazare (Ed.), *Outpatient psychiatry: Diagnosis and treatment*. Baltimore: Williams and Wilkens, 1979.

Lidz, R. Emotional factors in hyperthyroidism. *Psychosomatic Medicine*, 1949, 11, 2–9.

Lindemann, E. Symptomatology and management of acute grief. *American Journal of Psychiatry*, 1944, 101, 141–148.

Maddison, D. The consequences of conjugal bereavement. *Nursing Times*, 1969, 65, 50–52.

Maddison, D., and Viola, A. The health of widows in the year following bereavement. *Journal of Psychosomatic Research*, 1968, 12, 297–306.

Maddison, D., and Walker, W. Factors affecting the outcome of conjugal bereavement. *British Journal of Medical Psychology*, 1967, 113, 1057–1067.

McDermott, N., and Cobb, S. A psychiatric survey of 50 cases of bronchial asthma. *Psychosomatic Medicine*, 1939, 1, 201–204.

Parkes, C. M. Effects of bereavement on physical and mental health—A study of the case records of widows. *British Medical Journal*, 1964, 2, 274–279.

Parkes, C. M. Bereavement and mental illness: Part I—A clinical study of two griefs of bereaved psychiatric patients. *British Journal of Medical Psychology*, 1965, 38, 1–12.

Parkes, C. M. The first year of bereavement. *Psychiatry*, 1970, 33, 444–467.

Parkes, C. M. *Bereavement: Studies of grief in adult life*. New York: International Universities Press, 1972.

Parkes, C. M. Bereavement counseling: Does it work? *British Medical Journal*, 1980, 281, 3–6.

Parkes, C. M., Benjamin, B., and Fitzgerald, R. G. Broken heart: A statistical study of increased mortality among widowers. *British Medical Journal*, 1969, 1, 740–743.

Parkes, C. M., and Brown, R. J. Health after bereavement: A controlled study of young Boston widows and widowers. *Psychosomatic Medicine*, 1972, 34, 449–461.

Parkes, C. M., and Weiss, R. S. *Recovery from bereavement*. New York: Basic Books, 1983.

Raphael, B. *The anatomy of bereavement*. New York: Basic Books, 1983.

Rees, W. D., and Lutkins, S. G. Mortality of bereavement. *British Medical Journal*, 1967, 4, 13–16.

Siggins, L. Mourning: A critical survey of the literature. *International Journal of Psycho-Analysis*, 1966, 47, 14.

Stein, Z., and Susser, M. W. Widowhood and mental illness. *British Journal of Preventive and Social Medicine*, 1969, 23, 106–110.

Stroebe, M. S., and Stroebe, W. Who suffers more? Sex differences in health risk of the widowed. *Psychological Bulletin*, 1983, 93, 279–301.

Stroebe, M. S., Stroebe, W., Gergen, K., and Gergen, M. The broken heart: Reality or myth? *Omega*, 1981–82, 12, 87–105.

Worden, J. W. *Grief counseling and grief therapy: A handbook for the mental health practitioner*. New York: Springer, 1982.

Young, M., Benjamin, B., and Wallis, C. Mortality of widows. *Lancet*, 1963, 2, 454–456.

22 Disenfranchised Grief

Kenneth J. Doka

KENNETH DOKA is associate professor of gerontology at the College of New Rochelle, New York. This selection is the introductory chapter from his edited book, *Disenfranchised Grief*. In his book, individual chapters deal with various types of disenfranchised grief. This introductory chapter defines the concept and discusses some of the special problems linked to it.

INTRODUCTION

Ever since the publication of Lindemann's classic article, "Symptomatology and Management of Acute Grief" (1944), the literature on the nature of grief and bereavement has been growing. In the few decades following this seminal study, there have been comprehensive studies of grief reactions (for example, Glick, Weiss, and Parkes 1974, Bowling and Cartwright 1982, Parkes and Weiss 1983), detailed descriptions of atypical manifestations of grief (for example, Volkan 1970), theoretical and clinical treatments of grief reactions (for instance, Bowlby 1980, Worden 1982), and considerable research considering the myriad variables that affect grief (for example, Raphael 1983, Rando 1984). But most of this literature has concentrated on grief reactions in socially recognized and sanctioned roles: those of the parent, spouse, or child.

There are circumstances, however, in which a person experiences a sense of loss but does not have a socially recognized right, role, or capacity to grieve. In these cases, the grief is disenfranchised.[1] The person suffers a loss but has little or no opportunity to mourn publicly.

Up until now, there has been little research touching directly on the phenomenon of disenfranchised grief. In her comprehensive review of grief reactions, Raphael notes the phenomenon:

> *There may be other dyadic partnership relationships in adult life that show patterns similar to the conjugal ones, among them, the young couple intensely, even secretly, in*

love; the defacto relationships; the extra-marital relationship; and the homosexual couple . . . less intimate partnerships of close friends, working mates, and business associates, may have similar patterns of grief and mourning. (p. 227)

Focusing on the issues, reactions, and problems in particular populations, a number of studies have noted special difficulties that these populations have in grieving. For example, Kelly (1977) and Kimmel (1978, 1979), in studies of aging homosexuals, have discussed the unique problems of grief in such relationships. Similarly, studies (Heinemann et al. 1979, Geiss, Fuller, and Rush 1986) of the reactions of significant others of AIDS victims have considered bereavement. Other studies have considered the special problems of unacknowledged grief in prenatal death (Corney and Horton 1974, Wolff, Neilson, and Schiller 1970, Peppers and Knapp 1980, Kennell, Slyter, and Klaus 1970, Helmrath and Steinitz 1978), ex-spouses (Doka 1986, Scott 1985), therapists' reactions to a client's suicide, and pet loss. Finally, studies of families of Alzheimer's victims (Kay et al. 1985) and mentally retarded adults (Lipe-Goodson and Goebel 1983, Clyman et al. 1980, Edgerton, Bollinger, and Herr 1984) also have noted distinct difficulties of these populations in encountering varied losses which are often unrecognized by others.

Others have tried to draw parallels between related unacknowledged losses. For example, in a personal account, Horn (1979) compared her loss of a heterosexual lover with a friend's loss of a homosexual partner. Doka (1987) discussed the particular problems of loss in nontraditional relationships, such as extramarital affairs, homosexual relationships, and cohabiting couples.

This chapter attempts to integrate the literature on such losses in order to explore the phenomenon of disenfranchised grief. It will consider both the nature of disenfranchised grief and its central paradoxical problem: the very nature of this type of grief exacerbates the problems of grief, but the usual sources of support may not be available or helpful.

THE NATURE OF DISENFRANCHISED GRIEF

Disenfranchised grief can be defined as the grief that persons experience when they incur a loss that is not or cannot be openly acknowledged, publicly mourned, or socially supported. The concept of disenfranchised grief recognizes that societies have sets of norms—in effect, "grieving rules"—that attempt to specify who, when, where, how, how long, and for whom people should grieve. These grieving rules may be codified in personnel policies. For example, a worker may be allowed a week off for the death of a spouse or child, three days for the loss of a parent or sibling. Such policies reflect the fact that each society defines who has a legitimate right to grieve, and these definitions

of right correspond to relationships, primarily familial, that are socially recognized and sanctioned. In any given society these grieving rules may not correspond to the nature of attachments, the sense of loss, or the feelings of
survivors. Hence the grief of these survivors is disenfranchised. In our society,
this may occur for three reasons.

1. The Relationship Is Not Recognized

In our society, most attention is placed on kin-based relationships and roles.
Grief may be disenfranchised in those situations in which the relationship between the bereaved and deceased is not based on recognizable kin ties. Here the
closeness of other non-kin relationships may simply not be understood or appreciated. For example, Folta and Deck (1976) noted, "While all of these studies tell us that grief is a normal phenomenon, the intensity of which
corresponds to the closeness of the relationship, they fail to take this (i.e.,
friendship) into account. The underlying assumption is that closeness of relationship exists only among spouses and/or immediate kin" (p. 239). The roles
of lovers, friends, neighbors, foster parents, colleagues, in-laws, stepparents
and stepchildren, caregivers, counselors, co-workers, and roommates (for example, in nursing homes) may be long-lasting and intensely interactive, but
even though these relationships are recognized, mourners may not have full
opportunity to publicly grieve a loss. At most, they might be expected to support and assist family members.

Then there are relationships that may not be publicly recognized or socially
sanctioned. For example, nontraditional relationships, such as extramarital affairs, cohabitation, and homosexual relationships have tenuous public acceptance and limited legal standing, and they face negative sanction within the
larger community. Those involved in such relationships are touched by grief
when the relationship is terminated by the death of the partner, but others in
their world, such as children, may also experience a grief that cannot be acknowledged or socially supported.

Even those whose relationships existed primarily in the past may experience grief. Ex-spouses, past lovers, or former friends may have limited contact
or they may even engage in interaction in the present. Yet the death of that significant other can still cause a grief reaction because it brings finality to that
earlier loss, ending any remaining contact or fantasy of reconciliation or rein-
volvement. And again these grief feelings may be shared by others in their
world such as parents and children. They too may mourn the loss of "what
once was" and "what might have been." For example, in one case a twelve-
year-old child of an unwed mother, never even acknowledged or seen by the
father, still mourned the death of his father since it ended any possibility of a
future liaison. But though loss is experienced, society as a whole may not perceive that the loss of a past relationship could or should cause any reaction.

2. The Loss Is Not Recognized

In other cases, the loss itself is not socially defined as significant. Perinatal deaths lead to strong grief reactions, yet research indicates that many significant others still perceive the loss to be relatively minor (Raphael 1983). Abortions too can constitute a serious loss (Raphael 1972), but the abortion can take place without the knowledge or sanctions of others, or even the recognition that a loss has occurred. It may very well be that the very ideologies of the abortion controversy can put the bereaved in a difficult position. Many who affirm a loss may not sanction the act of abortion, while some who sanction the act may minimize any sense of loss. Similarly, we are just becoming aware of the sense of loss that people experience in giving children up for adoption or foster care (Raphael 1983), and we have yet to be aware of the grief-related implications of surrogate motherhood.

Another loss that may not be perceived as significant is the loss of a pet. Nevertheless, the research (Kay et al. 1984) shows strong ties between pets and humans, and profound reactions to loss.

Then there are cases in which the reality of the loss itself is not socially validated. Thanatologists have long recognized that significant losses can occur even when the object of the loss remains physically alive. Sudnow (1967) for example, discusses "social death," in which the person is alive but is treated as if dead. Examples may include those who are institutionalized or comatose. Similarly, "psychological death" has been defined as conditions in which the person lacks a consciousness of existence (Kalish 1966), such as someone who is "brain dead." One can also speak of "psychosocial death" in which the persona of someone has changed so significantly, through mental illness, organic brain syndromes, or even significant personal transformation (such as through addiction, conversion, and so forth), that significant others perceive the person as he or she previously existed as dead (Doka 1985). In all of these cases, spouses and others may experience a profound sense of loss, but that loss cannot be publicly acknowledged for the person is still biologically alive.

3. The Griever Is Not Recognized

Finally, there are situations in which the characteristics of the bereaved in effect disenfranchise their grief. Here the person is not socially defined as capable of grief; therefore, there is little or no social recognition of his or her sense of loss or need to mourn. Despite evidence to the contrary, both the very old and the very young are typically perceived by others as having little comprehension of or reaction to the death of a significant other. Often, then, both young children and aged adults are excluded from both discussions and rituals (Raphael 1983).

Similarly, mentally disabled persons may also be disenfranchised in grief. Although studies affirm that the mentally retarded are able to understand the concept of death (Lipe-Goodson and Goebel 1983) and, in fact, experience grief (Edgerton, Bollinger, and Herr 1984), these reactions may not be perceived by others. Because the person is retarded or otherwise mentally disabled, others in the family may ignore his or her need to grieve. Here a teacher of the mentally disabled describes two illustrative incidences:

> *In the first situation, Susie was 17 years old and away at summer camp when her father died. The family felt she wouldn't understand and that it would be better for her not to come home for the funeral. In the other situation, Francine was with her mother when she got sick. The mother was taken away by ambulance. Nobody answered her questions or told her what happened. "After all," they responded, "she's retarded." (H. Goldstein, private communication)*

THE SPECIAL PROBLEMS OF DISENFRANCHISED GRIEF

Though each of the types of grief mentioned earlier may create particular difficulties and different reactions, one can legitimately speak of the special problem shared in disenfranchised grief.

The problem of disenfranchised grief can be expressed in a paradox. The very nature of disenfranchised grief creates additional problems for grief, while removing or minimizing sources of support.

Disenfranchising grief may exacerbate the problem of bereavement in a number of ways. First, the situations mentioned tend to intensify emotional reactions. Many emotions are associated with normal grief. Bereaved persons frequently experience feelings of anger, guilt, sadness and depression, loneliness, hopelessness, and numbness (Lindemann 1944, Worden 1982). These emotional reactions can be complicated when grief is disenfranchised. Although each of the situations described is in its own way unique, the literature uniformly reports how each of these disenfranchising circumstances can intensify feelings of anger, guilt, or powerlessness (see, for example, Kelly 1977, Geis, Fuller, and Rush 1986, Peppers and Knapp 1980, Doka 1985, 1986, Miller and Roll 1985).

Second, both ambivalent relationships and concurrent crises have been identified in the literature as conditions that complicate grief (Worden 1982, Raphael 1983, Rando 1984). The conditions can often exist in many types of disenfranchised grief. For example, studies have indicated the ambivalence that can exist in cases of abortion (Raphael 1972), among ex-spouses (Doka 1986, Scott 1985), significant others in nontraditional roles (Doka 1987, Horn 1979), and among families of Alzheimer's disease victims (Doka 1985). Similarly, the literature documents the many kinds of concurrent crises that can trouble the disenfranchised griever. For example, in cases of cohabiting couples, either heterosexual or homosexual, studies have often found that survivors experience legal and financial problems regarding inheritance, ownership, credit, or leases (for example, Kimmel 1978, 1979, Doka 1987, Horn 1979). Likewise, the death of a parent may leave a mentally disabled person not only bereaved but also bereft of a viable support system (Edgerton, Bollinger, and Herr 1984).

Although grief is complicated, many of the factors that facilitate mourning are not present. The bereaved may be excluded from an active role in caring for the dying. Funeral rituals, normally helpful in resolving grief, may not help here. In some cases the bereaved may be excluded from attendance. In other cases they may have no role in planning those rituals or in deciding whether even to have them. Or in cases of divorce, separation, or psychosocial death, rituals may be lacking altogether.

In addition, the very nature of the disenfranchised grief precludes social support. Often there is no recognized role in which mourners can assert the right to mourn and thus receive such support. Grief may have to remain private. Though they may have experienced an intense loss, they may not be given time off from work, have the opportunity to verbalize the loss, or receive the expressions of sympathy and support characteristic in a death. Even traditional sources of solace, such as religion, are unavailable to those whose relationships (for example, extramarital, cohabiting, homosexual, divorced) or acts (such as abortion) are condemned within that tradition.

Naturally, there are many variables that will affect both the intensity of the reaction and the availability of support. All the variables—interpersonal, psychological, social, physiological—that normally influence grief will have an impact here as well. And while there are problems common to cases of disenfranchised grief, each relationship has to be individually considered in light of the unique combination of factors that may facilitate or impair grief resolution.

IMPLICATIONS

Despite the shortage of research on and attention given to the issue of disenfranchised grief, it remains a significant issue. Millions of Americans are involved in losses in which grief is effectively disenfranchised. For example, there are more than 1 million couples presently cohabiting (Reiss 1980). There are estimates that 3 percent of males and 2–3 percent of females are exclusively homosexual, with similar percentages having mixed homosexual and heterosexual encounters (Gagnon 1977). There are about a million abortions a year; even though many of the women involved may not experience grief reactions, some are clearly "at risk."

Disenfranchised grief is also a growing issue. There are higher percentages of divorced people in the cohorts now aging. The AIDS crisis means that more homosexuals will experience losses in significant relationships. Even as the disease spreads within the population of intravenous drug users, it is likely to create a new class of both potential victims and disenfranchised grievers among the victims' informal liaisons and nontraditional relationships.[2] And as Americans continue to live longer, more will suffer from severe forms of chronic brain dysfunctions (Atchley 1985). As the developmentally disabled live longer, they too will experience the grief of parental and sibling loss. In short, the proportion of disenfranchised grievers in the general population will rise rapidly in the future.

It is likely that bereavement counselors will have increased exposure to cases of disenfranchised grief. In fact, the very nature of disenfranchised grief and the unavailability of informal support make it likely that those who experience such losses will seek formal supports. Thus there is a pressing need for research that will describe the particular and unique reactions of each of the different types of losses; compare reactions and problems associated with these losses; describe the important variables affecting disenfranchised grief reactions;[3] assess possible interventions; and discover the atypical grief reactions, such as masked or delayed grief that might be manifested in such cases. Also needed is education sensitizing students to the many kinds of relationships and subsequent losses that people can experience and affirming that where there is loss there is grief.

Notes

1. A term suggested by Austin Kutscher (private communication).

2. One can also speak of "disenfranchising deaths." In some cases the cause of death creates such shame and embarrassment that even those in recognized survivor roles (such as spouse, child, or parent) may be reluctant to avail themselves of social support or may feel a sense of social reproach over the circumstances of death. Death from a dreaded disease like AIDS and certain situations surrounding suicide and homicide are illustrations of disenfranchising death. Each carries a stigma that may inhibit even survivors in recognizably legitimate roles from seeking and receiving social support.

3. As has been stated, some of these variables will be common to all losses. Others, such as the degree to which a loss is socially recognized, publicly sanctioned, openly acknowledged, or replaceable, may be unique to certain types of disenfranchised grief.

References

Atchley, R. 1985. *Social Forces and Aging.* 4th ed. Belmont, Calif.: Wadsworth.

Bowlby, J. 1980. *Attachment and Loss: Loss, Sadness and Depression*, vol. 3. New York: Basic Books.

Bowling, A., and A. Cartwright. 1982. *Life After a Death: A Study of the Elderly Widowed.* New York: Tavistock.

Clyman, R., C. Green, J. Rowe, C. Mikkelson, and L. Ataide. 1980. "Issues Concerning Parents After the Death of Their Newborn." *Critical Care Medicine* 8, 215–18.

Corney, R. J., and F. T. Horton. 1974. "Pathological Grief Following Spontaneous Abortion." *American Journal of Psychiatry* 131, 825–27.

Doka, K. 1985. "Crypto Death and Real Grief." Paper presented to a symposium of the Foundation of Thanatology, New York, March.

———. 1986. "Loss upon Loss: Death After Divorce." *Death Studies* 10, 441–49.

———. 1987. "Silent Sorrow: Grief and the Loss of Significant Others." *Death Studies* 11, 455–69.

Edgerton, R. B., M. Bollinger, and B. Herr. 1984. "The Cloak of Competence: After Two Decades." *American Journal of Mental Deficiency* 88, 345–51.

Folta, J., and G. Deck. 1976. "Grief, the Funeral and the Friend." In *Acute Grief and the Funeral*, edited by V. Pine, A. H. Kutscher, D. Peretz, R. C. Slater, R. DeBellis, A. I. Volk, and D. J. Cherico. Springfield, Ill.

Gagnon, J. 1977. *Human Sexuality*. Glenview, Ill.: Scott, Foresman.

Geis, S., R. Fuller, and J. Rush. 1986. "Lovers of AIDS Victims: Psychosocial Stresses and Counseling Needs." *Death Studies* 10, 43–54.

Glick, I., R. Weiss, and C. M. Parkes. 1974. *The First Years of Bereavement*. New York: Wiley.

Heinemann, A., et al. 1983. "A Social Service Program for AIDS Clients." Paper presented to the Sixth Annual Meeting of the Forum for Death Education, Chicago, October.

Helmrath, T. A., and G. M. Steinitz. 1978. "Parental Grieving and the Failure of Social Support." *Journal of Family Practice* 6, 785–90.

Horn, R. 1979. "Life Can Be a Soap Opera." In *Perspectives on Bereavement*, edited by I. Gerber, A. Weiner, A. Kutscher, D. Battin, A. Arkin, and I. Goldberg. New York: Arno Press.

Kalish, R. 1966. "A Continuum of Subjectively Perceived Death." *The Gerontologist* 6, 73–76.

Kay, W. J. et al., eds. 1984. *Pet Loss and Human Bereavement*. New York: Arno Press.

Kelly, J. 1977. "The Aging Male Homosexual: Myth and Reality." *The Gerontologist* 17, 328–32.

Kennell, J., M. Slyter, and M. Klaus. 1970. "The Mourning Response of Parents to the Death of a Newborn Infant." *New England Journal of Medicine* 283, 344–49.

Kimmel, D. 1978. "Adult Development and Aging: A Gay Perspective." *Journal of Social Issues* 34, 113–31.

———. 1979. "Life History Interview of Aging Gay Men." *International Journal of Aging and Human Development* 10, 237–48.

Lindemann, E. 1944. "Symptomatology and Management of Acute Grief." *American Journal of Psychiatry* 101, 141–49.

Lipe-Goodson, P. S., and B. I. Goebel. 1983. "Perception of Age and Death in Mentally Retarded Adults." *Mental Retardation* 21, 68–75.

Miller, L., and S. Roll. 1985. "A Case Study in Failure: On Doing Everything Right in Suicide Prevention." *Death Studies* 9, 483–92.

Parkes, C. M., and R. Weiss. 1983. *Recovery from Bereavement*. New York: Basic Books.

Peppers, L., and R. Knapp. 1980. *Motherhood and Mourning*. New York: Praeger.

Rando, T. 1984. *Grief, Dying and Death: Clinical Interventions for Caregivers*. Champaign, Ill.: Research Press.

Raphael, B. 1972. "Psychosocial Aspects of Induced Abortion." *Medical Journal of Australia* 2, 35–40A.

———. 1983. *The Anatomy of Bereavement*. New York: Basic Books.

Reiss, I. 1980. *Family Systems in America*. New York: Holt, Rinehart and Winston.

Scott, S. 1985. "Grief Reactions to the Death of a Divorced Spouse." Paper presented to the Seventh Annual Meeting of the Forum for Death Education and Counseling, Philadelphia, April.

Sudnow, D. 1967. *Passing On: The Social Organization of Dying*. Englewood Cliffs, N.J.: Prentice-Hall.

Volkan, V. 1970. "Typical Findings in Pathological Grief." *Psychiatric Quarterly* 44, 231–50.

Wolff, J., P. Neilson, and P. Schiller. 1970. "The Emotional Reaction to a Stillbirth." *American Journal of Obstetrics and Gynecology* 101, 73–76.

Worden, W. 1982. *Grief Counseling and Grief Therapy*. New York: Springer.

CHILDREN AND DEATH

Contents

THE SELECTION BY NAGY is based on her study of the development of children's thinking about death, in which she asked children between the ages of three and ten about their conceptions of death. She presents an interesting description of how those conceptions evolve over time. As the study was done a number of years ago on a sample of Hungarian children, the reader may want to ask why Nagy's observations about those aged three to five seem to generalize to contemporary American children better than do her observations about those aged five to nine. What role could American TV play?

The article by Bluebond-Langner is divided into two quite separate parts. The first focuses on the experience of being a terminally ill child. It is a study of changes in self-concept as the child progresses through the illness. The second part of the article analyzes the experience of being a well sibling in the home of a child who is terminally ill. The focus here is on changes over time in the relationship between the two siblings and on the

225

interactions among the well siblings and the parents. The well siblings often indicate in various ways that they are not happy with the lack of attention paid to them, but they also do seem to understand why the sick sibling is getting most of the attention.

The selection by Pynoos deals with the traumatic impact on children who have witnessed the death of a parent as a result of homicide or suicide. (What Lindemann would describe as a morbid grief reaction is common under such circumstances.)

Raphael examines differences in the bereavement experience for parents who lose children of different ages, including those lost under a variety of different circumstances prior to birth. The loss of an unborn child is often associated with disenfranchised grief, and it may be useful to link this discussion to Doka's article in the previous section.

23 The Child's Theories ❧
Concerning Death

Maria Nagy

MARIA NAGY was a Hungarian psychologist. She was the author of *The Child and Death* (in Hungarian). She began her career in Hungary, but shortly after World War II moved to the United States, where she held a number of teaching and research positions in clinical psychology. She did some very influential work on the development of children's conceptions of death. The selection below is taken from her article with the same name. In Hungary she asked children aged three to ten, "What is death?" She found that those under age five did not view death as irreversible, those between five and nine often personified death, and those over age nine generally had what we would consider an adult conception of death. In this article, she presents evidence in support of these three stages in the development of children's conceptions of death.

IF WE WISH TO INVESTIGATE EXPERIMENTALLY the child's attitude towards death, the theme must necessarily be divided into detailed questions. Among the questions connected with death, in the present study I wish to deal with only one. *What does the child think death to be, what theory does he construct of the nature of death?* . . .

What is death? Among the children from 3–10 the replies given to this question can be ranged in three groups. As the different sorts of answers can be found only at certain ages, one can speak of stages of development. The child of less than five years does not recognize death as an irreversible fact. In death it sees life. Between the ages of five and nine death is the most often personified and thought of as a contingency. And in general only after the age of nine is it recognized that death is a process happening in us according to certain laws. . . .

From *Journal of Genetic Psychology*, Volume 73, pp. 3–27, 1948. Reprinted with permission of the Helen Dwight Reid Educational Foundation. Published by Heldref Publications, 1319 Eighteenth St., N.W., Washington, D.C. 20036–1802. Copyright © 1948.

1. FIRST STAGE: THERE IS NO DEFINITIVE DEATH

In the first stage the child does not know death as such. He attributes life and consciousness to the dead. There are two variations of this affirmation, which I discuss the one after the other. According to one group, death is a departure, a sleep. This entirely denies death. The other group already recognizes the fact of death but cannot separate it from life. For that reason it considers death either gradual or temporary.

a. Death a departure, a sleep. *B. Jolan* (3,11)[1] "The dead close their eyes because the sand gets into them."

The child had heard something about the eyes of the dead being closed. It explained this by an exterior cause. The dead person voluntarily, defensively, closes its eyes.

Sch. Tomy (4, 8): "It can't move because it's in the coffin."

"If it weren't in the coffin, could it?"

"It can eat and drink."

Like the first with the closing of the eyes, here too the immobility is the consequence of exterior compulsive circumstances. It doesn't move because the coffin does not permit it. He considers the dead as still capable of taking nourishment.

Sch. Juliska (5, 10) had already seen a dead person. "Its eyes were closed, it lay there, so dead. No matter what one does to it, it doesn't say a word."

"After ten years will it be the same as when it was buried?"

"It will be older then, it will always be older and older. When it is 100 years old it will be exactly like a piece of wood."

"How will it be like a piece of wood?"

"That I couldn't say. My little sister will be five years old now. I wasn't alive yet when she died. She will be so big by this time. She has a small coffin, but she fits in the small coffin."

"What is she doing now, do you think?"

"Lying down, always just lies there. She's still so small, she can't be like a piece of wood. Only very old people."

In the beginning she sees the matter realistically. The dead person cannot speak. The closed eyes do not necessarily mean the cessation of sight. The dead person is compared to a piece of wood. In all probability she wanted thus to express immobility. Later it comes out that young people grow in the grave. The growth is not great. She says her sister is five years old because she herself is five.

B. Irén (4, 11): "What happens there under the earth?"

"He cries because he is dead."

---

[1]The age is significant. The child was past 3 years and 11 months old.

"But why should he cry?"

"Because he is afraid for himself."

She feels that death is bad. Perhaps she has had the experience of seeing the dead mourned. She transfers this sentiment to the dead themselves. They also mourn for themselves.

V. Juliska (5, 3): "What is your father doing now under the earth?"

"He lies there. Scratches the earth, to come up. To get a little air."

She knows of the reclining state of the dead. She imagines that in the earth it must be difficult to breathe. The dead person scratches the earth away, to get air. . . .

F. Robi (9, 11): "I was six years old. A friend of my father's died. They didn't tell me, but I heard. Then I didn't understand. I felt as when Mother goes travelling somewhere—I don't see her any more."

He feels the same about news of death as about travelling. The dead person resembles the absent, in that he sees neither of them.

Summary. As we see, in general these children do not accept death. To die means the same as living on, under changed circumstances.

Death is thus a departure. If someone dies no change takes place in him. Our lives change, inasmuch as we see him no longer, he lives with us no longer.

This, however, does not mean that the children have no disagreeable sentiments in relation to death, because for them the most painful things about death is just the separation itself.[2]

To the child the association Death=Departure exists also in the inverse sense. If anyone goes away it thinks him dead. Jaehner states that his children thought that whenever their father went away they were going to bury him, as they already knew the connection between death and burial.

Most children, however, are not satisfied, when someone dies, that he should merely disappear, but want to know where and how he continues to live. As all the children questioned knew of funerals, they connected the facts of absence and funerals. In the cemetery one lives on. Movement is to a certain degree limited by the coffin, but for all that the dead are still capable of growth. They take nourishment, they breathe. They know what is happening on earth. They feel it, if someone thinks of them, and they even feel sorry for themselves. Thus the dead live in the grave. Most children, however, feel too—and have therefore an aversion for death—that that life is limited, not so complete as our life. Some of them consider this diminished life exclusively restricted to sleep. While here they identify death with dreams, from seven years on they liken it to sleep. But as the child's sense of reality increases, the more it feels and knows the difference between the two. . . .

[2]As control I asked 30 older children what was the most terrible thing about death, and they all answered that it was the separation.

Finally I must answer the question, what impels the children to the denial of death. What endeavour brings about the identification of death with departure, or with sleep. In early infancy, that is, under five, its desires guide the child even at the price of modifying the reality. Opposition to death is so strong that the child denies death, as emotionally it cannot accept it.

b. Death is gradual, temporary. There are among children of five and six those who no longer deny death, but who are still unable to accept it as a definitive fact. They acknowledge that death exists but think of it as a gradual or temporary thing.

L. Bandika (5, 6): "His eyes were closed."

"Why?"

"Because he was dead."

"What is the difference between sleeping and dying?"

"Then they bring the coffin and put him in it. They put the hands like this when a person is dead."

"What happens to him in the coffin?"

"The worms eat him. They bore into the coffin."

"Why does he let them eat him?"

"He can't get up any longer, because there is sand on him. He can't get out of the coffin."

"If there weren't sand on him could he get out?"

"Certainly, if he wasn't very badly stabbed. He would get his hand out of the sand and dig. That shows that he still wants to live."

In the beginning the child sees realistically. He does not say, like the previous children, that "he closes his eyes," but that the eyes were closed. He sees only exterior differences between sleep and death. This would again be evidence of a denial of death, if immediately afterwards he had not begun to speak of worms. He does not state that the dead cannot move, merely that the sand hinders them in moving. On the other hand, he attributes a desire for life to the dead person—though only when he is not "very badly killed." Thus there are degrees of death. . . .

Pr. Ibolya (5): "His eyes were shut."

"Why?"

"Because he couldn't open them. Because he is in the coffin. Then, when he wakes up, then they take him out of the coffin. They put somebody else in."

"When they take him out of the coffin what happens to him?"

"If I die my heart doesn't beat."

In death the action of the heart stops. On the other hand, she states too that death is sleep. But not eternal sleep, because the dead person awakens. . . .

Summary. As we see, the children of the second group already accept death to a certain extent. The distinction between life and death is, however, not complete. If they think of death as gradual, life and death are in simultaneous relation; if it is temporary, life and death can change with one another repeatedly.

These conceptions are of a higher order than that which entirely denies death. Here, namely, the distinction between the two processes has already begun. Furthermore, beside their desires the feeling for reality also plays a rôle. Thus occurs the compromise solution, that while death exists it is not definitive. . . .

2. SECOND STAGE: DEATH = A MAN

In the second stage the child personifies death. This conception is to be found in the whole of childhood, but seems characteristic between the ages of five and nine. The personification of death takes place in two ways. Death is imagined as a separate person, or else death is identified with the dead. When death is imagined as a separate person we again find two conceptions. Either "the reaper" idea is accepted, or a quite individual picture is formed of the death-man. . . .

Br. Marta (6, 7): "Carries off bad children. Catches them and takes them away."

"What is he like?"

"White as snow. Death is white everywhere. It's wicked. It doesn't like children."

"Why?"

"Because it's bad-hearted. Death even takes away men and women too."

"Why?"

"Because it doesn't like to see them."

"What is white about it?"

"The skeleton. The bone–skeleton."

"But in reality is it like that, or do they only say so?"

"It really is, too. Once I talked about it and at night the real death came. It has a key to everywhere, so it can open the doors. It came in, messed about everywhere. It came over to the bed and began to pull away the covers. I covered myself up well. It couldn't take them off. Afterwards it went away."

"You only pretend it was there. It wasn't really there."

"I was ill then. I didn't go to the kindergarten. A little girl always came up. I always quarreled with her. One night it came. I always took raisins, though it was forbidden."

"Did you tell your mother?"

"I didn't dare to tell my mother, because she is anyhow afraid of everything."

"And your father?"

"Papa said it was a tale from the benzine tank. I told him it wasn't any fairy-tale."

"In the description of the skeleton-man his color is important. He carries people off because he is bad-hearted. So dying is considered a bad thing. Death was seen in feverish dreams. Since then she is convinced that it exists. Talk of death causes its magical advent. Death came too because she had done wrong. So there is a relationship between sin and death.

K. Karoly (7, 8): "Death is a living being and takes people's souls away. Gives them over to God. Death is the king of the dead. Death lives in the cemetery and can be seen only when he carries off some person's soul. There is a soul in death."

"How do you mean that?"

"He can go where he likes."

"What is death like?"

"White. Made of a skeleton. It's covered with a white sheet."

"How do you know it's like that?"

"Because once I saw a play and I saw it there."

"And in reality death is like that?"

"Alive he couldn't be drawn, because there isn't any such man who is made only of a skeleton. Who wants to can't see him and who doesn't want to sees him."

"How do you know it's like that?"

"It has already been experienced."

"People didn't just make it up? It's truly so?"

"It's really like that."

Death is king and in the service of God. Only the dying can see him. The ability to move about derives from the soul. He considers death impossible to draw.

P. Géza (8, 6): "Death comes when somebody dies, and comes with a scythe, cuts him down and takes him away. When death goes away it leaves footprints behind. When the footprints disappeared it came back and cut down more people. And then they wanted to catch it, and it disappeared."

Death is so much a person that it even leaves footprints. Like a child, it teases people. He wants to exterminate death. . . .

Summary. In the second stage of development, in general between five and nine, the children personify death in some form. Two-thirds of the children belonging to this group imagine death as a distinct personality. Either they believe in the reality of the skeleton-man, or individually create quite their own idea of the death-man. They say the death-man is invisible. This means two things. Either it is invisible in itself, as it is a being without a body, or it is only that we do not see him because he goes about in secret, mostly at night. They also state that death can be seen for a moment before, by the person he carries off.

Compared with the first stage, where death is denied, here we find an increase in the sense of reality as contrary to their desires. The child already accepts the existence of death, that is, its definitiveness. On the other hand, he has such an aversion to the thought of death that he casts it away. From a process which takes place in us death grows to a reality outside us. It exists but is remote from us. As it is remote our death is not inevitable. Only those die whom the death-man catches and carries off. Whoever can get away does not die.

Of the children in the second stage of development again one-third thought of death as a person and identified it with the dead. These children use the word death for the dead. In this conception, too, is evident a desire to keep death at a distance. Death is still outside us and is also not general.

It is surprising how little the literature on this subject deals with the personification of death, though the tendency to personify is in general well known at certain stages of a child's development. Only E. Stern mentions it concerning 10-year-olds but does not see its universal significance nor deal with its motives.

3. THIRD STAGE: DEATH—THE CESSATION OF CORPORAL ACTIVITIES

In general it is only after the age of nine that the child reaches the point of recognizing that in death is the cessation of corporal life. When he reaches the point where death is a process operating within us he recognizes its universal nature.

F. Eszter (10): "It means the passing of the body. Death is a great squaring of accounts in our lives. It is a thing from which our bodies cannot be resurrected. It is like the withering of flowers."

Death is the destruction of the body. She mixes the natural explanation with the moral, also considers death a reckoning.

Cz. Gyula (9, 4): "Death is the termination of life. Death is destiny. Then we finish our earthly life. Death is the end of life on earth."

He expresses its regularity by the word destiny.

F. Gàbor (9, 11): "A skull portrays death. If somebody dies they bury him and he crumbles to dust in the earth. The bones crumble later, and so the skeleton remains altogether, the way it was. That is why death is portrayed by a skeleton. Death is something that no one can escape. The body dies, the soul lives on."

He knows that the portrayal of death is not death itself. Indeed, he also explains why the skeleton became the symbol of death. Death is universal.

Sz. Tamàs (9, 4): "What is death? Well, I think it is a part of a person's life. Like school. Life has many parts. Only one part of it is earthly. As in school we go on to a different class. To die means to begin a new life. Everyone has to die once, but the soul lives on."

It is comprehensible; he sees eternal mystery beyond the physical changes.

Summary

I investigated how children from 3 to 10 think of death. I employed written compositions, drawings, and discussion alike in collecting the data, and 484 protocols from 378 children were at my disposition. In the present study the material has not been fully worked up; I only desired to answer the question of what death is to the child, what theories he constructs as to the nature of death. I found three stages of development. The first is characteristic of children between three and five. They deny death as a regular and final process. Death is a departure, a further existence in changed circumstances. There are ideas too that death is temporary. Indeed distinction is made of degrees of death.

The child knows itself as a living being. In his egocentric way he imagines the outside world after his own fashion, so in the outside world he also imagines everything, lifeless things and dead people alike, as living. Living and lifeless are not yet distinguished. He extends this animism to death too.

In the second stage, in general between the ages of five and nine, death is personified, considered a person. Death exists but the children still try to keep it distant from themselves. Only those die whom the death-man carries off. Death is an eventuality. There also occur fantasies, though less frequently, where death and the dead are considered the same. In these cases they consistently employ the word death for the dead. Here death is still outside us and not universal. The egocentric, otherwise called anthropocentric, view, therefore, plays a rôle not only in the birth of animism, but in the formation of artificialism too. Every event and change in the world derives from man. If in general death exists, it is a person, the death-man, who "does" it. We get no answer, naturally, as to why, if death is bad for people, he does it.

Finally, in the third stage, in general around nine years, it is recognized that death is a process which takes place in us, the perceptible result of which is the dissolution of bodily life. By then they know that death is inevitable. At this age not only the conception as to death is realistic, but also their general view of the world. Negatively this means that animistic and artificialistic tendencies are not characteristic and egocentrism is also much less.

As we see, the theory the child makes of death faithfully reflects at each stage a general picture of its world. To conceal death from the child is not possible and is also not permissible. Natural behaviour in the child's surroundings can greatly diminish the shock of its acquaintance with death.

24 Worlds of Dying Children and Their Well Siblings

Myra Bluebond-Langner

MYRA BLUEBOND-LANGNER is professor of anthropology at Rutgers University, Camden, New Jersey. She is a recipient of the Margaret Mead Award given by the American Anthropology Association and the Society for Applied Anthropology. In addition to presenting an analysis of the place of illness and death in the lives of the healthy siblings of children at the end stages of life, this article presents a summary of the major points made in her earlier book, *The Private Worlds of Dying Children*.

INTRODUCTION

A child is dying of kidney disease, of cystic fibrosis, of cancer. We refer to the child as a "victim of chronic or terminal illness." But that child, that dying child, is not necessarily the only victim of chronic or terminal illness. The victims of chronic or terminal illness are not limited to the diagnosed patient. The destructive effects of such diseases spread to the families of those afflicted. New events and activities become part of the everyday lives of these families: time consuming care of the patient, trips to the hospital, the absence of family members during hospitalizations. A constant concern for the ill patient settles in for the duration. New feelings develop as well. Who would not occasionally resent the way in which one's life has been complicated by capricious chance? Yet what right do the healthy family members have to feel such feelings, to think such thoughts? They do not look forward to permanent disability or to death. So begins for the family, for each and every member of that family, a cycle of feelings that includes anxiety, guilt, neglect, denial, anger, and depression.

I want to call your attention to some of the other "victims"—the well siblings of terminally ill children dying of cancer and cystic fibrosis. I want to explore with you the place that illness and death have in their worlds. But before doing that, I think it is important to acquaint you with the world of the terminally ill child. For it is through observation and interaction with the dying

From *Death Studies*, Vol. 13, pp. 1–16, by Myra Bluebond-Langner. Copyright © 1989 by Hemisphere Publishing Corporation, Bristol, PA. Reprinted by permission.

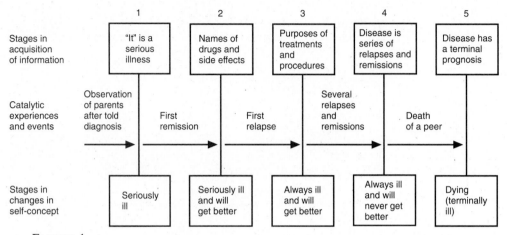

FIGURE 1

child that the well sibling comes to know of disease and death. I will limit my remarks to the terminal phases of the illness. I will not discuss the behaviors one sees in earlier phases of the illness (e.g., diagnostic, relapses, exacerbations). The behaviors one sees before the child is terminal are very different from what one sees during the terminal phases. Later I will discuss some of those differences. For now, let us turn to the world of the terminally ill child.

TERMINALLY ILL CHILDREN

While all terminally ill children become aware of the fact that they are dying before death is imminent, the acquisition and assimilation of information is a prolonged process. It is a process that involves not only learning about the disease, but also experiences in that disease world and changes in self-concept. In situations where the children are told their diagnosis and prognosis, I refer to the process as one of internalization. In situations where the children are not told, I refer to the process as one of discovery. The process, however, remains the same in both situations and is outlined in Figure 1.

In the first stage in the acquisition of information, the children learn that they have a serious illness. In the second stage, they learn the name of the drugs and their side effects. In the third stage they become aware of the purposes of various treatments and procedures. In the fourth stage, they are able to take all of these isolated bits and pieces of information and put them into a larger perspective, the cycle of relapses and remissions. At this point, however, the children do not incorporate death into the cycle. It is only when they reach the fifth stage that the children come to see the disease as having a terminal prognosis.

At the same time that the children pass through these stages in the acquisition of information, their view of themselves also changes. They move from a view of themselves as seriously ill to a view of themselves as ill and going to get better, to a view of themselves as always ill and going to get better, to a view of themselves as always ill and never going to get better, and finally, to a view of themselves as dying.

For children to pass through these stages though, certain significant experiences have to take place. The first stage follows upon observation of their parents and the reactions of others to the news of the diagnosis. The second stage comes with the first remission; the third with the first relapse; the fourth, after a series of relapses and remissions; and the fifth, on the death of a peer.

As you consider this processs, it is important to bear in mind that information is cumulative, such that if a child is at stage 2 and another child dies, he or she will not necessarily see the disease or himself or herself as having a terminal prognosis. Also, experience in the disease world is the most critical factor in the child's coming to understand the disease. As you may have noticed, I have not mentioned age in this process. The children that we are going to be talking about are children between the ages of 5 and 12, all of whom became aware of the fact that they were dying before death was imminent. While their awareness of death did not vary by age, the way that they expressed it sometimes did.

If I had time, what I would like to do at this point is to detail each of the stages for you. But given the constraints of time, I'm going to jump to stage 4. At this point, the child, like the parents, comes to see the disease as something from which he or she will probably not recover. While the world is becoming increasingly closed to these children, they are still very much concerned about maintaining contact. The child is keenly aware of people's exits and entrances. And perhaps that is why the death of a peer can have the impact that it does. It is as if in a matter of sentences the child assimilates a great deal of information and comes to the conclusion that he or she is dying. For example, a nurse had come into Tom's room while he was sleeping to check his IV. On hearing her by his bed, Tom spoke.

TOM: Jennifer died last night. I have the same thing, don't I?

NURSE: But they are going to give you different medicines.

TOM: What happens when they run out?

NURSE: Well maybe they will find more before then.

This kind of conversation, of which I will give several examples, I refer to as a *disclosure of awareness conversation*. The conversation follows the same format regardless of what the other person in the interaction might say. The child begins by mentioning someone who has died or is in danger of dying. He or she then attempts to establish the cause of death either through a statement or a hypothesis. Finally, the child compares himself or herself to the deceased. For example:

SCOTT: You know Lisa?

MYRA: [Nods.]

SCOTT: The one I played ball with. [Pause.] How did she die?

MYRA: She was sick, sicker than you are now.

SCOTT: I know that. What happened?

MYRA: Her heart stopped beating.

SCOTT [Hugging and crying]: I hope that never happens to me, but . . .

If the children recently discovered their prognosis, they talked about how different their condition was from that of the deceased, as in this conversation between a child I will call Benjamin and myself.

BENJAMIN: Dr. Richards told me to ask you what happened to Sylvia. [Dr. Richards had said no such thing.]

MYRA: What do you think happened to Sylvia?

BENJAMIN: Well, she didn't go to another hospital. Home?

MYRA: No. She was sick, sicker than you are now, and she died.

BENJAMIN: She had nosebleeds. I had nosebleeds, but mine stopped.

Benjamin repeated this conversation with everyone he saw that day.

A more abstract version of a disclosure conversation occurred between a child I will call Stuart and myself after Stuart had been visited by a woman whose child had died 6 months earlier.

STUART: Do you drive to the hospital?

MYRA: No, I walk.

STUART: Do you walk at night?

MYRA [Noting the look on his face]: You wouldn't?

STUART: No, you would get shot. [Silence.] An ambulance would come and take you to the funeral home. And they would drain the blood out of you and wait 3 days and bury you.

MYRA: That's what happens when you die?

STUART: I saw them do it to my grandmother.

MYRA: I thought you told me you were here [in the hospital] when your grandmother died? [He was.]

STUART [Quickly]: It was my grandmother. They wait 3 days to see if you're alive. I mean, they draw the blood after they wait 3 days. [*Note*: the child had been in the hospital 3 days. They had drawn blood, done a bone marrow, and told the parents that things were not good, but that they would try one more experimental drug.] That's what happens when you die. I'm going to get a new medicine put in me tonight.

If the child had known the prognosis for some time, he or she would talk about how much he or she was like the deceased, as in this conversation between a child I will call Mary, her mother, and an occupational therapy student when they were packing to go home.

OTS: What should I do with these, Mary? [Holding up the paper dolls that Mary, on an earlier occasion, said looked the way she did before she became ill.]

MARY [Who hadn't said anything the entire time that they were packing to go home]: Put them in their grave in the Kleenex box.

MOTHER: Well that's the first thing you offered to do since the doctors said that we could go home.

MARY: I'm burying them. [Carefully arranges them between sheets of Kleenex.]

There were many children who did not engage in such full-blown disclosure of awareness conversations, but they made their awareness known in other ways. One way was through simple declarative statements like "I'm not going to be here for your birthday," "I'm never going back to school again," or "They're not buying me a coat to grow into this winter." Interestingly, these statements accomplish the same things as the longer conversation. To say, for example, "I'm not getting a coat to grow into," or "I'm never going back to school," is to say, "I'm not like other children. When you are dead or you die, you don't go to school, and people don't buy you coats to grow into."

These statements are a telegraphic form of the disclosure of awareness conversations. There is a mention of death, but it is one's own. The death is implied rather than stated. The comparison this time is not to other deceased children, but rather to one's self, to the world of healthy children.

In the examples I have given, you may have noticed a lack of references to heaven. Very few of the children mentioned heaven when they spoke to me. That does not mean that heaven was not a part of their world. It just was not part of the world as they communicated it to me. I guess I don't bring out the heaven in people. Perhaps that is the clergy's job. But whatever it was, heaven did not come through in their discussions with me. This raises some important methodological issues. For example, while the responses we receive from children reflect their views of death, they also reflect their views of the interviewer. When I spoke with the children they tended not to take death further than the grave. Grave imagery was far more prevalent than heaven imagery. Their view of death was expressed in terms of what they would miss here on earth.

It is also important to note the context in which the disclosure of awareness conversations arose. The conversations always seemed to come up when one least expected them, when one was least prepared—passing by a child's room on the way to do something else, for example.

A quality of "out of nowhere" was characteristic of many of the statements the children made with regard to death—not only their more direct serious statements, but also those tinged with gallows humor. For example, one child on waking from a nap said, "Fooled you, I'm not dead yet." Another child, when asked if he could be made more comfortable because he had IVs going in both arms, said, "No, I'm practicing for my coffin."

In general, death and disease imagery increased as other topics decreased. The children spoke far less about the efficacy of various drugs in the end stages of life than they did in the early part of the disease when remissions were achieved. Notably absent from these children's conversations was any long-range future orientation. They did not talk about what they were going to be when they grew up, and they became angry when other people did. The furthest into the future that they would seem to go was the next holiday or event.

While the children's long-range future orientation diminished, they were still very much concerned about the amount of time that they had left. Staff often remarked on the activity and urgency that so often followed the death of a patient. Some children verbalized it on those days with statements like, "Don't waste time," or "I can't waste time." These children were having their time cut short and they knew it.

There was also a general lack of interest in typical childhood paraphernalia. Often what interest there was (when they were not too debilitated to pay attention) was filled with death and disease imagery. As one play therapist remarked, "Give 'em crayon, draws graves." One of the most popular books was *Charlotte's Web*, especially the chapter where Charlotte dies. Children buried toys in graves and often refused to play with toys from other diseased children. Among many of the children it was as if a taboo had developed around the names of diseased children and their belongings.

Perhaps what was most remarkable in all of these children was an overall shift in behavior from strategies that we would view as engaging people to strategies that we would view as disengaging people. There were frequent displays of anger, banal chit-chat, withdrawal. Children and adults said that these kinds of behaviors came about when things became unbearable. They provided individuals with an excuse for leaving and thereby a way of returning.

MYRA: Jeffrey, why do you always yell at your mother?

JEFFREY: Then she won't miss me when I'm gone.

MYRA [To Jeffrey's mother]: Why does Jeffrey always yell at you?

MOTHER: Look, Myra, he knows when I can't take it anymore in that room, and he knows that if he yells, I'll leave. He also knows I'll come back.

It was as if these disengaging or distancing behaviors were almost a kind of rehearsal for the final separation. As the people at St. Christopher's Hospice in London say, "Withdrawal is not necessarily a hostile act."

The behaviors that children display in the fifth stage reflect a variety of views of death. Imbedded in each of the aforementioned actions and statements are views of death as separation, mutilation, loss of identity, the result of a biological process that is inevitable and irreversible. Death comes across as many things, even contradictory things at once. For example, one 5-year-old concerned about separation who talked about worms eating him and refused to play with toys from deceased children was the same 5-year-old who knew that the drugs had run out and demanded that time not be wasted. So too, the 9-year-old girl who drew pictures of herself on blood red crosses knew that it was the medication that was making her liver bad. She was the same 9-year-old who could not bear to have her mother leave her for a moment and carefully avoided the names of the deceased children and their belongings.

I mention and underscore these seeming contradictions because they raise important questions about the development of children's views of death. In each of these cases, we find views of death that one would expect for children their age as well as ones we would not. I regret that time does not permit me to develop this point. So let me just give you an idea to reflect on later. When a child is dying, his or her experiences are very different from other children of the same age, and hence the accepted developmental model of children's view of death is not as applicable for the dying child as it would be for healthy children. Let us turn now from the world of the dying child to the world of the well sibling.

WELL SIBLINGS

The well siblings of terminally ill children live in houses of chronic sorrow. The signs of sorrow, illness, and death are everywhere, whether or not they are spoken of. The signs are written on parent's faces: "My mother always looks tired now," and "Even my dad's crying a lot." The signs are there in hushed conversations: "You learn everything by listening in on the [phone] extension." The signs of illness and death are there in the time the parents do not have to share with the well sibling: "My mom used to come watch me play ball;

she doesn't anymore." The sorrow comes through in outbursts of anger, short tempers and irritability: "My parents fight all the time now, one minute she's [child's mother] all lovey-dovey and the next minute, whammo, do this, do that." Illness makes for interrupted schedules. As one child said, "Who can plan?" Plans must often be changed. On hearing that the family wouldn't be going on a camping trip as planned, the younger brother of a terminally ill child said, "So what else is new?" And sometimes life-styles are changed. Many researchers have reported the financial strain that chronic illness places on a family budget. Some have listed financial strain among the top three sources of stress. For the well siblings, there is often less contact with peers: "I can't have my friends over because they may have a cold and give it to my brother." Finally, the signs of illness, of death and sorrow are there on their ill brother's or sister's face: "He can't do much now on account of his low platelets," "She just lies there now with the oxygen in her nose," and "Why is it she even looks dead now?" These children are living in a situation quite unlike their peers', quite unlike the situation that most adults find themselves in.

What happens to the well siblings in this situation? Many experience a change in their role in the family, a change in status. During hospitalizations, the well siblings often are shifted from place to place, from a relative's house to a neighbor's house, to home again for an evening. Some well siblings see themselves as the less favored child in the family. Often the well sibling parents the parent: "I must take care of Mommy now." In some families, the well sibling is the caretaker of the ill sibling, baby-sitting or helping with the therapy or equipment. Some become what Goffman (1) calls "nonpersons." They are there, but they are not there. They overhear conversations, but are not part of them. The well sibling may accompany the child to the clinic or to the hospital, but is not present during the examinations.

When a brother or sister is dying, the well siblings often find themselves not getting what one usually expects from one's parents, what they themselves once received from their parents. The well siblings experience difficulty receiving the kind of care, attention, support and nurturing that they once knew: "Nobody has time for me right now. I must always wait." But when a sibling is dying, a parent's attention is elsewhere. The well children often feel alone, unsupported, neglected; or the flip side, overprotected. As one boy said to me, "I can't turn around without her on me. Where are you going? What are you doing? When will you be back? Who is going with you?"

Well siblings often feel confused. They are confused about the information that they are receiving about their sibling's status. They receive information from a variety of sources—the ill brother or sister, the parent, their own observations. Some of the information is correct, some incorrect. Often the information is incomplete. The well sibling's knowledge of the disease may be limited to what he or she was told when the ill sibling was diagnosed, a time when the child was young and, hence, told very little. Because of the parents' reluctance to speak about the ill child's condition as the disease progressed, the well sibling's information might not have been updated.

Well siblings also feel confused about the shifts in their parents' emotions. Some well siblings feel confused about who they are and who they are supposed to be. Sometimes they feel like they should be sometimes like the dying child, sometimes like a parent, and sometimes, as one boy said, "just blend into the woodwork."

It is not unusual to hear well siblings express feelings of betrayal, that their parents were not honest with them: "I wish they'd tell me the truth. I can take it."

It is important to point out, however, that not all children feel betrayed. Many of the children said that they did not want to know, at least not from their parents, how really ill their brother or sister was. They feel it would be too hard to hear it from their parents.

Well siblings often feel rejected. Several saw their parent's preoccupation with the ill sibling as a rejection of them: "Nobody cares about me and my needs anymore," or

The gifts don't make up for the hurts and other things inside of me. It doesn't make anything, you know. You may smile on the outside, but on the inside, it hurts. It doesn't take care of the pain or anything.

The feelings and the experiences that I have just described exist not because parents do not want to do what is right for their well children, but because often they can't. The demands, physically, emotionally, not to mention financially, of caring for a terminally ill child—be it at home or in the hospital—are great. The demands are most keenly felt around the area of attention, which to children is the hallmark of love. Parents spoke of wanting to give the well siblings more attention, but not being able to. Well siblings spoke of wanting more attention, of not getting enough, but also knowing why they could not have more attention. The well siblings and the parents are in a bind: "It's tough when she gets extra attention, but she has to get extra attention so that she'll live," "My mother tries to make up the attention she gives him, but she can't make up for it all," or "Dad treats him better because he doesn't have much of a life. He's going to die. But what about me? You know, I could get hit by a car or something."

It's important to bear in mind for the well siblings of children suffering from chronic and terminal illness the feelings of betrayal, of anger, of rejection, and of lack of attention were not necessarily there throughout the course of the illness. My recent research with families of children with cystic fibrosis (2, 3) shows that for long periods of time, these families appear very much like other families. They are not homes of chronic sorrow. The feelings that are there in the terminal stages are not necessarily there in the earlier stages of the disease. And when they are, they are either muted or expressed quite directly. For example, I recall walking into the clinic waiting room and seeing the two well brothers of a CF patient, who was doing rather well, telling their mother that they were hungry and asking her if she would either take them to get something to eat or let them go on their own. The mother asked them to wait until Zöe, their sister, had been examined. The brothers replied, almost in chorus, "If Zöe wanted something to eat, you'd go get it for her right away."

In the final stages of the disease, though, the siblings feel less justified in making some of these same demands. For example, when one mother asked her son, "You feel like you want more, most of the attention?" he responded, "No, I don't want most of the attention. I know Ellen has CF, and she needs most of the attention." Nonetheless, he demonstrated his desire for attention in other ways. Like many well brothers of cystic fibrosis patients, he put on a great deal of weight and he was behind in his school work.

That the majority of parents are able to give their children, well and ill, so much of what they needed for so long, up until the terminal period, is due in large measure to the strategies that these families adopt to contain the intrusion that such a disease makes into their lives. While time does not permit a discussion of these strategies, suffice it to say, that these were strategies for dealing with a chronic illness and they were no longer used, no longer could be used, once the child's condition became terminal.

Returning to the terminal period, but shifting from the well sibling's relation to the parents to the well sibling's relationship with the ill brother or sister, we notice that the well brother also has difficulty getting what he once did from his ill brother or sister. Throughout the course of the illness, siblings struggle to maintain themselves in a relationship of give and take. As the disease progresses, as the child's physical condition deteriorates and hospitalizations become more frequent, elements of the sibling relationship (companionship, mutual aid, support, self-definition, communication) become problematic. During hospitalization, the well sibling is often left without a companion. Contact is neither regular nor in a familial context. Mutual aid declines. Siblings often find that they cannot give reciprocally to one another. Ill siblings often refuse gestures of help from their well siblings. For example, while Jake lay dying, complaining of his back hurting him and not being able to breathe, his brothers offered to rub his back. He pushed them away saying, "No, no, not you. Only Mommy now." The ill child's alliances shift from a closeness to both the parent and the sibling to a closeness with the parent divorced from that of the sibling.

Using the sibling as a means of self-definition also becomes problematic. One's sibling is like a mirror image, but what a distorted image stares back. Feelings of protection and worry replace those of identification.

LENNY: I think about her all the time.

MYRA: Even in school?

LENNY: [Nods.]

MYRA: What do you do in school?

LENNY: I just think about her.

Communication is often distorted as particular subjects are avoided: "We talk about everything except the CF," or "I don't want to talk about her CF because it might upset her."

Ironically, however, if once the siblings know the prognosis they do not begin to talk to each other, a distance is created in the relationship that can last until the patient's death: "We [my ill brother and I] weren't that close. We didn't talk. But my sister, she talked to him a lot. That made them very close." Now add to all the well sibling's feelings the normal feelings of jealousy, rivalry, hostility that are there in any sibling relationship, feelings that have been heightened by the disease, and add for good measure the feelings of guilt that come from seeing and acknowledging that one's peer—one's brother or sister—is dying, and the behaviors seen in well siblings become far more understandable. The well sibling is struggling with thoughts and fears that are not so easily managed, and often he or she struggles alone. The conflicting thoughts and feelings are well expressed in the following interchange among a therapist, a well child named Karen, whose sister, Linda, has cystic fibrosis and whose brother, Chip, died of cystic fibrosis, and their mother.

KAREN [Who is at this point in the discussion, crying]: I remember I used to like running around, and Chip would say, you know, "You quit running," and complain about what I was doing and stuff.

THERAPIST: It was hard for you to do normal things because they would bother Chip, is that right? Did you feel like a bad person for doing that?

KAREN: [Nods.]

THERAPIST: Do you still feel like maybe you hurt Chip? Does that still make you feel bad?

KAREN: [Nods.]

THERAPIST: Have you ever said that before, Karen?

KAREN: No. I worry about Linda because I don't want her to die. Because, you know, she's almost my best friend and she'll play with me.

THERAPIST: She's your best friend?

KAREN: Uh-huh. And sometimes she won't play with me 'cause she doesn't feel good and I get sad and stuff, you know.

MOTHER: Karen, you know Chip had those bad, bad headaches because he wasn't getting the oxygen that he was supposed to be getting. And really your running around had nothing to do with his headaches. It was just his lungs were so bad.

KAREN [Almost inaudibly]: I know that, but I still think it's my fault.

Ultimately, then, these children must face the death of their brothers and sisters. Their first words, on hearing of that death, often provide us with important clues as to what these children are thinking and feeling. In some cases, they may be the only clue that we get for a long time. It is not unusual to hear something like, "Good, now I can have all of his toys." Or in the words of another child, "I wanted my own room anyway."

If we step back for a moment and unpack those statements, I think we will hear some other things in their somewhat shocking remarks. We hear anger, "You left me." We also hear jealousy, "You had more than I did." And like so many adults arguing over the deceased's possessions, we also hear a desire to hold onto something. There are also the sounds of pain and loss. As one child who no longer played with the toys that he eagerly took at his brother's death put it, "I don't want them [toys] without John here. It's no fun." There are heightened feelings of loneliness. Siblings will often talk about how quiet the house has become since their brother or sister died.

Running through their statements is a great deal of ambivalence, ambivalence that was there throughout the entire relationship and throughout the entire illness. These ambivalent feelings are coupled with feelings of guilt. As one brother put it, "I'm glad it was him and not me. I know that's not nice, but I can't help it." Or in the words of another, "Do you think I'm cold-blooded? I couldn't stand him that way, just lying there with oxygen in his nose yelling, 'Rub me, rub me.'" Some siblings feel responsible: "I gave her that pneumonia."

It is important to bear in mind that many of the children felt that they could not express their feelings to their parents, that their parents were already too upset, and they did not want to upset them anymore. This is not to say that the well siblings' feelings do not come out in other ways.

John Gilenski, psychologist and priest at Oakland Children's Hospital, has found that the two most common ways the children exhibit their feelings are through sleep disorders and acting out (personal communication). He also has found that many children also engage in little adult behaviors. Other behaviors that have been reported for well siblings include: acting like the deceased, experiencing psychosomatic illnesses, fearing illness, fearing losing control, regressing, being unable to separate, refusing to mention the deceased, losing appetite or overeating, bed-wetting, and feeling depressed. I mention these behaviors not because they are going to happen (the frequency and prevalence of these phenomena are not known), but because they are things that serve to put us on warning, things that we should be looking at, that we may want to watch for in bereaved siblings.

In conclusion, how can we help the dying child and his or her siblings? What can we do? I think the most important thing we can do is to take our cues from the child, to tell the child what he or she wants to know, on his or her terms. The issue is not whether to tell, but rather when to tell, why you are telling, and who should do the telling.

I am reminded of that famous sex education story, which you probably know. After a hard day at school, Johnny sits down at the kitchen table to enjoy a glass of milk with his mom. Munching on a cookie, Johnny asks, "Where did I come from?" Mom opens her eyes real wide, takes a good strong, stiff drink of milk, and begins a lecture on the facts of life. Johnny eats a few more cookies, swallows the last of his milk, and comments, "Oh. Stevie said he came from New York."

The child has different needs, different concerns, at different times. The challenge before us is to recognize these different needs, these different concerns, at the time he brings them to us.

References

1. Goffman, E. (1959). *The presentation of self in everyday life.* Garden City, New York: Anchor, Doubleday.

2. Bluebond-Langner, M. (1978). *The private worlds of dying children.* Princeton: Princeton University.

3. Bluebond-Langner, M. (1985). Living with cystic fibrosis: A family affair. In D. Schidlow (Ed.), *Cystic fibrosis: Soma and psyche.* New Jersey: McNeil Laboratories.

25 Children Traumatized by
Witnessing Acts of Personal
Violence: Homicide, Rape, or
Suicide Behavior

Robert S. Pynoos

ROBERT PYNOOS is associate professor in the Department of Psychiatry and
Biobehavioral Sciences at the UCLA School of Medicine. He is also director
of the Program on Trauma, Violence, and Sudden Bereavement at the
UCLA Neuropsychiatric Institute. In this article, Pynoos discusses the traumatic psychological impact on children of witnessing extreme acts of violence such as homicide, rape, or the suicide of a parent. Pynoos argues that
there has been a substantial increase in exposure to such violence over the last
20 years, and he discusses some of the unique features and consequences of
children witnessing such dire events.

CHILDREN WHO WITNESS EXTREME ACTS OF VIOLENCE represent a population at
significant risk of developing anxiety, depressive, phobic, conduct, and post-
traumatic stress disorders, and are in need of both clinical and research attention. Our focus in this chapter is on the traumatic consequences for the child
witness to any of three types of violence likely to have great personal impact on
a child: the murder of a parent, the rape of a mother, and the suicidal act of a
parent. The violent injury or death of a parent, in itself, imposes a severe stress
on the child and serves as a psychic organizer profoundly altering the child's
view of the world. We have found that the added burden of actually witnessing
a portion of such an event will frequently produce an acute post-traumatic
stress disorder in the child.

We will first review background data describing the extent of childhood
exposure to violent acts in the United States, and discuss the psychological
stresses on the child witness. We will then summarize our clinical observations
of the children's responses: the immediate effect of the violence on the children,

the early efforts at mastery, the resultant symptomatology or behavior, the issue of accountability, the influence of mediating factors on recovery, and the potential long-term consequences of the trauma.

Freud (1918) offered one of the first theories of psychic trauma. In doing so, he specifically called attention to the child witness. From adult retrospective reporting and reconstruction of childhood experiences, he argued that young children, in observing parental intercourse, may experience a traumatic situation. The child assumes this is an act of violence, and feels helpless in the face of the danger to the mother. Because of the parents' lack of concern, Freud suggested, younger children are more likely to be exposed, and cannot escape the passive viewing.

The recent studies of psychic trauma in children have centered on those children who were victims of physical and sexual abuse or kidnapping. Terr (1983) and Green (1983) suggest that such direct victims of violence can suffer long-lasting ill effects. The conditions of these traumatized children resemble the post-traumatic stress disorder (PTSD) described in the third edition of the *Diagnostic and Statistical Manual of Mental Disorders (DSM-III)*, American Psychiatric Association (1980), as validated by Horowitz et al. (1980) for traumatized adults; although Terr (1979) first reported differences in the childhood presentation that may require revised criteria. Nearly 80 percent of the over 100 uninjured child witnesses we studied also exhibited a characteristic pattern of PTSD.

Child witnesses to a parent's homicide, rape, or suicidal behavior demonstrate symptomatology fulfilling the four major *DSM-III* criteria for PTSD:

1. The perceived presence of a distressing, traumatic event; children will often describe it as so upsetting as never to be forgotten.
2. The reexperiencing of the occurrence; in young children this frequently takes the form of traumatic play and dreams, as well as intrusive images or sounds.
3. Psychic numbing or affective constriction; children may exhibit subdued or mute behavior, on commonly adopt an unemotional or third-person, nearly journalistic attitude toward the event.
4. Incident-specific phenomena that were previously not present; children are as likely as adults to suffer from startle reactions and avoidant behavior linked to trauma-specific reminders, and they may be especially susceptible to sleep disturbances (Frederick 1983). In addition, developmental factors affect the clinical picture and course of recovery, influencing the child's capacity to cope with the distress and to contend with traumatic anxiety (Eth and Pynoos 1984).

As recognized with adults, post-traumatic stress disorders are apparently more severe and longer lasting when a stressor is of "human design" (American Psychiatric Association 1980), especially in cases of human-induced violence (Frederick 1980). The PTSD symptoms in these child witnesses are likely to persist, and the children will benefit from prompt psychiatric assistance. We think our work with this group of children is of special importance because the psychological needs of the child witness are commonly neglected by the family, school, law enforcement agencies, and mental health profession.

EXPOSURE TO VIOLENCE

Within the past 20 years, the rate of violent crime in the United States has increased dramatically in relationship to other Western countries, reaching what may be deemed "an epidemic of violence" (West 1984). As of 1980, the reported number of homicides per year was 23,967 (Centers for Disease Control 1984), and the number of reported aggravated assaults exceeded 265,000. Of the homicides, approximately 40 percent were the result of domestic violence, and the vast majority of the victims were in the 20–39, child-rearing age group. The Sheriff's Homicide Division of Los Angeles County estimates that dependent children witness between 10 to 20 percent of the approximately 2,000 annual homicides in their jurisdiction. If a similar exposure rate applies to other urban areas, then several thousand children per year witness a murder, and, commonly, the victim is one of their parents.

Recent population surveys have drawn attention to the previously unappreciated extent of domestic violence in our society (Straus et al. 1980). Spouse beating and child abuse not only account for the largest number of direct victims, they also result in an even larger number of child witnesses (Pfouts et al. 1982). Early efforts to account for the intergenerational transmission of spouse beating and child abuse had focused primarily on childhood victims becoming adult perpetrators. However, the most comprehensive epidemiologic survey of marital aggression within a large sample of a general population (Kalmuss 1984) indicates that childhood witnessing of domestic violence is in fact the most significant predictor. The findings also suggest intergenerational transmission is role-specific rather than sex-specific. Kalmuss concludes that: "Observing one's father hitting one's mother increases the likelihood that sons will be victims as well as perpetrators, and that daughters will be perpetrators as well as victims of severe marital aggression" (p. 17).

In an examination of homicidally aggressive young children, Lewis et al. (1983, 151) found that the most significant factor contributing to violence is "to have a father who behaves violently, often homicidally." They also note that some of these children also appear at an increased risk of suicidal behavior. Although they specifically mention the importance of being a witness, unfortunately they do not designate which of the evaluated children fall into this category. However, they did conclude that "witnessing and being a victim of irrational violence engenders a kind of rage and frustration that, when directed inward, expresses itself as suicidal behavior. When directed outward and displaced from the father, it manifests itself as homicidal aggression" (p. 152).

In 1980, there were over 77,000 reported rapes outside of marriage in the United States (Centers for Disease Control 1984). In contrast to homicide, rape is seriously underreported. Recent household surveys indicate that, at a minimum, there is a 10:1 ratio of unreported to reported rapes, with an estimated actual annual incidence of approximately 800,000 rapes. As in cases of homicide, 40 percent of all rape victims are in the 20 to 39-year-old, child-bearing age group, and over 40 percent of all rapes occur in the home. If, estimating *conservatively*, a child is in the home when a rape occurs in one out of five instances, then as many as 25,000 children are exposed to this form of violence each year. In Los Angeles County alone, Sgt. Beth Dickerson (Chair, California Association of Sexual Assault Investigators) estimates that children are in the home when a rape occurs as much as 50 percent of the time and that the child (or children) directly view the assault in approximately 10 percent of the cases reported to the Sheriff's office.

In addition to rape outside of marriage, Russell (1982) has recently concluded, from a survey of households, that 14 percent of all married women in the United States report experiencing marital rape at least once in their lifetimes. Further, she found that in 11 percent of the cases in her survey one or more of the woman's children knew about or witnessed the attack(s). Given the high incidence of children present during the sexual assault of their mothers, the literature on rape and rape treatment is surprisingly silent on the subject (Silverman 1978; Burgess and Holmstrom 1979; Crenshaw 1979).

Suicide and suicidal behavior are also violent acts, and present a major source of childhood exposure to violence. There is evidence of an epidemic increase in the prevalence of suicide attempts in the United States as well as in other Western countries during the past two decades, though the rate of completed suicide has remained stationary (Weissman 1974). As with homicide and rape, the epidemiologic characteristics of attemptors put young children at a particularly high risk of exposure to the violent behavior. In 1980, there were 27,000 reported completed suicides in the United States (Centers for Disease Control 1984). Using the most conservative ratio of 8:1 attempts to completions, the Centers for Disease Control estimates that there were, at least, 216,000 attempts. Of these, 120,000 occurred in the 20 to 39-year-old age group, and accounted for 24,000 reported hospitalizations for suicide behavior. As Weissman concludes in her review of the epidemiology of suicide attempts, the annual incidence rates as derived from known studies suggest a far greater ratio of attempts to completed suicides than the 8:1 ratio projected in earlier studies. Indeed, in a 1964 door-to-door survey in the city of Los Angeles, Mintz concluded that 75,000 Los Angeles residents (or 3.9 percent of the city's population) had a history of attempted suicide. He, therefore, estimated there were 5,000,000 suicide attemptors in the United States at that time.

Older studies implied that suicide attempts were made by single individuals with no dependent children. More recent evidence reveals a notable increase in married women among the attemptors (Aitkins et al. 1969), and indicates that having children does not serve as a deterrent, as once believed (Kozak and Gibbs 1979). Weissman (1974) notes studies using general population comparisons now show a statistical excess of separated or divorced persons of both sexes among the attemptors. As she concludes, their high number is "consistent with clinical observations that attempts take place in the context of interpersonal disorganization and a breakdown of personal resources" (p. 740).

Given the increase in parental suicide behavior, the likelihood of a child witnessing this form of violence has, itself, probably increased dramatically in the past two decades, so that many thousands of children each year are directly or indirectly exposed to the suicide behavior of a parent. It is surprising, then, how little attention is made of this fact in the current discussion of the increasing rate of suicidal ideation and behavior in childhood. Those studies of childhood suicide behavior that do mention this risk factor (Shaffer and Fisher 1981; Pfeffer et al. 1983) do not, in particular, address the child witness. Nor do Cain and Fast (1972) discuss any specific consequences for the child witness in their classic report on the long-term effects on children when a parent commits suicide.

In summary, there is ample epidemiologic evidence to suggest that each year many thousands of children in the United States witness extreme acts of violence involving at least one of their parents.

THE TRAUMA OF THE CHILD WITNESS

Psychic trauma occurs when an individual is exposed to an overwhelming event and is rendered helpless in the face of intolerable danger, anxiety, or instinctual arousal. Freud (1926, 168) noted that, in a traumatic situation, "external and internal, real and instinctual dangers converge." There are a number of unique features that define traumatic witnessing and distinguish it from the trauma of direct victimization.

The helplessness of the child witness is determined by the passivity imposed by having to watch or listen to the sights and sounds surrounding the violence and the physical mutilation it creates. The uninjured child witness is unprotected from the full emotional impact of the violence, and may suffer immediately all of the painful symptoms of a post-traumatic stress disorder. In contrast, the injured child victim may immediately become self-absorbed with the pain or internally perceived impact of the physical damage. From that moment on, the child's set of memories may be much more involved with internal sensations; and the child's first preoccupation may focus on physical recovery. The different experiences of the uninjured and injured child participant may significantly influence the subsequent symptomatic constellations and their time course. This distinction may help to explain the vulnerability of the direct victim to the later development of dissociative symptoms and even multiple personality disorders (Putnam 1984), in contrast to the absence of such subsequent psychopathology in uninjured child witnesses.

Child witnesses do not display traumatic amnesia or disavowal. None of the children we interviewed indicated having felt any disbelief about the reality of what they witnessed. Instead, they seem similar to adult viewers of Lazarus et al.'s study (1965) who, knowing they were watching a real injurious accident, were unprotected from the full emotional impact of and physiological response to watching the event, in contrast to the controls, who were told it was staged or an intellectual exercise.

The perceived danger to the child witness does not depend on fear of self-harm, but on the personal meaning of the threat of the victim's injury or loss. The greater the personal impact on the child, the greater the likelihood a traumatic state will occur. Therefore, it is not surprising that child witnesses to parental homicide, rape, or suicidal behavior all report feeling emotionally overwhelmed by the danger to their parent.

Certainly, all of these children describe having had an enormously intense perceptual, affective, and physiological experience. Two major examples of persistent physiological changes are the high frequency of sleep disturbances, including night terrors and somnambulism, and startle reactions to specific perceptual traumatic reminders. Experimental evidence indicates that, in adults, unwelcome intrusive imagery and autonomic physiological reactions can persist after watching a disturbing event (Horowitz 1970; Kolb and Mutalipassi 1982). Our experience would suggest that these phenomena are common in children as well.

The intrusive imagery and associated affect may markedly interfere with the child's capacity to learn. As one child described, "I hear everything at school, and then it's gone because what I saw happen to my Mommy comes right back to me." Gardner (1971) has previously reported that the experience of violence can chronically diminish precise learning in children.

We have found four common psychological methods employed by children for limiting traumatic anxiety in the immediate weeks or months after an occurrence. By using *denial-in-fantasy* the child tries to mitigate painful reality by imaginatively reversing the outcome. By the *inhibition of spontaneous thought* the child works to avoid reminders of the event. In *fixation to the trauma*, evidenced by incomplete, usually unemotional, journalistic recountings of the event the child hopes to make the event more tolerable by means of reiteration. Finally, by becoming preoccupied with *fantasies of future harm* the child avoids directly addressing the actual trauma by supplanting the memories of the event with new fears. These strategies of emotional coping may persist or remit, only to reappear with traumatic reminders.

The child witness may be mentally involved with continued cognitive reappraisals of the action of all participants and witnesses. To offset his or her traumatic helplessness, the child must consider, if only in fantasy, alternate actions that could have prevented the occurrence, interrupted the violence before harm was done, reversed the physical harm, or gained safe retaliation. Developmental considerations are important determinants of these cognitive efforts (Eth and Pynoos 1984); and subsequent developmental maturity may bring about revisions.

Child witnesses differ from victims in their set of observations. They can monitor simultaneously the assailant, the victim, others at the scene, and their own activity as well. As a result, they may, more easily than victims, identify with or imagine themselves directly involved in the event in any of three roles: the assailant committing the violence, the victim being harmed, and a third person intervening. Important predisposing factors may be in operation. Specific psychodynamic issues may be especially at work. The choice may be influenced by being of the same sex as the parent-victim or assailant. On the other hand, for example, being seen as a special child of one parent may prove the more determining factor. Even in the initial interview, there may be evidence of the child's early identification; the particular choice may appear to be fixed or fluid, conflicted or readily adopted.

Inner plans of action (Lifton 1979) are most likely whenever activity has appeared ineffectual in a catastrophic situation (Lazarus 1966). What is remarkable about the inner plans of action of the child witness is the dominance of fantasies of third-party intervention, either directly by the child or by another person. As a result of the child's fantasies of effective third-party intervention, the child may identify with the actions of the police, paramedics, or doctors to prevent violence or undo injuries, or with the judge, lawyers, and jailers to mete out punishment and revenge. The child may then develop new career interests that may entail a life of continued efforts to intervene successfully.

The descriptive account of post-traumatic stress disorders in *DSM-III* suggests that a more prolonged course can be expected if the stressor is of human design. As we have observed, struggles over assigning human accountability may add considerably to the child's traumatic burden after witnessing an extreme act of violence. Blame may be easy to assign, as in the case of a stranger assailant, or cause an intense conflict of loyalty, if a parent is to be held at fault. Intervention fantasies may also serve as a continuing source of self-blame for not having done more or of having been a coward. For the child witness, therefore, post-traumatic guilt is connected to imagined failures to intervene.

The fact of the violent occurrence, in itself, challenges the child's trust in adult restraint. Furthermore, it may prompt fantasies of revenge or an identification with the aggressor that can seriously jeopardize the child's confidence in his or her own impulse control. Uncharacteristic aggressive, reckless, or self-destructive behavior or prominent inhibitions may suddenly appear. Unconscious reenactment behavior may also endanger the child and others because it, too, may involve some repetition of violence.

Adult experimental studies (Feshbach 1955) have suggested that conscious aggressive fantasy expression after an insult, in contrast to nonexpression, reduces impulse tension and offers substitute goal satisfaction. However, the young child may need firm support to voice these frighteningly violent revenge fantasies, and, in doing so, may need assurances of safety against fantasies of retaliation.

Furthermore, because these children are preoccupied with the danger to the parent and with the need for intervention, they may not entertain a realistic appraisal of their own personal jeopardy. They may afterwards ignore, leave unacknowledged, or suppress any fear they might have experienced for their own safety. If their sense of fear is not adequately restored, they may be vulnerable to trauma-related dangerous situations, perhaps because of an inability or unwillingness to recognize a situation that requires personal protection.

On the other hand, there is an excitement that attends being witness to violence and danger. Thrilling situations, as characterized by Balint (1959, 23), all entail placing oneself in a dangerous situation that arouses fear. One is hopeful or confident that "the fear can be tolerated and mastered, the danger will pass, and that one will be able to return unharmed to safety." Child witnesses may be drawn to thrill seeking as one way to reassure themselves of their capacity to tolerate the shock of the traumatic occurrence. The popularity of extremely violent horror movies in part attests to the younger generation's preoccupation with the thrill of witnessing violence.

Finally, it is important to note that homicide, rape, and suicide behavior are not the collective violent acts of war, gang fights, or civil unrest, during which a general threat of harm may be perceived to be present. They are, instead, the isolated acts of individuals prompted by private motivations. Viewing such an event can cause profound changes in the child's sense of the safety and security of future intimate human relationships. As Terr (1983) notes, this change in future orientation may be one of the most significant markers of childhood trauma.

CLINICAL OBSERVATIONS

In this section we discuss our clinical observations of children who have witnessed a homicide. . . . Four key factors govern the onset and course of the child's post-traumatic stress disorder. First, there is the phenomenology of PTSD, that is, those symptoms that unavoidably result from a traumatic state. Second, there are the child's early efforts to master the anxiety or avoid its renewal, including efforts to assure that the violence will not recur. Third, there are the many possible mediating influences that enhance or adversely affect trauma resolution. Fourth, there are the demands of trauma mastery, which may significantly influence current and future developmental tasks by hindering normal progression or prematurely propelling the child into more mature roles. . . .

Homicide

It is hard to imagine a more harrowing experience than that of a child witnessing the murder of a parent. To date, we have evaluated over 50 such child witnesses, divided about equally in age among preschoolers, school children, and adolescents. Several Los Angeles agencies have served as subject referral sources, including the Police and Sheriff's Department, the District Attorney's Office, the Victim–Witness Assistance Program, and Child Protective Services. The homicides were the results of prolonged and brutal beatings, bloody stabbings, and massively disfiguring gunshot wounds. The assailants were identified as the other parent (35 percent), a friend or other relative (30 percent), or a stranger (35 percent).

We were able to conduct our initial interviews with the children within weeks of the event, and to follow them throughout the course of the acute traumatic response and subsequent criminal proceedings. All the children were haunted by the horrifying loss of impulse control in the assailant, the mutilation of the victim, and the helplessness of the victim and witness.

At the core of the child witness's trauma is the continued intrusion of the central violent action when physical harm was inflicted: the final blow with a fist, the plunge of a knife, or the blast of a shotgun. The child endures an intense perceptual experience. All sensory modalities are involved: the sight, sound, and smell of gunfire; the screams or sudden silence of the victim; the splash of blood and tissue on the child's clothes; the grasp of a dying parent; and the eventual police sirens. In addition, the child is aware of autonomic arousal and other bodily sensations. One young boy lamented, "It was awful, my heart hurt; it was beating so loud." The child may have been sharply attentive to a last, intense verbal exchange. One 13-year-old boy was haunted by the memory of his mother yelling at her estranged husband, "Go ahead, shoot me, show the kids what a big man you are." Special details may be imbued with traumatic meaning. One teenage daughter was preoccupied with the thought that her mother was wearing one of the teenager's dresses, borrowed that morning. Worst moments are not easily forgotten, as, for instance, when a dying father used a special nickname to call out to his young daughter.

Intrusion of traumatic references to the homicide is nearly universally present in projective drawings or storytelling tasks done within weeks of the event; and, as has been described in case reports, these references also directly appear in the child's play (Schetky 1978; Pruett 1979). In one such case (Bergen 1958), a 4-year-old girl whose mother was knifed to death carefully painted her hands red and acted out a game of being stabbed with a paint brush. School-age children may involve their schoolmates in their retelling or trauma-related games. One 7-year-old girl, who witnessed her father strangle her mother and then carry the body to the bedroom, forced all her friends to play the Mommy Game: "In the Mommy Game, you play dead, and I pick you up."

In order to mitigate the pain of the reality of the event the child may alter the fatal outcome in fantasy, while simultaneously giving an accurate description of what occurred. This process is often most apparent in the child's projective storytelling or traumatic play. One 7-year-old girl gave a careful description of her stuntman father's fatal shooting, while simultaneously drawing and telling the story of a clown who is saved by the sudden appearance of a net after being maliciously made to fall from a high wire. In this case, as in most others, the fantasied reversal of the violent outcome depends on outside intervention, thus highlighting the witness role. Addressing such denial-in-fantasy and its underlying meaning provides an important way to assist the child to be more sure of his or her capacity to cope with the intense affect associated with the violent death.

In homicide, there is little escape for the child witness from having to assign human responsibility for the loss of life. Human accountability only adds to the child's anguish and difficulty in achieving trauma mastery. As one 12-year-old girl said, "I'm mad at the way she did go. Because that hurt. I just wanted her to die naturally, not die because someone shot her." . . .

In therapeutic consultation, many children express particular relief at drawing or acting out their fantasy of punishment or revenge. Afterwards, we have often observed an increase in the child's overall affective expression, and only in retrospect to discern that a constriction of affect had been present. However, the child needs help to distinguish these impulses from the murderous act of the assailant, since fear of these fantasies and impulses may possibly lead to unrecognized inhibitions in the child's life. One woman, who as a child witnessed her mother's murder, continues to fear becoming rich because she might use all her money to hire a "hit man" to assassinate the killer.

Any of the child's convictions about the safety of interpersonal relationships may be shattered. Children have described having afterwards envisioned the need to live alone in an impenetrable fortress when they grow up. Other children have stated that they would never marry for fear that a marital argument would once again be fatal.

Since the judicial proceedings adjudicate blame, there is a necessary link between judicial outcome and trauma resolution (Pynoos and Eth 1984). If, for example, an arrest is not made, the child may never achieve psychological closure. One seven-year-old boy saw his father stabbed by a stranger who was never apprehended. Years later, he continues to fear for his own life, carries a switch-blade, and seeks to avenge his father's murder.

A parent's murder precipitates an irreversible upheaval in the child's life. As

Barkas (1978) describes, family and friends undergo a prolonged period of suffering. During this interval, the surviving parent may be in a traumatized and grief-stricken state, and emotionally unavailable to aid the child. In parent-parent homicide, the child can lose both parents, one by death and the other by incarceration. The child may be uprooted to live with relatives and may have to change schools. They may not only have to contend with their own intensely ambivalent feelings toward the homicidal parent, but also the embittered and revengeful feelings of the deceased parent's family of origin. Even among the deceased parent's family members there may be an implicit prohibition against any reference to the violent death (Lister 1982). Finally, they must endure the rigors of the legal proceedings that follow a homicide (Pynoos and Eth 1984).

All these additional, externally imposed stresses hinder the child's recovery from the initial traumatic impact of the homicide. Yet, as one assists the child to feel more efficacious in addressing the traumatic event, an enhanced sense of competence in facing difficult, immediate life tasks may also be exhibited. One of the most important of these is grief work. . . .

References

Aitkins R, Buglass D, Kreitman NJ: The changing pattern of attempted suicide in Edinburgh, 1962–67. British Journal of Preventive Social Medicine 23:111–115, 1969

American Psychiatric Association: Diagnostic and Statistical Manual of Mental Disorders, 3rd ed. Washington, DC, American Psychiatric Association, 1980

Balint, M: Thrills and Regression. New York, International Universities Press, 1959

Barkas JL: Victims. London, Peel Press, 1978

Baudry R: The evolution of the concept of character in Freud's writings. J Am Psychoanal Assoc 31:3–32, 1983

Bencke T: Men on Rape. New York, St Martin's Press, 1982

Bergen M: Effect of severe trauma on a 4-year-old child. Psychoanal Study Child 13:407–429, 1958

Bowlby J: On knowing what you aren't supposed to know and feeling what you are not supposed to feel. Can J Psychiatry 24:403–408, 1979

Burgess AW, Holmstrom LL: Rape: Crisis and Recovery. Bowie, Md, Robert J Brady Co, 1979

Cain A, Fast I: Children's disturbed reactions to parent suicide: distortion and guilt, communication and identification, in Survivors of Suicide. Edited by Cain A. Springfield, Ill, Charles C Thomas, 1972

Centers for Disease Control: Violent crime: Summary of morbidity. Atlanta, Violence Epidemiology Branch, 1984

Crenshaw T: Counseling of family and friends, in Rape: Helping the Victim. Edited by Halpern S. Medical Economic Company, 1979

Eth S, Pynoos R: Children who witness the homicide of a parent. Paper presented at the annual meeting of the American Psychiatric Association, New York, May 1983

Eth S, Pynoos R: Developmental perspectives on psychic trauma in childhood, in Trauma and Its Wake. Edited by Figley CR. New York, Brunner/Mazel, 1984

Feshbach S: The drive-reducing function of fantasy behavior. Journal of Abnormal and Social Psychology 50:3–11, 1955

Frederick C: Effects of natural versus human-induced violence upon victims. Evaluation and Change, Special Issue: 71–75, 1980

Frederick C: Violence and disasters: immediate and long-term consequences, in Helping Victims of Violence. Edited by Ministry of Welfare and Cultural Affairs. The Hague, Government Publishing Office, 1983

Freud S: From the history of an infantile neurosis, in The Standard Edition of the Complete Psychological Works of Sigmund Freud, vol. 17. Edited by James Strachey. London, Hogarth Press, 1918

Freud S: Inhibitions, symptoms and anxiety, in The Standard Edition of the Complete Psychological Works of Sigmund Freud, vol 20. Edited by James Strachey. London, Hogarth Press, 1926

Freud S: Moses and monotheism, in The Standard Edition of the Complete Psychological Works of Sigmund Freud, vol 23. Edited by James Strachey. London, Hogarth Press, 1937

Gardner GR: Aggression and violence—the enemies of precision learning in children. Am J Psychiatry 128:445–450, 1971

Green A: Dimensions of psychological trauma in abused children. J Am Acad Child Psychiatry 22:231–237, 1983

Horowitz MJ: Image Formation and Cognition. New York, Appleton-Century-Crofts, 1970

Horowitz MJ, Wilner M, Kultreider N, et al: Signs and symptoms of post-traumatic stress disorder. Arch Gen Psychiatry 37:85–92, 1980

Kalmuss D: The intergenerational transmission of marital aggression. Journal of Marriage and the Family 46:11–19, 1984

Kolb L, Mutalipassi L: The conditioned emotional response: a subclass of the chronic and delayed post-traumatic stress disorder. Psychiatric Annals 12:979–987, 1982

Kozak CM, Gibbs J: Dependent children and the suicide of married parents. Suicide Life Threat Behav 9:67–75, 1979

Lazarus RS: Psychological Stress and the Coping Process. New York, McGraw-Hill, 1966

Lazarus RS, Opton EM Jr, Nomikos MS, et al: The principle of short-circuiting of threat: further evidence. J Pers 33:622–635, 1965

Lewis DO, Shanok SS, Grant M, et al: Homicidally aggressive young children: neuropsychiatric and experiential correlates. Am J Psychiatry 140:148–153, 1983

Lifton RJ: The Broken Connection. New York, Simon and Schuster, 1979

Lister ED: Forced silence: a neglected dimension of trauma. Am J Psychiatry 139:867–872, 1982

Mintz R: Prevalence of persons in the city of Los Angeles who have attempted suicide: a pilot study. Bulletin of Suicidology 7:9–16, 1970

Pfeffer C, Plutchik R, Mizruchi MS: Suicidal and assaultive behavior in children: classification, measurement, and interrelations. Am J Psychiatry 140: 154–157, 1983

Pfouts J, Schopler J, Henley HC: Forgotten victims of family violence. Social Work 27:367–368, 1982

Pruett KR: Home treatment for two infants who witnessed their mother's murder. J Am Acad Child Psychiatry 18:647–657, 1979

Putnam FW, Post RM, Guroff JJ, et al: One hundred cases of multiple personality disorder. Presented at the annual meeting of the American Psychiatric Association, Los Angeles, May 1984

Pynoos R, Eth S: The child as witness to homicide. Journal of Social Issues 40:269–290, 1984

Pynoos R, Eth S: Witness to violence: the child interview. J Am Acad Child Psychiatry (in press)

Pynoos R, Gilmore K, Shapiro T: Children's response to parental suicide behavior. Presented at the annual meeting of the American Academy of Child Psychiatry, Dallas, 1981

Russell D: Rape in Marriage. New York, Macmillan, 1982

Shaffer D, Fisher P: The epidemiology of suicide in children and young adolescents. J Am Acad Child Psychiatry 20:545–565, 1981

Shetky PH: Preschoolers' responses to murder of their mothers by their fathers: a study of four cases. Bull Am Acad Psychiatry Law 6:45–57, 1973

Silverman D: Sharing the crisis of rape: counseling the mates and family members of victims. Am J Orthopsychiatry 1:166–173, 1978

Strauss M, Gelles R, Steinmetz S: Behind Closed Doors: Violence in the American Family. New York, Anchor Books, 1980

Terr L: Children of Chowchilla: study of psychic trauma. Psychoanal Study Child 34:547–623, 1979

Terr L: Chowchilla revisited: the effects of psychic trauma four years after a school bus kidnapping. Am J Psychiatry 140:1543–1550, 1983

Weissman M: The epidemiology of suicide attempts. Arch Gen Psychiatry 30:737–746, 1974

Wells A: No more victims: Carolyn Craven talks about rape, and about what women and men can do to stop it. Self-Determination Quarterly Journal 2:2, 1978

West LJ: The epidemic of violence. Presented at the annual meeting of the American Psychiatric Association, Los Angeles, May 1984

26 The Death of a Child ❧

Beverley Raphael

BEVERLEY RAPHAEL is professor of psychiatry on the Faculty of Medicine at
the University of Newcastle (in Australia). She is author of *Management of
Bereavement* and *The Anatomy of Bereavement*, the book our selection is taken
from. In this selection, Raphael explores variations in the nature of bereavement associated with the loss of a child at various ages starting prior to the
actual birth. She considers the special nature of bereavement in connection
with miscarriage, induced abortion, stillbirth, neonatal death, death during
the childhood years, death of the adolescent, and death of the adult child.
Case study material is presented in connection with her analysis of parental
bereavement in each of these different contexts.

A CHILD IS MANY THINGS: a part of the self, and of the loved partner; a representation of the generations past; the genes of the forebears; the hope of the future; a source of love, pleasure, even narcissistic delight; a tie or a burden; and
sometimes a symbol of the worst parts of the self and others.

The loss of a child will always be painful, for it is in some way a loss of part
of the self. The death is likely to be complex: the death of babies and children
are not expected in Western society, are even denied. In any society, the death
of a young child seems to represent some failure of family or society and some
loss of hope. . . .

DEATHS

The death of the child is always untimely. In most developed societies, he is expected to reach adult life. So, inevitably, the parent will feel cheated of the
child's life, the child's future. Often the death is sudden and unexpected, from
accident, injury, or medical emergency. Much less frequently, it is caused by
progressive, debilitating, or malignant conditions with opportunities for pre-
parative, anticipatory grief. Many of the slowly progressive conditions have
congenital factors in their etiology so that the death may be complicated by the

extra burden of shame and guilt such illnesses bring. Malignant disease in childhood brings images of horror: the fantasies of small and helpless bodies being taken over by cancer. All the deaths of childhood are abhorrent and so especially stressful. Futhermore, there is societal expectation that children should not die. Parents are likely to feel they somehow failed, that society will condemn them when death does occur. When the death is a consequence of accident, say drowning, burns, or poisoning, or there has already been a background of ambivalent neglect, then the condemnation may be profound. The parent's condemnation of the self or partner is likely to be even more judgmental, so guilt is prominent.

Although the death may be understood intellectually, it is nevertheless difficult to accept, because it "should not have happened" in the parents' minds. There may be much preoccupation with possible causes, both to settle issues of fault and blame and to attempt to gain control in the future to prevent such a thing happening again. Magical thinking is often prominent in the interpretation of possible causes or in the development of protective ritual with other children subsequently.

The death of a child is evocative for the whole social group. The tragedy of lost life and future, the fears for other children and the self, make these deaths particularly significant.

BEREAVEMENT AT DIFFERENT STAGES OF DEVELOPMENT

Miscarriage

The woman who spontaneously miscarries may experience significant grief, may mourn the lost, hoped-for child. This loss is poorly recognized by others, especially if the pregnancy is lost in early weeks or months before the fetus is considered viable. The special meaning of the pregnancy to her, whether it is wanted or not, will influence her level of grief. A later pregnancy, when the baby's movements have been felt, is more likely to be seen as the loss of a person, a baby, even if it has not reached the legal limit of twenty weeks for being considered so. If the pregnancy is accompanied by a desperate hope for childbirth, then its loss will be most painfully felt and perhaps be considered as a personal failure. Fearfulness is common after miscarriage, even where there is a sense of relief that the baby will not come after all. The grief may appear immediately or may be delayed until the time the baby's movements would have been felt, or some other trigger reminds the mother of the loss, such as the date the baby would have been born. Sadness is the predominant affect, although there may be anger if the mother feels it should not have happened, either because she wanted the baby so much, or because she perceived medical or personal care as failing. There may be guilt if her wish not to have the baby had been significant at some point, especially if it had reached the level of thinking or planning for an abortion. The woman may have little support for her feelings in such instances, since she is expected to be relieved. Where the pregnancy had been gained after a long period of infertility, it may seem that all hopes are dashed. Despair is substantial. Long after the event, the woman may dwell on the details, allocating blame to herself or others for what went wrong. Her failure to rest, undue activity, sexual intercourse, or medical mismanagement may all be seen as at fault. The whole episode may become a focus of unresolved grief.

In her mourning for the lost pregnancy, the woman may have many fantasies about the state of development, the sex, any abnormality, damage to, or disposal of the fetus. An opportunity to share these thoughts and feelings is often of great value to her in assisting her to relinquish the dead baby and her hopes for it. She may seek rationalizations about the loss, such as "it would have been abnormal anyway," which are only partly reassuring, for they carry the covert message that her body produces bad and damaged things. Nevertheless, with support, such issues are usually worked through.

The loss is significant to the woman and will be stated as such by her. For her it is not "nothing," "just a scrape," or "not a life." It is the beginning of a baby. Years later, she may recall it not just as a miscarriage but also as a baby that was lost.

Sandra, age twenty-four, spoke of her grief after miscarrying.

> "They said it was nothing . . . just a miscarriage. I was only a few weeks overdue. I had seen those pictures, and I know it was only tiny, but it was my baby, and it counted as a real baby.
>
> "I wanted to see it, but really all there was was blood. They said I couldn't see anything in that. When I got home I cried and cried and they couldn't understand. Jim tried to comfort me. He kept on saying it would be alright because we could have another baby right away. But that was another baby—it wasn't the same at all. It was this baby I was crying for, and there'd never be another one just the same as it. Jim said we hadn't really been ready for it anyway, that it was just as well. That only made me feel worse, as though we'd got rid of it. Then I wanted it all the more, just to show it that we loved it and cared for it. Some days I would think of how it would have been—a little boy or a little girl.
>
> "Anyway, my tears went. I was a bit sad again now and then. Each month I used to think, now the baby would have been this big; now I would have been feeling the movements; now it would have been due. I felt a failure until I became pregnant again and then it faded. Really, I got over it alright when you look back. But it wasn't 'nothing.' For me I really did lose a baby—not just a miscarriage."

The father may also feel some sadness, but it is likely to be less intense than the mother's, unless he had particular hopes and fantasies invested in the pregnancy. First pregnancies have a unique significance for both the uniqueness of the fantasized baby and the changes it induces for the first time in the woman's body. Pregnancies lost to the couple whose fertility is unproven are also a more painful loss. The grief from previous miscarriages may also be reawakened with new losses. In each instance, the grief and mourning need recognition, perhaps support, to facilitate resolution. . . .

Termination by Induced Abortion

The reaction to induced abortion highlights the dilemma of loss of a pregnancy. Here is a pregnancy, at least to some degree "unwanted." The decision to terminate is often conflictual, forced on the girl or woman by social circumstances, her needs of the moment, or the wishes of others. The pregnancy that ends in termination may, in the first place, have been more likely to be a consequence of unresolved conflicts, such as those discussed previously. The girl's personality may be vulnerable because of earlier deprivations, and, in some instances, she may have characteristics that are self-destructive or accident prone. The pregnancy itself, and the choice of termination as a solution, may indicate the girl lacks necessary support from her family and social group (Raphael 1972a). It is only in relatively recent years that termination has become socially acceptable as a solution to unwanted pregnancy in some societies. However, stigma, shame, and secrecy may still remain. Religious background may make the choice even more conflictual if the girl has had a strong Catholic upbringing. Family moral values may reinforce the "wrong" of such a solution to her pregnancy.

For many, the abortion may consciously or unconsciously be equated with murder. Even women with attested liberal views and strong beliefs in the freedom of a woman to do what she will with her own body, are likely to nurse deep inside them something they deny—a feeling that they have somehow "killed" the baby. The termination may be the obvious, the only, solution seen as appropriate for the pregnancy. And the procedure may be simple, painless, and conducted under the best medical conditions. Yet for many women there will be grief to follow and often an undue burden of guilt as well. It is particularly difficult for the woman that she seeks on one hand to be rid of the pregnancy, yet at the same time mourns its loss. Often she is expected to feel grateful that she had been able to obtain the termination, as well she may. Those to whom she might turn for support give her a covert message that her affects should be of pleasure and relief rather than sadness, failing to recognize that the two may coexist. The woman may have required a high level of defensive denial of her tender feelings for the baby to allow her to make the decision for termination. This denial often carries her through the procedure and the hours immediately afterward, so that she seems cheerful, accepting, but unwilling to talk at that time when supportive counseling may be offered by the clinic. She is notorious in avoiding follow-up because she wishes no painful reminders of her loss, such as the place or people with whom it occurred.

In the decision-making process before termination, many clinics offer the opportunity for counseling for the decision. Most young women are afraid to face their ambivalence about the decision at this stage for fear the abortion will be denied them, or because they fear they will not have the strength to carry it through if they do. Often they are far along the pathway of decision making because of the pressures others place on them, especially their mothers, families, and boyfriends. When the decision is strongly influenced in this way, making the girl's ambivalence even higher, she is more likely to do badly afterward in psychological terms. . . .

Not every woman who presents for termination may have done so as a result of conflict about pregnancy. Contraceptive practice may have failed, or termination may be the method of that society for fertility control. Ambivalence toward the pregnancy may not be great, and the choice to terminate it may be clear and simple for the woman. In these circumstances, grief may be minimal, simply resolved, unlikely to lead to pathological outcomes. Just what proportion of women presenting for termination resolve the issue easily is not really known. Most studies are simple short-term follow-ups with little recognition of some of the complexities that may be involved in outcome. There is often little recognition of grief and mourning in the surveys, which ask if the woman is pleased with her decision, which in most cases she is. Most studies suggest that the younger age group (especially first pregnancies), those persuaded to termination by others, those lacking social support, those having it under socially negative or illegal circumstances, are most likely to be at risk. To this list would be added those for whom the pregnancy represents an attempted, yet failed, solution to conflict.

The pattern of grief and mourning is not dissimilar to that for spontaneous abortion, except that suppression and inhibition of grief and mourning are much more likely. The first appearance of sadness is often noted six weeks or so after the termination, when defenses are down or the loss of the baby is obvious because of the failure of anticipated body changes. Anger is more likely to be directed toward the self or toward those who are seen as pressing the girl to have the termination. Guilt is not shown. There are many anxious, querying rationalizations that it was "the only thing to do, so why should I feel like this?" Thoughts about what the baby might have been like and fears about possible negative effects on future pregnancies may appear. Many women are curious about what has happened to the fetus, but this does not necessarily block mourning. Some grief and mourning may appear when the baby would have been born. The woman may find herself depressed and tearful some months later "for no good reason," she says—then she remembers that this is when the aborted baby would have been born. . . .

Stillbirth

When there is a stillbirth, the loss is not a chosen one. It seems to come tragically when the fulfillment of pregnancy seems at hand. It may be quite unexpected, often sudden. Hopes built during the months of pregnancy are dashed. The psychology of stillbirth has been recently reviewed by Kirkley-Best and Kellner (1982).

The relationship of the mother to the baby that is stillborn may fall anywhere on the spectrum. Some of these pregnancies will have been unwanted, the attachments highly ambivalent, and abortion contemplated. Some will have experienced transient ambivalence, the baby wanted sometimes and not others. Some babies will have been longed for, ardently desired. The father's developing attachment to the baby is likely to be similar to the mother's. He may be present at the baby's birth.

The baby's death may occur with some forewarning. Either through congenital abnormality or intrauterine event, it may become obvious that the baby will not be viable, or that it has already died. This is immensely painful for the parents, particularly if they must wait for the natural onset of labor to produce the dead baby. Some anticipatory grieving may commence when the death is discovered or when diagnosis is made of a nonviable deformity such as anencephaly. The knowledge of the baby's death may come to the parents in such a way. However, on many occasions, the mother senses something wrong—cessation of movements, unexpected sensations, something not quite right—that leads her to have the matter investigated. She may have kept this concern to herself or shared it with her husband. This may be the beginning of her working through her loss.

In some instances, it may be that "a dull, sad quietness pervades the labor ward as the baby emerges, and its floppy body is hurriedly wrapped in a sheet and whisked away" (*British Medical Journal*, January 1977, p. 126). In others, when the stillbirth is unexpected, there may be "frantic efforts at resuscitation as the silence becomes increasingly oppressive, raising everyone's anxiety, especially the mother's" (p. 126). The cause of the death may be difficult to ascertain and even more difficult to explain to the distressed mother. The borderline between natural causes and some sort of medical mismanagement may be a narrow one in some instances. The doctor's sense of guilt and failure may add to the mother's belief that the baby should not have died. It may be easier for her to believe that someone is to blame than to face some of her own feelings of guilt and failure. In her fantasy, the death is likely to be seen as a punishment for the ambivalence in her relationship with the baby, for the times she did not fully want or love it, for past misdeeds, such as abortions. And congenital abnormalities, birth trauma, intrauterine defects might all be interpreted by her as evidence of her damaging and destructive body and womb.

The mother's comprehension of the death, and her mourning for the baby she has lost, are often further complicated by the fact that she has been prevented from seeing and touching the baby. Medical assistants and hospital systems are frequently extremely reluctant to let her have any sight or contact at all, in the mistaken belief that this policy will aid in her recovery. But the majority of mothers are more anxious to see their babies, to touch, hold, name them, and take part in the arrangements for the burial. They may find photos of the baby helpful, especially as evidence that the whole pregnancy produced something: a baby that was real and can be remembered. . . .

Lena, age thirty, told of her experience: "I wanted this baby so desperately. We'd tried so hard to get pregnant again. I'd had two miscarriages, so we were specially careful. I hardly dared hope. But when I got to sixteen weeks, twenty weeks, I started to believe that it might be all right. I started to think about the baby. Joe was so thrilled. We didn't mind if it was a boy or a girl—as long as it was all right. I was scared to get clothes or even to get the room ready—I had been so disappointed before. I didn't want to tempt fate. When it started to move we'd lie in bed at night feeling it. Joe was so proud. I was scared. I didn't know how I'd be as a mother. I was so worried something might go wrong. I kept hearing stories of women who had deformed babies and hadn't realized anything was wrong. I worried so much about that that the doctor got a scan—just to be sure. I could see the baby and there wasn't anything wrong. It was a wonderful feeling. I took the 'pictures' home to Joe and said, 'That's our baby's first photo—we'll put it in the book.'

"When I got to thirty-six weeks, I started to feel strange, worried—I was sure something was wrong. They kept telling me the baby had to be alright—nothing could happen now. Then my water broke. Everything started to happen at once. Joe came home and took me to the hospital. They listened to the baby and they all seemed worried, but they kept telling me it would be fine. I knew things were terribly wrong. Then everything happened so quickly. The baby came. I was in a daze—full of drugs they gave me. I kept calling out 'Where's my baby, I want my baby—my baby's dead isn't it?' They all said 'Sh,' 'sh,' and gave me another injection. But I saw them taking her away—all wrapped up in a blanket.

"The next few days were like a nightmare. There were drips in my arms. I kept asking about the baby, but no one told me anything. I was so drugged. I slept most of the time. Sometimes when I woke Joe was there beside me. He looked terrible. I'd say to him, 'Our baby's dead isn't she?' and all he'd say was 'Shush, shush,' just like the rest of them, and keep telling me I was very sick and had to rest.

"Then I seemed to come out of it. The doctor came and told me: 'Your baby was born dead Mrs. King. We don't know why, but it was probably for the best—it might not have lived long anyway. You'll be well enough to go home soon.' Then I said 'I want to see my baby, Doctor.' He said, 'No you can't Mrs. King—it's no good, the baby's dead. It will only give you bad memories to take away. It would be better if you put it out of your mind.' Then he hurried away as though he was ashamed or something—maybe so he wouldn't see me cry. They kept telling me not to cry or they'd have to give me something to settle me down. I was upsetting the other women. The nurses couldn't bear me crying. They didn't seem to know how I felt. When Joe came in at visiting hours, I told him I had to see the baby. He said, 'It's no good, Love, I've had to bury her. We couldn't put you through that.' I felt as though I could die—she was gone—as though there had never been anything there—like a puff of smoke—phantom pregnancy. It was nothing. All I had was nothing. That's all there was. All

those months of longing and fear, all those years of wanting my baby—all gone for nothing. . . .

Neonatal Death

Many of the characteristics of the bereavement following neonatal death are similar to those following stillbirth, except in neonatal death the parents have some opportunity, even if limited, to know and attach to the real child. The two conditions have been studied together by many workers, under the heading "perinatal death" (see, for example, Peppers and Knapp 1980). Although the bonding to the sick neonate may be inhibited by the threat to the child's life, its prematurity or illness, in most instances, with modern obstetric practices, the attachment to the real baby has time to consolidate.

When the parents realize their newborn child has some life-threatening condition they experience the typical responses to loss. Initially there may be shock, numbness, and disbelief, particularly if there has been nothing to foreshadow the threat. Then there follows an acute longing for the baby, more pronounced in mothers. Where there is a period of illness the baby is usually cared for in a neonatal intensive care unit where the parents are actively involved in its care. The mother's bonding will be enhanced by the tactile contact and seeing her child, but she may have already commenced anticipatory grieving for it. The extent of her anticipatory grief may be determined by the degree of forewarning of the baby's death or serious condition, with the more sudden and unexpected deaths of otherwise healthy neonates being associated with the greatest shock effects for both parents. Whatever his condition, there is an intense longing to hold and cuddle the baby, which is likely to be quite impossible because of his physical condition. As anticipatory grief and mourning progress, the parents may find themselves withdrawing from the child. The dilemma and distress of the parents in such instances is most sensitively described in Wendy Bowie's story of the life and death of her firstborn (Bowie 1977). . . .

According to Helmrath and Steinitz (1978), the acute grief may last six months to a year, but paternal grief is likely to have a much more rapid resolution. This may cause difficulties, but on the other hand, the relationship between the couple may be deepened or improved. Patients describe many problems in their family and social field following the death (Clyman et al. 1980). The parents may be preoccupied with their own distress. There may be difficulties in explaining to the children what has happened, in understanding their different grief and mourning, and in responding to their questions and needs. There is the problem of what to do with the things they got for the baby. This may only be resolved as they gradually mourn the loss and feel able to relinquish them. Parents often feel very unsupported by family and friends. Few can let them talk of the baby and their fears and sadness as they need to, to mourn their loss. Parents often feel they require ongoing assistance, but this may not be readily available to them. In Clyman's subjects 80 percent felt they needed continuing follow-up because of "inability to resume previous responsibilities." Yet for many, such support is not available. . . .

Unresolved grief may be more common with this type of bereavement. It often occurs when the loss of the child reawakens a parent's unresolved feelings of helplessness, inadequacy, as well as irrational guilt. The mother may resort to maladaptive behavior of the dependent, learned-helplessness type. This may be difficult for others to handle. Other forms of pathological outcome have not been systematically studied but appear to be very similar to those following stillbirth (Peppers and Knapp 1980).

> *Margaret was twenty-two when she lost her baby.*
>
> *"Our baby was so small. He was premature, six weeks premature and just so tiny. At first I thought he wouldn't live at all when I came into labor so early. But the doctors told me that they had saved babies smaller than this, so that there was every hope that he would be all right. The intensive care nursery was a strange place—like somewhere from outer space. There were all those tiny little things looking more like mice or tiny monkeys than real babies. And there was our Justin, he was one of them.*
>
> *"Bill and I would go there all the time. They'd let us touch him through that little plastic cabinet, but he looked so fragile—all those tubes and his skinny little arms. We loved him very much, although when we first knew we were having him, we hadn't really wanted him at all. Then we got used to the idea and it was terrible to think of anything happening to him. When he was born too soon, I was really frightened. I felt God was punishing me for not wanting him in the first place. . . . When he was so sick, all I wanted to do was hold him close, breathe my warmth and life into him. But I couldn't do that. I would touch him, and look into his little face and hope that all my love would somehow make him better.*
>
> *"He wasn't growing, so even though they kept telling me he was all right, I didn't really believe them in my heart.*
>
> *"The day he died seemed like any other day, warm and sunny. It just didn't seem possible that a little baby like that should die. He hadn't had any life yet—how could God let it happen? I couldn't cry at first—I felt dry, drained, as though there wasn't a tear left in me. For a long time I tried to believe he was still there at the hospital.*
>
> *"Then there was the empty room at home, and it all came over me like a great tidal wave of grief. I was so sad, so empty, I thought I'd never feel whole again. I used to think about the funeral, and think about him. It was such a tiny casket. He was such a little person to die."* . . .

Death in the Childhood Years

Death in the childhood years takes on a new significance. The child in these years is known and related to as a real person. The family unit is established in its own particular system. There will be many shared pasts to be lost when the child dies, as well as hoped-for futures. . . .

The deaths Deaths are not common in this age group. The two main causative elements are accidental deaths (by far the commonest) and malignant disease. A third smaller group includes the congenitally fatal conditions such as cystic fibrosis or fulminating infection or disease.

Accidental deaths in this age range are complex and traumatic. Motor vehicle accidents are likely to involve other family members in many instances, unless the child is hit as a pedestrian. The shocking unexpected nature of these deaths, their "killing" aspects all lead to great problems of adjustment which will be heightened if the parent was in any way involved. If the mother or father was driving the car in which the child was killed or, as sometimes happens, backed the car out of the garage over the young child and fatally injured him, guilt and recrimination are overwhelming. Blame from the other parent and family members is also very great. Other very traumatic accident situations occur, such as drowning and burns. While many of these deaths are truly accidental, in others there seems some elements of unconscious or even perhaps conscious parental rejection. . . .

Deaths from malignant disease in childhood involve a different type of stress. There is likely to be a process of gradual adaptation to the reality of the child's illness and fatal prognosis. Although childhood malignancy, especially leukemia, is viewed with abhorrence, nevertheless it is seen as a disease state, not the outcome of personal action. Some parents actively seek to blame some factor in themselves or others, but this usually occurs when there are other sources of guilt, perhaps in ambivalence to the child or over past perceived sins for which the child's illness is seen as a punishment. Malignant disease is seen as untimely in this age group. The child and parent are cheated of life by something that they feel should not have happened. This theme is common to bereavements within the childhood age range, for it is assumed in present-day society that children should not die. Deaths from leukemia create special problems, for this condition, which was previously seen as inevitably fatal may now achieve prolonged remission (perhaps cure?). Parents and children may feel they dare not hope for the child's survival, yet the evidence is clear that he is not dying. Such diseases may lead to an orientation of "living each day as it comes," not investing in the unpredictable future.

Where death occurs from some inherited disorder there may be an extra element to it. There is likely to be a sense of shame—inadequacy at having produced the damaged child—for the "bad," destructive genetic inheritance. Guilty feelings about such disorders in the family are also likely to complicate the anticipatory grief and mourning as well as the subsequent bereavements.

Experience and behavior Where the death is sudden, a typical pattern of adult grief and mourning may follow. There will be a large element of shock, however, in accidental deaths, and all these deaths will be perceived as untimely, making them especially difficult for the bereaved to accept. Where the parents do not see the body the death may be even more unreal. Extreme anger about the accident—a hatred of the driver of the car, for example, a desire to hit out and get revenge—may dominate the parents' response. This may be directed toward other agencies or toward the husband or wife. A traumatic neurosis effect is common if the parent was present at the death or in any way involved.

> *Mr. and Mrs. L were at home when they heard a loud crash. Mrs. L suddenly realized Melissa, her four-year-old, was not playing in the house where she had been a moment earlier. She ran, but said she felt almost paralyzed because she "knew it was her; she was hit." Vividly etched in her memory, replayed in slow motion are the details of the scene as she passed through her front door and out onto the street—the gathering crowd, the blood, the small still body.*
>
> *This replayed constantly, in repetitive cognitions, with periods of repression over the two years following the death. There was all the helplessness, dread, and panic she felt at that moment—powerless rage at God and the driver. Her life had become disorganized and purposeless. She had not mourned but had become fixed in that time and place, neither having her child nor relinquishing her.*

The parents' thoughts are filled with "if only." All the events leading up to the death are gone over, revised. What could have been done differently, actions that might have contributed, omissions, are all sought in these attempts at mastery, and perhaps also allocation of blame. The bereaved parent may become locked into the angry "if only" stage of separation from the dead child. There is yearning for the child, restless searching, helplessness, but no real acceptance. There may be little overt grief, just restless agitated distress. In other instances, some level of acceptance is achieved but only with guilty recriminations, sometimes bordering on the delusional. It is as though such parents recognize a connection between their ambivalence to the child and the death, and seek atonement in their *mea culpa*. For many of these parents the grief becomes pathological and chronic, continuing many years after the death with little abatement. They may be preoccupied with the image and the presence of the lost child, keeping his room untouched, visiting the grave daily, and talking to him.

> *Mrs. S told of how the only place she "felt all right, whole" after her son of three was run over, was by the grave. She would visit daily, or on alternate days, and leave flowers. She could feel him there with her, and she no longer felt distressed. She would tend the grave, feeling reassured that she was mothering, protecting him. She would tell him she loved him. Her interest in her other children became vague and secondary. Her husband's support enabled her to keep up this ritual, which she said was "all that kept me from going mad."* . . .

Death of the Adolescent

Deaths in younger adolescents are likely to have very similar outcomes to those of the childhood years. Resolution may be complicated, however, because of the heightened ambivalence and struggles for independence that occur at this time. The deaths are often accidental and may be the consequence of premature attempts to be involved with adult pursuits, such as car driving, bike riding, and drinking. There has often been a family conflict in the background. Deaths from illness during adolescence have many of the patterns described for children. All of these deaths seem particularly bitter, since the young person was just stepping onto the threshold of life.

Deaths of older adolescents perhaps reflect most clearly some of the issues for the family. Typically the death occurs in a motor vehicle accident of some kind. It is sudden and unexpected. It frequently occurs on a background of substantial family conflict. Alcohol is often involved. The child is an emotional focus for parental conflict where ambivalence is high; or perhaps is a greatly loved child still living at home, with a role of fulfilling parental hopes. He or she may be out with other young people in a car, or alone on a motorbike, when fatally injured. (Some injuries are not fatal, of course, but may for many reasons become a source of grief, as when there is severe disability.) There has often been an argument beforehand about whether or not the adolescent should go. The whole outing may have been intended as an act of defiance of parental wishes, or simply for the thrill of risk taking. Police officers bring the message of the death. The shocked mother and father may have to identify the body. Sometimes the mother is prevented from seeing it, so that she has an additional problem in accepting the reality and finality of her loss. Grief appears for the mother, but the father is frequently "strong and silent," suppressing his feelings. Maternal grief continues unabated, often for many years. There is great anger: anger at the son for deserting her in this way, though it is usually denied; anger at those involved with the accident; anger at the husband because of the arguments and noninvolvement in the circumstances that led up to the death. The bereaved feels cheated and rages at the world because all her hopes are lost. She cannot replace this child. She feels she has nothing. Her background may be one of deprivation, so that all her earlier losses are reawakened. She resents her husband because he is there and not the son, and he does not seem to grieve. She is often bitter toward her surviving children, in the early days at least, because they are there and "the most loved one" is not. She may alienate their support. She may take over one of them as an emotional replacement. But nothing assuages the pain. She grieves. She visits the grave. She enshrines his room, his possessions. She hates others who have not lost their children. She turns away his friends because she cannot bear to see them in his place. She hangs onto his memory, idealizing him, bitter toward the world. She will not give up her grief, for she feels she has nothing else. She may continue thus for years, her grief unabated, or eventually and very slowly time may heal to some degree.

This sad picture is not inevitable. Some parents do painfully, yet slowly, resolve such losses. They are more likely to do so if there are other children and the investment in the dead child was not too neurotically overdetermined. The extent of chronic grief as opposed to resolution is unknown, for no systematic studies have been undertaken. However, the follow-up of bereaved parents whose late adolescent children were killed in a major rail disaster confirmed that this group was very severely affected, particularly the mothers (Singh and Raphael 1981).

> *Alan was seventeen and had been working a year when he finally bought his motor-bike. His mother, Mary, was apprehensive about its dangers. She had always been anxious and overprotective toward him. Her relationship with his father was fraught with provocations, alcohol, and verbal and physical violence. She had asked Alan not to go out that night, but his father had abused her and Alan had laughingly said he'd be all right. The night went on and he failed to return. She worried and would not sleep, but kept reasoning to herself that he would be with his mates.*
>
> *At 3:00 A.M., the police arrived to inform her that "there had been an accident," and they "thought it was her son involved. Did she have a picture of him." Her husband, Wal, finally woke. Identification proved that it was indeed Alan. He had run his bike into a car on the opposite side of the road. Blood alcohol levels were high. Mary wept profusely in the hours and days that followed, bemoaning her fate and the death of her son. Her doctor gave her heavy sedation, but to little avail. Wal took to drinking more, as he felt useless at home and heartbroken in his own way about Alan's death. He was deeply hurt and felt his wife gave him no support but was instead "wallowing in self-pity."*
>
> *Mary's grief continued unabated until she was referred for psychiatric assessment two years later following an overdose of barbiturates which she had been using excessively over that time. Some specific work promoting mourning by going with her to the grave, going over photos and memories, helped lessen some of the intensity of her grief. She progressed slowly to a baseline of some periods of depression and many sad memories. She did not return to her premorbid level of functioning.*

Deaths during adolescence are common. They are often traumatic and on the background of ambivalence. It is likely the bereaved parents are a high-risk group requiring further research assessment and preventive management.

Suicide is an increasingly common cause of death in this age range. It too occurs on a family background high in ambivalence, with open hostility and unresolved dependence. The death itself brings shame, stigma, and guilt. Complicated, maybe pathological, bereavements seem a likely outcome for the survivors. This painful legacy has been described in the case of a younger child (Whitis 1968), and findings are similar in this age group.

Death of the Adult Child

The older parent who experiences the death of an adult child is likely to be deeply disturbed by it. Such a person is likely to feel that his or her own death would have been far preferable to that of the son or daughter. The parent adjusts, for there has usually been a degree of separation from the adult child already. Nevertheless, grief is intense. The parent may also be expected to take on parenting roles for the child's children at a time when emotional resources seem drained. Despite their own grief many parents do this successfully. There is little known of the patterns of grief and mourning in this group. They seem from clinical experience to follow the usual pattern of shock, separation pain, and mourning. The deaths are difficult to adjust to because they are untimely. Like other deaths they may be harder to resolve if ambivalence and dependence levels were unduly high. One study of parents who had lost sons in the 1969–70 war of attrition in Israel, found that most resolved this loss reasonably well, and that good family relationships and education beforehand facilitated this (Purisman and Maoz 1977).

Sometimes parents in this older age group will be resentful of the child's family who have "taken" him from them. There may be competition for the role of the most bereaved between, for example, the mother of a son and his younger widow, each claiming her loss is the greater. Resentment may arise at the needs of the surviving in-laws, fear of their dependency and that of the grandchildren. Survivor guilt may be another problem faced by these bereaved parents. They feel they should not have survived, fantasize dying instead, yet are glad to be alive and guilty at that feeling.

> *Helen and Ross, both age fifty, were grief stricken when their daughter Jenny, age twenty-five, died from malignant melanoma. The condition had been rapidly fatal over the six-month period following diagnosis. At that time they moved closer to where Jenny lived with her husband Stan and two young children, girls of five and three. Helen helped care for the children as Jenny's illness progressed, but, as she confessed to Ross, it was all she could do to attend to the children's needs, so great was her distress at her daughter's condition. She constantly thought of Jenny and prayed for her cure, although as the weeks progressed she could see this was impossible.*
>
> *Following Jenny's death she and Ross moved in with Stan. There was often friction between them, yet they felt bound to "do the best they could" for the children. Helen loved them but at another level resented the sacrifice she and Ross were now forced to make for them, and, as she kept telling herself, "for Jenny." She was recurrently depressed over the next two years until they moved back to their own home when Stan remarried. Helen felt that it was only then that she and Ross could really "let go" their grief for their daughter. They had "done their duty," but now faced the terrible loss it meant for them.*

CONCLUSIONS

Whatever the age, the death of the child is seen as untimely by his parents. They often feel that their care has somehow failed, no matter how loving and adequate it was. In mourning the child the parent will go back to the child's earliest beginnings, his conception. Yet it will be difficult to give the child up. Patterns of chronic grief are common and irrational guilt may prevail. In losing the child the parent loses not only the relationship but a part of the self and a hope for the future. Even when mourned, the child is not forgotten. He is always counted as one of the children. And such a loss may alter, forever, the course of the parents' life and even of the parents' relationship to one another. As Sanders (1979/80) points out, for adults, the death of a child when compared to the death of a spouse or parent, evokes the highest intensities of bereavement and the widest range of reactions. Sanders's study showed death anxiety to be higher for this group, with despair prominent. Somatic symptoms were multiple. Their lives seemed not to make sense. Sanders suggests that most of the parents "gave the appearance of individuals who have suffered a physical blow [which] left them with no strength or will to fight, hence *totally vulnerable*" (p. 317).

References

Bowie, W. K. 1977. Story of a first-born. *Omega* 8 (1): 1–17.

British Medical Journal 1(January): 126. 1977. Annotation: Grief and stillbirth.

Clyman, R.; Green, C.; Rowe, J.; Mikkelsen, C.; and Ataide, L. 1980. Issues concerning parents after the death of their newborn. *Critical Care Medicine* 8 (4): 215–18.

Helmrath, T. A., and Steinitz, E. M. 1978. Parental grieving and the failure of social support. *Journal of Family Practice* 6: 735–90.

Kirkley-Best, E., and Kellner, K. R. 1982. The forgotten grief: A review of the psychology of stillbirth. *American Journal of Orthopsychiatry* 52: 420–29.

Peppers, L. G., and Knapp, R. J. 1980. *Mothering and Mourning*. New York: Praeger.

Purisman, R., and Maoz, B. 1977. Adjustment and bereavement: Some considerations. *British Journal of Medical Psychology* 50: 1–9.

Raphael, B. 1972a. Psychosocial aspects of induced abortion: Part I. *Medical Journal of Australia* 2: 35–40.

Sanders, C. M. 1979–80. A comparison of adult bereavement in the death of a spouse, child, and parent. *Omega* 10 (4): 303–21.

Singh, B. S., and Raphael, B. 1981. Post-disaster morbidity of the bereavement. *Journal of Nervous and Mental Disease* 169 (4): 208–12.

Whitis, P. R. 1968. The legacy of a child's suicide. *Family Process* 7 (2): 159–68.

EUTHANASIA AND
MEDICAL ETHICS

Contents

WE CONSIDER FOUR ARTICLES IN PART VII. The first two deal with the
contemporary debates over voluntary active euthanasia and assisted suicide. In the first of these articles, Brock outlines the main arguments that
have been made by advocates of voluntary active euthanasia. In the original
article, Brock also reviews a number of arguments that can be made against
this point of view.

The article by Callahan presents the major arguments that are made by
those who oppose voluntary active euthanasia. Toward the end of that essay, he discusses—and rejects—the argument made by some that euthanasia and assisted suicide are compatible with the practice of medicine. He
believes that it is a mistake to conclude that a physician is the appropriate
person to make the decision as to when the quality of life is so low that it
justifies ending life. He argues that "too often in human history killing has
seemed the quick, efficient way to put aside that which burdens us." This is

an indirect reference to the Nazi program for killing—the topic of the selection by Lifton.

Lifton's article relates how Hitler and the Nazis began by killing children who were considered defective and continued on to killing adult mental patients, a barbaric program that escalated into a systematic killing of all "non-Aryans," which meant all gypsies, Poles, Russians, and especially all Jews (in the millions), and eventually anyone who opposed their dictatorial policies. The Nazis' deliberate policy of extermination of entire peoples has been called "the worst crime in the history of mankind."

The article by Gaylin provides a good context for a discussion of the ethical implications of the modern medical technologies that make it possible to keep alive (for months and years) those who are brain dead. In theory, at least, these living bodies could be used as blood banks, for body parts, to test new drugs, and to practice a variety of medical procedures. Most readers will not feel comfortable about using bodies in these ways. This may suggest that we do not fully accept the conclusions that the brain-dead are really dead; alternatively, it may reflect our feelings about the appropriate and inappropriate uses of corpses.

27 Voluntary Active Euthanasia ﾖ

Dan W. Brock

DAN W. BROCK is professor of philosophy and biomedical ethics and director of the center for Biomedical Ethics in the School of Medicine at Brown University. He is author of *Deciding for Others: The Ethics of Surrogate Decision Making* (with Allen Buchanan) and *Life and Death: Philosophical Essays in Biomedical Ethics*. This selection is taken from an essay in which Brock presents and analyzes the central ethical arguments for voluntary active euthanasia. In a part of the essay not reprinted here, he goes on to analyze the potential bad consequences of permitting euthanasia.

SINCE THE CASE OF KAREN QUINLAN first seized public attention fifteen years ago, no issue in biomedical ethics has been more prominent than the debate about forgoing life-sustaining treatment. Controversy continues regarding some aspects of that debate, such as forgoing life-sustaining nutrition and hydration, and relevant law varies some from state to state. Nevertheless, I believe it is possible to identify an emerging consensus that competent patients, or the surrogates of incompetent patients, should be permitted to weigh the benefits and burdens of alternative treatments, including the alternative of no treatment, according to the patient's values, and either to refuse any treatment or to select from among available alternative treatments. This consensus is reflected in bioethics scholarship, in reports of prestigious bodies such as the President's Commission for the Study of Ethical Problems in Medicine, The Hastings Center, and the American Medical Association, in a large body of judicial decisions in courts around the country, and finally in the beliefs and practices of health care professionals who care for dying patients.[1]

More recently, significant public and professional attention has shifted from life-sustaining treatment to euthanasia—more specifically, voluntary active euthanasia—and to physician-assisted suicide. Several factors have contributed to the increased interest in euthanasia. In the Netherlands, it has been openly practiced by physicians for several years with the acceptance of the country's highest court.[2] In 1988 there was an unsuccessful attempt to get the question of whether it should be made legally permissible on the ballot in Cal-

From "Voluntary Active Euthanasia." *Hastings Center Report*, Volume 22 (March–April), pp. 10–22. Copyright © 1992 by The Hastings Center, Briarcliff Manor, NY.

ifornia. In November 1991 voters in the state of Washington defeated a widely publicized referendum proposal to legalize both voluntary active euthanasia and physician-assisted suicide. Finally, some cases of this kind, such as "It's Over, Debbie," described in the *Journal of the American Medical Association*, the "suicide machine" of Dr. Jack Kevorkian, and the cancer patient "Diane" of Dr. Timothy Quill, have captured wide public and professional attention.[3] Unfortunately, the first two of these cases were sufficiently problematic that even most supporters of euthanasia or assisted suicide did not defend the physicians' actions in them. . . . My primary aim . . . is not to argue for euthanasia, but to identify confusions in some common arguments, and problematic assumptions and claims that need more defense or data in others. The issues are considerably more complex than either supporters or opponents often make out; my hope is to advance the debate by focusing attention on what I believe the real issues under discussion should be.

In the recent bioethics literature some have endorsed physician-assisted suicide but not euthanasia.[4] Are they sufficiently different that the moral arguments for one often do not apply to the other? A paradigm case of physician-assisted suicide is a patient's ending his or her life with a lethal dose of a medication requested of and provided by a physician for that purpose. A paradigm case of voluntary active euthanasia is a physician's administering the lethal dose, often because the patient is unable to do so. The only difference that need exist between the two is the person who actually administers the lethal dose—the physician or the patient. In each, the physician plays an active and necessary causal role.

In physician-assisted suicide the patient acts last (for example, Janet Adkins herself pushed the button after Dr. Kevorkian hooked her up to his suicide machine), whereas in euthanasia the physician acts last by performing the physical equivalent of pushing the button. In both cases, however, the choice rests fully with the patient. In both the patient acts last in the sense of retaining the right to change his or her mind until the point at which the lethal process becomes irreversible. How could there be a substantial moral difference between the two based only on this small difference in the part played by the physician in the causal process resulting in death? Of course, it might be held that the moral difference is clear and important—in euthanasia the physician kills the patient whereas in physician-assisted suicide the patient kills him- or herself. But this is misleading at best. In assisted suicide the physician and patient together kill the patient. To see this, suppose a physician supplied a lethal dose to a patient with the knowledge and intent that the patient will wrongfully administer it to another. We would have no difficulty in morality or the law recognizing this as a case of joint action to kill for which both are responsible.

If there is no significant, intrinsic moral difference between the two, it is also difficult to see why public or legal policy should permit one but not the other; worries about abuse or about giving anyone dominion over the lives of others apply equally to either. As a result, I will take the arguments evaluated below to apply to both and will focus on euthanasia.

My concern here will be with *voluntary* euthanasia only—that is, with the case in which a clearly competent patient makes a fully voluntary and persistent request for aid in dying. Involuntary euthanasia, in which a competent patient explicitly refuses or opposes receiving euthanasia, and nonvoluntary euthanasia, in which a patient is incompetent and unable to express his or her wishes about euthanasia, will be considered here only as potential unwanted side-effects of permitting voluntary euthanasia. I emphasize as well that I am concerned with *active* euthanasia, not withholding or withdrawing life-sustaining treatment, which some commentators characterize as "passive euthanasia." Finally, I will be concerned with euthanasia where the motive of those who perform it is to respect the wishes of the patient and to provide the patient with a "good death," though one important issue is whether a change in legal policy could restrict the performance of euthanasia to only those cases.

A last introductory point is that I will be examining only secular arguments about euthanasia, though of course many people's attitudes to it are inextricable from their religious views. The policy issue is only whether euthanasia should be permissible, and no one who has religious objections to it should be required to take any part in it, though of course this would not fully satisfy some opponents.

THE CENTRAL ETHICAL ARGUMENT FOR VOLUNTARY ACTIVE EUTHANASIA

The central ethical argument for euthanasia is familiar. It is that the very same two fundamental ethical values supporting the consensus on patients' rights to decide about life-sustaining treatment also support the ethical permissibility of euthanasia. These values are individual self-determination or autonomy and individual well-being. By self-determination as it bears on euthanasia, I mean people's interest in making important decisions about their lives for themselves according to their own values or conceptions of a good life, and in being left free to act on those decisions. Self-determination is valuable because it permits people to form and live in accordance with their own conception of a good life, at least within the bounds of justice and consistent with others doing so as well. In exercising self-determination people take responsibility for their lives and for the kinds of persons they become. A central aspect of human dignity lies in people's capacity to direct their lives in this way. The value of exercising self-determination presupposes some minimum of decisionmaking capacities or competence, which thus limits the scope of euthanasia supported by self-determination; it cannot justifiably be administered, for example, in cases of serious dementia or treatable clinical depression.

Does the value of individual self-determination extend to the time and manner of one's death? Most people are very concerned about the nature of the last stage of their lives. This reflects not just a fear of experiencing substantial suffering when dying, but also a desire to retain dignity and control during this last period of life. Death is today increasingly preceded by a long period of significant physical and mental decline, due in part to the technological interventions of modern medicine. Many people adjust to these disabilities and find meaning and value in new activities and ways. Others find the impairments and burdens in the last stage of their lives at some point sufficiently great to make life no longer worth living. For many patients near death, maintaining the quality of one's life, avoiding great suffering, maintaining one's dignity, and insuring that others remember us as we wish them to become of paramount importance and outweigh merely extending one's life. But there is no single, objectively correct answer for everyone as to when, if at all, one's life becomes all things considered a burden and unwanted. If self-determination is a fundamental value, then the great variability among people on this question makes it especially important that individuals control the manner, circumstances, and timing of their dying and death.

The other main value that supports euthanasia is individual well-being. It might seem that individual well-being conflicts with a person's self-determination when the person requests euthanasia. Life itself is commonly taken to be a central good for persons, often valued for its own sake, as well as necessary for pursuit of all other goods within a life. But when a competent patient decides to forgo all further life-sustaining treatment then the patient, either explicitly or implicitly, commonly decides that the best life possible for him or her with treatment is of sufficiently poor quality that it is worse than no further life at all. Life is no longer considered a benefit by the patient, but has now become a burden. The same judgment underlies a request for euthanasia: continued life is seen by the patient as no longer a benefit, but now a burden. Especially in the often severely compromised and debilitated states of many critically ill or dying patients, there is no objective standard, but only the competent patient's judgment of whether continued life is no longer a benefit.

Of course, sometimes there are conditions, such as clinical depression, that call into question whether the patient has made a competent choice, either to forgo life-sustaining treatment or to seek euthanasia, and then the patient's choice need not be evidence that continued life is no longer a benefit for him or her. Just as with decisions about treatment, a determination of incompetence can warrant not honoring the patient's choice; in the case of treatment, we then transfer decisional authority to a surrogate, though in the case of voluntary active euthanasia a determination that the patient is incompetent means that choice is not possible.

The value or right of self-determination does not entitle patients to compel physicians to act contrary to their own moral or professional values. Physicians are moral and professional agents whose own self-determination or integrity should be respected as well. If performing euthanasia became legally permissible, but conflicted with a particular physician's reasonable understanding of his or her moral or professional responsibilities, the care of a patient who requested euthanasia should be transferred to another.

Most opponents do not deny that there are some cases in which the values of patient self-determination and well-being support euthanasia. Instead, they commonly offer two kinds of arguments against it that in their view outweigh or override this support. The first kind of argument is that in any individual case where considerations of the patient's self-determination and well-being do support euthanasia, it is nevertheless always ethically wrong or impermissible. The second kind of argument grants that in some individual cases euthanasia may *not* be ethically wrong, but maintains nonetheless that public and legal policy should never permit it. The first kind of argument focuses on features of any individual case of euthanasia, while the second kind focuses on social or legal policy. In the next section I consider the first kind of argument.

EUTHANASIA IS THE DELIBERATE KILLING OF AN INNOCENT PERSON

The claim that any individual instance of euthanasia is a case of deliberate killing of an innocent person is, with only minor qualifications, correct. Unlike forgoing life-sustaining treatment, commonly understood as allowing to die, euthanasia is clearly killing, defined as depriving of life or causing the death of a living being. While providing morphine for pain relief at doses where the risk of respiratory depression and an earlier death may be a foreseen but unintended side effect of treating the patient's pain, in a case of euthanasia the patient's death is deliberate or intended even if in both the physician's ultimate end may be respecting the patient's wishes. If the deliberate killing of an innocent person is wrong, euthanasia would be nearly always impermissible.

In the context of medicine, the ethical prohibition against deliberately killing the innocent derives some of its plausibility from the belief that nothing in the currently accepted practice of medicine is deliberate killing. Thus, in commenting on the "It's Over, Debbie" case, four prominent physicians and bioethicists could entitle their paper "Doctors Must Not Kill."[5] The belief that doctors do not in fact kill requires the corollary belief that forgoing life-sustaining treatment, whether by not starting or by stopping treatment, is allowing to die, not killing. Common though this view is, I shall argue that it is confused and mistaken.

Why is the common view mistaken? Consider the case of a patient terminally ill with ALS disease. She is completely respirator dependent with no hope of ever being weaned. She is unquestionably competent but finds her condition intolerable and persistently requests to be removed from the respirator and allowed to die. Most people and physicians would agree that the patient's physician should respect the patient's wishes and remove her from the respirator, though this will certainly cause the patient's death. The common understanding is that the physician thereby allows the patient to die. But is that correct?

Suppose the patient has a greedy and hostile son who mistakenly believes that his mother will never decide to stop her life-sustaining treatment and that even if she did her physician would not remove her from the respirator. Afraid that his inheritance will be dissipated by a long and expensive hospitalization, he enters his mother's room while she is sedated, extubates her, and she dies. Shortly thereafter the medical staff discovers what he has done and confronts the son. He replies, "I didn't kill her, I merely allowed her to die. It was her ALS disease that caused her death." I think this would rightly be dismissed as transparent sophistry—the son went into his mother's room and deliberately killed her. But, of course, the son performed just the same physical actions, did just the same thing, that the physician would have done. If that is so, then doesn't the physician also kill the patient when he extubates her?

I underline immediately that there are important ethical differences between what the physician and the greedy son do. First, the physician acts with the patient's consent whereas the son does not. Second, the physician acts with a good motive—to respect the patient's wishes and self-determination—whereas the son acts with a bad motive—to protect his own inheritance. Third, the physician acts in a social role through which he is legally authorized to carry out the patient's wishes regarding treatment whereas the son has no such authorization. These and perhaps other ethically important differences show that what the physician did was morally justified whereas what the son did was morally wrong. What they do *not* show, however, is that the son killed while the physician allowed to die. One can either kill or allow to die with or without consent, with a good or bad motive, within or outside of a social role that authorizes one to do so.

The difference between killing and allowing to die that I have been implicitly appealing to here is roughly that between acts and omissions resulting in death.[6] Both the physician and the greedy son act in a manner intended to cause death, do cause death, and so both kill. One reason this conclusion is resisted is that on a different understanding of the distinction between killing and allowing to die, what the physician does is allow to die. In this account, the mother's ALS is a lethal disease whose normal progression is being held back or blocked by the life-sustaining respirator treatment. Removing this artificial intervention is then viewed as standing aside and allowing the patient to die of her underlying disease. I have argued elsewhere that this alternative account is deeply problematic, in part because it commits us to accepting that what the greedy son does is to allow to die, not kill.[7] Here, I want to note two other reasons why the conclusion that stopping life support is killing is resisted.

The first reason is that killing is often understood, especially within medicine, as unjustified causing of death; in medicine it is thought to be done only accidentally or negligently. It is also increasingly widely accepted that a physician is ethically justified in stopping life support in a case like that of the ALS patient. But if these two beliefs are correct, then what the physician does cannot be killing, and so must be allowing to die. Killing patients is not, to put it flippantly, understood to be part of physicians' job description. What is mistaken in this line of reasoning is the assumption that all killings are *unjustified* causings of death. Instead, some killings are ethically justified, including many instances of stopping life support.

Another reason for resisting the conclusion that stopping life support is often killing is that it is psychologically uncomfortable. Suppose the physician had stopped the ALS patient's respirator and had made the son's claim, "I didn't kill her, I merely allowed her to die. It was her ALS disease that caused her death." The clue to the psychological role here is how naturally the "merely" modifies "allowed her to die." The characterization as allowing to die is meant to shift felt responsibility away from the agent—the physician—and to the lethal disease process. Other language common in death and dying contexts plays a similar role; "letting nature take its course" or "stopping prolonging the dying process" both seem to shift responsibility from the physician who stops life support to the fatal disease process. However psychologically helpful these conceptualizations may be in making the difficult responsibility of a physician's role in the patient's death bearable, they nevertheless are confusions. Both physicians and family members can instead be helped to understand that it is the patient's decision and consent to stopping treatment that limits their responsibility for the patient's death and that shifts that responsibility to the patient.

Many who accept the difference between killing and allowing to die as the distinction between acts and omissions resulting in death have gone on to argue that killing is not in itself morally different from allowing to die.[8] In this account, very roughly, one kills when one performs an action that causes the death of a person (we are in a boat, you cannot swim, I push you overboard, and you drown), and one allows to die when one has the ability and opportunity to prevent the death of another, knows this, and omits doing so, with the result that the person dies (we are in a boat, you cannot swim, you fall overboard, I don't throw you an available life ring, and you drown). Those who see no moral difference between killing and allowing to die typically employ the strategy of comparing cases that differ in these and no other potentially morally important respects. This will allow people to consider whether the mere difference that one is a case of killing and the other of allowing to die matters morally, or whether instead it is other features that make most cases of killing worse than most instances of allowing to die. Here is such a pair of cases:

Case 1. *A very gravely ill patient is brought to a hospital emergency room and sent up to the ICU. The patient begins to develop respiratory failure that is likely to re-*

quire intubation very soon. At that point the patient's family members and long-standing physician arrive at the ICU and inform the ICU staff that there had been extensive discussion about future care with the patient when he was unquestionably competent. Given his grave and terminal illness, as well as his state of debilitation, the patient had firmly rejected being placed on a respirator under any circumstances, and the family and physician produce the patient's advance directive to that effect. The ICU staff do not intubate the patient, who dies of respiratory failure.

Case 2. *The same as Case 1 except that the family and physician are slightly delayed in traffic and arrive shortly after the patient has been intubated and placed on the respirator. The ICU staff extubate the patient, who dies of respiratory failure.*

In Case 1 the patient is allowed to die, in Case 2 he is killed, but it is hard to see why what is done in Case 2 is significantly different morally than what is done in Case 1. It must be other factors that make most killings worse than most allowings to die, and if so, euthanasia cannot be wrong simply because it is killing instead of allowing to die.

Suppose both my arguments are mistaken. Suppose that killing is worse than allowing to die and that withdrawing life support is not killing, although euthanasia is. Euthanasia still need not for that reason be morally wrong. To see this, we need to determine the basic principle for the moral evaluation of killing persons. What is it that makes paradigm cases of wrongful killing wrongful? One very plausible answer is that killing denies the victim something that he or she values greatly—continued life or a future. Moreover, since continued life is necessary for pursuing any of a person's plans and purposes, killing brings the frustration of all of these plans and desires as well. In a nutshell, wrongful killing deprives a person of a valued future, and of all the person wanted and planned to do in that future.

A natural expression of this account of the wrongness of killing is that people have a moral right not to be killed.[9] But in this account of the wrongness of killing, the right not to be killed, like other rights, should be waivable when the person makes a competent decision that continued life is no longer wanted or a good, but is instead worse than no further life at all. In this view, euthanasia is properly understood as a case of a person having waived his or her right not to be killed.

This rights view of the wrongness of killing is not, of course, universally shared. Many people's moral views about killing have their origins in religious views that human life comes from God and cannot be justifiably destroyed or taken away, either by the person whose life it is or by another. But in a pluralistic society like our own with a strong commitment to freedom of religion, public policy should not be grounded in religious beliefs which many in that society reject. I turn now to the general evaluation of public policy on euthanasia.

WOULD THE BAD CONSEQUENCES OF EUTHANASIA
OUTWEIGH THE GOOD?

The argument against euthanasia at the policy level is stronger than at the level of individual cases, though even here I believe the case is ultimately unpersuasive, or at best indecisive. The policy level is the place where the main issues lie, however, and where moral considerations that might override arguments in favor of euthanasia will be found, if they are found anywhere. It is important to note two kinds of disagreement about the consequences for public policy of permitting euthanasia. First, there is empirical or factual disagreement about what the consequences would be. This disagreement is greatly exacerbated by the lack of firm data on the issue. Second, since on any reasonable assessment there would be both good and bad consequences, there are moral disagreements about the relative importance of different effects. In addition to these two sources of disagreement, there is also no single, well-specified policy proposal for legalizing euthanasia on which policy assessments can focus. But without such specification, and especially without explicit procedures for protecting against well-intentioned misuse and ill-intentioned abuse, the consequences for policy are largely speculative. Despite these difficulties, a preliminary account of the main likely good and bad consequences is possible. This should help clarify where better data or more moral analysis and argument are needed, as well as where policy safeguards must be developed.

Potential Good Consequences of Permitting Euthanasia

What are the likely good consequences? First, if euthanasia were permitted it would be possible to respect the self-determination of competent patients who want it, but now cannot get it because of its illegality. We simply do not know how many such patients and people there are. In the Netherlands, with a population of about 14.5 million (in 1987), estimates in a recent study were that about 1,900 cases of voluntary active euthanasia or physician-assisted suicide occur annually. No straightforward extrapolation to the United States is possible for many reasons, among them, that we do not know how many people here who want euthanasia now get it, despite its illegality. Even with better data on the number of persons who want euthanasia but cannot get it, significant moral disagreement would remain about how much weight should be given to any instance of failure to respect a person's self-determination in this way.

One important factor substantially affecting the number of persons who would seek euthanasia is the extent to which an alternative is available. The widespread acceptance in the law, social policy, and medical practice of the right of a competent patient to forgo life-sustaining treatment suggests that the number of competent persons in the United States who would want euthanasia if it were permitted is probably relatively small.

A second good consequence of making euthanasia legally permissible benefits a much larger group. Polls have shown that a majority of the American public believes that people should have a right to obtain euthanasia if they want it.[10] No doubt the vast majority of those who support this right to euthanasia will never in fact come to want euthanasia for themselves. Nevertheless, making it legally permissible would reassure many people that if they ever do want euthanasia they would be able to obtain it. This reassurance would supplement the broader control over the process of dying given by the right to decide about life-sustaining treatment. Having fire insurance on one's house benefits all who have it, not just those whose houses actually burn down, by reassuring them that in the unlikely event of their house burning down, they will receive the money needed to rebuild it. Likewise, the legalization of euthanasia can be thought of as a kind of insurance policy against being forced to endure a protracted dying process that one has come to find burdensome and unwanted, especially when there is no life-sustaining treatment to forgo. The strong concern about losing control of their care expressed by many people who face serious illness likely to end in death suggests that they give substantial importance to the legalization of euthanasia as a means of maintaining this control.

A third good consequence of the legalization of euthanasia concerns patients whose dying is filled with severe and unrelievable pain or suffering. When there is a life-sustaining treatment that, if forgone, will lead relatively quickly to death, then doing so can bring an end to these patients' suffering without recourse to euthanasia. For patients receiving no such treatment, however, euthanasia may be the only release from their otherwise prolonged suffering and agony. This argument from mercy has always been the strongest argument for euthanasia in those cases to which it applies.[11]

The importance of relieving pain and suffering is less controversial than is the frequency with which patients are forced to undergo untreatable agony that only euthanasia could relieve. If we focus first on suffering caused by physical pain, it is crucial to distinguish pain that *could* be adequately relieved with modern methods of pain control, though it in fact is not, from pain that is relievable only by death.[12] For a variety of reasons, including some physicians' fear of hastening the patient's death, as well as the lack of a publicly accessible means for assessing the amount of the patient's pain, many patients suffer pain that could be, but is not, relieved.

Specialists in pain control, as for example the pain of terminally ill cancer patients, argue that there are very few patients whose pain could not be adequately controlled, though sometimes at the cost of so sedating them that they are effectively unable to interact with other people or their environment. Thus, the argument from mercy in cases of physical pain can probably be met in a large majority of cases by providing adequate measures of pain relief. This should be a high priority, whatever our legal policy on euthanasia—the relief of pain and suffering has long been, quite properly, one of the central goals of medicine. Those cases in which pain could be effectively relieved, but in fact is not, should only count significantly in favor of legalizing euthanasia if all reasonable efforts to change pain management techniques have been tried and have failed.

Dying patients often undergo substantial psychological suffering that is not fully or even principally the result of physical pain.[13] The knowledge about how to relieve this suffering is much more limited than in the case of relieving pain, and efforts to do so are probably more often unsuccessful. If the argument from mercy is extended to patients experiencing great and unrelievable psychological suffering, the numbers of patients to which it applies are much greater.

One last good consequence of legalizing euthanasia is that once death has been accepted, it is often more humane to end life quickly and peacefully, when that is what the patient wants. Such a death will often be seen as better than a more prolonged one. People who suffer a sudden and unexpected death, for example by dying quickly or in their sleep from a heart attack or stroke, are often considered lucky to have died in this way. We care about how we die in part because we care about how others remember us, and we hope they will remember us as we were in "good times" with them and not as we might be when disease has robbed us of our dignity as human beings. As with much in the treatment and care of the dying, people's concerns differ in this respect, but for at least some people, euthanasia will be a more humane death than what they have often experienced with other loved ones and might otherwise expect for themselves.

Some opponents of euthanasia challenge how much importance should be given to any of these good consequences of permitting it, or even whether some would be good consequences at all. But more frequently, opponents cite a number of bad consequences that permitting euthanasia would or could produce. . . . [*Space limitations here prevent enumerating and evaluating these potential bad consequences, but the reader is referred to the original paper from which this selection is drawn for a discussion of them.* —Editors]

References

1. President's Commission for the Study of Ethical Problems in Medicine and Biomedical and Behavioral Research, *Deciding to Forego Life-Sustaining Treatment* (Washington, D.C.: U.S. Government Printing Office, 1983); The Hastings Center, *Guidelines on the Termination of Life-Sustaining Treatment and Care of the Dying* (Bloomington: Indiana University Press, 1987); *Current Opinions of the Council on Ethical and Judicial Affairs of the American Medical Association—1989: Withholding or Withdrawing Life-Prolonging Treatment* (Chicago: American Medical Association, 1989); George Annas and Leonard Glantz, "The Right of Elderly Patients to Re-

fuse Life-Sustaining Treatment," *Millbank Memorial Quarterly* 64, suppl. 2 (1986): 95–162; Robert F. Weir, *Abating Treatment with Critically Ill Patients* (New York: Oxford University Press, 1989); Sidney J. Wanzer et al. "The Physician's Responsibility toward Hopelessly Ill Patients," *NEJM* 310 (1984): 955–59.

2. M.A.M. de Wachter, "Active Euthanasia in the Netherlands," *JAMA* 262, no. 23 (1989): 3315–19.

3. Anonymous, "It's Over, Debbie," *JAMA* 259 (1988): 272; Timothy E. Quill, "Death and Dignity," *NEJM* 322 (1990): 1881–83.

4. Wanzer et al., "The Physician's Responsibility toward Hopelessly Ill Patients: A Second Look," *NEJM* 320 (1989): 844–49.

5. Willard Gaylin, Leon R. Kass, Edmund D. Pellegrino, and Mark Siegler, "Doctors Must Not Kill," *JAMA* 259 (1988): 2139–40.

6. Bonnie Steinbock, ed., *Killing and Allowing to Die* (Englewood Cliffs, N.J.: Prentice Hall, 1980).

7. Dan W. Brock, "Forgoing Food and Water: Is It Killing?" in *By No Extraordinary Means: The Choice to Forgo Life-Sustaining Food and Water*, ed. Joanne Lynn (Bloomington: Indiana University Press, 1986), pp. 117–31.

8. James Rachels, "Active and Passive Euthanasia," *NEJM* 292 (1975): 78–80; Michael Tooley, *Abortion and Infanticide* (Oxford: Oxford University Press, 1983). In my paper, "Taking Human Life," *Ethics* 95 (1985): 851–65, I argue in more detail that killing in itself is not morally different from allowing to die and defend the strategy of argument employed in this and the succeeding two paragraphs in the text.

9. Dan W. Brock, "Moral Rights and Permissible Killing," in *Ethical Issues Relating to Life and Death*, ed. John Ladd (New York: Oxford University Press, 1979), pp. 94–117.

10. P. Painton and E. Taylor, "Love or Let Die," *Time*, 19 March 1990, pp. 62–71; *Boston Globe*/Harvard University Poll, *Boston Globe*, 3 November 1991.

11. James Rachels, *The End of Life* (Oxford: Oxford University Press, 1986).

12. Marcia Angell, "The Quality of Mercy," *NEJM* 306 (1982): 98–99; M. Donovan, P. Dillon, and L. Mcguire, "Incidence and Characteristics of Pain in a Sample of Medical-Surgical Inpatients," *Pain* 30 (1987): 69–78.

13. Eric Cassell, *The Nature of Suffering and the Goals of Medicine* (New York: Oxford University Press, 1991).

28 When Self-Determination Runs Amok

Daniel Callahan

DANIEL CALLAHAN is the director of The Hastings Center (located in Briar-cliff Manor, New York), a research organization devoted to ethical problems of medicine. He is author of *What Kind of Life: The Limits of Medical Progress* and *Setting Limits: Medical Goals in an Aging Society*. In this essay, Callahan presents a number of arguments against acceptance of voluntary active euthanasia. He makes an effort to answer a number of the main arguments that have been made by those who favor acceptance of this practice.

THE EUTHANASIA DEBATE is not just another moral debate, one in a long list of arguments in our pluralistic society. It is profoundly emblematic of three important turning points in Western thought. The first is that of the legitimate conditions under which one person can kill another. The acceptance of voluntary active euthanasia would morally sanction what can only be called "consenting adult killing." By that term I mean the killing of one person by another in the name of their mutual right to be killer and killed if they freely agree to play those roles. This turn flies in the face of a long-standing effort to limit the circumstances under which one person can take the life of another, from efforts to control the free flow of guns and arms, to abolish capital punishment, and to more tightly control warfare. Euthanasia would add a whole new category of killing to a society that already has too many excuses to indulge itself in that way.

The second turning point lies in the meaning and limits of self-determination. The acceptance of euthanasia would sanction a view of autonomy holding that individuals may, in the name of their own private, idiosyncratic view of the good life, call upon others, including such institutions as medicine, to help them pursue that life, even at the risk of harm to the common good. This works against the idea that the meaning and scope of our own right to lead our own lives must be conditioned by, and be compatible with, the good of the community, which is more than an aggregate of self-directing individuals.

From "When Self-Determination Runs Amok," *Hastings Center Report*, Volume 22 (March–April), pp. 52–55. Copyright © 1992 by The Hastings Center, Briarcliff Manor, NY.

The third turning point is to be found in the claim being made upon medicine: it should be prepared to make its skills available to individuals to help them achieve their private vision of the good life. This puts medicine in the business of promoting the individualistic pursuit of general human happiness and well-being. It would overturn the traditional belief that medicine should limit its domain to promoting and preserving human health, redirecting it instead to the relief of that suffering which stems from life itself, not merely from a sick body.

I believe that, at each of these three turning points, proponents of euthanasia push us in the wrong direction. Arguments in favor of euthanasia fall into four general categories, which I will take up in turn: (1) the moral claim of individual self-determination and well-being; (2) the moral irrelevance of the difference between killing and allowing to die; (3) the supposed paucity of evidence to show likely harmful consequences of legalized euthanasia; and (4) the compatibility of euthanasia and medical practice.

Self-determination

Central to most arguments for euthanasia is the principle of self-determination. People are presumed to have an interest in deciding for themselves, according to their own beliefs about what makes life good, how they will conduct their lives. That is an important value, but the question in the euthanasia context is, What does it mean and how far should it extend? If it were a question of suicide, where a person takes her own life without assistance from another, that principle might be pertinent, at least for debate. But euthanasia is not that limited a matter. The self-determination in that case can only be effected by the moral and physical assistance of another. Euthanasia is thus no longer a matter only of self-determination, but of a mutual, social decision between two people, the one to be killed and the other to do the killing.

How are we to make the moral move from my right of self-determination to some doctor's right to kill me—from *my* right to *his* right? Where does the doctor's moral warrant to kill come from? Ought doctors to be able to kill anyone they want as long as permission is given by competent persons? Is our right to life just like a piece of property, to be given away or alienated if the price (happiness, relief of suffering) is right? And then to be destroyed with our permission once alienated?

In answer to all those questions, I will say this: I have yet to hear a plausible argument why it should be permissible for us to put this kind of power in the hands of another, whether a doctor or anyone else. The idea that we can waive our right to life, and then give to another the power to take that life, requires a justification yet to be provided by anyone.

Slavery was long ago outlawed on the ground that one person should not have the right to own another, even with the other's permission. Why? Because it is a fundamental moral wrong for one person to give over his life and fate to another, whatever the good consequences, and no less a wrong for another person to have that kind of total, final power. Like slavery, dueling was long ago banned on similar grounds: even free, competent individuals should not have the power to kill each other, whatever their motives, whatever the circumstances. Consenting adult killing, like consenting adult slavery or degradation, is a strange route to human dignity.

There is another problem as well. If doctors, once sanctioned to carry out euthanasia, are to be themselves responsible moral agents—not simply hired hands with lethal injections at the ready—then they must have their own *independent* moral grounds to kill those who request such services. What do I mean? As those who favor euthanasia are quick to point out, some people want it because their life has become so burdensome it no longer seems worth living.

The doctor will have a difficulty at this point. The degree and intensity to which people suffer from their diseases and their dying, and whether they find life more of a burden than a benefit, has very little directly to do with the nature or extent of their actual physical condition. Three people can have the same condition, but only one will find the suffering unbearable. People suffer, but suffering is as much a function of the values of individuals as it is of the physical causes of that suffering. Inevitably in that circumstance, the doctor will in effect be treating the patient's values. To be responsible, the doctor would have to share those values. The doctor would have to decide, on her own, whether the patient's life was "no longer worth living."

But how could a doctor possibly know that or make such a judgment? Just because the patient said so? I raise this question because, while in Holland at the euthanasia conference reported by Maurice de Wachter elsewhere in this issue, the doctors present agreed that there is no objective way of measuring or judging the claims of patients that their suffering is unbearable. And if it is difficult to measure suffering, how much more difficult to determine the value of a patient's statement that her life is not worth living?

However one might want to answer such questions, the very need to ask them, to inquire into the physician's responsibility and grounds for medical and moral judgment, points out the social nature of the decision. Euthanasia is not a private matter of self-determination. It is an act that requires two people to make it possible, and a complicit society to make it acceptable.

Killing and allowing to die

Against common opinion, the argument is sometimes made that there is no moral difference between stopping life-sustaining treatment and more active forms of killing, such as lethal injection. Instead I would contend that the notion that there is no morally significant difference between omission and commission is just wrong. Consider in its broad implications what the eradication of the distinction implies: that death from disease has been banished, leaving only the acts of physicians in terminating treatment as the cause of death. Biology, which used to bring about death, has apparently been displaced by human agency. Doctors have finally, I suppose, thus genuinely become gods, now doing what nature and the deities once did.

What is the mistake here? It lies in confusing causality and culpability, and in failing to note the way in which human societies have overlaid natural causes with moral rules and interpretations. Causality (by which I mean the direct physical causes of death) and culpability (by which I mean our attribution of moral responsibility to human actions) are confused under three circumstances.

They are confused, first, when the action of a physician in stopping treatment of a patient with an underlying lethal disease is construed as *causing* death. On the contrary, the physician's omission can only bring about death on the condition that the patient's disease will kill him in the absence of treatment. We may hold the physician morally responsible for the death, if we have morally judged such actions wrongful omissions. But it confuses reality and moral judgment to see an omitted action as having the same causal status as one that directly kills. A lethal injection will kill both a healthy person and a sick person. A physician's omitted treatment will have no effect on a healthy person. Turn off the machine on me, a healthy person, and nothing will happen. It will only, in contrast, bring the life of a sick person to an end because of an underlying fatal disease.

Causality and culpability are confused, second, when we fail to note that judgments of moral responsibility and culpability are human constructs. By that I mean that we human beings, after moral reflection, have decided to call some actions right or wrong, and to devise moral rules to deal with them. When physicians could do nothing to stop death, they were not held responsible for it. When, with medical progress, they began to have some power over death—but only its timing and circumstances, not its ultimate inevitability—moral rules were devised to set forth their obligations. Natural causes of death were not thereby banished. They were, instead, overlaid with a medical ethics designed to determine moral culpability in deploying medical power.

To confuse the judgments of this ethics with the physical causes of death—which is the connotation of the word *kill*—is to confuse nature and human action. People will, one way or another, die of some disease; death will have dominion over all of us. To say that a doctor "kills" a patient by allowing this to happen should only be understood as a moral judgment about the licitness of his omission, nothing more. We can, as a fashion of speech only, talk about a doctor *killing* a patient by omitting treatment he should have provided. It is a fashion of speech precisely because it is the underlying disease that brings death when treatment is omitted; that is its cause, not the physician's omission. It is a misuse of the word *killing* to use it when a doctor stops a treatment he believes will no longer benefit the patient—when, that is, he steps aside to allow an eventually inevitable death to occur now rather than later. The only deaths that human beings invented are those that come from direct killing—when, with a lethal injection, we both cause death and are morally responsible for it. In the case of omissions, we do not cause death even if we may be judged morally responsible for it.

This difference between causality and culpability also helps us see why a doctor who has omitted a treatment he should have provided has "killed" that patient while another doctor—performing precisely the same act of omission on another patient in different circumstances—does not kill her, but only allows her to die. The difference is that we have come, by moral convention and conviction, to classify unauthorized or illegitimate omissions as acts of "killing." We call them "killing" in the expanded sense of the term: a culpable action that permits the real cause of death, the underlying disease, to proceed to its lethal conclusion. By contrast, the doctor who, at the patient's request, omits or terminates unwanted treatment does not kill at all. Her underlying disease, not his action, is the physical cause of death; and we have agreed to consider actions of that kind to be morally licit. He thus can truly be said to have "allowed" her to die.

If we fail to maintain the distinction between killing and allowing to die, moreover, there are some disturbing possibilities. The first would be to confirm many physicians in their already too-powerful belief that, when patients die or when physicians stop treatment because of the futility of continuing it, they are somehow both morally and physically responsible for the deaths that follow. That notion needs to be abolished, not strengthened. It needlessly and wrongly burdens the physician, to whom should not be attributed the powers of the gods. The second possibility would be that, in every case where a doctor judges medical treatment no longer effective in prolonging life, a quick and direct killing of the patient would be seen as the next, most reasonable step, on grounds of both humaneness and economics. I do not see how that logic could easily be rejected.

CALCULATING THE CONSEQUENCES

When concerns about the adverse social consequences of permitting euthanasia are raised, its advocates tend to dismiss them as unfounded and overly speculative. On the contrary, recent data about the Dutch experience suggests that such concerns are right on target. From my own discussions in Holland, and from the articles on that subject in this issue and elsewhere, I believe we can now fully see most of the *likely* consequences of legal euthanasia.

Three consequences seem almost certain, in this or any other country: the inevitability of some abuse of the law; the difficulty of precisely writing, and then enforcing, the law; and the inherent slipperiness of the moral reasons for legalizing euthanasia in the first place.

Why is abuse inevitable? One reason is that almost all laws on delicate, controversial matters are to some extent abused. This happens because not everyone will agree with the law as written and will bend it, or ignore it, if they can get away with it. From explicit admissions to me by Dutch proponents of euthanasia, and from the corroborating information provided by the Remmelink Report and the outside studies of Carlos Gomez and John Keown, I am convinced that in the Netherlands there are a substantial number of cases of nonvoluntary euthanasia, that is, euthanasia undertaken without the explicit permission of the person being killed. The other reason abuse is inevitable is that the law is likely to have a low enforcement priority in the criminal justice system. Like other laws of similar status, unless there is an unrelenting and harsh willingness to pursue abuse, violations will ordinarily be tolerated. The worst thing to me about my experience in Holland was the casual, seemingly indifferent attitude toward abuse. I think that would happen everywhere.

Why would it be hard to precisely write, and then enforce, the law? The Dutch speak about the requirement of "unbearable" suffering, but admit that such a term is just about indefinable, a highly subjective matter admitting of no objective standards. A requirement for outside opinion is nice, but it is easy to find complaisant colleagues. A requirement that a medical condition be "terminal" will run aground on the notorious difficulties of knowing when an illness is actually terminal.

Apart from those technical problems there is a more profound worry. I see no way, even in principle, to write or enforce a meaningful law that can guarantee effective procedural safeguards. The reason is obvious yet almost always overlooked. The euthanasia transaction will ordinarily take place within the boundaries of the private and confidential doctor-patient relationship. No one can possibly know what takes place in that context unless the doctor chooses to reveal it. In Holland, less than 10 percent of the physicians report their acts of euthanasia and do so with almost complete legal impunity. There is no reason why the situation should be any better elsewhere. Doctors will have their own reasons for keeping euthanasia secret, and some patients will have no less a motive for wanting it concealed.

I would mention, finally, that the moral logic of the motives for euthanasia contain within them the ingredients of abuse. The two standard motives for euthanasia and assisted suicide are said to be our right of self-determination, and our claim upon the mercy of others, especially doctors, to relieve our suffering. These two motives are typically spliced together and presented as a single justification. Yet if they are considered independently—and there is no inherent reason why they must be linked—they reveal serious problems. It is said that a competent, adult person should have a right to euthanasia for the relief of suffering. But why must the person be suffering? Does not that stipulation already compromise the principle of self-determination? How can self-determination have any limits? Whatever the person's motives may be, why are they not sufficient?

Consider next the person who is suffering but not competent, who is perhaps demented or mentally retarded. The standard argument would deny euthanasia to that person. But why? If a person is suffering but not competent, then it would seem grossly unfair to deny relief solely on the grounds of incompetence. Are the incompetent less entitled to relief from suffering than the competent? Will it only be affluent, middle-class people, mentally fit and savvy about working the medical system, who can qualify? Do the incompetent suffer less because of their incompetence?

Considered from these angles, there are no good moral reasons to limit euthanasia once the principle of taking life for that purpose has been legitimated. If we really believe in self-determination, then any competent person should have a right to be killed by a doctor for any reason that suits him. If we believe in the relief of suffering, then it seems cruel and capricious to deny it to the incompetent. There is, in short, no reasonable or logical stopping point once the turn has been made down the road to euthanasia, which could soon turn into a convenient and commodious expressway.

EUTHANASIA AND MEDICAL PRACTICE

A fourth kind of argument one often hears both in the Netherlands and in this country is that euthanasia and assisted suicide are perfectly compatible with the aims of medicine. I would note at the very outset that a physician who participates in another person's suicide already abuses medicine. Apart from depression (the main statistical cause of suicide), people commit suicide because they find life empty, oppressive, or meaningless. Their judgment is a judgment about the value of continued life, not only about health (even if they are sick). Are doctors now to be given the right to make judgments about the kinds of life worth living and to give their blessing to suicide for those they judge wanting? What conceivable competence, technical or moral, could doctors claim to play such a role? Are we to medicalize suicide, turning judgments about its worth and value into one more clinical issue? Yes, those are rhetorical questions.

Yet they bring us to the core of the problem of euthanasia and medicine. The great temptation of modern medicine, not always resisted, is to move beyond the promotion and preservation of health into the boundless realm of general human happiness and well-being. The root problem of illness and mortality is both medical and philosophical or religious. "Why must I die?" can be asked as a technical, biological question or as a question about the meaning of life. When medicine tries to respond to the latter, which it is always under pressure to do, it moves beyond its proper role.

It is not medicine's place to lift from us the burden of that suffering which turns on the meaning we assign to the decay of the body and its eventual death. It is not medicine's place to determine when lives are not worth living or when the burden of life is too great to be borne. Doctors have no conceivable way of evaluating such claims on the part of patients, and they should have no right to act in response to them. Medicine should try to relieve human suffering, but only that suffering which is brought on by illness and dying as biological phenomena, not that suffering which comes from anguish or despair at the human condition.

Doctors ought to relieve those forms of suffering that medically accompany serious illness and the threat of death. They should relieve pain, do what they can to allay anxiety and uncertainty, and be a comforting presence. As sensitive human beings, doctors should be prepared to respond to patients who ask why they must die, or die in pain. But here the doctor and the patient are at the same level. The doctor may have no better an answer to those old questions than anyone else; and certainly no special insight from his training as a physician. It would be terrible for physicians to forget this, and to think that in a swift, lethal injection, medicine has found its own answer to the riddle of life. It would be a false answer, given by the wrong people. It would be no less a false answer for patients. They should neither ask medicine to put its own vocation at risk to serve their private interests, nor think that the answer to suffering is to be killed by another. The problem is precisely that, too often in human history, killing has seemed the quick, efficient way to put aside that which burdens us. It rarely helps, and too often simply adds to one evil still another. That is what I believe euthanasia would accomplish. It is self-determination run amok.

29 The Nazi "Euthanasia" Program

Robert Jay Lifton

ROBERT JAY LIFTON is professor of psychiatry at Yale University. His books include *Death in Life: Survivors of Hiroshima* (which won the National Book Award in Science in 1969), *Home from the War, Explorations in Psychohistory*, and *The Nazi Doctors*, the book the current selection is drawn from. The Nazi "euthanasia" program was not a program that involved euthanasia as decent citizens ordinarily define it; rather, this was the name given to a program for systematically killing people the Nazis classified as undesirables, with the cooperation of a substantial number of medical doctors. This selection is not included as an example of euthanasia, but rather because the unspeakable Nazi atrocities are so frequently mentioned in contemporary debates about euthanasia.

The state organism . . . [is] a whole with its own laws and rights, much like one self-contained human organism . . . which, in the interest of the welfare of the whole, also—as we doctors know—abandons and rejects parts or particles that have become worthless or dangerous.

ALFRED HOCHE

Either one is a doctor or one is not.

A FORMER NAZI DOCTOR

HITLER'S INVOLVEMENT—THE FIRST "MERCY KILLING"

Hitler had an intense interest in direct medical killing. His first known expression of intention to eliminate the "incurably ill" was made to Dr. Gerhard Wagner at the Nuremberg Party rally of 1935. Karl Brandt, who overheard that remark, later testified that Hitler thought that the demands and upheavals of war would mute expected religious opposition and enable such a project to be implemented smoothly. Hitler was also said to have stated that a war effort requires a very healthy people, and that the generally diminished sense of the value of human life during war made it "the best time for the elimination of the incurably ill." And he was reportedly affected by the burden imposed by the mentally ill not only on relatives and the general population but on the medical profession. In 1936, Wagner held discussions with "a small circle of friends" (specifically, high-ranking officials, some of them doctors) about killing "idiotic children" and "mentally ill" people, and making films in "asylums and idiot homes" to demonstrate the misery of their lives. This theoretical and tactical linking of war to direct medical killing was maintained throughout.

By 1938, the process had gone much further. Discussions moved beyond high-level political circles; and at a national meeting of leading government psychiatrists and administrators, an SS officer gave a talk in which he stated that "the solution of the problem of the mentally ill becomes easy if one eliminates these people."

Toward the end of 1938, the Nazi regime was receiving requests from relatives of newborns or very young infants with severe deformities and brain damage for the granting of a mercy killing. These requests had obviously been encouraged, and were channeled directly to the Chancellery—that is, to Hitler's personal office. Whatever the plans for using war as a cover, the program for killing children was well under way by the time the war began. And from the beginning, this program circumvented ordinary administrative channels and was associated directly with Hitler himself.

The occasion for initiating the actual killing of children, and of the entire "euthanasia" project, was the petition for the "mercy killing" (*Gnadentod*, really "mercy death") of an infant named Knauer, born blind, with one leg and part of one arm missing, and apparently an "idiot." Subsequent recollections varied concerning who had made the petition and the extent of the deformity, as the case quickly became mythologized.

In late 1938 or early 1939, Hitler ordered Karl Brandt, his personal physician and close confidant, to go to the clinic at the University of Leipzig, where the child was hospitalized, in order to determine whether the information submitted was accurate and to consult with physicians there: "If the facts given by the father were correct, I was to inform the physicians in [Hitler's] name that they could carry out euthanasia." Brandt was also empowered to tell those physicians that any legal proceedings against them would be quashed by order of Hitler.

Brandt reported that the doctors were of the opinion "that there was no justification for keeping [such a child] alive"; and he added (in his testimony at the Nuremberg Medical Trial) that "it was pointed out [presumably by the doctors he spoke to] that in maternity wards in some circumstances it is quite natural for the doctors themselves to perform euthanasia in such a case without anything further being said about it." The doctor with whom he mainly consulted was Professor Werner Catel, head of the Leipzig pediatrics clinic and a man who was soon to assume a leading role in the project. All was to be understood as a responsible medical process, so that—as Brandt claimed was Hitler's concern—"the parents should not have the impression that they themselves were responsible for the death of this child." . . . On returning to Berlin, Brandt was authorized by Hitler, who did not want to be publicly identified with the project, to proceed in the same way in similar cases: that is, to formalize a program with the help of the high-ranking Reich leader Philip Bouhler, chief of Hitler's Chancellery. This "test case" was pivotal for the two killing programs—of children and of adults.

The two programs were conducted separately, though they overlapped considerably in personnel and in other ways.

THE KILLING OF CHILDREN

It seemed easier—perhaps more "natural" and at least less "unnatural"—to begin with the very young: first, newborns; then, children up to three and four; then, older ones. Similarly, the authorization—at first, oral and secret and to be "kept in a very narrow scope, and cover only the most serious cases"—was later to become loose, extensive, and increasingly known. A small group of doctors and Chancellery officials held discussions in which they laid out some of the ground rules for the project. Then a group of medical consultants known to have a "positive" attitude to the project was assembled, including administrators, pediatricians, and psychiatrists.

The sequence was typical: the order to implement the biomedical vision came from the political leadership (in this case Hitler himself); the order was conveyed to a leading doctor within the regime, who combined with high-ranking administrators to organize a structure for the project; and prominent academic administrative doctors sympathetic to the regime were called in to maintain and administer this *medicalized* structure. It was decided that the program was to be secretly run from the Chancellery, though the health division of the Reich Interior Ministry was to help administer it. And for that purpose an organization was created: the Reich Committee for the Scientific Registration of Serious Hereditary and Congenital Diseases (*Reichsausschuss zur wissenschaftlichen Erfassung von erb- und anlagebedingten schweren Leiden*). The name conveyed the sense of a formidable medical-scientific registry board, although its leader, Hans Hefelmann, had his degree in agricultural economics. That impression was maintained in a strictly confidential directive (of 18 August 1939) by the minister of the interior to non-Prussian state governments. The directive stated that, "for the clarification of scientific questions in the field of congenital malformation and mental retardation, the earliest possible registration" was required of all children under three years of age in whom any of the following "serious hereditary diseases" were "suspected": idiocy and mongolism (especially when associated with blindness and deafness); microcephaly; hydrocephaly; malformations of all kinds, especially of limbs, head, and spinal column; and paralysis, including spastic conditions.

Midwives were required to make these reports at the time of birth (with a portion of the report filled in by a doctor, if present), and doctors themselves were to report all such children up to the age of three. District medical officers were responsible for the accuracy of the reports, and chief physicians of maternity clinics and wards were all notified that such reports were required. The reports took the form of questionnaires that originated in the Reich Health Ministry. At first simple, they were expanded considerably in June 1940 by participating doctors to go beyond specific illness or condition and to include: details about the birth; elements of family history, especially concerning hereditary illness and such things as excessive use of alcohol, nicotine, or drugs; a further evaluation of the condition (by a physician) indicating possibilities for improvement, life expectancy, prior institutional observation and treatment, details of physical and mental development, and descriptions of convulsions and related phenomena. The wording of the questionnaire and the essential absence of a traditional medical history and record led many physicians and district medical officers to assume, at least at first, that affected children would merely be registered for statistical purposes. (Hefelmann later testified that the diseases were broadly described in order to disguise the reason for the duty to report.)

Three central medical experts were then required to make their either-or judgments without examining the children or even reading their medical records, but solely on the basis of the questionnaire. They recorded their decisions on a small form with the names of the three experts printed on the left side; on the right side, under the word "treatment" (*Behandlung*), were three columns, making a small space available parallel to each individual expert's name. If an expert decided upon "treatment"—meaning the killing of the child—he put a plus sign (+) in the left column. If he decided against killing the child, he put a minus sign (–) in the middle column. If he thought a definite decision should not yet be made, he wrote in the right-hand column the phrase "temporary postponement" or the word "observation" and then initialed this opinion. The same form was passed in sequence to the three experts, so that the second one receiving it would know the opinion of the first, and the third would know the opinion of the first two. A unanimous opinion was necessary for a child to be killed—an outcome favored by the reporting arrangement. . . .

Before being killed, children were generally kept for a few weeks in the institution in order to convey the impression that they were being given some form of medical therapy. The killing was usually arranged by the director of the institution or by another doctor working under him, frequently by innuendo rather than specific order. It was generally done by means of luminal tablets dissolved in liquid, such as tea, given to the child to drink. This sedative was given repeatedly—often in the morning and at night—over two or three days, until the child lapsed into continuous sleep. The luminal dose could be increased until the child went into coma and died. For children who had difficulty drinking, luminal was sometimes injected. If the luminal did not kill the child quickly enough—as happened with excitable children who developed considerable tolerance to the drug because of having been given so much of it—a fatal morphine-scopolamine injection was given. The cause of death was listed as a more or less ordinary disease such as pneumonia, which could even have the kind of kernel of truth we have noted. . . .

THE KILLING OF ADULTS

Extending the project from children to adults meant rendering medical killing an official overall policy—a policy Hitler enunciated in his "Führer decree" of October 1939. A few months earlier, he had called in Leonardo Conti, secretary for health in the Interior Ministry, as well as the head of the Reich Chancellery, Hans Lammers, and told them (as recalled by the latter) that "he considered it to be proper that the 'life unworthy of life' of severely mentally ill persons be eliminated by actions [*Eingriffe*] that bring about death." Hitler went on to cite "as examples . . . cases in which the mentally ill could only be bedded on sand or sawdust because they continually befouled themselves," and in which "patients put their own excrement into their mouths, eating it and so on." Hitler pointed out that in this way "a certain saving in hospitals, doctors, and nursing personnel could be brought about." The caricatured mentally ill would come to symbolize all that threatened the purity of the *Volk*.

The decree itself was brief:

> *Reich Leader Bouhler and Dr. Brandt are charged with the responsibility for expanding the authority of physicians, to be designated by name, to the end that patients considered incurable according to the best available human judgment [*menschlichem Ermessen*] of their state of health, can be granted a mercy death [*Gnadentod*].*

Actually issued in October, the decree was backdated to 1 September, so that it could relate directly to the day of the outbreak of the Second World War. While the backdating is usually attributed to Hitler's conviction that a wartime atmosphere would render the German population more amenable to such a project, there was a deeper psychological relationship between "euthanasia" and war. As the fanatical Dr. Pfannmüller in the Nazi program put it: "The idea is unbearable to me that the best, the flower of our youth must lose its life at the front in order that feebleminded and irresponsible asocial elements can have a secure existence in the asylum."

The Nazis viewed their biomedical vision as having a heroic status parallel to that of war. Hitler's concept that the state in itself was nothing, and existed only to serve the well-being of the *Volk* and the race, applied also to the major enterprises of the state, especially its transcendent enterprise of war. Rather than medical killing being subsumed to war, the war itself was subsumed to the vast biomedical vision of which "euthanasia" was a part. Or, to put the matter another way, the deepest impulses behind the war had to do with the sequence of sterilization, direct medical killing, and genocide.

Yet Hitler and other Nazi leaders were aware that they were embarking on a draconian, though in their eyes necessary, measure for which the German public and even the official state bureaucracy were not quite ready. Hence, the decree was written on Hitler's private stationery, as though he "considered the death of many thousands of sick persons as his private matter, not . . . a decision of the head of state." Or, we may say, he understood himself to be a prophet whose racial vision outdistanced the state's structure, making it necessary for him to avoid the bureaucratic apparatus and proceed directly to the matter at hand.

His way of doing that was to go straight to the doctors. Inevitably, he ended up creating an elaborate new bureaucracy, one that was both medical and murderous. In his decision to turn the program over to Karl Brandt rather than to Conti (who, as health minister and Reich Health Leader, was the logical person to run it), Hitler was choosing his own "escort physician and close confidant." Probably similar personal reasons determined his selection of Philip Bouhler, chief of Hitler's Chancellery and considered absolutely loyal to him, to run the program with Brandt. An additional reason for this arrangement was said to be the fear that radical district leaders (*Gauleiter*) might otherwise, "ruthlessly and without medical consultation," take over much of the control of the project—as they indeed eventually did. For Hitler, this was a conscious choice of "party discipline" over a state apparatus that still made some demands for legal procedure and fiscal accountability; it was also a choice of procedure most protective of secrecy. Above all, these arrangements suggest how far the impulse toward killing mental patients had already taken hold among Nazi leaders, and their determination to keep the project in medical channels.

Not only Brandt and Bouhler, but also Dr. Herbert Linden of the Health Ministry and Dr. Grawitz, chief physician of the SS, were active in choosing doctors for leadership roles. Their criteria included the closeness of these doctors to the regime, high recognition in the profession, and known sympathy for "euthanasia" or at least a radical approach to eugenics, probably in about that order. Included were several doctors who had been associated with the children's program (Unger, Heinze, and Pfannmüller), but also a group of psychiatrists of some prominence in academic circles, notably Professor Werner Heyde of Würzburg, Professor Carl Schneider of Heidelberg, Professor Max de Crinis of Berlin, and Professor Paul Nitsche from the Sonnenstein state institution. Others, like Friedrich Mennecke, were primarily Nazified psychiatrists. Heyde became Brandt's representative and directed the program, with Nitsche his assistant and eventual replacement.

At these early meetings, Brandt was introduced as the medical leader of the project, and Hitler's decree was read and sometimes displayed ("I believe I saw Adolf Hitler's signature on it," Mennecke later testified). It was carefully explained that there was no official law, because Hitler thought such a law could only feed enemy propaganda; that the authorization to Bouhler and Brandt in the Hitler decree was the equivalent of a law; and that doctors participating would be immune from legal consequences. One participant later insisted that the emphasis was on killing only hopeless mental patients: "Those cases . . . we in psychiatry know as burned-out ruins (*ausgebrannte Ruinen*). But many of those present knew of Hitler's views on eliminating genetically inferior people in general. Although the phrase "life unworthy of life" was liberally invoked, another doctor could feel "not quite clear on where the line was to be drawn." There was stress on constructing a careful medical sequence of evaluation before any patient would be put to death. And the entire project was to be "unconditionally kept secret." In those important early meetings, just one doctor—Max de Crinis—refused . . . to participate fully. The general response was that "nobody mentioned any misgivings."

What was secret was the actual killing project, not the idea. Some months earlier (April 1939), an article had appeared in a semi-official Nazi magazine, estimating that it would probably be desirable to exterminate one million people.

Organizing for Killing

Unlike the children's "euthanasia" program, the T4 program, with its focus on adult chronic patients, involved virtually the entire German psychiatric community and related portions of the general medical community. The camouflage organization created for the medical killing was the Reich Work Group of Sanatoriums and Nursing Homes (*Reichsarbeitsgemeinschaft Heil- und Pflegeanstalten*, or RAG) operating from the Berlin Chancellery at its Tiergarten 4 address—hence, the overall code name "T4" for the adult project. Questionnaires were worked out by the leadership group of psychiatrists and administrators and distributed, with the help of the Health Ministry, not only to psychiatric institutions but to all hospitals and homes for chronic patients. The limited space provided for biographical and symptomatic categories, as well as the covering letter, gave the impression that a statistical survey was being undertaken for administrative and possibly scientific purposes. All the more so because the questionnaire for patients was accompanied by an institutional questionnaire, which focused on such matters as annual budget, number of beds, and number of doctors and nurses. But the sinister truth was suggested by the great stress put on a "precise description" of the working ability of the patients, as well as by the juxtaposition of the following four categories:

1. Patients suffering from specified diseases who are not employable or are employable only in simple mechanical work. The diseases were schizophrenia, epilepsy, senile diseases, therapy-resistant paralysis and other syphilitic sequelae, feeblemindedness from any cause, encephalitis, Huntington's chorea, and other neurological conditions of a terminal nature.
2. Patients who have been continually institutionalized for at least five years.
3. Patients who are in custody as criminally insane.
4. Patients who are not German citizens, or are not of German or kindred blood, giving race and nationality.

There are added instructions about filling in the section on work, including that of noting "patients in the higher diet categories [who] perform no work though they might be able to do so." . . . By mid-1940, these report forms were required not only on patients who came under the four categories but on all inmates of these institutions.

The process was haphazard from the start. It was required that forms be returned quickly, and one institutional doctor had to fill out fifteen hundred questionnaires in two weeks. Early confusion about the purpose of the form led some doctors to exaggerate the severity of patients' conditions, as a way of protecting them from what was assumed to be a plan to release them from institutions in order to send them to work. The extent to which psychiatrists could continue to disbelieve what was happening—especially when they did not *want* to believe it—is suggested by a leading professor of psychiatry's later description of his response to a rumor he had heard that patients were being "euthanized":

> *I considered the rumor completely unbelievable. . . . Thinking that the questionnaire did not give the slightest cause to suppose such an action, . . . I imagined the intended action was a way of separating the curable patients, or those able to work, from those who were incurable, in order to provide better food for the first group and to provide the second group . . . only the amount of food necessary to keep them alive. . . . [My staff] was persuaded by my argument, and we all worked innocently on the questionnaire project.*

The "expert evaluation" differed from the children's program in that the three medical (usually psychiatric) authorities, drawn from among the leaders of the project, did their reviewing independently. Of every questionnaire collected, four or five photocopies were made in the Reich Interior Ministry, one for each of these three "experts" (*Gutachter*), the other one or two for the later death procedure, with the original usually kept in the central files. Each of the experts wrote in a special thick black frame at the lower left-hand corner of the form, "+" in red pencil, meaning death; "–" in blue pencil, meaning life; or "?," sometimes with a comment, which was most often "worker." He then initialed the mark. If anything, their work was even more mercurial and superficial than the initial filling out of the forms. Each doctor was sent at least 100 photocopied questionnaires at a time; during one seventeen-day period, Pfannmüller was required to complete 2,109 such evaluations. And once more they did no examinations, had no access to medical histories, and made their decision solely on the basis of the questionnaire. . . .

Psychiatric Transfer: "White Coats and SS Boots"

Transportation arrangements were a caricature of psychiatric transfer. The organization created for this function, the Common Welfare Ambulance Service Ltd. (*Gemeinnützige Krankentransport*, or *Gekrat*), sent out "transport lists" to the hospitals from which it was to collect patients; issued instructions that patients were to be accompanied by their case histories and personal possessions as well as lists of valuables held for them; and specified that those patients for whom lengthy transport could be dangerous to their lives should not be transferred (a show of medical propriety and an actual means of avoiding the awkward situation of a patient dying en route).

SS personnel manned the buses, frequently wearing white uniforms or white coats in order to appear to be doctors, nurses, or medical attendants. There were reports of "men with white coats and SS boots," the combination that epitomized much of the "euthanasia" project in general.

To hide patients from the public, bus windows were covered with dark paint or fixed curtains or blinds. The destination of the buses was specifically kept secret from the medical staff of the institution from which they were loaded, and of course from the patients themselves. SS guards on the buses carried special documents enabling them to pass unchallenged through all checkpoints. The initial practice of taking patients directly to the killing centers was after some time discontinued in favor of "observation institutions" or "transit institutions"—often large state hospitals near killing centers—where patients spent brief periods before being sent to their deaths. These observation institutions, which were suggested by Heyde and may have enhanced scheduling arrangements, provided an aura of medical check against mistakes, while in fact no real examination or observation was made. In addition, they seemed to have been part of an impulse toward bureaucratic mystification that further impaired the autonomous existence and the traceability of a patient and, to a considerable extent, of his or her family as well.

The bureaucratic mystification was furthered by letters sent to the family: first, notification of transfer "because of important war-related measures"; and then a second letter upon the patient's reaching the killing center announcing his or her "safe" arrival, and adding that "at this time . . . Reich defense reasons" and "the shortage of personnel brought about by the war" made visits or inquiries of any kind impossible, although the family would "immediately" be informed of changes in a patient's condition or in the visiting policy. The second letter was signed, with a false name, by either the killing doctor or the chief of the killing center. The third letter, sent—under a false name by the Condolence-Letter Department—just days or perhaps weeks later, was a notification of the patient's death.

"The Syringe Belongs in the Hand of a Physician"

That death generally occurred within twenty-four hours of the patient's arrival at the killing center. Under T4 policy, a doctor had to do the actual killing, in accordance with the motto enunciated by Dr. Viktor Brack, head of the Chancellery's "Euthanasia" Department II: "The syringe belongs in the hand of a physician." Rather than a syringe, however, it was usually a matter of opening a gas cock.

There were six main killing centers—Hartheim, Sonnenstein, Grafeneck, Bernburg, Brandenburg, and Hadamar. Typically they were converted mental hospitals or nursing homes; at least one had been a prison. They were in isolated areas and had high walls—some had originally been old castles—so that what happened within could not be readily observed from without. "The unloading of the buses could be done in a way [so that] neither the screams of the patients nor any other occurrences could penetrate to the outside world."

Hitler himself is said to have decided upon the use of carbon monoxide gas as the killing method, on the so-called medical advice of Dr. Heyde. The decision followed upon an experiment conducted in early 1940 at Brandenburg, then being converted from a prison into a killing center. Killing by injection (using various combinations of morphine, scopolomine, curare, and prussic acid [cyanide]) was directly compared with killing by means of carbon monoxide gas. Karl Brandt, "a very conscientious man [who] took his responsibility very seriously," requested the experiment; and he and Conti administered the injections themselves "as a symbolic action in which the most responsible physicians in the Reich subjected themselves to the practical carrying through of the Führer's order."

The four or six injected patients ("six at the most") "died only slowly," and some had to be injected again. In contrast, the gas worked perfectly. The first Nazi gas chamber had been constructed under the supervision of Christian Wirth, of the SS Criminal Police, lent to the T4 staff. The arrangement included a fake shower room with benches, the gas being inserted from the outside into water pipes with small holes through which the carbon monoxide could escape. Present were two SS chemists with doctoral degrees, one of whom operated the gas. The other, August Becker, told how eighteen to twenty people were led naked into the "shower room": through a peephole he observed that very quickly "people toppled over, or lay on the benches"—all without "scenes or commotion." The room was ventilated within five minutes; SS men then used special stretchers which mechanically shoved the corpses into crematory ovens without contact. The technical demonstration was performed before a select audience of the inner circle of physicians and administrators of the medical killing project. Having been shown the technique, Dr. Irmfried Eberl, newly appointed head of the Brandenburg institution, took over "by himself and on his own responsibility." Both Brack and Brandt expressed their satisfaction with the experiment, the latter stressing that "only doctors should carry out the gassings."

I have referred to those initial gassings as both experiments and demonstrations, since later testimony—for instance, Brandt's remarkable statements at the Nuremberg Medical Trial—make clear that they were both. Brandt said that the original plan was to kill people by injecting narcotics, until it was realized that these would cause lack of consciousness but that death would not occur for some time. An alternative suggestion was made by a psychiatrist (presumably Heyde) to use carbon monoxide gas (which, in turn, led to the demonstration just described). Brandt recalled not liking the idea because he felt that "this whole question can only be looked at from a medical point of view," and that "in my medical imagination carbon monoxide had never played a part." Killing by gas, that is, made it much more difficult to maintain a medical aura. Brandt was able to change his mind when he recalled a personal experience of carbon monoxide poisoning in which he lost consciousness "without feeling anything," and realized that carbon monoxide "would be the most humane form of death." Yet he remained troubled because that method required "a whole change in medical conception," and gave the matter extensive thought "in order to put my own conscience right." He brought up to Hitler the difference of opinion about the two methods, and later remembered the Führer asking, "Which is the more humane way?" "My answer was clear," Brandt testified—and other leading physicians in the program agreed. Brandt concluded this segment of testimony with a meditation on medical breakthrough:

> This is just one example of [what happens] when major advances in medical history are being made. There are cases of an operation being looked on at first with contempt, but then later on one learned it and carried it out. Here the task required by state authority was added to the medical conception of this problem, and it was necessary to find with good conscience a basic method that could do justice to both of these elements.

Allowing for self-serving elements and for retrospective father-son mythology in his early relationship to Hitler, Brandt's description takes us to the heart of the doctors' embrace of medicalized killing.

30 Harvesting the Dead

Willard Gaylin

WILLARD GAYLIN, a psychiatrist, is past president of The Hastings Center. In this essay he discusses possible uses of the bodies of those who have experienced brain death. While the modern technological ability to keep these bodies alive opens up a number of potentially useful medical uses for them, it is clear from this essay that such possibilities also raise a number of troublesome ethical issues.

NOTHING IN LIFE IS SIMPLE ANYMORE, not even the leaving of it. At one time there was no medical need for the physician to consider the concept of death; the fact of death was sufficient. The difference between life and death was an infinite chasm [bridged] in an infinitesimal moment. Life and death were ultimate, self-evident opposites.

With the advent of new techniques in medicine, those opposites have begun to converge. We are now capable of maintaining visceral functions without any semblance of the higher functions that define a person. We are, therefore, faced with the task of deciding whether that which we have kept alive is still a human being, or, to put it another way, whether that human being that we are maintaining should be considered "alive."

Until now we have avoided the problems of definition and reached the solutions in silence and secret. When the life sustained was unrewarding—by the standards of the physician in charge—it was discontinued. Over the years, physicians have practiced euthanasia on an ad hoc, casual, and perhaps irresponsible basis. They have withheld antibiotics or other simple treatments when it was felt that a life did not warrant sustaining, or pulled the plug on the respirator when they were convinced that what was being sustained no longer warranted the definition of life. Some of these acts are illegal and, if one wished to prosecute, could constitute a form of manslaughter, even though it is unlikely that any jury would convict. We prefer to handle all problems connected with death by denying their existence. But death and its dilemmas persist.

New urgencies for recognition of the problem arise from two conditions: the continuing march of technology, making the sustaining of vital processes possible for longer periods of time; and the increasing use of parts of the newly dead to sustain life for the truly living. The problem is well on its way to being resolved by what must have seemed a relatively simple and ingenious method. As it turned out, the difficult issues of euthanasia could be evaded by redefining death.

In an earlier time, death was defined as the cessation of breathing. Any movie buff recalls at least one scene in which a mirror is held to the mouth of a dying man. The lack of fogging indicated that indeed he was dead. The spirit of man resided in his *spiritus* (breath). With increased knowledge of human physiology and the potential for reviving a nonbreathing man, the circulation, the pulsating heart, became the focus of the definition of life. This is the tradition with which most of us have been raised.

There is of course a relationship between circulation and respiration, and the linkage, not irrelevantly, is the brain. All body parts require the nourishment, including oxygen, carried by the circulating blood. Lack of blood supply leads to the death of an organ; the higher functions of the brain are particularly vulnerable. But if there is no respiration, there is no adequate exchange of oxygen, and this essential ingredient of the blood is no longer available for distribution. If a part of the heart loses its vascular supply, we may lose that part and still survive. If a part of the brain is deprived of oxygen, we may, depending on its location, lose it and survive. But here we pay a special price, for the functions lost are those we identify with the self, the soul, or humanness, i.e., memory, knowledge, feeling, thinking, perceiving, sensing, knowing, learning, and loving.

Most people are prepared to say that when all of the brain is destroyed the "person" no longer exists; with all due respect for the complexities of the mind/brain debate, the "person" (and personhood) is generally associated with the functioning part of the head—the brain. The higher functions of the brain that have been described are placed, for the most part, in the cortex. The brain stem (in many ways more closely allied to the spinal cord) controls primarily visceral functions. When the total brain is damaged, death in all forms will ensue because the lower brain centers that control the circulation and respiration are destroyed. With the development of modern respirators, however, it is possible to artificially maintain respiration and with it, often, the circulation with which it is linked. It is this situation that has allowed for the redefinition of death—a redefinition that is being precipitously embraced by both scientific and theological groups.

The movement toward redefining death received considerable impetus with the publication of a report sponsored by the Ad Hoc Committee of the Harvard Medical School in 1968. The committee offered an alternative definition of death based on the functioning of the brain. Its criteria stated that if an individual is unreceptive and unresponsive, i.e., in a state of irreversible coma;

if he has no movements or breathing when the mechanical respirator is turned off; if he demonstrates no reflexes; and if he has a flat electroencephalogram for at least twenty-four hours, indicating no electrical brain activity (assuming that he has not been subjected to hypothermia or central nervous system depressants), he may then be declared dead.

What was originally offered as an optional definition of death is, however, progressively becoming *the* definition of death. In most states there is no specific legislation defining death;[1] the ultimate responsibility here is assumed to reside in the general medical community. Recently, however, there has been a series of legal cases which seem to be establishing brain death as a judicial standard. In California in May of [1974] an ingenious lawyer, John Cruikshank, offered as a defense of his client, Andrew D. Lyons, who had shot a man in the head, the argument that the cause of death was not the bullet but the removal of his heart by a transplant surgeon, Dr. Norman Shumway. Cruikshank's argument notwithstanding, the jury found his client guilty of voluntary manslaughter. In the course of that trial, Dr. Shumway said: "The brain in the 1970s and in the light of modern day medical technology is the sine qua non—the criterion for death. I'm saying anyone whose brain is dead is dead. It is the one determinant that would be universally applicable, because the brain is the one organ that can't be transplanted."

This new definition, independent of the desire for transplant, now permits the physician to "pull the plug" without even committing an act of passive euthanasia. The patient will first be defined as dead; pulling the plug will merely be the harmless act of halting useless treatment on a cadaver. But while the new definition of death avoids one complex problem, euthanasia, it may create others equally difficult which have never been fully defined or visualized. For if it grants the right to pull the plug, it also implicitly grants the privilege *not* to pull the plug, and the potential and meaning of this has not at all been adequately examined.

These cadavers would have the legal status of the dead with none of the qualities one now associates with death. They would be warm, respiring, pulsating, evacuating, and excreting bodies requiring nursing, dietary, and general grooming attention—*and could probably be maintained so for a period of years.* If we chose to, we could, with the technology already at hand, legally avail ourselves of these new cadavers to serve science and mankind in dramatically useful ways. The autopsy, that most respectable of medical traditions, that last gift of the dying person to the living future, could be extended in principle beyond our current recognition. To save lives and relieve suffering—traditional motives for violating tradition—we could develop hospitals (an inappropriate word because it suggests the presence of living human beings), banks, or farms

---

[1]Kansas and Maryland have recently legislated approval for a brain definition of death.

of cadavers which require feeding and maintenance, in order to be harvested. To the uninitiated the "new cadavers" in their rows of respirators would seem indistinguishable from comatose patients now residing in wards of chronic neurological hospitals.

PRECEDENTS

The idea of wholesale and systematic salvage of useful body parts may seem startling, but it is not without precedent. It is simply magnified by the technology of modern medicine. Within the confines of one individual, we have always felt free to transfer body parts to places where they are needed more urgently, felt free to reorder the priorities of the naturally endowed structure. We will borrow skin from the less visible parts of the body to salvage a face. If a muscle is paralyzed, we will often substitute a muscle that subserves a less crucial function. This was common surgery at the time that paralytic polio was more prevalent.

It soon becomes apparent, however, that there is a limitation to this procedure. The person in want does not always have a second-best substitute. He may then be forced to borrow from a person with a surplus. The prototype, of course, is blood donation. Blood may be seen as a regeneratable organ, and we have a long-standing tradition of blood donation. What may be more important, and perhaps dangerous, we have established the precedent in blood of commercialization—not only are we free to borrow, we are forced to buy and, indeed, in our country at least, permitted to sell. Similarly, we allow the buying or selling of sperm for artificial insemination. It is most likely that in the near future we will allow the buying and selling of ripened ova so that a sterile woman may conceive her baby if she has a functioning uterus. Of course, once *in vitro* fertilization becomes a reality (an imminent possibility), we may even permit the rental of womb space for gestation for a woman who does manufacture her own ova but has no uterus.

Getting closer to our current problem, there is the relatively long-standing tradition of banking body parts (arteries, eyes, skin) for short periods of time for future transplants. Controversy has arisen with recent progress in the transplanting of major organs. Kidney transplants from a near relative or distant donor are becoming more common. As heart transplants become more successful, the issue will certainly be heightened, for while the heart may have been reduced by the new definition of death to merely another organ, it will always have a core position in the popular thinking about life and death. It has the capacity to generate the passion that transforms medical decisions into political issues.

The ability to use organs from cadavers has been severely limited in the past by the reluctance of heirs to donate the body of an individual for distribution.

One might well have willed one's body for scientific purposes, but such legacies had no legal standing. Until recently, the individual lost control over his body once he died. This has been changed by the Uniform Anatomical Gift Act. This model piece of legislation, adopted by all fifty states in an incredibly short period of time, grants anyone over eighteen (twenty-one in some states) the right to donate en masse all "necessary organs and tissues" simply by filling out and mailing a small card.

Beyond the postmortem, there has been a longer-range use of human bodies that is accepted procedure—the exploitation of cadavers as teaching material in medical schools. This is a long step removed from the rationale of the transplant—a dramatic gift of life from the dying to the near dead; while it is true that medical education will inevitably save lives the clear and immediate purpose of the donation is to facilitate training.

It is not unnatural for a person facing death to want his usefulness to extend beyond his mortality; the same biases and values that influence our life persist in our leaving of it. It has been reported that the Harvard Medical School has no difficulty in receiving as many donations of cadavers as they need, while Tufts and Boston Universities are usually in short supply. In Boston, evidently, the cachet of getting into Harvard extends even to the dissecting table.

The way is now clear for an ever-increasing pool of usable body parts, but the current practice minimizes efficiency and maximizes waste. Only a short period exists between the time of death of the patient and the time of death of his major parts.

USES OF THE NEOMORT

In the ensuing discussion, the word *cadaver* will retain its usual meaning, as opposed to the new cadaver, which will be referred to as a *neomort*. The "ward" or "hospital" in which it is maintained will be called a *bioemporium* (purists may prefer *bioemporion*).

Whatever is possible with the old embalmed cadaver is extended to an incredible degree with the neomort. What follows, therefore, is not a definitive list but merely the briefest of suggestions as to the spectrum of possibilities.

Training Uneasy medical students could practice routine physical examinations—auscultation, percussion of the chest, examination of the retina, rectal and vaginal examinations, et cetera—indeed, everything except neurological examinations, since the neomort by definition has no functioning central nervous system.

Both the student and his patient could be spared the pain, fumbling, and embarrassment of the "first time."

Interns also could practice standard and more difficult diagnostic procedures, from spinal taps to pneumoencephalography and the making of arteriograms, and residents could practice almost all of their surgical skills—in other words, most of the procedures that are now normally taught with the indigent in wards of major city hospitals could be taught with neomorts. Further, students could practice more exotic procedures often not available in a typical residency—eye operations, skin grafts, plastic facial surgery, amputation of useless limbs, coronary surgery, etc.; they could also practice the actual removal of organs, whether they be kidneys, testicles, or what have you, for delivery to the transplant teams.

Testing The neomort could be used for much of the testing of drugs and surgical procedures that we now normally perform on prisoners, mentally retarded children, and volunteers. The efficacy of a drug as well as its toxicity could be determined beyond limits we might not have dared approach when we were concerned about permanent damage to the testing vehicle, a living person. For example, operations for increased vascularization of the heart could be tested to determine whether they truly do reduce the incidence of future heart attack before we perform them on patients. Experimental procedures that proved useless or harmful could be avoided; those that succeed could be available years before they might otherwise have been. Similarly, we could avoid the massive delays that keep some drugs from the marketplace while the dying clamor for them.

Neomorts would give us access to other forms of testing that are inconceivable with the living human being. We might test diagnostic instruments such as sophisticated electrocardiography by selectively damaging various parts of the heart to see how or whether the instrument could detect the damage.

Experimentation Every new medical procedure demands a leap of faith. It is often referred to as an "act of courage," which seems to me an inappropriate terminology now that organized medicine rarely uses itself as the experimental body. Whenever a surgeon attempts a procedure for the first time, he is at best generalizing from experimentation with lower animals. Now we can protect the patient from too large a leap by using the neomort as an experimental bridge.

Obvious forms of experimentation would be cures for illnesses which would first be induced in the neomort. We could test antidotes by injecting poison, induce cancer or virus infections to validate and compare developing therapies.

Because they have an active hematopoietic system, neomorts would be particularly valuable for studying diseases of the blood. Many of the examples that I draw from that field were offered to me by Dr. John F. Bertles, a hematologist at St. Luke's Hospital Center in New York. One which interests him is the utilization of marrow transplants. Few human–to–human marrow transplants have been successful, . . . the kind of immunosuppression techniques that require research could most safely be performed on neomorts. Even such research as the recent experimentation at Willowbrook—where mentally retarded children were infected with hepatitis virus (which was not yet culturable outside of the human body) in an attempt to find a cure for this pernicious disease—could be done without risking the health of the subjects.

Banking While certain essential blood antigens are readily storable (e.g., red cells can now be preserved in a frozen state), others are not, and there is increasing need for potential means of storage. Research on storage of platelets to be used in transfusion requires human recipients, and the data are only slowly and tediously gathered at great expense. Use of neomorts would permit intensive testing of platelet survival and probably would lead to a rapid development of a better storage technique. The same would be true for white cells.

As has been suggested, there is great wastage in the present system of using kidney donors from cadavers. Major organs are difficult to store. A population of neomorts maintained with body parts computerized and catalogued for compatibility would yield a much more efficient system. Just as we now have blood banks, . . . we could have banks for all the major organs that may someday be transplantable—lungs, kidney, heart, ovaries. Beyond the obvious storage uses of the neomort, there are others not previously thought of because there was no adequate storage facility. Dr. Marc Lappe of the Hastings Center has suggested that a neomort whose own immunity system had first been severely repressed might be an ideal "culture" for growing and storing our lymphoid components. When we are threatened by malignancy or viral disease, we can go to the "bank" and withdraw our stored white cells to help defend us.

Harvesting Obviously, a sizable population of neomorts will provide a steady supply of blood, since they can be drained periodically. When we consider the cost-benefit analysis of this system, we would have to evaluate it in the same way as the lumber industry evaluates sawdust—a product which in itself is not commercially feasible but which supplies a profitable dividend as a waste from a more useful harvest.

The blood would be a simultaneous source of platelets, leukocytes, and red cells. By attaching a neomort to an IBM cell separator, we could isolate cell types at relatively low cost. The neomort could also be tested for the presence of hepatitis in a way that would be impossible with commercial donors. Hepatitis as a transfusion scourge would be virtually eliminated.

Beyond the blood are rarer harvests. Neomorts offer a great potential source of bone marrow for transplant procedures, and I am assured that a bioemporium of modest size could be assembled to fit most transplantation antigen requirements. And skin would, of course, be harvested—similarly bone, corneas, cartilage, and so on.

Manufacturing In addition to supplying components of the human body, some of which will be continually regenerated, the neomort can also serve as a manufacturing unit. Hormones are one obvious product, but there are others. By the injection of toxins, we have a source of antitoxin that does not have the complication of coming from another animal form. Antibodies for most of the major diseases can be manufactured merely by injecting the neomort with the viral or bacterial offenders.

Perhaps the most encouraging extension of the manufacturing process emerges from the new cancer research, in which immunology is coming to the fore. With certain blood cancers, great hope attaches to the use of antibodies. To take just one example, it is conceivable that leukemia could be generated in individual neomorts—not just to provide for *in vivo* (so to speak) testing of anti-leukemic modes of therapy but also to generate antibody immunity responses which could then be used in the living.

COST-BENEFIT ANALYSIS

If seen only as the harvesting of products, the entire feasibility of such research would depend on intelligent cost-benefit analysis. Although certain products would not warrant the expense of maintaining a community of neomorts, the enormous expense of other products, such as red cells with unusual antigens, would certainly warrant it. Then, of course, the equation is shifted. As soon as one economically sound reason is found for the maintenance of the community, all of the other ingredients become gratuitous by-products, a familiar problem in manufacturing. There is no current research to indicate the maintenance cost of a bioemporium or even the potential duration of an average neomort. Since we do not at this point encourage sustaining life in the brain-dead, we do not know the limits to which it could be extended. This is the kind of technology, however, in which we have previously been quite successful.

Meantime, a further refinement of death might be proposed. At present we use total brain function to define brain death. The source of electroencephalogram activity is not known and cannot be used to distinguish between the activity of higher and lower brain centers. If, however, we are prepared to separate the concept of "aliveness" from "personhood" in the adult, as we have in the fetus, a good argument can be made that death should be defined not as cessation of total brain function but merely as cessation of cortical function. New tests may soon determine when cortical function is dead. With this proposed extension, one could then maintain neomorts without even the complication and expense of respirators. The entire population of decorticates residing in chronic hospitals and now classified among the incurably ill could be redefined as dead.

But even if we maintained the more rigid limitations of total brain death it would seem that a reasonable population could be maintained if the purposes warranted it. It is difficult to assess how many new neomorts would be available each year to satisfy the demand. There are roughly 2 million deaths a year in the United States. The most likely sources of intact bodies with destroyed brains would be accidents (about 113,000 per year), suicides (around 24,000 per year), homicides (18,000), and cerebrovascular accidents (some 210,000 per year). Obviously, in each of these categories a great many of the individuals would be useless—their bodies either shattered or scattered beyond value or repair.

And yet, after all the benefits are outlined, with the lifesaving potential clear, the humanitarian purposes obvious, the technology ready, the motives pure, and the material costs justified—how are we to reconcile our emotions? Where in this debit-credit ledger of limbs and livers and kidneys and costs are we to weigh and enter the repugnance generated by the entire philanthropic endeavor?

Cost-benefit analysis is always least satisfactory when the costs must be measured in one realm and the benefits in another. The analysis is particularly skewed when the benefits are specific, material, apparent, and immediate, and the price to be paid is general, spiritual, abstract, and of the future. It is that which induces people to abandon freedom for security, pride for comfort, dignity for dollars.

William May, in a perceptive article,[2] defended the careful distinctions that have traditionally been drawn between the newly dead and the long dead. "While the body retains its recognizable form, even in death, it commands a certain respect. No longer a human presence, it still reminds us of that presence which once was utterly inseparable from it." But those distinctions become obscured when, years later, a neomort will retain the appearance of the newly dead, indeed, more the appearance of that which was formerly described as living.

Philosophers tend to be particularly sensitive to the abstract needs of civilized man; it is they who have often been the guardians of values whose abandonment produces pains that are real, if not always quantifiable. Hans Jonas, in his *Philosophical Essays*, anticipated some of the possibilities outlined here, and defended what he felt to be the sanctity of the human body and the unknowability of the borderline between life and death when he insisted that "Nothing less than the maximum definition of death will do—brain death plus heart

---

[2]"Attitudes Toward the Newly Dead," *The Hastings Center Studies*, volume 1, number 1, 1973.

death plus any other indication that may be pertinent—before final violence is allowed to be done." And even then Jonas was only contemplating *temporary* maintenance of life for the collection of organs.

The argument can be made on both sides. The unquestionable benefits to be gained are the promise of cures for leukemia and other diseases, the reduction of suffering, and the maintenance of life. The proponents of this view will be mobilized with a force that may seem irresistible.

They will interpret our revulsion at the thought of a bioemporium as a bias of our education and experience, just as earlier societies were probably revolted by the startling notion of abdominal surgery, which we now take for granted. The proponents will argue that the revulsion, not the technology, is inappropriate.

Still there will be those, like May, who will defend that revulsion as a quintessentially human factor whose removal would diminish us all, and extract a price we cannot anticipate in ways yet unknown and times not yet determined. May feels that there is "a tinge of the inhuman in the humanitarianism of those who believe that the perception of social need easily overrides all other considerations and reduces the acts of implementation to the everyday, routine, and casual."

This is the kind of weighing of values for which the computer offers little help. Is the revulsion to the new technology simply the fear and horror of the ignorant in the face of the new, or is it one of those components of humanness that barely sustain us at the limited level of civility and decency that now exists, and whose removal is one more step in erasing the distinction between man and the lesser creatures—beyond that, the distinction between man and matter?

Sustaining life is an urgent argument for any measure, but not if that measure destroys those very qualities that make life worth living.

SUICIDE

Contents

ORDINARILY, WE TEND TO THINK OF DEATH as a biological or adventitious event. Suicide falls outside that pattern, and for that reason it is generally the most enigmatic of all modes of death. In the last 25 years, there has been a great expansion of interest and effort in suicide prevention; the number of books and articles written about suicide has increased enormously and a whole new field of specialization—suicidology—has arisen. Numerous suicide prevention centers have been established. But still, suicide is a ubiquitous and intransigent issue and suicidal deaths remain the most cryptic of all.

The first article in Part VIII is by the nineteenth-century French sociologist Émile Durkheim. This article illustrates the type of sociological explanations he advocated. His method of analysis and his techniques for doing sociological research played an important role in the emergence of sociology as a distinct discipline. In his 1897 book, *Le Suicide,* Durkheim discusses four different kinds of suicide. In this selection, he deals with only one form: what he calls egoistic suicide (the others were fatalistic suicide, anomic suicide, and altruistic suicide). Egoistic suicide, according to Durkheim, is caused by a lack of social integration into society. He argues that suicide rates vary inversely with the degree of social integration of society in the religious sphere (e.g., being Catholic as opposed to Protestant), the domestic sphere (e.g., being married as opposed to being single), and the political sphere (e.g., being at war as opposed to being at peace).

The article by McIntosh is a contemporary example of research on suicide in the Durkheimian tradition. It is based on aggregate data and it makes use of demographic categories to account for variations in suicide rates. This article presents data with respect to trends in suicide rates for various demographically-defined segments of the population. When discussing this article it would make sense to spend some time considering the debate about the reliability and validity of data on suicide rates, potential sources of bias, and the consequences of change in the ways in which decisions are made as to whether or not to classify certain categories of deaths as suicides.

The article by Stillion and McDowell presents a useful model for the analysis of the various different types of factors that, together, contribute to suicidal behavior. Their model makes use of causative (or risk) factors that they group into four broad categories: biological, psychological, cognitive, and environmental. They believe that these four categories of risk factors contribute to the level of suicidal ideation, which in turn may lead directly to suicidal behavior or to the triggering events and warning signs that generally precede suicidal behavior.

The selection by Shneidman represents an effort to distill into a short article what he views as the primary cause of suicide, psychological pain. He argues that the main single cause of suicide is psychache. The focus of the article is on showing how this explanation differs from other less-focused approaches. His explanation, with its emphasis on the hurt, anguish, and psychological pain that he calls psychache, can be distinguished from explanations that emphasize sociological categories (e.g., gender, age) or psychiatric categories (e.g., depression, schizophrenia, alcoholism, etc.). Why do some people who experience psychache commit suicide and others do not? He argues that an important factor is differences between individuals in their thresholds for tolerating the psychological pain associated with life.

31 Egoistic Suicide ❦

Émile Durkheim

ÉMILE DURKHEIM (1858–1917) is one of the founding fathers of sociology. In 1897 he published one of his most important books, *Le Suicide* (*Suicide*). This book presents one of the first modern examples of the use of the statistical method in social research. His other major books include *The Elementary Forms of the Religious Life, Division of Labor in Society*, and *The Rules of the Sociological Methods*. The selection included here is from the section of *Le Suicide* that deals with "egoistic" suicide, one of several different types of suicide that Durkheim discusses in this book. It illustrates a mode of empirical analysis that has influenced many researchers over the decades since his death. Empirical studies of suicide in the Durkheimian tradition continue to be influential today.

OF ALL THE GREAT STATES OF GERMANY, Bavaria has by far the fewest suicides. There have been barely 90 per million inhabitants yearly since 1874, while Prussia has 133 (1871–75), the duchy of Baden 156, Wurttemberg 162, Saxony 300. Now, Bavaria also has most Catholics, 713.2 to 1,000 inhabitants. On the other hand, if one compares the different provinces of Bavaria, suicides are found to be in direct proportion to the number of Protestants and in inverse proportion to that of Catholics (See Table 1). Not only the proportions of averages to one another confirm the law but all the numbers of the first column are higher than those of the second and those of the second higher than those of the third without exception.

It is the same with Prussia (See Table 2).

There are only two slight irregularities among the 14 provinces thus compared, so far as detail is concerned; Silesia, which because of its relatively high number of suicides should be in the second category, is only in the third, while on the contrary Pomerania would be more in its place in the second than in the first column.

Switzerland forms an interesting study from this same point of view. For as both French and German populations exist there, the influence of the confession is observable separately on each race. Now, its influence is the same on

Table 1 Bavarian Provinces (1867–75)*

Provinces w. Catholic Minority (less than 50%)	Suicides Per Million Inhabitants	Provinces w. Catholic Majority (50 to 90%)	Suicides Per Million Inhabitants	Provinces w. More Than 90% Catholic	Suicides Per Million Inhabitants
Rhenish Palatinate	167	Lower Franconia	157	Upper Palatinate	64
Central Franconia	207	Swabia	118	Upper Bavaria	114
Upper Franconia	204			Lower Bavaria	19
Average	192	Average	135	Average	75

* The population below 15 years has been omitted.

both. Catholic cantons show four and five times fewer suicides than Protestant, of whichever nationality (See Table 3).

Confessional influence is therefore so great as to dominate all others. . . .

But if religion preserves men from suicide only because and in so far as it is a society, other societies probably have the same effect. From this point of view let us consider the family and political society.

If one consults only the absolute figures, unmarried persons seem to commit suicide less than married ones. Thus in France, during the period 1873–78, there were 16,264 suicides of married persons while unmarried persons had only 11,709. The former number is to the second as 132 to 100.[1] As the same proportion appears at other periods and in other countries, certain authors had once taught that marriage and family life multiply the chances of suicide. Certainly, if in accordance with current opinion one regards suicide primarily as an act of despair caused by the difficulties of existence, this opinion has all the appearance of probability. An unmarried person has in fact an easier life than a married one. Does not marriage entail all sorts of burdens and responsibilities? To assure the present and future of a family, are not more privations and sufferings required than to meet the needs of a single person?[2] Nevertheless, clear as it seems, this a priori reasoning is quite false and the facts only seem to support it because of being poorly analyzed. . . .

Really to appreciate the figures given in Table 3, we must remember that a very large number of unmarried persons are less than 16 years old, while all married persons are older. Up to 16 years the tendency to suicide is very slight,

[1] Durkheim's figure of 132 appears to be a misprint. The figure works out to 139.—Ed.
[2] See Wagner. Die Gesetzmässigkeit, etc., p. 177.

TABLE 2 Prussian Provinces (1883–90)

Provinces with More Than 90% Protestant	Suicides Per Million Inhabitants	Provinces with from 89 to 68% Protestant	Suicides Per Million Inhabitants
Saxony	309.4	Hanover	212.3
Schleswig	312.9	Hesse	200.3
		Bradenburg and Berlin	296.3
Pomerania	171.5		
		E. Prussia	171.3
Average	264.6	Average	220.0

Provinces with from 40 to 50% Protestant	Suicides Per Million Inhabitants	Provinces with from 32 to 28% Protestant	Suicides Per Million Inhabitants
W. Prussia	123.9	Posen	96.4
Silesia	260.2	Rhineland	100.3
Westphalia	107.5	Hohenzollern	90.1
Average	163.6	Average	95.6

due to age, without considering other factors. In France only one or two suicides per million inhabitants are found at this time of life; at the following period there are twenty times as many. The inclusion of many children below 16 among unmarried persons thus unduly reduces the average aptitude of the latter, since the reduction is due to age, not celibacy. If they seem to contribute fewer suicides, it is not because they are unmarried but because many of them are yet immature. So, if one tries to compare the two populations to determine the influence of marital status and that alone, one must rid oneself of this disturbing element and compare with married persons only the unmarried above 16. When this subtraction is made, it appears that between 1863–68 there were on the average 173 suicides in a million unmarried persons above 16 years and 154.5 for a million married persons. The ratio of the first to the second number is that of 112 to 100. . . .

Great political upheavals are sometimes said to increase the number of suicides. But Morselli has conclusively shown that facts contradict this view. All the revolutions which have occurred in France during this century reduced the number of suicides at the moment of their occurrence. In 1830, the total fell to 1,756 from 1,904 in 1829, amounting to a sudden drop of nearly 10 per cent. In 1848 the drop is no less; the annual figure changes from 3,647 to 3,301. Then,

Table 3

French Cantons		German Cantons		Total of Cantons of All Nationalities	
Catholics	83 suicides per million inhabitants	Catholics	87 suicides	Catholics	86.7 suicides
				Mixed	212.0 suicides
Protestants	453 suicides per million	Protestants	293 suicides	Protestants	326.3 suicides

during the years 1848–49, the crisis which has just shaken France spreads through Europe; everywhere suicides decrease, and this decrease is more and more perceptible the more serious and prolonged the crisis. This appears in the following table:

	Denmark	Prussia	Bavaria	Kingdom of Saxony	Austria
1847	345	1,852	217	—	611 (in 1846)
1848	305	1,649	215	398	—
1849	337	1,527	189	328	452

In Germany public feeling ran much higher than in Denmark and the struggle lasted longer even than in France, where a new government was immediately formed; accordingly, the decrease is prolonged in the German states up to 1849. For that year, the decrease is 13 per cent in Bavaria, 18 per cent in Prussia; in Saxony, in a single year from 1848 to 1849, it is likewise 18 per cent. . . .

Great national wars have the same effect as political disturbances. In 1866 war breaks out between Austria and Italy, and suicides drop 14 per cent in both countries.

	1865	1866	1867
Italy	678	588	657
Austria	1,464	1,265	1,407

In 1864 it was the turn of Denmark and Saxony. In the latter state suicides, which numbered 643 in 1863, fell to 545 in 1864 (16 per cent), only to return to

619 in 1865. As to Denmark, since we do not know the number of suicides for 1863, we cannot compare that of 1864 with it; but we do know that the figure for the second year (411) is the lowest since 1852. And as there is a rise to 451 in 1865, this figure of 411 very probably betokens a considerable drop.

The war of 1870–1871 had the same results in France and Germany:

	1869	1870	1871	1872
Prussia	3,186	2,963	2,723	2,950
Saxony	710	657	653	687
France	5,114	4,157	4,490	5,275

This decrease might perhaps be considered due to the drafting of a part of the civilian population in war-time and the fact that it is very hard to keep track of suicides in an army in the field. But women as well as men contribute to this decrease. . . .

We have thus successively set up the three following propositions:

Suicide varies inversely with the degree of integration of religious
    society.
Suicide varies inversely with the degree of integration of domestic
    society.
Suicide varies inversely with the degree of integration of political society.

This grouping shows that whereas these different societies have a moderating influence upon suicide, this is due not to special characteristics of each but to a characteristic common to all. Religion does not owe its efficacy to the special nature of religious sentiments, since domestic and political societies both produce the same effects when strongly integrated. This, moreover, we have already proved when studying directly the manner of action of different religions upon suicide. Inversely, it is not the specific nature of the domestic or political tie which can explain the immunity they confer, since religious society has the same advantage. The cause can only be found in a single quality possessed by all these social groups, though perhaps to varying degrees. The only quality satisfying this condition is that they are all strongly integrated social groups. So we reach the general conclusion: suicide varies inversely with the degree of integration of the social groups of which the individual forms a part.

But society cannot disintegrate without the individual simultaneously detaching himself from social life, without his own goals becoming preponderant over those of the community, in a word without his personality tending to surmount the collective personality. The more weakened the groups to which he belongs, the less he depends on them, the more he consequently depends only on himself and recognizes no other rules of conduct that what are founded on his private interests. If we agree to call this state egoism, in which the individual ego asserts itself to excess in the face of the social ego and at its expense, we may call egoistic the special type of suicide springing from excessive individualism.

But how can suicide have such an origin?

First of all, it can be said that, as collective force is one of the obstacles best calculated to restrain suicide, its weakening involves a development of suicide. When society is strongly integrated, it holds individuals under its control, considers them at its service and thus forbids them to dispose wilfully of themselves. Accordingly it opposes their evading their duties to it through death. But how could society impose its supremacy upon them when they refuse to accept this subordination as legitimate? It no longer then possesses the requisite authority to retain them in their duty if they wish to desert; and conscious of its own weakness, it even recognizes their right to do freely what it can no longer prevent. So far as they are the admitted masters of their destinies, it is their privilege to end their lives. They, on their part, have no reason to endure life's sufferings patiently. For they cling to life more resolutely when belonging to a group they love, so as not to betray interests they put before their own. The bond that unites them with the common cause attaches them to life and the lofty goal they envisage prevents their feeling personal troubles so deeply. There is, in short, in a cohesive and animated society a constant interchange of ideas and feelings from all to each and each to all, something like a mutual moral support, which instead of throwing the individual on his own resources, leads him to share in the collective energy and supports his own when exhausted.

But these reasons are purely secondary. Excessive individualism not only results in favoring the action of suicidogenic causes, but it is itself such a cause. It not only frees man's inclination to do away with himself from a protective obstacle, but creates this inclination out of whole cloth and thus gives birth to a special suicide which bears its mark. This must be clearly understood for this is what constitutes the special character of the type of suicide just distinguished and justifies the name we have given it. What is there then in individualism that explains this result?

It has been sometimes said that because of his psychological constitution, man cannot live without attachment to some object which transcends and survives him, and that the reason for this necessity is a need we must have not to perish entirely. Life is said to be intolerable unless some reason for existing is involved, some purpose justifying life's trials. The individual alone is not a sufficient end for his activity. He is too little. He is not only hemmed in spatially; he is also strictly limited temporally. When, therefore, we have no other object than ourselves we cannot avoid the thought that our efforts will finally end in nothingness, since we ourselves disappear. But annihilation terrifies us. Under these conditions one would lose courage to live, that is, to act and struggle, since nothing will remain of our exertions. The state of egoism, in other words, is supposed to be contradictory to human nature and, consequently, too uncertain to have chances of permanence.

32 Epidemiology of Suicide in the United States

John L. McIntosh

JOHN MCINTOSH is professor of psychology at Indiana University at South Bend. He is author, co-author, or co-editor of several books on suicide, including *Suicide and Its Aftermath*, *Suicide and the Older Adult*, and *Elder Suicide*. He is past president of the American Association of Suicidology. This article is an example of a contemporary study in the Durkheimian tradition. It presents an overview of major demographic factors linked to differences in suicide rates and, over time, trends in these rates. McIntosh considers differences based on gender, race, ethnicity, age, marital status, time of year, and day of week.

AN AMERICAN DIES BY HIS OR HER OWN HAND on the average of every 17 minutes (1986, data calculated from figures in National Center for Health Statistics [NCHS]; 1988a) or approximately 85 self-inflicted deaths per day. The more than 30,000 suicides in 1986 (30,904) represent a rate of 12.8 per 100,000 population. In other words, if a representative sample of 100,000 Americans had been chosen on January 1 of 1986 and followed through the year, by the end of the day on December 31 about 12 or 13 would have died by suicide. This number of deaths places suicide currently as the eighth leading cause of death in the United States. The present chapter will focus on the epidemiological factors associated with these 30,000 annual suicide deaths.

Trends in suicide rates for the United States indicate increases over the last several decades (see Figure 1). These increases have been slight, however. As observed for most cultures, suicide rates tend to remain somewhat stable over time. . . . The United States ranks among those cultures with moderate levels of suicide, and this has not changed over time. Although the number of suicides has steadily increased (see bottom of Figure 1), the change in number has only slightly outpaced increases in the number of individuals in the country.

Suicide, the fatal self-inflicted act, is only one dimension of the entire spectrum of self-destructive behaviors. It is conservatively estimated that in addi-

From John L. McIntosh, 1991. "Epidemiology of Suicide in the United States." Pp. 55–69 in *Life Span Perspectives of Suicide*, edited by Antoon A. Leenaars. Copyright © 1991 by Plenum Publishing Corporation. Reprinted by permission.

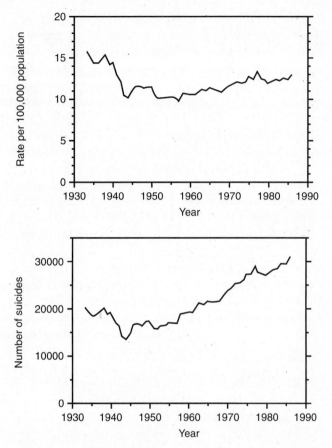

FIGURE 1 U.S. suicide rates and number of suicides,
1933 to 1986.

tion to the deaths occurring each year there are at least 600,000 nonfatal suicide attempts or "parasuicides" ("suicide-like") in the United States. Furthermore, the loved ones of those who die by their own hand, individuals called "suicide survivors," also pay a heavy emotional toll in altered grief and bereavement processes. Although these two groups (attempters and survivors) are also immensely important in the total picture of suicidal behavior and in their own right (e.g., Dunne, McIntosh & Dunne-Maxim, 1987; Kreitman, 1977), this chapter will focus on the epidemiology (i.e., characteristics, levels, and trends) of those whose deaths are by suicide.

Before proceeding to the major demographic factors associated with elevated suicide risk, it is important to realize that the figures discussed thus far and in the information to follow are derived from official statistics for suicide mortality. This means that the numbers and rates presented result from the compilation (by the NCHS) of individual deaths for which the official cause of death was designated as suicide. Only in the case of this definitive classification would the death be included in the official statistics reported by NCHS in its many reports and annual volumes of *Vital Statistics of the United States*.

Official statistics have a longstanding history in the study of suicide, including most famously the classic work of sociologist Émile Durkheim (1897/1951). This long history notwithstanding, these official data have frequently been criticized and questioned as indices of the actual levels and number of suicides that occur (Atkinson, 1978, Chapter 3; Douglas, 1967, Chapter 12; Lester, 1972). Among the criticisms that have been leveled against the accuracy of official suicide data are bias and stigma resulting in underreporting and even blatant and intentional misclassification; variability in classification depending on several factors such as the training of the medical examiner or coroner, the use of different definitions, or the lack of a clear, generally accepted definition of suicide.

These and other criticisms and shortcomings of official figures should be taken seriously such that the consumer of suicide data realizes that numbers and rates are imperfect. At the same time, although the imperfect nature of suicide data has been generally accepted, others (e.g., Sainsbury & Barraclough, 1968; Sainsbury & Jenkins, 1982) have argued that the bias so often attributed to suicide classifications may not be as great as claimed. In any event, official suicide statistics are the most reliably and consistently maintained indices of suicide levels, trends, and high-risk factors that exist. If properly recognized as an indication of the most conservative estimates of actual suicide occurrence (Allen, 1984), they provide a useful index of the extent to which suicide is a mental health problem within a particular culture and its subgroups.

MAJOR DEMOGRAPHIC FACTORS IN SUICIDE

Within its large literature (e.g., Farberow, 1972; McIntosh, 1985a), suicide has been studied in association with a large number of factors. Many of these factors have proven unreliable or the data or methodologies associated with them have been poor (e.g., weather conditions, time of day, occupations, socioeconomic levels, etc.). This chapter will focus on the major factors for which U.S. data are both consistent and more reliable. Such factors are most often derived from the official mortality data (and the death certificates from which they are taken) mentioned above and include: sex/gender, race/ethnicity, age, marital status, temporal factors (day of week, monthly visitations), geographic differences (states, regions), and the method employed in the suicide. Official statistics, on which this presentation will rely, are published after data collection and reliability checks have been made that necessitate a time-lag. Generally, official suicide figures are available for the United States from NCHS that are approx-

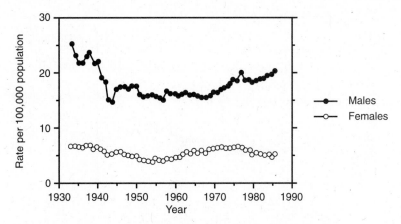

FIGURE 2 U.S. male and female suicide rates, 1933 to 1986.

imately 2 to 3 years old. Thus, until approximately September of 1989, the most current suicide data available are for the year 1986 (NCHS, 1988a,b).

Sex/Gender

One of the single most important factors with respect to suicide is the sex or gender of the individual. Males as a group kill themselves more than three times more often than do females both in numbers as well as for rates. For example, in 1986 there were on the average 66 male and 18 female suicides each day. In that same year the male rate of suicide was 20.6 per 100,000 population compared to 5.4 for females (a ratio of 3.8). The number of male suicides was 24,226 whereas for females the figure was 6,678 (a ratio of 3.6). Predictions in recent years (e.g., Neuringer, 1982) have suggested that because of the women's movement, increased numbers of women in the work force, and increased stress for women, female suicide rates would increase and become closer to those for males. In reality, however, differences between the sexes have actually *increased* rather than decreased since the early 1970s (e.g., McIntosh & Jewell, 1986; Steffensmeier, 1984). There was a slight tendency toward decreased differences during the 1960s, but the rates were at their closest ratio in 1971 at 2.46. Since that time female rates have been either stable or displayed a slight tendency toward decline whereas male rates have increased (see Figure 2).

Race/Ethnicity

Race Suicide, as measured by either rates or numbers, is a white phenomenon when compared to nonwhites as a whole. For example, whites committed 28,347 of the 1986 suicides for a rate of 13.9 per 100,000 population. By contrast, nonwhites accounted for 2,467 suicides for a rate of 6.7 (a ratio of 2.1 for

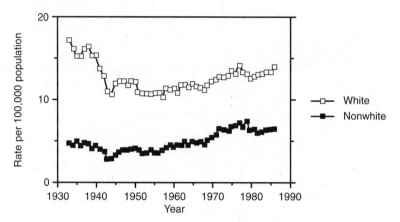

FIGURE 3 U.S. white versus nonwhite suicide rates, 1933 to 1986.

rates). On an average day in 1986, 78 whites and 7 nonwhites died by their own hand. Although some suggestions of increases in nonwhite races of suicide and a lessening of racial differences in suicide have been made, the data show no real change in this white predominance (e.g., McIntosh, 1989) (see Figure 3).

When considering race and sex, males are at highest risk within each racial grouping. In 1986 white males had a suicide rate of 22.3 while white females' rate was 5.9. Among nonwhites the rates were 11.1 and 2.7 for males and females, respectively. As can be seen, overall racial differences of 2:1 (white:nonwhite) are consistent for both males and females. Clearly the group at highest risk therefore is white males and the lowest risk is among nonwhite females.

Ethnicity Little attention has been given to ethnic differences in suicide other than among blacks and Native Americans (American Indians). There is evidence, however, that there is tremendous diversity among the various ethnic groups that comprise the nonwhite as a whole population. It is likely that some differences would also exist among white ethnic groups if data were available, but presently only partial data (only 18 states report such data) for Hispanics (who may be of any race but are most often white) are available. Rates of suicide are not available annually for the specific ethnic groups in the United States, but in 1986 blacks accounted for 1,892 of the 2,467 nonwhite suicides while Native Americans, Chinese-Americans, Japanese-Americans, Filipino-Americans, and other Asian or Pacific Islanders committed 218, 65, 81, 36, and 173 suicides, respectively. McIntosh (1985b, 1986, 1987a) reported age-adjusted suicide rates for these groups for the years 1979 to 1981. Age-adjusted suicide rates control for the differences in the distributions of the populations of the groups by age. McIntosh found that the highest rates were among Native Americans (18.1), followed by whites (16.7), Hispanics from 10 south-

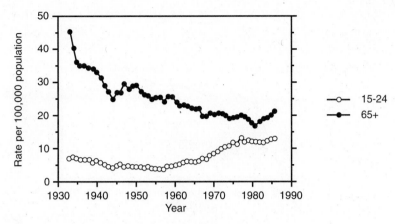

FIGURE 4 Suicide among U.S. young (15–24) and old (65+),
1933 to 1986.

western, midwestern, and eastern states (10.8), Japanese-Americans (10.7), Chinese-Americans (10.6), blacks (9.0), and Filipino-Americans (4.9).

Age

Suicide rates have shown increases with increasing age for as long as U.S. figures have been kept (and indeed in many other cultures as well). There have been two major trends in suicide rates by age that have slightly altered that characterization, however (see Figure 4). First, as highly publicized, there has been an increase in suicide rates among the young. Although the media and research literature have focused on the 15 to 24 age group, these increases have been seen for all age groups younger than 45 years of age. Among 15- to 24-year-olds there has been an increase of approximately 200% from the mid-1950s to the early 1980s. For example, in 1953 the suicide rate for those 15 to 24 was 4.4 compared to 13.1 in 1986 (an increase of 198%).

The second major trend with respect to age and suicide has been the decline in suicide among all age groups older than 45 and especially those older than age 65. This trend has received far less attention but for the elderly has occurred over a longer time period and has been as dramatic as the youth increases, simply in the opposite direction. For instance, suicide rates for those 65 and older were 45.3 per 100,000 population in 1933, declined to 26.2 for 1953, and to 21.5 in 1986. The decline from 1933 to 1986 has therefore been 52%. Despite these large declines, however, the suicide rate for older adults remains at a level more than 50% above those for the 15 to 24 age group (21.5 vs. 13.1 in 1986).

There are reasons then to target both the young and old as high risks for suicide. Among the young we see (1) a pattern of increased suicide risk over the last several decades (even though a slowing in this trend may have already oc-

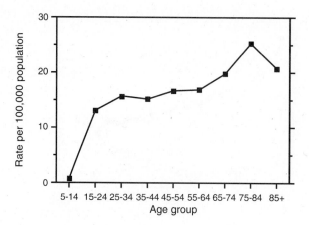

FIGURE 5   U.S. suicide rates by age groups, 1986.

curred and declines are predicted to continue until the mid-1990s, e.g., [Holinger, Offer, & Zola, 1988]) to levels greatly elevated over earlier times and currently at levels similar to those for the nation as a whole, (2) suicide is a higher ranking cause of death than for any other age group or the nation as a whole (3rd in 1986 behind accidents and homicide compared to 13th for those 65 and older), (3) suicide accounts for a much higher proportion of deaths than in the nation as a whole and other age groups (suicides were 12.8% of deaths for those 15–24 in 1986 compared to 1.5% in the nation as a whole and 0.4% for those 65 years of age and older), and (4) there annually have been more than 5,000 young people 15 to 24 years of age who officially committed suicide (5,120 in 1986 and an additional 255 younger than the age of 15).

Among the elderly, on the other hand, although suicide ranks relatively low among the many causes from which older adults die and represents a much smaller proportion of deaths compared to young people, there are several reasons that demand attention to the phenomenon of elderly suicide. Despite long-term declines in elderly suicide (1) suicide rates for older adults have increased each year through 1986 from their lowest point ever recorded in 1981 (from 17.1 to 21.5, respectively; an increase of 25.7%), (2) several writers have predicted long-term increases in elderly suicide (e.g., Manton, Blazer, & Woodbury, 1987; Pollinger-Haas & Hendin, 1983), (3) the elderly remain the highest risk group for suicide by age, and (4) the elderly commit greater proportions of the suicides than their proportion in the population (20.3% of suicides and 12.1% of the U.S. population, U.S. Bureau of the Census, 1988, compared to 16.2% and 16.6%, respectively, for those 15–24 years of age).

The net result of these two trends in suicide rates is a slight tendency toward characterizing the U.S. rates by age as bimodal. That is, suicide rates increase with age reaching an early life peak followed by slight decreases in successive age groups and an increase again to a second, highest peak after age

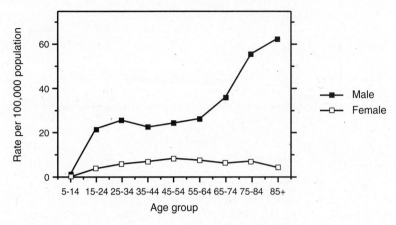

FIGURE 6 U.S. suicide rates by age and gender, 1986.

65 (see Figure 5). Although still not pronounced, this bimodal pattern in U.S. suicide is perhaps closer to characterizing current U.S. rates by age than is the earlier unimodal pattern with rates strictly increasing with age to a peak in older adulthood.

The factor of sex is also important when looking at suicide risk and age. Male suicide rates follow the increases with age (or more recent bimodal pattern) described above at even higher rates than for the nation as a whole (see Figure 6). Female rates, on the other hand, increase with advancing age until "middle age" (the mid-40s to mid-50s) and then decline thereafter in older age groups. Therefore, after age 65 male and female suicide rates are most divergent because male rates continue to increase in old age whereas female rates decline throughout older adulthood. The smallest differences between the sexes across the life span are in middle age when female rates reach their peak.

The age characterization of suicide as increasing with age and peaking in old age is particularly true when white suicide is studied (as well as among Chinese-, Japanese-, and Filipino-Americans) (see Figure 7). Among non-whites as a whole, however, and particularly blacks, Native Americans, and Hispanics, suicide rates are highest in young adulthood and decline to low levels in old age (e.g., McIntosh, 1985b, 1986, 1987a; McIntosh & Santos, 1981).

Marital Status

The majority of suicides occur among the married population. However, when taking into account the number of individuals in this group within the total population (i.e., by calculating suicide rates), the married are actually the lowest risk group for suicide. For example, in 1986 the married committed 13,526 of the 30,637 suicides above the age of 15. Those who were single and never married represented 8,921 suicides followed by 5,049 for the divorced,

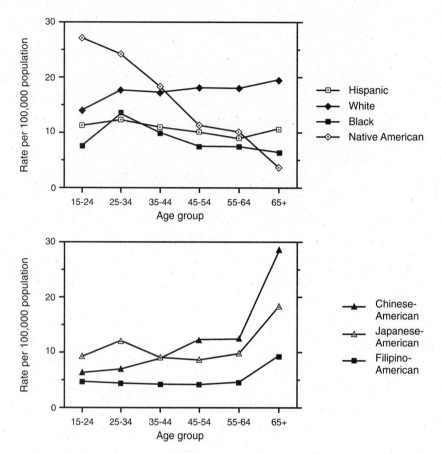

FIGURE 7   U.S. suicide rates by ethnic groups and age,
1979 to 1981 average.

and 2,925 among the widowed. When rates are calculated, highest risk is among the divorced with lower rates among the widowed and single and lowest rates for the married (see Figure 8). With few exceptions these levels of risk are seen among those of both sexes (e.g., McIntosh, 1987b). It might also be kept in mind that the married category includes those who are married but separated. It is likely that this subgroup has higher risk than the married, spouse-present category, and inclusion of the separated in the calculation of rates probably increases the overall rate of the married population.

Methods

Suicide in the United States is most often committed with firearms. In 1986 firearms were utilized in 18,153 of the 30,904 suicides (58.7%) compared with 4,606 by hanging (14.9%), 3,070 by solid and liquid poisons (9.9%), and 2,966

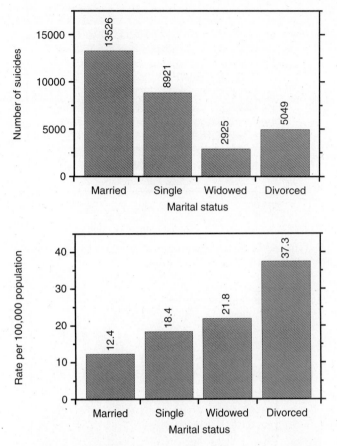

FIGURE 8 U.S. suicide rates and number of suicides by
marital status (15+ years of age), 1986.

by gas poisoning (9.6%). Indeed, the use of firearms is now ranked first among
both males (64.1%) and females (39.5% vs. 25.3% by solid and liquid poisons)
and have increased among all age, sex, and race groups over time (e.g., Mc-
Intosh & Santos, 1982, 1985–1986).

Temporal Factors

Although winter is often thought to be associated with high suicide risk (e.g.,
McIntosh, Hubbard, & Santos, 1985), the highest time of year for suicide is
consistently observed in spring (see Figure 9). In general, fall has most often
been second in suicide risk followed by summer and winter. Although these
differences are relatively consistent they are usually small from one season or
month to another. The same could be said for the small but consistent differences by day of the week. Monday and Tuesday are nearly always the highest

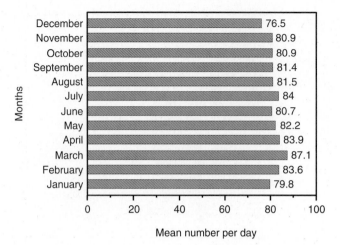

FIGURE 9 U.S. mean number of suicides by months, 1984 to 1986 average.

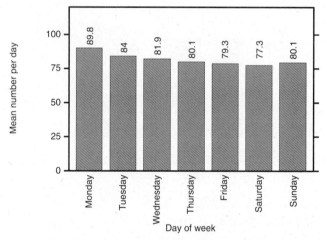

FIGURE 10 U.S. mean number of suicides by day of week, 1984 to 1986 average.

days for suicides, with Wednesday, Thursday, Friday, and Sunday lower (but similar) and lowest risk of all for Saturdays (see Figure 10).

Geographic Differences: States and Regions

Suicide rates are highest in the western divisions of the United States (see Table 1 and Figure 11). The Mountain Region has the highest rates and among the 8

TABLE 1 Rates and Rankings of Suicide for Each State, 1986[a]

Rank	State	Rate	Rank	State	Rate
1	Nevada	24.1 [M][b]	27	Georgia	13.0 [SA]
2	Montana	21.7 [M]	27	New Hampshire	13.0 [NE]
3	New Mexico	19.4 [M]	29	Tennessee	12.9 [ESC]
4	Arizona	19.3 [M]	29	Iowa	12.9 [WNC]
5	Wyoming	19.1 [M]	—	U.S. Total	12.8
6	Idaho	17.7 [M]	31	Minnesota	12.8 [WNC]
7	Colorado	17.6 [M]	32	Wisconsin	12.5 [ENC]
8	Oregon	16.7 [P]	33	Alabama	12.4 [ESC]
9	Florida	16.0 [SA]	34	Michigan	12.3 [ENC]
10	Washington	15.3 [P]	35	North Carolina	12.2 [SA]
11	Alaska	14.8 [P]	35	Pennsylvania	12.2 [MA]
12	California	14.7 [P]	35	Maryland	12.2 [SA]
12	Utah	14.7 [M]	38	Washington, D.C.	12.0 [SA]
14	Oklahoma	14.6 [WSC]	39	Indiana	11.7 [ENC]
15	South Dakota	14.3 [WNC]	40	Ohio	11.6 [ENC]
15	Nebraska	14.3 [WNC]	41	South Carolina	11.4 [SA]
17	Missouri	14.2 [WNC]	42	Maine	11.1 [NE]
17	Louisiana	14.2 [WSC]	42	Mississippi	11.1 [ESC]
17	West Virginia	14.2 [SA]	44	Illinois	11.0 [ENC]
17	Kentucky	14.2 [ESC]	45	North Dakota	10.8 [WNC]
21	Virginia	14.1 [SA]	45	Hawaii	10.8 [P]
22	Vermont	14.0 [NE]	47	Rhode Island	10.2 [NE]
23	Texas	13.6 [WSC]	48	Connecticut	9.6 [NE]
23	Kansas	13.6 [WNC]	49	Massachusetts	9.2 [NE]
25	Arkansas	13.5 [WSC]	50	New Jersey	7.6 [MA]
26	Delaware	13.3 [SA]	50	New York	7.6 [MA]

[a] From the National Center for Health Statistics (1988b, pp. 45–46, Table 18) (data are by place of residence).
[b] Region: Mountain [M]; Pacific [P]; West South Central [WSC]; South Atlantic [SA]; West North Central [WNC]; East South Central [ESC]; East North Central [ENC]; New England [NE]; Middle Atlantic [MA].

states that comprise this region were the top 7 in the United States in 1986 with the 8th tied for 12th. The Pacific states had the next highest rates, and all but 1 of its 5 states were in the top 13 in 1986. Central and southern states had lower rates, with lowest rates in the New England and Middle Atlantic states. These distributions of suicide by geographic regions and states have also been observed generally for the young (Seiden, 1984) and elderly (McIntosh, 1988).

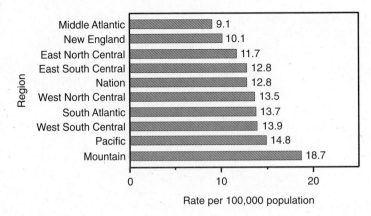

FIGURE 11   U.S. suicide rates by geographic regions, 1986.

Other Factors

A final factor that has been consistently observed to be associated with high risk of suicide but is not included in the characteristics and information that appears on death certificates and therefore in official national data is the presence of mental illness. Numerous studies have observed that virtually all mental illnesses increase the risk of suicide when compared to the nation as a whole (Lester, 1972, 1983, Chapters 17 and 18, respectively; Miles, 1977). Particularly high risk of suicide is observed in the categories of depression (Sainsbury, 1986), alcoholism (Murphy, 1986), and schizophrenia (Roy, 1986).

CONCLUSIONS

Based on the most consistent data, therefore, the modal suicide victim is an elderly white male who commits suicide with a firearm. Although those with the opposite demographic characteristics may also consider and commit suicide, individuals with these modal and other psychological (e.g., hopelessness, helplessness), physical (e.g., illness, pain), and social circumstances (e.g., social isolation, loneliness) should be targeted for special suicide prevention efforts.

References

Allen, N. H. (1984). Suicide statistics. In C. L. Hatton & S. M. Valente (Eds.), *Suicide: Assessment and intervention* (2nd ed., pp. 17–31). Norwalk, CT: Appleton-Century-Crofts.

Atkinson, J. M. (1978). *Discovering suicide: Studies in the social organization of sudden death*. Pittsburgh: University of Pittsburgh Press.

Douglas, J. D. (1967). *The social meanings of suicide.* Princeton, NJ: Princeton University Press.

Dunne, E. J., McIntosh, J. L., & Dunne-Maxim, K. (Eds.). (1987). *Suicide and its aftermath: Understanding and counseling the survivors.* New York: W. W. Norton.

Durkheim, É. (1951). *Suicide.* New York: Free Press. (Original work published 1897)

Farberow, N. L. (1972). *Bibliography on suicide and suicide prevention, 1897–1957, 1958–1970* (DHEW Publication No. (HSM) 72-9080). Washington, DC: United States Government Printing Office.

Holinger, P. C., Offer, D., & Zola, M. A. (1988). A prediction model of suicide among youth. *Journal of Nervous and Mental Disease, 176,* 275–279.

Kreitman, N. (1977). *Parasuicide.* New York: Wiley.

Lester, D. (1972). *Why people kill themselves: A summary of research findings on suicidal behavior.* Springfield, IL: Charles C Thomas.

Lester, D. (1983). *Why people kill themselves: A 1980s summary of research findings on suicidal behavior* (2nd ed.). Springfield, IL: Charles C. Thomas.

Manton, K. G., Blazer, D. G., & Woodbury, M. A. (1987). Suicide in middle age and later life: Sex and race specific life tables and cohort analysis. *Journal of Gerontology, 42,* 219–227.

McIntosh, J. L. (1985a). *Research on suicide: A bibliography.* Westport, CT: Greenwood Press.

McIntosh, J. L. (1985b, November). *Suicide among minority elderly.* Paper presented at annual meeting of the Gerontological Society of America, New Orleans, LA.

McIntosh, J. L. (1986, April). *Cross-ethnic suicide: U.S. trends and levels.* Paper presented at the annual meeting of the American Association of Suicidology, Atlanta, GA.

McIntosh, J. L. (1987a, May). *Hispanic suicide in ten U.S. states.* Paper presented at the joint meeting of the American Association of Suicidology and the International Association for Suicide Prevention, San Francisco, CA.

McIntosh, J. L. (1987b, May). *Marital status and suicide: Recent U.S. data.* Paper presented at the joint meeting of the American Association of Suicidology and the International Association for Suicide Prevention, San Francisco, CA.

McIntosh, J. L. (1988, April). *Geographic changes in U.S. elderly suicide.* Paper presented at the annual meeting of the American Association of Suicidology, Washington, DC.

McIntosh, J. L. (1989). Trends in racial differences in United States suicide statistics. *Death Studies, 13,* 275–286.

McIntosh, J. L., Hubbard, R. W., & Santos, J. F. (1985). Suicide facts and myths: A study of prevalence. *Death Studies, 9,* 267–281.

McIntosh, J. L., & Jewell, B. L. (1986). Sex difference trends in completed suicide. *Suicide and Life-Threatening Behavior, 16,* 16–27.

McIntosh, J. L., & Santos, J. F. (1981). Suicide among minority elderly: A preliminary investigation. *Suicide and Life-Threatening Behavior, 11,* 151–166.

McIntosh, J. L., & Santos, J. F. (1982). Changing patterns in methods of suicide by race and sex. *Suicide and Life-Threatening Behavior, 12,* 221–233.

McIntosh, J. L., & Santos, J. F. (1985–1986). Methods of suicide by age: Sex and race differences among the young and old. *International Journal of Aging and Human Development, 22,* 123–139.

Miles, C. P. (1977). Conditions predisposing to suicide: A review. *Journal of Nervous and Mental Disease, 164*, 231–246.

Murphy, G. E. (1986). Suicide in alcoholism. In A. Roy (Ed.), *Suicide* (pp. 89–96). Baltimore: Williams & Wilkins.

National Center for Health Statistics. (1988a; and annual volumes, 1937–1985). *Vital Statistics of the United States, 1986* (and other annual volumes). *Volume II—Mortality*. Washington, DC: U.S. Government Printing Office.

National Center for Health Statistics. (1988b). Advance report of final mortality statistics, 1986. *NCHS Monthly Vital Statistics Report, 37*(6, Suppl.).

Neuringer, C. (1982). Suicidal behavior in women. *Crisis, 3*, 41–49.

Pollinger-Haas, A., & Hendin, H. (1983). Suicide among older people: Projections for the future. *Suicide and Life-Threatening Behavior, 13*, 147–154.

Roy, A. (1986). Suicide in schizophrenia. In A. Roy (Ed.), *Suicide* (pp. 97–112). Baltimore: Williams & Wilkins.

Sainsbury, P. (1986). Depression, suicide, and suicide prevention. In A. Roy (Ed.), *Suicide* (pp. 73–88). Baltimore: Williams & Wilkins.

Sainsbury, P., & Barraclough, B. (1968). Difference in suicide rates. *Nature, 220*, 1252.

Sainsbury, P., & Jenkins, J. S. (1982). The accuracy of officially reported suicide statistics for purposes of epidemiological research. *Journal of Epidemiology and Community Health, 36*, 43–48.

Seiden, R. H. (1984). Death in the West—A regional analysis of the youthful suicide rate. *Western Journal of Medicine, 140*, 969–973.

Steffensmeier, R. H. (1984). Suicide and the contemporary woman: Are male and female suicide rates converging? *Sex Roles, 10*, 613–631.

U.S. Bureau of the Census. (1987). Marital status and living arrangements: March 1986. *Current Population Reports*, Series P-20, No. 418.

U.S. Bureau of the Census. (1988). United States population estimates, by age, sex, and race: 1980 to 1987. *Current Population Reports*, Series P-25, No. 1022.

33 Examining Suicide from a Life Span Perspective ❧

Judith M. Stillion and Eugene E. McDowell

JUDITH STILLION is professor of psychology and associate vice chancellor at Western Carolina University. She is also a past president of the Association for Death Education and Counseling. EUGENE MCDOWELL is professor of psychology and director of the Asheville Graduate Center of the University of North Carolina. Stillion and McDowell are coauthors of *Suicide Across the Life Span*. In this article, the authors present a suicide-trajectory model derived from a life span perspective. The model includes four risk factors: biological, environmental, psychological, and cognitive. These factors in various combinations lead to the development of what the authors call suicidal ideation, which, in turn, may lead to warning signs and eventually to suicide attempts. They argue that their model can be used to help assess a person's potential for suicide.

SUICIDE IS A BEHAVIOR THAT IS AS OLD AS HUMANKIND. The earliest recorded suicides in Western culture were the deaths of Samson and Saul around 1000 B.C. From that time on, humans have considered suicide, pondered its meaning, written treatises about it (e.g., *Summa Theologica*, circa 1270; *Biathanatos*, 1647; *Le Suicide*, 1897), and in other ways struggled to understand this behavior, which seems to violate the most basic of instincts: the instinct for survival itself. In the struggle to understand what appears to be a violation of the essence of the human condition, researchers have attempted to place suicidal behaviors within categories—for example, anomic, egoistic, altruistic, and fatalistic (1)—and types (e.g., cluster suicides, copycat suicides). They have also studied the emotional and psychological states of suicidal people and the environments that predispose to suicidal behavior. As evidence accumulated from each of these approaches, it became increasingly clear that suicidal behavior is one of the most complex behaviors in the human repertoire. Because this is true, no simple categorization or typology has proved to be very helpful. Indeed, Shneidman (2), the father of suicidology in the United States, recently concluded that "classifications [of suicide] taken singly or together, have either an

From *Death Studies*, 1991, Vol. 15, pp. 327–354, Judith M. Stillion and Eugene E. McDowell, Hemisphere Publishing, Bristol, PA. Reprinted with permission.

arbitrary, esoteric, or ad hoc quality to them. They do not seem impressively definitive. I know for a fact the best known of them is of practically no use in the clinic, where the task is saving lives" (p. 29).

One factor influencing suicide that has been overlooked until very recently is age and concomitant developmental level of at-risk individuals. Not only do the rate and patterns of suicide (e.g., ratio of male to female) differ among different age levels, but the types of suicide as well as the variables influencing suicidal behavior also vary by age. Therefore, any new attempt to understand suicidal behavior must rely on a model that takes into account the complexity of suicidal behavior and serves as a helpful framework in making sense of what is known about suicide by age group across the life span. The purpose of this article is to introduce a developmental model of suicidal behavior, grounding it in research wherever possible, and using it to illuminate the commonalities and differences in suicide across the life span.

MODEL OF THE SUICIDE TRAJECTORY

Suicidal behavior has at least four categories of causal factors: biological, psychological, cognitive, and environmental. Although any individual's suicidal behavior may reflect different weightings of these categories, each of them must be examined to understand any suicide completely. The four roots constitute major categories of risk factors, which, when they accumulate enough negative force, may result in suicide ideation in any human being. The ideation may lead to the emission of warning signs and/or triggering events that may eventuate into suicidal behavior. Figure 1 shows the interaction of these factors in what can be called the suicide trajectory. Research has illuminated the role that each risk factor plays in promoting suicidal behavior.

Biological Risk Factors

There are three lines of research into the biological roots of suicide that illuminate the role that biological risk factors play in suicidal behaviors. The first is research on the functioning of the brain at the cellular level. The second is research into possible genetic bases of suicidal behavior. The third is research into behaviors associated with gender (i.e., with being male or female).

Suicidal behavior is intimately related to clinical depression. Although many suicides are committed by people who are not clinically depressed, and there are many clinically depressed people who do not attempt suicide, the link between the two is sufficiently strong to justify a brief review of research on the biology of depression.

Over the past 20 years, a number of researchers have been working to show that depression is related to the level of certain neurotransmitters in the brain of depressed individuals (3–5). A deficiency of one neurotransmitter,

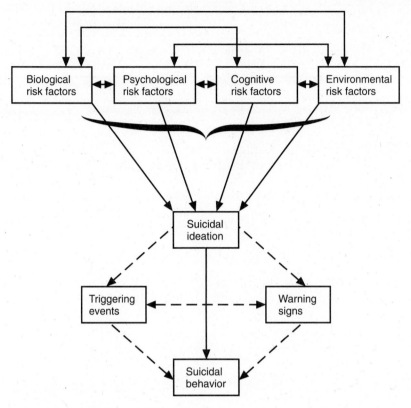

FIGURE 1 The Suicide Trajectory.

serotonin, has been found in the brain of some people who have completed suicide and in the cerebrospinal fluid of suicide attempters (6). Because serotonin
has been shown to be instrumental in regulating emotion, some researchers
have suggested that a deficiency of serotonin may be implicated in both depression and suicide attempts, especially impulsive suicide attempts. One researcher found that serotonin, as measured by one of its main metabolic
products (5-HIAA), was correlated both with depression and with the seriousness of suicide attempts. Furthermore, this researcher showed that, among patients who had been hospitalized in conjunction with a suicide attempt, those
who had less 5-HIAA were 10 times more likely to have died from suicide a
year later than were those who had higher levels of the substance (7). Other
lines of research into the biology of depression have implicated the neurotransmitters acetylcholine and norepinephrine (3–5). Although this intriguing
work has already led to the development of some drugs to treat neurotransmitter deficiencies, it does not address the question of how the deficiencies
arise.

The second line of research into the biological aspects of suicidal behavior
raises the possibility of a genetic basis. As in many studies designed to tease out

TABLE 1 Suicide Rates for Selected Countries by Sex and Age Group

Sex and age	United States 1984	Australia 1985	Austria 1986	Canada 1985	Denmark[a] 1985	France 1985
Males						
15–24 years	20.5	24.0	31.0	25.2	17.0	17.0
25–34 years	24.9	26.6	48.6	27.0	38.7	35.2
35–44 years	22.6	22.5	53.3	24.7	38.5	36.5
45–54 years	23.7	21.5	54.2	26.4	56.6	45.4
55–64 years	27.2	22.0	52.5	26.5	55.3	48.0
65–74 years	33.5	24.8	72.8	28.5	57.7	61.4
75 and older	49.1	27.4	106.5	28.4	83.4	120.5
Total[c]	19.7	18.2	42.1	20.5	35.1	33.1
Females						
15–24 years	4.4	4.9	9.7	4.0	8.1	4.7
25–34 years	6.1	4.7	14.3	6.6	14.3	10.6
35–44 years	7.7	6.1	18.5	8.0	28.6	14.6
45–54 years	9.2	8.7	20.2	9.0	34.0	17.7
55–64 years	8.5	8.3	18.9	8.0	41.5	20.8
65–74 years	7.3	7.6	29.0	7.8	34.1	26.8
75 and older	6.0	9.7	31.5	5.3	24.6	27.5
Total[c]	5.4	5.1	15.8	5.4	20.6	12.7
Total	12.4	11.8	26.7	12.8	26.9	21.8

NOTE: Rate per 100,000 population. Includes deaths resulting indirectly from self-inflicted injuries. Except as noted, deaths classified according to the ninth revision of the *International Classification of Diseases* (ICD).

[a] Based on the eighth revision of the ICD.
[b] England and Wales only.
[c] Includes other age groups not shown separately.

the relative amount of nature or nurture in a behavior, this line of research has examined suicide among monozygotic twins and across generations in families. Blumenthal and Kupfer (8) reviewed the literature on family history and genetics as they relate to suicide. The authors concluded that the incidence of suicidal behavior among relatives of suicidal persons is higher than in the general population. One study reviewed showed that half of a sample of psychiatric inpatients who had a family history of suicide had attempted suicide themselves. They also reported 10 cases of identical twins in which both had committed suicide. Although this number is not impressive, they were not able to report a single case of fraternal twins in which both had committed suicide. Finally, these reviewers summarized a study of adoptees in Copenhagen. Included among the adoptees were 57 who had committed suicide. Of the 269

Table 1 Suicide Rates for Selected Countries by Sex and Age Group (cont.)

Italy 1983	Japan 1986	Netherlands 1985	Poland 1986	Sweden[a] 1985	United Kingdom[b] 1985	West Germany 1986
5.2	14.1	10.6	17.5	14.3	8.2	17.7
8.4	25.1	17.6	29.3	32.0	15.3	25.3
9.1	31.6	16.1	33.5	29.0	16.3	28.5
14.8	51.0	20.0	36.7	39.3	17.1	35.6
18.4	44.8	21.0	35.9	32.7	18.1	36.7
29.7	43.9	26.1	30.6	36.2	16.9	44.7
47.9	78.8	41.0	29.3	45.3	22.3	72.8
11.0	27.8	14.6	22.0	25.0	12.1	26.6
1.3	8.0	3.1	2.7	7.6	1.8	5.3
3.3	11.6	9.3	5.3	13.2	4.4	9.1
3.7	12.8	9.9	5.8	15.5	5.4	10.5
5.6	18.4	12.5	8.4	14.8	9.2	14.8
8.3	20.2	14.6	7.6	13.8	10.5	16.5
10.1	33.0	15.5	6.6	20.1	11.9	23.6
11.0	59.1	10.8	5.5	14.0	10.1	24.8
4.3	14.9	8.1	4.4	11.5	5.7	12.0
7.3	21.1	11.2	13.8	17.2	8.8	17.0

source: World Health Organization, Geneva, Switzerland, *World Health Statistics*, annual; and unpublished data.

identified biological relatives of the suicides, 12 (4.5%) had also committed suicide. No adopting relatives had committed suicide. Of the 57 nonsuicidal adoptees who were matched to the suicides, only 2 (0.7%) of their biological relatives and none of their adoptive relatives had committed suicide.

The third avenue of research into possible biological bases of suicide is found in the sex-differences literature. One clear behavioral difference between the sexes is the fact that, in all developed countries, males complete suicide at higher rates than do females. Table 1 shows the most recent suicide rates in 13 developed countries. It is clear from Table 1 that males in all reporting countries are two to five times more likely to commit suicide than females. Table 2 shows male and female suicide rates in the United States across a 26-year period. Once again, the sex differences remain more than three male deaths for every one fe-

TABLE 2 Deaths by Suicide in the United States, 1960–1986

Races	1960	1970	1980	1986
All races				
Both sexes	10.6	11.8	11.4	11.9
Male	16.6	17.3	18.0	19.3
Female	5.0	6.8	5.4	5.1
White				
Both sexes	11.1	12.4	12.1	12.7
Male	17.5	18.2	18.9	20.5
Female	5.3	7.2	5.7	5.4
Black				
Both sexes	4.7	6.1	6.4	6.6
Male	7.8	9.9	11.1	11.5
Female	1.9	2.9	2.4	2.4

NOTE: Table represents age-adjusted deaths per 100,000 population in specified group.
SOURCE: U.S. Bureau of the Census, Statistical abstract of the United States: 1989 (109th edition), Washington, DC, 1989, p. 80.

male death by suicide. When a behavior shows clear sex differences across both cultures and time, researchers may begin to suspect that it is based, at least in part, on genetic influences.

Because suicide is clearly an aggressive behavior, a possible explanation of the heightened male suicide rates may lie in the research on aggression. Examining the literature on sex differences leads to the observation that sex differences in aggression are among the most consistent findings (9–12). Not only do boys and men show more aggression than girls and women from a very early age, but such heightened aggression is also found in the males of other species (13–16). Given the facts that male aggression is greater than female aggression across species and from the very earliest ages at which it can be measured, the most logical inference is that there is a genetic or prenatal basis for heightened male aggression. Males may simply inherit a tendency toward higher aggressive activity. Such a tendency, when directed at the self, may help to explain the consistent sex difference in suicide rates.

Psychological Risk Factors

Psychological risk factors refer to feelings and behaviors that contribute to suicidal ideation. There are at least four general categories of psychological risk factors that emerge from the literature on suicide. These include depression, feelings of hopelessness and helplessness, low self-esteem, and poor coping behaviors.

Depression, whether based in biology or beginning as a result of environmental stimuli, is the psychological classification most often associated with suicidal behavior (17–23). People who are depressed suffer from low self-esteem and show varying levels of hopelessness and helplessness. Although many studies have shown that depression, hopelessness, and low self-esteem are positively interrelated, at least three studies have shown that hopelessness is the factor that could best predict the level of lethality of a suicide attempt (24–26). Taken together, these studies indicate that people who dislike themselves and are generally depressed may contemplate suicide, but the seriousness of such contemplation is greatly increased in people who also feel hopeless about the future.

The lack of healthy coping skills is the final psychological factor predisposing toward suicide. The use of alcohol and drugs as well as other avoidant behaviors that reflect poor coping abilities are frequent correlates in the lives of suicidal individuals (17, 27–28, 29).

Cognitive Risk Factors

Because humans use their intellectual capabilities to shape their self-concepts and their views of the world and to evaluate their past life choices and future options, cognitive risk factors play a growing role in suicidal behavior across the life span. Evidence is accumulating that suicidal individuals become more rigid and dichotomous in their thinking and narrow their cognitive focus to suicide as the best, and perhaps the only, answer to their problems. Beck and his associates (30–33) accumulated a body of work that shows that the thoughts of depressed people (who are often also suicidal) are marked by four types of cognitive distortions: rigidity of thought, selective abstraction, overgeneralization, and inexact labeling. Rigidity of thought is shown in the narrowing of the cognitive focus of suicidal individuals, which results in their inability to consider more positive alternatives and to learn new coping techniques. Selective abstraction occurs when people focus only on the bad or negative events and surroundings in their lives and ignore the positive ones. Overgeneralization is the tendency to apply negative thoughts to all current and future possibilities, to see little or no hope anywhere. Finally, inexact labeling occurs when individuals interpret a situation negatively, place a negative all-encompassing label on themselves as a result of their negative interpretations, and react to the label from then on rather than to the realities of the situation. Once begun, all of these cognitions are strengthened by the phenomenon that Meichenbaum (34) called "negative self-talk." Depressed and suicidal people tend to reinforce their misery by giving themselves continuous messages relating to their inferiority, their hopelessness, and their helplessness, thus using their cognitive gift of language to reinforce their suicidal state.

Environmental Risk Factors

Many factors in the external environment can increase the risk of suicide. However, there are four categories of environmental factors that have clearly been shown to be related to suicidal behavior. These include negative experiences in the family, loss, negative life events, and the presence of firearms and other means of self-destruction.

Researchers into child and adolescent suicide have shown that turbulent home lives, the presence of child abuse, alcoholism, separation, and divorce are all correlated with increases in depression, self-destructive behavior, and suicide (17, 22, 35–39). Suicidal behavior is also more frequent among adults from broken or turbulent homes (40–42).

Loss is a clear factor increasing the risk of suicide, and cumulative loss increases it dramatically. The normal reaction to loss is grief, and one of the most typical characteristics of grief is depression. Thus, when a normal person loses something that is valued (e.g., loss of a relationship, death of a loved one), that person will generally experience mild to severe depression. If multiple losses occur in rapid succession, before an individual has time to work his or her way through the normal grieving process, their cumulative effect may predispose to suicide (23, 43).

Negative life events inevitably lead to loss. Examples of such events are accidents, losing one's job, not being promoted, failing examinations, and so on. Each of these negative events has the power to make people examine their prior assumptions. Generally, such examinations lead individuals to lose some of their faith in a just world, their self-esteem, their basic sense of trust, and positive outlook. Just as the loss of a relationship or the death of a loved one initiates a grief reaction, so also do important negative life events. Slater and Depue (44) found that "exit events" (e.g., separation, divorce, and death) differentiated suicidal depressed individuals from nonsuicidal depressed individuals more than any other type of loss.

Finally, easy access to instruments of destruction, especially firearms, is an environmental factor that increases the risk of suicide. Hudgens (45) pointed out that the rise in suicide during the last three decades can be accounted for almost entirely by the rise in deaths caused by handguns. He further maintained that suicide rates are lower in states that have strict handgun laws. The National Task Force on Suicide in Canada (46) echoed Hudgens's observations by calling for measures "to reduce the lethality and availability of instruments of suicide" (p. 41), including more stringent gun control.

Suicidal Ideation, Triggering Events, and Warning Signs

Suicidal ideation, triggering events, and warning signs form an interrelated triad that is present in many suicides. Suicidal ideation, including the making of specific plans, is an essential phase in all but the most impulsive of suicides. There is a wide variation in the time periods during which suicidal individuals consider suicide. They may range from a few minutes to many years. However, suicidal ideation moves from the general to the specific, from considering suicide as a possible coping behavior to accepting it as the best coping behavior and accompanying that acceptance with detailed plans for carrying out the suicidal action. Once plans are formed, warning signs may be evidenced. The most common warning signs are verbal threats, self-injurious behaviors, and indications of closure such as saying good-bye or giving away prized possessions. These warning signs may precipitate a triggering event. For example, saying good-bye to a friend may cause the friend to become suspicious and call the authorities. The appearance of the authorities may trigger the suicide attempt. A negative life event may occur and become the triggering event, which may or may not be accompanied by warning signs. Triggering events, like warning signs, are not universally present in suicidal behavior; therefore, we have shown the categories connected by dotted lines in Figure 1. Triggering events are best conceptualized as "last-straw" phenomena; that is, they are not necessarily dramatic or particularly traumatic. They differ from regular negative life events in that they occur after the individual has already engaged in significant suicide ideation. Because of the amount of suicide ideation already experienced, even quite small occurrences may serve to trigger the final suicide attempt.

Summary of the Model

In summary, the model we propose is one that requires the user to examine systematically the individual's situation from four different categories of risk behaviors: biological, psychological, cognitive, and environmental. The model predicts that each of these categories will add its own weight to the suicidal equation. Furthermore, each of these categories may influence the others. (For example, the environmental factor of a turbulent home life may interact with a biological tendency toward depression to alter an individual's cognitive understanding of self and the world. As the individual begins to view himself or herself and the world in ever more narrow and negative terms, his or her depression is strengthened.) Working together synergistically, these negative risk factors increase the probability that suicide will come to be seen as a viable way of coping with life's conditions. Once the idea of suicide becomes firmly implanted, it is elaborated on until it becomes a detailed plan for self-destruction that may or may not be given away by warning signs. All that is lacking at this point is the final triggering event or the passage of enough time for consolidation of the plan to become final. When that happens, a suicide attempt is the result.

Models may be interesting and may seem intuitively to make sense. However, the ultimate test of a model is whether it helps concerned professionals to understand, to predict, and ultimately to control behavior. To this point only the commonalities in suicidal behavior have been examined. The first test of the model will be to see if it also sheds light on the differences in suicidal behavior. The remainder of this article deals with changes in the suicide trajectory across the life span. Listed in Table 3 are the age-related differences in the four categories of risk factors, warning signs, triggering events, and suicidal behavior, as well as the commonalities discussed in the preceding section of this article.

TESTING THE MODEL: DEVELOPMENTAL DIFFERENCES IN THE SUICIDE TRAJECTORY

It is well known that suicide rates differ across the life span and between the sexes. Table 4 lists the suicide rates for men and women among different age groups. As shown in Table 4, the suicide rate for men is significantly higher than that for women at all ages. The suicide rate for men increases generally with age, especially during the postretirement years. The suicide rate for women, which is always low relative to that of men, increases to age 50 and then gradually declines. Although the statistics reported in Table 4 do not include rates for children, there is evidence that suicide among 5- to 14-year-olds is a growing phenomenon. Suicide data for this age group were not reported until 1970. In that year, the official suicide rate for 5- to 14-year-olds was 0.3 per 100,000 population. In 1986, the last year for which official statistics for this age group were available, the reported suicide rate for children was 0.8 per 100,000 (23).

Childhood

Table 3 shows that, during the childhood years (ages 5–14), there are two risk factors for suicide that may be rooted in biology. The first is a tendency toward impulsivity. Although childhood suicide almost always results from a history of problems, the act itself tends to be more impulsive in childhood than in any other age period (38, 47). A child who has suffered from abuse or neglect over a long period of time will jump in front of a car without warning. Another child may run from the room in the midst of a parental argument, find the father's gun, and shoot himself or herself almost in one movement. Hyperactivity also seems to play a role in childhood suicide, adding to the apparent impulsivity of the act (48). Hyperactive children are unable to sit for a long time or to consider in detail the repercussions of an action (49). They have a bias for action and seem to move almost anxiously from one situation to another. Hyperactivity by itself does not predispose a child to suicide. However, if the predisposition to depression is there or if there are sufficient other psychological, cognitive, or environmental risk factors present, hyperactive children may have less protection against suicide than others who can contemplate more fully alternative solutions to problems.

There are two major psychological factors that increase children's risk of suicide. The first, explained well by Erikson (61), is a sense of inferiority. Children who feel inferior to others develop poor self-concepts and low self-esteem. They frequently act out in ways that confirm their low opinion of themselves and increase the likelihood that they will receive negative feedback from significant others. In this way, they act so as to maintain or enhance their negative self-concepts, which may eventually lead to depression and possible suicide behavior. The second psychological risk factor specific to childhood is the expendable child syndrome. The expendable child experiences loss of love in the most extreme form. Parents of these children communicate very low regard for, hostility toward, and even hatred of them on a daily basis. These children believe they are unworthy and "expendable," that their deaths will not matter to anyone (50). It should be emphasized that young children are especially vulnerable to low self-esteem and to the expendable child syndrome. Unlike their older counterparts, their psychological resources are limited because they have had less opportunity to develop good coping behaviors.

The cognitive risk factor most closely associated with childhood suicide is an immature understanding of death. Many children in the concrete operations stage of cognitive development (ages 5 to 12) do not comprehend the finality of death (51). They tend to view death as a temporary and reversible state. Furthermore, there is evidence that suicidal children have less well-developed concepts of death than other children their age, which are especially evident in a crisis situation (38, 52). Investigators have found that many suicidal children are likely to view death as a transient and pleasant state (53). It is not unusual for suicidal children, who have lost loved ones, to view death as a vehicle for a happy reunion. It seems that lack of understanding of the finality of death plus the belief that death is a gateway to a happier situation are cognitions that increase the risk of suicide. Another cognitive characteristic of young children is an inability to see the multiple dimensions of a situation. Concrete operational thinking resembles in many ways the rigid thought patterns associated with suicide at later ages (22, 54). Children simply are not able to envision multiple possibilities for the future and are, therefore, likely to experience excessive hopelessness when they are in a negative life situation. In addition to their cognitive limitations, children also lack the life experiences of adults. These years of experience teach us that problem situations often do turn out well.

TABLE 3 Commonalities and Differences in the Suicide Trajectory Across the Life Span

Age Group	Biological Risk Factors	Psychological Risk Factors	Cognitive Risk Factors
Life cycle commonalities	Genetic predisposition to depression, maleness	Depression, helplessness, hoplessness, low self-esteem, lack of coping skills	Rigidity of thought, overgeneralization, selective abstraction, inexact labeling
Childhood (5–14 years)	Impulsivity, hyperactivity	Inferiority, expendable child syndrome	Immature views of death, concrete operational thinking
Adolescence (15–24 years)	Puberty, hormonal changes	Identity crisis, fluctuating mood states	Formal operational thinking, idealistic thinking, increased egocentrism, illusion of invulnerability, imaginary audience
Young adulthood (25–34 years)	Postpartum depression	Lack of intimate relationships	Reevaluation of life choice (catch 30)
Middle adulthood (35–64 years)	Menopause (W), climacteric (M), decline in physical abilities and attractiveness	Loss of youthful dreams, increased inferiority, feelings of stagnation and self-absorption	Change in time perspective, midlife evaluation
Old age (65 years and older)	Physical decline, organic mental decline, chronic illness, chronic pain	Increased passivity, loneliness, feelings of despair	Declining learning, declining retrieval, growing acceptance of death

NOTE: W = women; M = men; AIDS = acquired immune deficiency syndrome.

Environmental Risk Factors	Warning Signs	Triggering Events	Suicidal Behaviors
Negative experiences in the family, loss, negative life events, presence of firearms and other means of self-destruction	Verbal threats, self-injurious behavior	"Final straw" life event	Higher rate for males; males use more lethal methods
Abuse and neglect, parental conflict, family role definitions, inflexible family structure, parental suicidal behavior, repeated failure	Truancy, poor school performance, increased anxiety, sleep disturbance, aggression, low frustration tolerance, poor impulse control	Minor life events	Impulsive, highly lethal; males attempt and complete more suicides; greatest incidence of failed suicides; lowest completion rate
Parental conflict, drug or alcohol abuse, poor peer relationships, anomic families	Self-mutilation, change in habits, truancy, poor school performance, preparation for death	Suicides by peers, suicides by famous people, failure experiences, problems with peers, parents, opposite sex, siblings	Largest rate of increase in past 30 years; most dramatic sex difference in attempts; vulnerable to cluster and copycat suicides
Presence of children (W), marital problems (W), occupational problems (M), drug and alcohol abuse (M), AIDS	Precipitous multiple life changes	Occupational setback, marital difficulty, AIDS diagnosis	Small reduction in rate in past 5 years; peak suicide rate for Blacks and American Indians
Deaths of significant others, empty nest, fewer activities, fewer interpersonal activities, accumulation of negative life events, alcoholism			Peak suicide rate for women
Widowhood, retirement, inactivity, financial problems, cumulative loss, negative social attitudes toward elderly	Physicians' visits, putting affairs in order	Terminal illness	Highest rate of all groups; largest sex difference in completions; highest male completion rate; highest lethality level

Table 4 Suicide Rates Per 100,000 Population for
Different Age Groups of Males and Females

Age (years)	Males	Females
15–24	21.7	4.4
25–34	25.5	5.9
35–44	23.0	7.6
45–54	24.4	8.8
55–64	26.7	8.4
65–74	35.5	7.2
75–84	54.8	7.5
85 and older	61.6	4.7

SOURCE: U.S. Bureau of the Census (1989). *Statistical Abstracts of the United States* (109th Edition) Washington, DC, 1989, p. 80.

The major environmental risk factors associated with childhood suicide are centered in the family and the school. Many studies have shown that suicidal children are more likely than others to be victims of child abuse and neglect (22, 38, 39, 54–56). In addition, parental conflict, unclear role definitions, and inflexible structure often characterize the families of suicidal children (47, 57, 58). Several studies and clinical observations show that suicidal children have many negative experiences at school as well as at home. They tend to perform poorly at school, both academically and socially (21, 38, 59).

Warning signs in childhood include truancy and poor school performance. Children may also demonstrate depression differently from adults. Depressed children may manifest increased anxiety, sleep disturbance, aggressive behavior, low frustration tolerance, and poor impulse control.

More so than at any other period of life, triggering events may be minor occurrences. Because impulsive children are at higher risk for suicide, a seemingly tiny incident may trigger an act of self-destruction.

Unlike all other periods except old age, in childhood boys both attempt and complete suicide more often than do girls. Children are more likely than those in other age groups to fail in their suicide attempts, and they have the lowest overall suicide rate.

Adolescence

The risk factors that are specific to the adolescent years (ages 15–24) are presented in Table 3 also. In the biological sphere, the onset of puberty, triggered by increased production of hormones, brings about sexual maturation. The process of maturation occurs over a period of years but has its most dramatic effects in the early part of adolescence. These biological changes add their weight to the tumult of this age period, increasing suicidal risk.

In the category of psychological risk factors, the establishment of a sense of identity is a major developmental task of adolescence (60). Teenagers who develop some consistent understanding of who they are and who they are becoming will have a foundation of competence for dealing with the stresses of this period. In contrast, adolescents who struggle with their identities are less well-prepared to cope with these challenges (61). Identity crisis is a significant psychological risk factor for suicide among adolescents. Young people in the midst of unsuccessful struggles to better understand their identities have few resources for dealing with other problems. A second psychological risk factor is the fluctuation of mood states. Moodiness is experienced by all adolescents; however, when it becomes extreme, the risk of suicide is increased. Although moodiness is partially rooted in the biological changes of this period, it is experienced as an emotional state and, therefore, classified as a psychological risk factor in our suicide trajectory.

Adolescents are also undergoing rapid change in the cognitive realm. As they become capable of formal operational thought, they begin to practice hypothetical and abstract thinking for the first time (51). They try out their newly acquired skills, imagining worlds that have never existed. For the first time, they understand at a personal level the implications of such constructs as equality and justice. This may result in idealistic thinking, tinged with a sense of tragedy, as they see the distance between their idealized worlds and what really exists. They may also have difficulty in accepting their own mortality; the result is an illusion of invulnerability, which contributes to higher risk taking among adolescents. In addition, adolescents experience a renewed period of egocentrism, because they believe that they are the first ones to really understand the world from their new perspective. This egocentrism fuels their sense of performing for an imaginary audience and increases their feelings of self-consciousness, making small embarrassments seem like major traumas. In this way, the pain of daily living is increased for adolescents. All of these factors may play a role in enhancing the risk of suicidal behavior.

The literature shows that there are a number of environmental events that impact on adolescent suicide. Leading the list is parental conflict and divorce. Families of suicide attempters in this age group are often highly conflicted and unresponsive to the adolescent's needs (17). In addition, homes of adolescent suicide attempters are more likely than the national average to be disrupted by parental separation and divorce (35, 36). Although there are many exceptions, families of suicidal adolescents are more likely to be anomic (i.e., not accepting of usual standards of conduct; 28). There is also a higher incidence of alcoholism and drug abuse among the parents of suicidal adolescents (62) and among the young people themselves (63). Finally, the unhappiness of suicidal adolescents does not end with the home environment. There is growing evidence that adolescent suicides often have a basis in poor peer relationships. Suicidal adolescents rarely have close friends and are often "nonjoiners" who tend to be invisible to peers and teachers (64).

Warning signs in adolescence include self-mutilation, such as tattooing oneself with a penknife, changes in habits, truancy, poor school performance, and behavior that implies preparation for death, such as giving away prized possessions. Because the teenage years are characterized by mood swings, spotting these warning signs may be difficult. It is not uncommon for people closest to a teenager to remark, after a suicide attempt, "I knew he was acting strangely, but I thought that was typical behavior for an adolescent."

Certain types of triggering events appear to be more common in adolescence than in other age periods. The suicides of other people trigger suicidal behavior more frequently among teenagers than among others. Perhaps this phenomenon is related to the fact that adolescents are trying out new identities and therefore are more likely to engage in imitation and modeling. Also the suicide of a peer or of a well-known public figure may be interpreted as permission giving by the adolescent. Finally, there is evidence that some young people take their lives as a gesture of heroic camaraderie with another suicide. Whatever its effect, it is clear that publicized acts of suicide trigger more copycat and cluster suicides among adolescents than among any other age group (65–67). Other triggering events common to adolescence include experiences of failure and interpersonal problems.

Suicide among adolescents has had the highest rate of increase of any age group during the past 30 years (23). As shown in Table 4, the adolescent suicide rate is presently very close to the average for adults. The attempt to completion ratio for suicidal adolescent girls is almost a mirror image of that for boys. Ninety percent of all suicide attempts in adolescence are by girls, whereas 80% of all completed suicides are by boys (17).

Young Adulthood

As shown in Table 3, there are several indicators of suicide risk among young adults (ages 25–34) that differ from those of other age groups. In the biological arena, a special risk for suicide—for a small percentage of women—is the experience of postpartum depression. It should be noted that women who suffer from depression after their first birth are at higher risk for depression after subsequent births. Thus, postpartum depression may also be a risk factor for some women during the first decade of middle adulthood.

In the category of psychological risk factors, young adults are working on the task of establishing intimacy and avoiding isolation (60). At this stage of life, there is a heightened risk of becoming psychologically isolated from others. The suicide statistics show higher rates of suicide among single people of both sexes. Young adulthood seems to be a critical time for forming bonds of intimacy with mates and friends, which will protect against isolation and the accompanying sense of loneliness.

In the cognitive arena, young adults tend to face the first in a series of re-evaluations of life choices. Whether called "the age 30 transition" or "catch 30" (68), this process calls for a cognitive examination of all aspects of life to date, including occupation, marital choice, and parenting decisions, and it frequently leads to a reconceptualization of life goals. The process involves feelings as well as cognitions, but it is included under this category because it is experienced and described essentially as a thought process.

Environmental variables that increase the risk for suicide in young adulthood include, for women, the presence of young children in the home and marital problems (69, 70). For men, the environmental risk factors appear to be related to occupational problems and to drug and alcohol abuse (71, 72). A new factor increasing the suicide rates among young adults is acquired immune deficiency syndrome (AIDS) (73).

Common triggering events among young adults include quarrels or physical fights with spouses and occupational setbacks. Recent research has shown that a new triggering event for young adults is a positive diagnosis of AIDS (74).

As shown in Table 4, the suicide rate for young adults is significantly higher than that for adolescents. Unlike their adolescent counterparts, however, young adults have shown a small reduction in their suicide rate over the past 5 years. Also young adulthood is the period in which suicide rates for blacks and American Indians reach their peak (75).

Middle Adulthood

During middle age, menopause for women and the climacteric for men represent important biological events that may heighten the suicide risk (23). Both of these involve changes in the ability to reproduce, which are triggered by the body's producing lower levels of hormones than at any time since puberty. Once again, individuals find their behavior and moods influenced by biology. Also equally important in a culture as youth oriented as ours, any decline in physical abilities or attractiveness is likely to increase feelings of anxiety, inferiority, and depression.

In the psychological arena, many middle-aged adults experience the loss of their youthful dreams when they realize they have gone as far as they are going to in their careers or that they will never achieve a perfect family or become famous in any way. Although some middle-aged adults are able to become reconciled to the vanishing of their hopes for outstanding accomplishment, others experience great pain and become highly vulnerable to depression and suicide (76, 77).

Another important psychological risk factor for suicide in middle age is the increasing movement toward interiority. Interiority can be healthy if it promotes positive self-knowledge and increased satisfaction with one's life pattern. However, often the tendency toward interiority results in unhealthy ego absorption. As responsibilities to the family of procreation decline, the amount of daily interaction with one's children and with the individuals they bring into one's life also declines, resulting in the danger of cathectic impoverishment (78). Middle-aged individuals need to struggle against this natural tendency toward cathectic impoverishment to be productive and happy during midlife. Those who fail to do so begin to slip toward the stagnation pole of Erikson's continuum and increase their risk of isolation, depression, and suicide (60).

Cognitively, middle-aged adults experience a shift in their time perspective (79). They tend to change their focus from the amount of time already lived to the amount of time left to live, a shift that may trigger higher anxiety. It may also contribute to the onset of despair as middle-aged adults give up their youthful dreams and become convinced that there is not enough time left to begin anew. Many middle-aged adults also engage in a major cognitive evaluation of their life choices and patterns, often with such intensity that the term *crisis* is appropriate (76).

Increased environmental risk factors for suicide during middle age include the deaths of significant others, the loss of parental and filial roles, lower levels of activity and involvement, and an accumulation of negative life events (44). Alcoholism plays more of a role in the suicide of adults between the ages of 35 and 64 than for any other age group (80). Alcohol abuse among the middle-aged seems to especially enhance depression and to exacerbate negative life events such as divorce, loss of employment, and illness (81).

As shown in Table 4, the suicide rate for men grows gradually during the middle-age years before the major increase in old age. In contrast, middle age is the peak age for suicides among women. From this age on, the rate of suicide among women actually decreases.

Elderly

There is reason to believe that suicidal risk in old age is greatly enhanced by biological factors. General physical and organic mental declines, combined with chronic illness and chronic pain, undoubtedly contribute both to the depression that is endemic to old age and to the high suicide rates among the elderly (82, 83).

In the psychological sphere, elderly people experience increased passivity and loneliness. The passivity may be rooted in a lack of meaning in life because of a reduction in purposeful activity. These feelings undoubtedly add to a growing sense of despair among a minority of older people. This sense of despair, the polar opposite to Erikson's sense of ego integrity, undermines both pleasure and meaning in life among some elderly individuals. One study found that suicide notes among the elderly, more than any other age group, often include references to loneliness and isolation (84).

Cognitive risk factors in old age include a decline in intellectual functioning, both in the rate of learning new material and the rate of retrieval of information. Confronted by the cliché "You can't teach an old dog new tricks," many elderly persons stop trying to learn new material and withdraw further from involvement with the world. There is also some evidence that elderly people cognitively and emotionally reach a point of acceptance of death (85).

Many environmental risk factors have been shown to be important contributors to elderly suicide. Widowhood, a major source of social isolation among the elderly, has been shown to increase the likelihood of suicide among this age group (86–88). Retirement and the concomitant reduction in activity and financial loss appears to be a special risk factor for elderly men (43, 86, 89–91). Many elderly people must cope with a rapid succession of losses, which does not allow sufficient time for resolution of the grief inherent in each loss. Although the experience of cumulative loss may happen at any time across the life cycle, it most commonly occurs during old age. When many losses are experienced within a relatively short period of time, the associated depression may become a chronic state. Indeed, depression has been found to be the most common of all illnesses among the elderly (92).

Warning signs among the elderly include visits to doctors' offices and visible indications of putting affairs in order. Studies have shown that 70% or more of elderly people who kill themselves visit a physician within 1 month of the suicide, and that as many as 10% consult a physician on the actual day of the suicide (93–95). Suicide among the elderly may be triggered by a diagnosis of terminal illness.

As shown in Table 4, elderly men have the highest suicide rate of any group. Also this age group has the largest sex difference in suicide rate. Suicide attempts among elderly people are generally well planned and highly lethal, indicating a seriousness of purpose more developed than in other age groups (96).

Summary of Applications of the Model

In the second portion of this article, we have explored developmental differences in the suicide-trajectory model. The life span development literature plus empirical findings from suicide research have been applied to the suicide trajectory to explain age differences in suicidal behavior. Application of the risk factors in the model to predictable stages in life span development can help promote more complete understanding and perhaps enhance prediction of suicidal behavior.

References

1. Durkheim, E. (1951). *Suicide* (J. A. Spaulding & G. Simpson, Trans.). Glencoe, IL: The Free Press. (Original work published 1897)

2. Shneidman, E. S. (1985). *Definition of suicide*. New York: Wiley.

3. Asberg, M., & Traskman, L. (1981). Studies of CSF 5-HIAA in depression and suicidal behavior. *Experiments in Medical Biology, 133,* 739–752.

4. Banki, C. M., & Arato, M. (1983). Amine metabolites, neuroendocrine findings, and personality dimension as correlates of suicidal behavior. *Psychiatry Research, 10,* 253–261.

5. Schildkraut, J. J. (1965). The catecholamine hypothesis of affective disorders. A review of supporting evidence. *American Journal of Psychiatry, 122,* 509–522.

6. Asberg, M., Nordstrom, P., & Traskman-Bendz, L. (1986, December). Cerebrospinal fluid studies in suicide. *Annals of the New York Academy of Sciences, 487,* 243–255.

7. Asberg, M., Traskman, L., & Thoren, P. (1976). 5-HIAA in the cerebrospinal fluid: A biochemical suicide predictor. *Archives of General Psychiatry, 33,* 1193–1197.

8. Blumenthal, S. J., & Kupfer, D. J. (1986). Generalizable treatment strategies for suicidal behavior. In J. J. Mann & M. Stanley (Eds.), *Psychobiology of suicidal behavior* (pp. 327–340). New York: New York Academy of Sciences.

9. Unger, R. K. (1979). Female and male psychological perspectives. New York: Harper & Row.

10. Maccoby, E. E., & Jacklin, C. N. (1974). *The psychology of sex differences*. Stanford, CA: Stanford University Press.

11. Hoyenga, K. B., & Hoyenga, K. T. (1979). *The question of sex differences*. Boston: Little, Brown.

12. Money, J., & Ehrhardt, A. (1972). *Man and woman, boy and girl*. Baltimore: Johns Hopkins University Press.

13. Goy, R. W., & Resko, J. A. (1972). Gonadal hormones and behavior of normal and pseudohermaphroditic non-human female primates. In E. Astwood (Ed.), *Recent progress in hormone research* (pp. 707–733). New York: Academic Press.

14. Rose, R. M., Gordon, T. P., & Bernstein, I. S. (1972). Plasma testosterone levels in the male rhesus: Influences of sexual and social stimuli. *Science, 178,* 643–645.

15. Svare, B., & Gandelman, R. (1975). Aggressive behavior of juvenile mice: Influence of androgen and olfactory stimuli. *Developmental Psychobiology, 8,* 405–415.

16. Mitchell, G. (1979). *Sex differences in non-human primates*. New York: Van Nostrand Reinhold.

17. Berman, A. L., & Carroll, T. A. (1984). Adolescent suicide: A critical review. *Death Education, 8,* 53–64.

18. Goldberg, E. L. (1981). Depression and suicide ideation in the young adult. *American Journal of Psychiatry, 138,* 35–40.

19. Linehan, M. M. (1981). A social behavioral analysis of suicide and parasuicide. Implications for clinical assessment and treatment. In J. F. Clarkin & H. I. Glazer (Eds.), *Depression: Behavioral and directive intervention strategies* (pp. 229–294). New York: Garland Press.

20. Rosenthal, P. A., & Rosenthal, S. (1984). Suicidal behavior by preschool children. *American Journal of Psychiatry, 141*, 520–525.

21. Pfeffer, C. R. (1981a). Suicidal behavior of children: A review with implications for research and practice. *American Journal of Psychiatry, 138*, 154–159.

22. Orbach, I. (1984). Personality characteristics, life circumstances, and dynamics of suicidal children. *Death Education, 8*, 37–52.

23. Stillion, J. M., McDowell, E. E., & May, J. H. (1989). *Suicide across the life span: Premature exits.* Washington, DC: Hemisphere.

24. Wetzel, R. D. (1976). Hopelessness, depression, and suicide intent. *Archives of General Psychiatry, 33*, 1069–1073.

25. Goldney, R. D. (1981). Attempted suicide in young women: Correlate of lethality. *British Journal of Psychiatry, 139*, 382–390.

26. Kazdin, A. E., French, N. H., Unis, A. S., Esveldt-Dawson, K., & Sherick, R. B. (1983). Helplessness, depression, and suicidal intent among psychiatrically disturbed inpatient children. *Journal of Consulting and Clinical Psychology, 51*, 504–510.

27. Eisenberg, L. (1980). Adolescent suicide: On taking arms against a sea of troubles. *Pediatrics, 66*, 315–321.

28. Garfinkel, B. D., Froese, A., & Hood, J. (1982). Suicide attempts in children and adolescents. *American Journal of Psychiatry, 139*, 1257–1261.

29. Shaffer, D. (1974). Suicide in childhood and early adolescence. *Journal of Child Psychology and Psychiatry, 15*, 275–291.

30. Beck, A. T. (1967). *Depression: Clinical, experimental, and theoretical aspects.* New York: Hoeber.

31. Beck, A. T., Kovacs, M., & Weissman, A. (1979). Assessment of suicide ideation: The scale for suicide ideators. *Journal of Consulting and Clinical Psychology, 47*, 343–352.

32. Beck, A. T., Rush, A., Show, B., & Emery, G. (1979). *Cognitive therapy of depression.* New York: Guilford Press.

33. Beck, A. T., Steer, R. A., Kovacs, M., & Garrison, B. (1985). Hopelessness and eventual suicide: A 10-year prospective study of patients hospitalized with suicidal ideation. *American Journal of Psychiatry, 142*, 559–563.

34. Meichenbaum, D. (1985). *Stress inoculation training.* Elmsford, NY: Pergamon.

35. McAnarney, E. R. (1979). Adolescent and the young adult suicide in the United States—a reflection of social unrest? *Adolescence, 14*, 765–774.

36. Walker, W. L. (1980). Intentional self-injury in school age children. *Journal of Adolescence, 3*, 217–228.

37. Tishler, C. L., McKenry, P. C., & Morgan, K. C. (1981). Adolescent suicide attempts: Some significant factors. *Suicide and Life-Threatening Behavior, 11*, 86–92.

38. Joffe, R. T., & Offord, D. R. (1983). A review: Suicidal behavior in childhood. *Canadian Journal of Psychiatry, 28*, 57–63.

39. Pfeffer, C. R. (1981b). The family system of suicidal children. *American Journal of Psychotherapy, 35*, 330–341.

40. Adam, K. S., Bouckoms, A., Streiner, D. L. (1982). Parental loss and family stability in attempted suicide. *Archives of General Psychiatry, 39*, 1081–1085.

41. Richman, J. (1981). Suicide and the family: Affective disturbances and their implications for understanding, diagnosis, and treatment. In M. R. Lansky (Ed.), *Family therapy and major psychopathology* (pp. 145–160). New York: Grune & Stratton.

42. Warren, L. W., & Tomlinson-Keasey, C. (1987). The context of suicide. *American Journal of Orthopsychiatry, 57,* 41–48.

43. McIntosh, J. L., Hubbard, R. W., & Santos, J. F. (1981). Suicide among the elderly: A review of issues with case studies. *Journal of Gerontological Social Work, 4,* 63–74.

44. Slater, J., & Depue, R. A. (1981). The contribution of environmental events and social support to serious suicide attempts in primary depressive disorder. *Journal of Abnormal Psychology, 40,* 275–285.

45. Hudgens, R. W. (1983). Preventing suicide. *New England Journal of Medicine, 308,* 897–898.

46. Health and Welfare Canada. (1987). *Suicide in Canada: Report of the National Task Force on Suicide in Canada.* Ottawa: Department of National Health and Welfare.

47. Kosky, P. (1982). Childhood suicidal behavior. *Journal of Child Psychology and Psychiatry and Allied Disciplines, 24,* 457–467.

48. Pfeffer, C. R., Plutchik, R., & Mizruchi, M. S. (1983). Suicidal and assaultive behavior in children: Classification, measurement, and intervention. *American Journal of Psychiatry, 140,* 154–157.

49. Derryberry, D., & Rothbart, M. K. (1984). Emotion, attention, and temperament. In C. E. Izard, J. Kagan, & R. B. Zajonc (Eds.), *Emotions, cognition and behavior* (pp. 132–167). Cambridge: Cambridge University Press.

50. Sabbath, J. C. (1969). The suicidal adolescent: The expendable child. *Journal of the American Academy of Child Psychiatry, 8,* 272–289.

51. Piaget, J., & Inhelder, B. (1969). *The psychology of the child.* New York: Basic Books.

52. Orbach, I., & Glaubman, H. (1979). The concept of death and suicidal behavior in young children: Three case studies. *Journal of the American Academy of Child Psychiatry, 18,* 668–678.

53. McIntire, M. S., Angle, C. R., & Struempler, L. J. (1972). The concept of death in midwestern children and youth. *American Journal of Diseases of Children, 123,* 527–532.

54. Pfeffer, C. R. (1986). *The suicidal child.* New York: Guilford Press.

55. Green, A. H. (1978). Self-destructive behavior in battered children. *American Journal of Psychiatry, 135,* 579–582.

56. Adams-Tucker, C. (1982). Proximate effects of sexual abuse in childhood: A report in 28 children. *American Journal of Psychiatry, 139,* 1252–1256.

57. Orbach, I., Gross, Y., & Glaubman, H. (1981). Some common characteristics of latency-age suicidal children: A tentative model based on case study analyses. *Suicide and Life-Threatening Behavior, 11,* 180–190.

58. Pfeffer, C. R. (1982). Intervention for suicidal children and their parents. *Suicide and Life-Threatening Behavior, 12,* 240–248.

59. Connell, H. M. (1972). Attempted suicide in school children. *Medical Journal of Australia, 1,* 686–690.

60. Erikson, E. H. (1980). *Identity and the life cycle*. New York: Norton.

61. Erikson, E. H. (1968). *Identity: Youth and crisis*. New York: Norton.

62. Jacobs, J. (1971). *Adolescent suicide*. New York: Wiley Interscience.

63. Curran, D. K. (1987). *Adolescent suicidal behavior*. Washington, DC: Hemisphere.

64. Topol, P., & Reznikoff, M. (1982). Perceived peer and family relationships, hopelessness, locus of control as factors in adolescent suicide attempts. *Suicide and Life-Threatening Behavior, 12*, 141–150.

65. Coleman, L. (1987). *Suicide clusters*. Boston: Faber & Faber.

66. Gould, M. S., & Shaffer, D. (1986). The impact of suicide in television movies: Evidence of imitation. *New England Journal of Medicine, 315*, 690–694.

67. Phillips, D. P., & Carstensen, L. L. (1986). Clustering of teenage suicides after television news stories about suicide. *New England Journal of Medicine, 315*, 685–689.

68. Sheehy, G. (1976). *Passages: Predictable crises of adult life*. New York: Dutton.

69. Brown, G. W., & Harris, T. (1978). *Social origins of depression*. London: Tavistock.

70. Stephens, J. B. (1985). Suicidal women and their relationships with husbands, boyfriends, and lovers. *Suicide and Life-Threatening Behavior, 15*, 77–89.

71. Illfeld, F. W. (1977). Current social stressors and symptoms of depression. *American Journal of Psychiatry, 134*, 161–166.

72. Maris, R. W. (1981). *Pathways to suicide: A survey of self-destructive behaviors*. Baltimore: Johns Hopkins University Press.

73. Fryer, J. (1987). AIDS and suicide. In J. D. Morgan (Ed.), *Suicide: Helping those at risk* (pp. 193–200). London, Ontario: King's College Press.

74. Marzuk, P. M., Tierney, H., Tardiff, K., Gross, E. M., Morgan, E. B., Hsu, M., & Mann, J. J. (1988). Increased risk of suicide in persons with AIDS. *Journal of the American Medical Association, 259*, 1333–1337.

75. National Center for Health Statistics. (1987, August 28). *Monthly vital statistics report* (Vol. 36, no. 5, DHHS Publication No. PHS 87-1120). Washington, DC: Government Printing Office.

76. Levinson, D. J., Darrow, C., Klein, E., Levinson, M., & McKee, B. (1978). *The seasons of a man's life*. New York: Knopf.

77. Viorst, J. (1986). *Necessary losses*. New York: Fawcett.

78. Peck, R. C. (1968). Psychological developments in the second half of life. In B. L. Neugarten (Ed.), *Middle age and aging: A reader in social psychology* (pp. 88–92). Chicago: University of Chicago Press.

79. Santrock, J. W. (1985). *Adult development and aging*. Dubuque, IA: William C. Brown.

80. Roy, A., & Linnoila, M. (1986). Alcoholism and suicide. In R. Maris (Ed.), *Biology of suicide* (pp. 162–191). New York: Guilford Press.

81. Dorpat, T. L., & Ripley, H. S. (1960). A study of suicide in the Seattle area. *Comprehensive Psychiatry, 1*, 349–359.

82. Dorpat, T. L., Anderson, W. F., & Ripley, H. S. (1968). The relationship of physical illness to suicide. In H. L. P. Resnik (Ed.), *Suicide: Diagnosis and management* (pp. 208–219). Boston: Little, Brown.

83. Miller, M. (1979). *Suicide after sixty: The final alternative.* New York: Springer.

84. Darbonne, A. R. (1969). Suicide and age: A suicide note analysis. *Journal of Consulting and Clinical Psychology, 33,* 46–50.

85. Wass, H. (1979). Death and the elderly. In H. Wass (Ed.), *Dying: Facing the facts* (pp. 182–203). Washington, DC: Hemisphere.

86. Benson, R. A., & Brodie, D. C. (1975). Suicide by overdose of medicines among the aged. *Journal of the American Geriatrics Society, 23,* 304–308.

87. Bock, E. W., & Webber, I. L. (1972, February). Suicide among the elderly: Isolating widowhood and mitigating alternatives. *Journal of Marriage and the Family, 34,* 24–31.

88. Butler, R. N., & Lewis, M. I. (1977). *Aging and mental health: Positive psychological approaches.* St. Louis: Mosby.

89. Breed, W., & Huffine, C. (1979). Sex differences in suicide among older White Americans: A role and developmental approach. In O. J. Kaplan (Ed.), *Psychopathology of aging* (pp. 289–309). New York: Academic Press.

90. Lyons, M. J. (1984). Suicide in later life: Some putative causes with implications for prevention. *Journal of Community Psychology, 12,* 379–388.

91. Miller, M. (1978). Note: Toward a profile of the older white male suicide. *The Gerontologists, 18,* 80–82.

92. Butler, R. N., & Lewis, M. I. (1982). *Aging and mental health: Positive psychological and biomedical approaches* (3rd ed.). St. Louis: Mosby.

93. Barraclough, B. M. (1971). Suicide in the elderly. In D. W. Kay & A. Walk (Eds.), *Recent developments in psychogeriatrics* (pp. 89–97). Kent, England: Headly Brothers.

94. Miller, M. (1978). Geriatric suicide: The Arizona study. *The Gerontologists, 18,* 488–495.

95. Rockwell, D., & O'Brien, W. (1973). Physicians' knowledge and attitudes about suicide. *Journal of the American Medical Association, 225,* 1347–1349.

96. McIntosh, J. L. (1985). Suicide among the elderly: Levels and trends. *American Journal of Orthopsychiatry, 35,* 288–293.

34 Suicide as Psychache ∿

Edwin S. Shneidman

EDWIN S. SHNEIDMAN is Professor of Thanatology Emeritus at the UCLA
Neuropsychiatric Institute. He was the founder of the American Association
of Suicidology. This selection is a brief article in which Shneidman makes
the argument that the cause of suicide is psychache; that is, psychological
pain or anguish in the psyche (mind). It is only when this psychological pain
becomes unbearable (and different people have different thresholds in this
respect) that suicide occurs. Where does this pain come from? He argues that
it comes from frustrated psychological needs. His main point is that the
cause is psychological as opposed to sociological or psychiatric (e.g., depression). He argues a major focus of suicidology in the years ahead should be on
ways to measure the levels and degrees of psychache.

AS I NEAR THE END OF MY CAREER IN SUICIDOLOGY, I think I can now say what
has been on my mind in as few as five words: *Suicide is caused by psychache* (sīk-
āk; two syllables). Psychache refers to the hurt, anguish, soreness, aching, psychological *pain* in the psyche, the mind. It is intrinsically psychological—the
pain of excessively felt shame, or guilt, or humiliation, or loneliness, or fear, or
angst, or dread of growing old or of dying badly, or whatever. When it occurs,
its reality is introspectively undeniable. Suicide occurs when the psychache is
deemed by that person to be unbearable. This means that suicide also has to do
with different individual *thresholds* for enduring psychological pain (Shneidman, 1985, 1992).

All our past efforts to relate or to correlate suicide with simplistic nonpsy-
chological variables, such as sex, age, race, socioeconomic level, case history
items (no matter how dire), psychiatric categories (including depression), etc.,
were (and are) doomed to miss the mark precisely because they ignore the one
variable that centrally relates to suicide, namely, intolerable psychological
pain; in a word, psychache.

By its very nature, psychological pain is tied to psychological needs. In
general, the broadest purpose of most human activity is to satisfy psychological needs. Suicide relates to psychological needs in that suicide is a specific way

From Edwin S. Shneidman, "Suicide as Psychache," *Journal of Nervous and Mental Disease*,
Vol. 181, No. 3, pp. 147–149. Copyright © Williams and Wilkins, 1993. Reprinted by permission of the publisher.

to stop the unbearable psychachical flow of the mind. Furthermore, what causes this pain is the blockage, thwarting, or frustration of certain psychological needs believed by that person (at that time and in those circumstances) to be vital to continued life.

Suicide is not adaptive, but adjustive in the sense that it serves to reduce the tension of the pain related to the blocked needs. Murray's (1938) monumental volume *Explorations in Personality* provides a comprehensive list of psychological needs, and their definitions: abasement, achievement, affiliation, aggression, autonomy, counteraction, defendance, deference, dominance, exhibition, harmavoidance, infavoidance, inviolacy, nurturance, order, play, rejection, sentience, succorance, and understanding.

There is an integral relationship between suicide and happiness—or rather the absence of it. Genuine happiness—contrary to the 19th and 20th century materialistic notions that narrowly identified happiness with the mere absence of pain and the presence of creature comforts—has a special magical quality (Spender, 1988). There is a mundane happiness of comfort, pain avoidance, and psychological anesthesia. But genuine, magical happiness has relatively little to do with creature comfort; rather, it is the kind of ecstasy and consuming exuberance that one can experience only in a benign childhood. To the extent that suicide relates to happiness, it relates in people of any age—not to lack of mundane happiness but the loss of childhood's magical joys.

A principal task for contemporary suicidology is to operationalize (and metricize) the key dimension of psychache. One way to begin is to ask the simple question, "How much do you hurt?" (Kropf, 1990).

One trenchant way to understand any individual is to rank order (or Q-sort) the prepotency among the 20 needs, that is, to define or characterize that individual's personality in terms of his or her weightings among all the needs. This can be done by assigning, for that individual, a number to each need, so that the total sum for the individual adds up to 100. This permits us to rate various individuals (or a single individual over time) by use of the constant sum method. The task is simple and takes only a few minutes. (Try it by rating yourself; and then rate a well-known public figure, have colleagues rate that same figure, rate your patients after each session, rate suicidal patients, and rate nonsuicidal patients.)

In relation to suicide, there are, within any individual, two sets of dispositions or sets of relative weightings among the 20 psychological needs. They are: a) those psychological needs that the individual lives with, that define his or her personality in its day-to-day intrapsychic and interpersonal functioning—the *modal* needs; and b) those few psychological needs, the frustration of what that individual simply cannot tolerate; the needs that person would die for—the *vital* needs. Within an individual, these two kinds of needs are psychologically consistent with each other. The vital needs come into play when the individual is under threat or duress. This special disposition of needs can be elicited by asking an individual about his precise reactions to the failures or losses or rejections or humiliations—the dark moments—previously in his life.

By means of an intensive psychological autopsy (Shneidman, 1977), it should be possible to identify (or label) every committed suicide in terms of the two or three prepotent needs the frustration of which played a major role in that death. (With 20 needs, we have a possible taxonomy of a few hundred different "types" of suicide.)

The prevention of suicide (with a highly lethal person) is then primarily a matter of addressing and partially alleviating those frustrated psychological needs that are driving that person to suicide. The rule is simple: Mollify the psychache.

In the progression to a suicidal outcome, I believe that we can distinguish seven components. They are:

1. The vicissitudes of life; those stresses, failures, rejections, and catabolic and social and psychological insults that are omnipresent by virtue of living.

2. Various approaches to understanding human behavior. Suicidal behavior (as is all behavior) is obviously multidimensional, which means, in practice, that its proper explication has to be multidisciplinary. The relevant fields for suicidology include biochemistry (and genetics), sociology, demography-epidemiology, psychology, psychiatry, linguistics, and so on. The reader should appreciate that *this* paper is limited to the psychological approach to suicide, without derogating the importance of other legitimate approaches.

3. The vicissitudes of life as they are perceptually funnelled through the human mind and apperceived (or appreciated) as ecstatic, pleasurable, neutral, inconsequential, or painful. If there is extreme psychache, a necessary condition for suicide is present. "I hurt too much."

4. The perception of the pain as unbearable, intolerable, and unacceptable, another necessary condition for suicide, in addition to psychache. "I won't put up with this pain."

5. The thought (or insight) that cessation of consciousness is the solution for the unbearable psychache, still another necessary condition. In a phrase, death is preferable to living, with death as a means of egression or escape. "I can kill myself."

6. A lowered threshold for enduring or sustaining the crippling psychache, a final necessary condition for suicide. A priori, people with more or less equal amounts of psychache might have radically different overt outcomes depending upon their different thresholds for tolerating or enduring

psychological pain. (In life, pain is ubiquitous and inescapable; suffering is optional.)

7. The suicidal outcome. "I hurt too much to live."

About now, the alert and restive reader might be asking, What about depression? As everyone knows, depression is a serious psychiatric syndrome, well recognized and relatively treatable. But depression is not the same as suicide. They are quite different. For one thing, they have enormously different fatality rates. One can live a long, unhappy life with depression—not true of an acutely suicidal state. Theoretically, no one has ever died of depression—it is not a legitimate cause of death on the death certificate—but many people, too many, have died of suicide. Vast numbers of people suffer from minor and major depressions. Depression seems to have physiological, biochemical, and probably genetical components. The use of medications in treatment is on target. It is, so to speak, a biological storm in the brain. Suicide, on the other hand, is a phenomenological event, a transient tempest in the mind. It is responsive to talk therapy and to changes in the environment. Suicide is not a psychiatric disorder. Suicide is a nervous dysfunction, not a mental disease. *All* persons who commit suicide—100% of them—are perturbed, but they are not necessarily clinically depressed (or schizophrenic, or alcoholic or addicted or psychiatrically ill). A suicidal crisis is best treated on its own terms. It is a deadly serious (temporary and treatable) psychache (Table 1).

Depression never causes suicide; rather, suicide results from severe psychache, coupled with dysphoria, constriction of perceptual range, and the idea of death as preferable to life. By themselves, the clinical symptoms of depression are debilitating, but, by their nature, not deadly. On the other hand, severe psychache by itself may be life threatening. Correlating suicide with DSM categories is irrelevant to the real action in the mind's main tent. Depression merits treatment for itself, but then to assert that suicide is essentially depression is either a logical mistake, a conceptual confusion, or a professional gambit. In any case, it is past time to make this correction.

Here, finally, after over 40 years of experience as a suicidologist, is a tight summary of my current beliefs about suicide.

1. The explanation of suicide in humankind is the same as the explanation of the suicide of any particular human. Suicidology, the study of human suicide, and a psychological autopsy (of a particular case) are identical in their goals: to nibble at the puzzle of human self-destruction.

2. The most evident fact about suicidology and suicidal events is that they are multidimensional, multifaceted, and multidisciplinary, containing, as they do, concomitant biological, sociological, psychological (interpersonal and intrapsychic), epidemiological, and philosophical elements.

TABLE 1 Symptoms of Depression: Characteristics of Suicide

Depression[a]	Suicide
1. Sadness	1. In great psychological pain (psychache)
2. Apathy	
3. Loss of appetite or increased appetite	2. Cannot stand the pain (lowered threshold for suffering)
4. Insomnia, or sleeping far more than usual	
5. Feeling physically agitated or slowed down	3. Sees ending life as an escape (death as solution)
6. Fatigue and lack of energy	4. Sees no possibilities other than death (constriction)
7. Feelings of worthlessness or great guilt	5. May or may not have symptoms of depression (suicide as a mental state)
8. Inability to concentrate or indecisiveness	
9. Thoughts of death or suicide	

[a] The source (for Depression) was *The New York Times*, August 5, 1992 (by permission).

3. From the view of the psychological factors in suicide, the key element in every case is psychological pain: psychache. All affective states (such as rage, hostility, depression, shame, guilt, affectlessness, hopelessness, etc.) are relevant to suicide only as they relate to unbearable psychological pain. If, for example, feeling guilty or depressed or having a bad conscience or an overwhelming unconscious rage makes one suicidal, it does so only because it is painful. No psychache, no suicide.

4. Individuals have different thresholds for enduring or tolerating pain; thus, the individual's decision not to bear the pain—the threshold for enduring it—is also directly relevant.

5. In every case, the psychological pain is created and fueled by frustrated psychological needs. These needs have been explicated by Murray (1938, chapter 3, pp. 142–242).

6. There are modal psychological needs with which the person lives (and which define the personality) and there are vital psychological needs whose frustration cannot be tolerated (which define the suicide). Within an individual, these two kinds of needs are psychologically consistent with each other, although not necessarily the same as each other.

7. The remediation (or therapy) of the suicidal state lies in addressing and mollifying the vital frustrated needs. The therapist does well to have this

template (of psychological needs) in mind so that the therapy can be tailor-made for that patient. Often, just a little bit of mollification of the patient's frustrated needs can change the vital balance sufficiently to save a life.

References

Kropf J (1990) An empirical assessment of Murray's personological formation of suicide. Unpublished doctoral dissertion. California School of Professional Psychology, Fresno, CA.

Murray H (1938) *Explorations in personality.* New York: Oxford University Press.

Shneidman ES (1977) The psychological autopsy. In L Gottschalk et al (Eds), *Guide to the investigation and reporting of drug abuse deaths.* Rockville, MD: ADAMHA.

Shneidman ES (1985) *Definition of suicide.* New York: Wiley.

Shneidman ES (1992) A conspectus of the suicidal scenario. In RW Maris et al (Eds), *Assessment and prediction of suicide.* New York: Guilford.

Spender S (1988) Introduction to the second edition. In P O'Connor, *Memoirs of a public baby.* New York: W. W. Norton.

PART NINE

VIOLENT DEATH, DISASTERS, AND MEGADEATH

Contents

PART IX BEGINS WITH AN ARTICLE by Witkin dealing with the epidemic of urban homicide that has swept across our nation in recent years. Witkin seeks to understand why it is that so many inner-city teenagers find it so easy to kill for offenses that in the past would have led to fist fights. He argues that these teenagers have been desensitized to violence. He discusses the important role of gun proliferation and the evidence that teenagers who kill with guns almost always get them illegally, suggesting that current gun control legislation is unlikely to have much impact. Other factors considered include lack of fear of the criminal justice system, gang participation, and drug consumption and dealing. At the end of the article, the author discusses some possible ways to deal with these problems. We urge the reader to ask how much impact these programs and strategies are likely to have. What other strategies might work?

The discussion of trends in homicide rates naturally leads to discussion of the death penalty and capital punishment. The article by Weisberg presents a very graphic description of what it is like to be put to death using each of the methods that are currently legal in the United States. One thing we learn is that it is not uncommon for there to be a discrepancy between the way the method is supposed to work and what actually happens. Another interesting aspect of this selection is the discussion of whether or not it would be a good idea to start televising executions.

The article by Zeisel and Gallup represents an effort to assess public sentiment on the issue of the death penalty by using national poll data. They trace shifts in sentiment over the 50-year period from 1936 to 1986, and include a very interesting overview of the strength of sentiment on this issue. The selection also includes a discussion of the reasons people give for favoring or opposing the death penalty, including their assessment of its deterrence value. The authors present evidence that sentiment in favor of the death penalty has been increasing in recent decades.

The selection by Erikson describes another form of violent death: death as the result of a natural disaster. The focus of this account is not on the experience of dying in a natural disaster, rather it is on the aftermath of a disaster in which there has been a great deal of loss of life and property. Of interest to Erikson was the destruction of the sense of community (Erikson uses the term communality). The disaster was the Buffalo Creek flood of 1972 that resulted when a dam burst in a West Virginia mountain hollow. When the survivors of the flood were forced to give up their ties with familiar places (relocation was necessary) and people, they experienced disorientation, demoralization, and the loss of a sense of community. They became very apathetic and were no longer able to care for one another in the way they did prior to the flood.

The article by Wiesel is taken from *Night*, his well-known book that describes his concentration camp experience as a child. This selection presents a moving and graphic description of the train trip to the concentration camp with his father, life in the camp, and the experience of being liberated at the end of the war. Most, if not all, readers of this article will be aware of the general outline of what went on in the Nazi concentration camps. The power of this selection is in the graphic first-person account of the experience, particularly the relationship between Elie Wiesel and his father during this experience.

The selection by Rummel deals with murder on a much more massive scale than that considered by Witkin. Rummel's article deals with what he refers to as megamurderers, national governments that are responsible for the deaths of 1 million or more people (excluding those who have died as the result of warfare). He estimates that over 142 million people have died during this century at the hands of 11 such governments. An attribute of all these states is absolute power. The list includes the Soviet Union, Communist China, Nazi Germany, Khmer Rouge Cambodia, Communist Vietnam, and Communist Yugoslavia. He also discusses states he describes as "kilomurderers" as well. The reference here is to nations that have killed tens or hundreds of thousands of innocent citizens. Here he includes such countries as Angola, Ethiopia, Chile, Croatia (1941–1944), Indonesia, Iran, and Uganda, among others. He argues that the vast majority of these deaths are caused by authoritarian regimes, but he does also point out that a substantial number of foreigners have been killed in cold blood by democratic states as well. In this category, he includes the deliberate targeting of civilian populations in Germany and Japan by allied bombers during World War II, the massacres of Filipinos during the period of American colonization at the turn of the century, and atrocities committed by Americans in Vietnam. In some important respects, this article is an update of Gil Elliot's 1972 book, *The Twentieth Century Book of the Dead*. The reader is urged to consult that book (or the selection from that book included in the third edition of this anthology) for a detailed accounting of the various ways in which millions of people have met violent and untimely deaths during this century.

35 Kids Who Kill ∾

Gordon Witkin

In this selection, GORDON WITKIN discusses the sources of youth violence
in the cities. He argues that today's youth are desensitized to violence—in
part by the violence they experience on an everyday basis, and in part by
Rambo-like images in the media that glorify violence. His explanations
emphasize the impact of poverty as well as the abuse and neglect many of
these children experience, but he gives particular attention to the role of
drugs, gangs, and the availability of guns. Witkin also has some ideas about
steps that can be taken to reduce the level of youth violence in the inner
cities.

KEVIN'S MOTHER WAS A DRUG ADDICT, his father a dope dealer. After being
taken from them by social workers in his native Massachusetts, Kevin★ went to
live with his grandparents in Texas. His grandfather, a security guard, let him
shoot a .22, and "firing it made me feel like I was on top." By his early teens,
he was firing a gun out windows at a nearby day-care center to show off and he
had joined a gang. He began carrying a .38-caliber revolver at 14 and obtained
guns by burglarizing nearby homes. "I wanted to carry a weapon because I
wasn't going to tolerate anything. I was scared and I was mad." At 15, Kevin
began working for a Jamaican drug trafficking posse and eventually became an
enforcer who did his work by shooting people in the arm.

One day, $2,000 of the Jamaicans' money was lost, and though Kevin says
he was innocent, the blame fell on him. Panicking, he confronted an acquaintance whom he suspected of the theft. "I figured if I shot him, the Jamaicans
wouldn't think I'd taken the money," he says. "He begged for his life five
times. I shot him in the face at point-blank range and killed him instantly.
Blood was everywhere, and some parts of his head were laying in the doorway.
I didn't have to kill him. If I'd just pulled the gun, I could have gotten my
money. But still I shot him. The man lost his life over nothing."

This is the stone-hearted ethos of an astonishingly large segment of the
teenage population. It saturates not only the gang-ridden environment of the
cities but the supposedly more benign suburban world as well. Everyday quar-

rels that used to result in flailing fists and bloody noses—over a bump on the shoulder, a misinterpreted glance, romantic complications or flashy clothes—now end, with epidemic frequency, in gunshots.

The reasons why are clear. Today's kids are desensitized to violence as never before, surrounded by gunfire and stuffed with media images of Rambos who kill at will. For many inner-city youngsters, poverty and hopelessness yield a "what the hell" attitude that provides the backdrop for gunplay. Family breakdowns further fuel the crisis; a survey of Baltimore public-school students showed that 59 percent of the males who came from one-parent or no-parent homes have carried a handgun. But by far the biggest difference in to-day's atmosphere is that the no-problem availability of guns in every nook of the nation has turned record numbers of everyday encounters into deadly ones.

The datelines change daily, but the stories are chillingly similar. In Wash-ington, D.C., 15-year-old Jermaine Daniel is shot to death by his best friend. In New Haven, Conn., Markiest Alexander, 14, is killed in a drive-by shoot-ing. In St. Louis, Leo Wilson, 16, is robbed of his tennis shoes and Raiders jacket and then shot dead. In New York, a 14-year-old boy opens up with a semiautomatic pistol in a Bronx schoolyard, wounding one youngster and nar-rowly missing another, apparently in a dispute over a girl.

Those outside the city are no less vulnerable. Within the past fortnight, in an exclusive neighborhood of Pasadena, Calif., police say two teenage boys passed a shotgun between them to shoot three young women to death at close range. Asked why, the suspects reportedly told police they'd had angry words with the victims but couldn't remember what the fight was about. In middle-class Lumberton, N.J., outside Philadelphia, a 14-year-old boy took a revolver from his father's gun cabinet in late February and fatally shot a basketball team-mate in the back of the head.

These tales from the streets were punctuated last month by some knee-weakening numbers from the government's National Center for Health Statis-tics, which analyzed youth firearm death rates from 1979 to 1988. The study showed that gun homicides felled 1,022 teens ages 15 to 19 in 1984; the number spiked to 1,641 in 1988. The picture was especially bleak for young black males 15 to 19, for whom firearm homicides climbed from 418 in 1984 to 955 in 1988. Their homicide rate in 1988 was more than 11 times the rate for their white counterparts. And research by James Alan Fox of Northeastern University shows that the number of black teenage gunmen who have killed has risen sharply, from 181 in 1984 to a record 555 in 1989.

"During every 100 hours on our streets we lose more young men than were killed in 100 hours of ground war in the Persian Gulf," lamented Louis Sullivan, secretary of the Department of Health and Human Services. "Where are the yellow ribbons of hope and remembrance for our youth dying in the streets?"

Amid the carnage, much of the political discussion seems sterile and off the point. . . . When Ronald Reagan endorsed the Brady bill, a modest measure that would require a seven-day waiting period to buy a gun, it was heralded by gun-control advocates. In fact, almost all teens who kill with guns *already* get them illegally, and nothing in the bill or George Bush's get-tough crime law will address the existing system that places more and more guns with greater and greater firepower in the hands of kids.

Some communities are taking small steps to halt the tragic cycle of teenage gun violence. But psychologist Charles Patrick Ewing, author of "When Children Kill," argues that the confluence of several trends is foreboding. Among them: the continuing proliferation of guns, increases in numbers of abused and neglected children, hefty juvenile poverty rates and a projected 7.7 percent increase in the population of 5-to-17-year-olds. Ewing predicts this will be "the bloodiest decade of juvenile violence we've ever seen."

THE EXPLOSION OF GUNS

John★ had two requirements for the homes he burglarized around Winston-Salem, N.C.: first, that they belonged to gun owners and, second, that the owners weren't home. For more than a year and a half, at the rate of a house a day, he batted nearly 1.000. John, now 15, traded many of the guns for marijuana and cocaine. Sometimes he sold the guns at school. Either way, they moved. "If somebody knows you have a gun—nobody is going to mess with you," he says.

John's days as a gun burglar ended when the police were tipped off to his activities. He was charged with 15 counts of breaking and entering and two counts of burglary. He spent 14 months at a camp for problem kids, must serve 660 hours of community service and must pay $2,212 in restitution. His court-appointed counselor says John's only remaining problem is truancy, but for John, temptation abounds. "You can get drugs and guns here real easy," he says of school.

It's the presence of so many guns that makes the current atmosphere so volatile. Arrests of kids under 18 for weapons violations jumped from 19,649 in 1976 to 31,577 in 1989. Firearm murders committed by youngsters in that same age bracket leaped from 444 in 1984 to 952 in 1989, according to the National Crime Analysis Program at Northeastern University.

Ask a streetwise kid how tough it is to get a gun, and a smile is often the response—"no problem." The best available estimates indicate that between 150 million and 200 million guns nationwide are in civilian hands. A 1989 poll reported that nearly 3 out of 5 Americans own guns. Domestic firearm production, after dipping in the early 1980s, grew steadily from 3.1 million in 1986 to 4.4 million in 1989.

A 20-state survey of 11,000 adolescents found that 41 percent of the boys could obtain a handgun if they wanted to. An extrapolation of surveys by the National School Safety Center suggested that 135,000 students carried guns to school daily in 1987. Officials at the center think that figure is higher today.

In cities with strong gun-control laws, like Boston, New York and Washington, weapons are imported and resold at a profit by traffickers who purchase them in states that until recently have had few gun-buying restrictions: Florida, Texas, Virginia, Georgia and Ohio. In Los Angeles, two men operating out of a van in a park east of downtown are thought to have sold more than 1,000 handguns over an eight-month period last year, largely to street-gang members, before being arrested. In suburban Chicago last fall, police say, a 16-year-old boy rented a gun from a fellow student for $100, then used it to kill his parents.

There is no mystery about how kids get guns. A survey of Baltimore public-school students showed the four most prevalent sources to be street corners, friends, drug dealers and thefts. Residential burglaries are lucrative pipelines, and mom and dad are often unknowingly a ready supply. A Florida school study found that 86 percent of the guns taken from students were from their homes.

And the trend is toward more powerful guns with higher-capacity magazines, like 9-mm semiautomatic pistols. "You ask a young kid what a '9' is, he knows what you're talking about," says Art Boissiere, 19, who grew up in a tough Oakland, Calif., neighborhood and considered carrying a gun himself. A popular 9-mm gun like a Tec-9 might sell for $300 to $700 on the street. Other, cheaper guns might go for as little as $50.

THE GANG CONNECTION

It began as a typical adolescent dispute—two Texas teenagers talking trash over broken car windows. "And then I pulled out the gun," says Victor,★ 15, whose 1984 Cutlass had been damaged. "And he said, 'You ain't going to shoot me,' and I just started shooting, because he didn't think I would. It would have looked stupid if I pulled the gun and then didn't shoot him. I would have looked dumb."

That's the last thing Victor wanted. He joined a gang at 13 "because I thought I'd be accepted better, and they seemed like family." Guns were everywhere. Soon, Victor was participating in drive-by shootings. "My friends would call me their 'little gangster,'" he says. "With the gun, I felt like I couldn't be stopped." Victor and his friends broke into homes and pawnshops to steal guns, sometimes running pickup trucks right through the front window of a store. Then he'd sell the guns—some 100 in all—to drug dealers and other unsavory acquaintances. In three months, Victor made about $6,000.

Then, in retaliation for a drive-by shooting Victor had taken part in, rival gang members broke the windows in that 1984 Cutlass. After he hunted down the supposed culprits, he fired nine shots, wounding two members. "I just got in the car and sped away," he says. "And then right after that, it started raining, right after I shot them. And it didn't seem like a day where it was going to rain."

Much of the fuel for the growth in youth violence flows from gangs and drugs. Not nearly as many teens would have guns if they hadn't raised the money by dealing drugs, nor would the streets be so violent these days in the absence of drug trade. While there has been progress in the war against casual drug use, some 1.7 million to 2.4 million Americans are still weekly cocaine users. But some authorities think the drug trade today is more deadly than ever precisely because traffickers are tussling over a shrinking pie.

Gangs are growing like a cancer. The Crips and the Bloods began in Southern California about 20 years ago but now have loose affiliations in 32 states and 113 cities. Not only have they absorbed the talents of local toughs, but they've given a twisted kind of haven to confused inner-city kids for whom gangs provide the security, acceptance and protection that are often missing in fragmented homes. The price of that kind of security is horrific. In the Los Angeles area, gangs doubled from 400 with 45,000 members in 1985 to 800 with 90,000 members in 1990. Gang-related killings last year accounted for 690 deaths, 35 percent of the county's homicides.

In this atmosphere, carrying a gun is just keeping up with the Joneses. "The gun is your best friend," says a 15-year-old gang member in south central L.A. One popular local saying: "I'd rather be judged by 12 than carried by six."

Using a gun is often a rite of passage for joining a gang or enhancing a reputation. Recently, a 14-year-old rode by an East L.A. schoolyard on his bike, randomly firing a semiautomatic at the nearly 2,000 children on the playground. "He just wanted to prove to his gang he was worthy," says Capt. Ray Gott of the L.A. County Sheriff's Department.

Los Angeles gang experts have identified three levels of gun-packing gang involvement. "The wannabes are starting to do target practice and get used to holding a gun. They may shoot, but in a lot of cases they won't aim," says Steve Valdivia, director of an outreach program called Community Youth Gang Services. "The next level is a gang-involved youth who wants to make his stripes. He's going to kill somebody. But he's not yet seen by his peers as a hard-core crazy person. If they get to that final level, they don't care about themselves or the victim—very random violence, very cold-blooded. These are the guys who will open a casket and shoot a dead body with a semiautomatic until it turns to ketchup. I know that has happened."

The spread of gangs basically followed the interstate highway system. They moved into Minneapolis from Chicago almost 10 years ago and have been building ever since. "The word got out that Minneapolis was easy pickings," says one gang member. "Moneyapolis." The police can identify more than 3,000 gang members, though no one knows for sure. And with the gangs came the guns. Hundreds of them. "They're coming up from Chicago every day," says Ramone,★ a member of the Bloods. "My gang holds them until we need them. I say I'm in trouble and they give me a gun." In Hennepin County, the number of juveniles tried as adults for carrying dangerous weapons—mostly guns—jumped from 14 in 1986–87 to 63 in 1990.

In cities like Austin, Texas, gang growth has come from both home-grown groups and infiltration by outsiders. Gang membership there has climbed from just 200 five years ago to some 2,800 today. Last September, after rival gang members taunted each other at a crowded downtown bus stop, a 16-year-old fired a 9-mm pistol, wounding two other teens and a 61-year-old man.

Fear of the criminal-justice system is largely absent in these teens because they realize the system is jammed and know that juvenile penalties lack real bite. In Austin, older gang members call their younger compadres "minutemen" because they'll only be in jail for a minute. Partly for that reason, the high-stakes hurly-burly of drug trafficking has also drawn scores of youths into gun ownership. Adults hire youngsters to run the drugs because the penalties are so much weaker if they're caught. The danger level, though, is no different. Clarence,★ a big-city Texas teen who was clearing $1,200 weekly dealing dope at 15, needed a gun "because people on the corner where I was selling were getting robbed, and you never knew who was coming for you." In February 1989, he saw his best friend get killed for dealing bad dope.

As many as 20 to 25 percent of the kids who shoot people are high themselves—on alcohol or drugs like crack or PCP, all of which are "disinhibitors" that may spur violent behavior. "One time I burst right into this guy's house and shot him," says Shooter, 17, of Los Angeles. "Man, was he surprised. But I wasn't thinking about anything bad happening, because I was doing PCP, and I was all kicked up. It was like he could have shot me, and it wouldn't have mattered."

LOWERING THE KILLING THRESHOLD

Arthur★ is busted now, spending a year at the Hennepin County Home School in Minnetonka, just outside Minneapolis. But he can still wax nostalgic about the small, profitable empire he ran with his younger brother and four others, none older than 16. Drugs gave them money; guns gave them power. "Everybody knew we had them," he says. "Everybody knew not to mess with us." Arthur's gang had some real firepower. "There were just so many coming in," he says. "We had six automatics. We had a .25; a .38; two 9-mm semiautomatic pistols, one of which was a Beretta; a .32 automatic; a 20-gauge shotgun. Some we got out of the newspapers. My brother Dennis★ went way out in some suburbs and picked them up. He bought an AK-47 [assault rifle] for $500. It seemed like we were the only ones who were out there with real artillery. You'd hear all that gunfire, and it was all us."

For some kids, drugs, gangs and guns are simply vehicles through which to satisfy more basic yearnings. Teens have always wanted power, attention, respect and a tough-guy reputation. But the prevailing gang ethos has lowered the threshold of violence and sanctioned the replacement of fists with firearms as the way to achieve those goals.

Often, the fast route to attention is through money or material goods. Sneakers, coats or cash—kids want it now, and the gun can get it. For Clarence, at 15, the motivation for dealing dope and carrying guns was this: "I wanted to get paid. I thought money was the world. I'd spend it on my girlfriend, or I'd take all my homeboys out. If you made money that day, you'd pay, and that made me feel like I was the big daddy, the big man with the master plan."

But Clarence also discovered that the gun provided a power and an image all its own. "If you had a gun, and you were with a girl, she'd be thinking, 'He's bad,'" says Clarence. "It made me feel macho, like nobody could touch me, like no one's going to mess with me."

Nothing inflames the extreme narcissism and hypersensitivity of teens more than disrespect—"dissin'," in the language of the streets. Teen killers cite it perhaps most often as the justification for their lethal acts. "If someone disrespects you or your homeboys, you've got to do something about it," says one Los Angeles teen. "You just can't have them doing that and hold your head up."

One byproduct of this arms race is that many basically good kids now carry guns simply because they're terrified or fed up—or both. "I had it for protection," says Derek of Washington, D.C., who bought a gun at age 17 after a friend was shot to death and Derek himself was robbed. "You lose your sense of dignity after a while, and I wasn't going to let that happen again. I figured the gun would prevent it." In a Boston program for kids caught with weapons, a teacher recently asked, "Is there any way to exist without a weapon?" "Yeah," snapped one teen. "Stay in the house."

THE SCHOOLS CRACK DOWN

Damon★ got angry in his Milwaukee school on Valentine's Day. Some friends were teasing him, slapping him in the face. So Damon, 12, decided to get even. "Wait until I get back," he said as he ran off the playground. "I'm going to cap all of you guys." When Damon returned, he stepped through the opening of the fenced-in playground and pulled from his jacket a silver .25 semiautomatic pistol. He fired it, again and again and again. In an instant, a mass of bluejeans and ponytails was screaming and running toward the school's metal doors. The boy Damon says was slapping him cowered behind a teacher. Damon pointed the gun at him. "I'm going to blow your head off," the teachers quoted Damon as saying. Damon fired five shots, hit nobody and then ran from the schoolyard. Why, he is asked, did he do it? "He slapped me in my face," says Damon, tears rolling down his cheeks. What was Damon thinking? "I don't remember thinking anything," he says. "I just did it."

A Seattle high school uses a breathalyzer to test students suspected of drinking; hundreds of Detroit students pass through metal detectors before entering school, and teachers at Fairfax Elementary School in Mentor, Ohio, signal students to duck from gunfire by yelling "earthquake drill." Welcome to the campus of '91, where "bullies," "deathtraps" and "hole diggers"—commonly known as guns—are often as much the rage as faddish haircuts, team jackets and Air Jordans.

School systems across the country are borrowing heavily from correctional institutions with dress codes, metal detectors and security forces patrolling the hallways. Not surprisingly, more and more schools, especially in America's troubled inner cities, now resemble prisons, with bars across windows, camera monitors and bolted doors. Some school systems are even requiring students to wear identification badges.

At Belvedere Junior High in Los Angeles, where campus aides patrol the hall to maintain order, visitors register name, time and destination with security personnel and are escorted by aides with two-way walkie-talkies. Signs, barely legible through the graffiti, warn against vandalism and trespassing. Seven students, some members of notorious local gangs, have been killed in the past year; two died in one weekend last month. Last fall, a 13-year-old gang member was shot just blocks from the school and died on a sidewalk as his friends gathered around. "This is my fifth year as principal," says Victoria Castro. "The first four years, I lost maybe two children to gang violence. Now we have driveby shootings onto campus. The only thing I keep hoping is that I have no actual incident on campus."

Even suburban schools are coming face to face with guns and crime. A recent study of Illinois high-school students found that 5.3 percent of them said they had brought a gun to school, and 1 in 12 students confessed to sometimes staying away out of fear.

COMMUNITIES RESPOND

Exasperated by the ever growing teenage body count, a variety of educators, psychologists, pediatricians and just plain folks are experimenting with ways of stopping the carnage. Among them:

Violence prevention Several programs attempt to teach children how to prevent violence; most prominent among them is a curriculum for adolescents used in Boston high schools and several other cities, developed by Deborah

Prothrow-Stith of the Harvard School of Public Health. The 10-session curriculum tries to reduce the allure of violence, make clear its consequences and show kids alternative avenues for dealing with anger. Most experts are encouraged but think the jury's still out on the curriculum's effectiveness.

Gun awareness Alarmed by a rise in gun deaths, schools in Dade County, Fla., inaugurated their own gun-safety program in the 1988–89 school year, in cooperation with the Center to Prevent Handgun Violence. The effort employs books, role-playing and videos to "deglamorize and deglorify the possession and use of guns," says coordinator Bill Harris. Early results are promising, but such programs are only a small piece of the puzzle. The National Rifle Association also runs several gun safety programs tailored to different age groups; one emphasis is the need to secure guns at home.

Offender diversion For the past four years, every Boston public-school student caught with a weapon has been sent to the Barron Assessment & Counseling Center for a five-to-10-day stay. Students there undergo a detailed psychological and educational assessment, and a plan is developed for working with them once they are either back in school or in some alternative setting. BACC students also participate in counseling, regular academic work, violence-prevention classes and trips to local detention facilities. The center has serviced more than 1,000 students, and the recidivism rate is about 5 percent. Director Franklin Tucker admits it would be helpful to have the kids for a longer time. But, adds staffer Richard Puckerin, BACC does provide its kids "a timeout, a chance to think and reflect."

Peers Teens on Target, an Oakland, Calif., program, is based on the idea that young people are better equipped than adults to attack their violence problem. Student volunteers are trained as violence-prevention "advocates," learning about guns, drugs and family violence, and then sent to schools to teach ways of preventing violence. Officials are enthusiastic; they are scraping up more money for the program.

Many believe getting the guns off the streets is the only answer. But the existing gun-control debate misses the mark. Gun-control measures that might help—like personalized combination locks on the gun's safety, allowing only the original owner to use the gun—aren't even part of the current political debate.

Some argue that focusing solely on the weapons obscures the underlying causes of teen gun violence—especially the sense of hopelessness that pervades many inner cities. Yet the national inclination not even to tackle systematically the immediate issue of violence and gun availability suggests there's even less hope that the larger issues will be addressed. And that means the uniquely American tragedy of teens killing teens is likely to continue its record run.

❧ 36 This Is Your Death

Jacob Weisberg

JACOB WEISBERG is a journalist. This article presents very graphic and somewhat grisly descriptions of what it would be like to view people being put to
death using each of the five means of execution used in the United States.
There is also a discussion of what the experience is like for the person being
executed by each of these methods. The author discusses the history of the
movement away from public viewing of executions and discusses recent calls
to begin televising executions—calls that the author does not support. While
the article spends little time discussing the death penalty debate, indirectly it
constitutes a strong plea against capital punishment.

THANKS TO THE DECISION of a California district judge last week, the American public has been spared the spectacle of criminals being executed on television. But the lawsuit, filed by KQED, the public television station in San
Francisco, still served a useful function. It reminded people not only that the
United States remains the only advanced democracy that executes criminals,
but that it is the only country in the world with a grotesque array of execution
techniques worth televising. A century ago Americans knew full well what it
meant for the state to hang someone from the end of a rope. Today, thanks to
the century-long search for a more "humane" method, we know little about
the range of practices that would be featured on the execution channel.

Of the five means of execution still extant in the United States, the oldest
is hanging, which was nearly universal before 1900. The gallows was last used
in Kansas in 1965 and remains an option in Delaware, Montana, and Washington State. If a hanging were ever televised, viewers would see the blindfolded
prisoner standing on a trap door with a rope fastened around his neck, the knot
under his left ear. So long as he is hooded, it is impossible to know for how long
after the trap door opens the victim suffers, or at what point he loses consciousness. But according to Harold Hillman, a British physiologist who has studied
executions, the dangling person feels cervical pain, and probably suffers from
an acute headache as well, a result of the rope closing off the veins of the neck.

In the opinion of Dr. Cornelius Rosse, the chairman of the Department of
Anatomy at the University of Washington School of Medicine, the belief that

fracture of the spinal cord causes instantaneous death is wrong in all but a small fraction of cases. The actual cause of death is strangulation or suffocation. In medical terms, the weight of the prisoner's body causes tearing of the cervical muscles, skin, and blood vessels. The upper cervical vertebrae are dislocated, and the spinal cord is separated from the brain, which causes death.

Clinton Duffy, the warden at San Quentin from 1942 to 1954, who participated in sixty hangings, described his first thus:

> *The man hit bottom and I observed that he was fighting by pulling on the straps, wheezing, whistling, trying to get air, that blood was oozing through the black cap. I observed also that he urinated, defecated, and droppings fell on the floor, and the stench was terrible. I also saw witnesses pass out and have to be carried from the witness room. Some of them threw up.*

It took ten minutes for the condemned man to die. When he was taken down and the cap removed, "big hunks of flesh were torn off" the side of his face where the noose had been, "his eyes were popped," and his tongue was "swollen and hanging from his mouth." His face had also turned purple. The annals of Walla Walla State Penitentiary in Washington, which was seeking to hire an executioner in 1988 when Charles Campbell obtained a stay of execution, are filled with horror stories: prisoners partially decapitated by overlong drops, or pleading with hangmen to take them up and drop them again.

Almost as rare as hanging—but still around—is the firing squad. Gary Gilmore, who was shot in Utah in 1977, was the last to die by this method, which remains an option only there and in Idaho. Gilmore was bound to a chair with leather straps across his waist and head, in front of an oval-shaped canvas wall. A black hood was pulled over his head. A doctor then located his heart with a stethoscope and pinned a circular white cloth target over it. Five shooters armed with .30-caliber rifles loaded with single rounds (one of them blank to spare the conscience of the executioners) stood in an enclosure twenty feet away. Each man aimed his rifle through a slot in the canvas and fired.

Though shooting through the head at close range causes nearly instantaneous death, a prisoner subjected to a firing squad dies as a result of blood loss caused by rupture of the heart or a large blood vessel, or tearing of the lungs. The person shot loses consciousness when shock causes a fall in the supply of blood to the brain. If the shooters miss, by accident or intention, the prisoner bleeds to death slowly, as Elisio J. Mares did in Utah in 1951. It took Gilmore two minutes to die.

It was to mitigate the barbarism of these primitive methods that New York introduced the electric chair in 1890 as a humane alternative. Eighty-three people have been electrocuted since the Supreme Court reinstated capital punishment in 1976, making the method the most common one now in use. It is probably the most gruesome to watch. After being led into the death chamber, the prisoner is strapped to the chair with belts that cross his chest, groin, legs, and arms. Two copper electrodes are then attached; one to his leg, a patch of which will have been shaved bare to reduce resistance to electricity, and another to his shaved head. The electrodes are either soaked in brine or treated with gel (Electro-Creme) to increase conductivity and reduce burning. The prisoner will also be wearing a diaper.

The executioner gives a first jolt of between 500 and 2,000 volts, which lasts for thirty seconds. Smoke usually comes out of the prisoner's leg and head. A doctor then examines him. If he's not dead, another jolt is applied. A third and fourth are given if needed to finish the job. It took five jolts to kill Ethel Rosenberg. In the grisly description of Justice Brennan:

> . . . the prisoner's eyeballs sometimes pop out and rest on [his] cheeks. The prisoner often defecates, urinates, and vomits blood and drool. The body turns bright red as its temperature rises, and the prisoner's flesh swells and his skin stretches to the point of breaking. Sometimes the prisoner catches on fire, particularly if [he] perspires excessively. Witnesses hear a loud and sustained sound like bacon frying, and the sickly sweet smell of burning flesh permeates the chamber.

An electrocuted corpse is hot enough to blister if touched. Thus autopsy must be delayed while internal organs cool. According to Robert H. Kirschner, the deputy chief medical examiner of Cook County, Illinois, "The brain appears cooked in most cases."

There is some debate about what the electrocuted prisoner experiences before he dies, but most doctors I spoke to believe that he feels himself being burned to death and suffocating, since the shock causes respiratory paralysis as well as cardiac arrest. According to Hillman, "It must feel very similar to the medieval trial by ordeal of being dropped in boiling oil." Because the energy of the shock paralyzes the prisoner's muscles, he cannot cry out. "My mouth tasted like cold peanut butter. I felt a burning in my head and my left leg, and I jumped against the straps," Willie Francis, a 17-year-old who survived an attempted execution in 1946, is reported to have said. Francis was successfully executed a year later.

Though all methods of execution can be botched, electrocutions go wrong frequently and dramatically, in part because the equipment is old and hard to repair. At least five have gone awry since 1983. If the electrical current is too weak, the prisoner roasts to death slowly. An instance of this was the May 4, 1990, killing of Jesse Joseph Tafero in Florida. According to witnesses, when the executioner flipped the switch, flames and smoke came out of Tafero's head, which was covered by a mask and cap. Twelve-inch blue and orange flames sprouted from both sides of the mask. The power was stopped, and Tafero took several deep breaths. The superintendent ordered the executioner to halt the current, then try it again. And again.

The affidavits presented for an internal inquiry into what went wrong describe the bureaucratization of the death penalty brilliantly. In the words of one of the officials:

> . . . while working in the Death Chamber, proceeding with the execution as scheduled, I received an indication from Mr. Barton to close my electric breaker. I then told the executioner to close his electric breaker. When the executioner completed the circuit, I noticed unusual fire and smoke coming from the inmate's headpiece. After several seconds, I received an indication to open the electrical breaker to stop the electrical flow. At this time, I noticed the body move as if to be gasping for air. After several seconds, I received the indication to close the breaker the second time, which I did. Again, I noticed the unusual fire and smoke coming from the headpiece. After several seconds, I received the third indication to close the breaker, and again, the fire and smoke came from the headpiece . . .

And so on. Apparently a synthetic sponge, soaked in brine, had been substituted for the natural one applied to Tafero's head. This reduced the flow of electricity to as little as one hundred volts, and ended up torturing the prisoner to death. According to the state prison medical director, Frank Kligo, who attended, it was "less than aesthetically attractive."

Advanced technology does not always make the death penalty less painful to undergo or more pleasant to watch. The gas chamber, which was invented by an army medical corps officer after World War I, was first introduced as a humane alternative to the electric chair in 1924 in Nevada. The original idea, which proved impracticable, was to surprise the prisoner by gassing him in his cell without prior warning. Seven states, including California, still use the gas chamber. The most recent fatality was Leo Edwards, a 36-year-old who was killed in Jackson County, Mississippi, in 1989.

Had KQED won its suit, millions of viewers would have joined a dozen live witnesses in seeing Robert Alton Harris, who murdered two teenage boys in San Diego in 1978, led into a green, octagonal room in the basement of San Quentin Penitentiary. Inside the chamber are two identical metal chairs with perforated seats, marked "A" and "B." The twin chairs were last used in a double execution in 1962. If Harris's execution goes ahead this year or next, two orderlies will fasten him into chair A, attaching straps across his upper and lower legs, arms, groin, and chest. They will also affix a long stethoscope to Haris's chest so that a doctor on the outside can pronounce death.

Beneath the chair is a bowl filled with sulfuric acid mixed with distilled water, with a pound of sodium cyanide pellets suspended in a gauze bag just above. After the door is sealed, and when the warden gives the signal, an executioner in a separate room flicks a lever that releases the cyanide into the liquid. This causes a chemical reaction that releases hydrogen cyanide gas, which rises through the holes in the chair. Like most death row prisoners, Harris is likely to have been reduced to a state of passive acquiescence by his years on death row, and will probably follow the advice of the warden to breathe deeply as soon as he smells rotten eggs. As long as he holds his breath nothing will happen. But as soon as he inhales, according to the testimony of Duffy, the former warden, Harris will lose consciousness in a few seconds. "At first there is evidence of extreme horror, pain, and strangling. The eyes pop. The skin turns purple and the victim begins to drool. It is a horrible sight," he testified.

In medical terms, victims of cyanide gas die from hypoxia, which means the cut-off of oxygen to the brain. The initial result of this is spasms, as in an epileptic seizure. Because of the straps, however, involuntary body movements are restrained. Seconds after he first inhales, Harris will feel himself unable to breathe, but will not lose consciousness immediately. "The person is unquestionably experiencing pain and extreme anxiety," according to Dr. Richard Traystman of Johns Hopkins. "The pain begins immediately and is felt in the arms, shoulders, back, and chest. The sensation is similar to the pain felt by a person during a heart attack, where essentially the heart is being deprived of oxygen." Traystman adds: "We would not use asphyxiation, by cyanide gas or by any other substance, in our laboratory to kill animals that have been used in experiments."

Harris will stop wriggling after ten or twelve minutes, and the doctor will pronounce him dead. An exhaust fan then sucks the poison air out of the chamber. Next the corpse is sprayed with ammonia, which neutralizes traces of the cyanide that may remain. After about half an hour, orderlies enter the chamber, wearing gas masks and rubber gloves. Their training manual advises them to ruffle the victim's hair to release any trapped cyanide gas before removing him.

Thanks to these grotesqueries, states are increasingly turning to lethal injection. This method was imagined for decades (by Ronald Reagan, among others, when he was governor of California in 1973), but was technically invented in 1977 by Dr. Stanley Deutsch, who at the time chaired the Anesthesiology Department at Oklahoma University Medical School. In response to a call by an Oklahoma state senator for a cheaper alternative to repairing the state's derelict electric chair, Deutsch described a way to administer drugs through an intravenous drip so as to cause death rapidly and without pain. "Having been anesthetized on several occasions with ultra short-acting barbiturates and having administered these drugs for approximately 20 years, I can assure you that this is a rapid, pleasant way of producing unconsciousness," Deutsch wrote to state senator Bill Dawson in February 1977. The method was promptly adopted in Oklahoma, and is now either the exclusive method or an option in half of the thirty-six states with death penalty laws. It is becoming the method of choice around the country because it is easier on both the witnesses and the prisoner.

A recent injectee was Lawrence Lee Buxton, who was killed in Huntsville, Texas, on February 26. Buxton was strapped to a hospital gurney, built with an extension panel for his left arm. Technicians stuck a catheter needle into Buxton's arm. Long tubes connected the needle through a hole in a cement block wall to several intravenous drips. The first, which was started immediately, dispensed harmless saline solution. Then, at the warden's signal, a curtain went up, which permitted the witnesses—reporters and friends of the soon-to-be deceased—to view the scene. Unlike some prisoners, Buxton did not have a long wait before the warden received a call from the governor's office, giving the final go-ahead.

According to Lawrence Egbert, an anesthesiologist at the University of Texas in Dallas who has campaigned against lethal injection as a perversion of medical practice, the first drug administered was sodium thiopental, a common barbiturate used as an anesthetic, which puts patients quickly to sleep. A normal dose for a long operation is 1,000 milligrams; Buxton got twice that. As soon as he lost consciousness, the executioner administered pavulon, another common muscle relaxant used in heart surgery. The dose was 100 milligrams, ten times the usual, which stops the prisoner's breathing. This would have killed him in about ten minutes; to speed the process, an equal dose of potassium chloride was subsequently administered. This is another drug commonly used in bypass surgery that relaxes the heart and stops it pumping. It works in about ten seconds. All witnesses heard was the prisoner take a deep breath, then a gurgling noise as his tongue dropped back in his mouth. Watt Espy, who has compiled a list of 17,718 executions in America, from the early period of drownings, burnings, sawings-in-half, pressings-to-death, and even the crucifixions of two mutinous Continental Army soldiers, compares lethal injection to the way a devoted owner treats "a faithful dog he's loved and cherished."

The only physical pain, if the killing is done correctly, "is the pain of the initial prick of the needle," according to Traystman. There are, however, some potential hitches. Since doctors are precluded by medical ethics from participating in executions, except to pronounce death, the injections are often performed by incompetent or inexperienced technicians. If a death worker injects the drugs into muscle instead of a vein, or if the needle becomes clogged, extreme pain can result. This is what happened when James Autry was killed in 1984 in Texas. *Newsweek* reported that he "took at least ten minutes to die and throughout much of that time was conscious, moving about, and complaining of pain." Many prisoners have damaged veins from injecting drugs intravenously, and technicians sometimes struggle to find a serviceable one. When Texas executed Stephen Morin, a former heroin addict, orderlies prodded his arms with catheters for forty-one minutes. Being strapped to a table for a lengthy period while waiting to die is a form of psychological torture arguably worse than most physical kinds. This is demonstrated by the fact that mock executions, which cause no physical pain, are a common method of torture around the world. The agony comes not from the prospect of pain, but from the expectation of death.

Televised executions would mark the reversal of the process described in Louis P. Masur's *Rites of Execution* and Robert Johnson's *Death Work*, whereby executions have been removed further and further from the community that compels them. Through the eighteenth century, executions were atavistic spectacles performed in full public view. In the nineteenth they were moved inside the prison yard and witnessed by only a few. In the twentieth century, executions moved deep inside the bowels of prisons, where they were performed ever more quickly and quietly to attract minimal notice. American death penalty opponents in the 1800s supported the abolition of public executions as a way-station to ending all executions. They thought that eliminating the grossest manifestations of public barbarism would inevitably lead to the end of capital punishment as an institution. The reform had the opposite effect, however. Invisible executions shocked the sensibilities of fewer people, and dampened the momentum of the reform movement.

Those abolitionists who now support televising executions have absorbed this historical lesson. They want to bring back the equivalent of public executions in order to shock the public into opposing all executions. They hope to accomplish with pictures what Arthur Koestler did with words in his 1955 tract *Reflections on Hanging*, the publication of which led to the abolition of the rope in Great Britain in 1969.

But advances in the art of killing may have deprived them of that tactic. The prospect of televised executions is likely to accelerate the trend away from grisly methods and toward ever more hermetic ways of dispatching wrongdoers. Had the KQED suit been successful, Henry Schwarzschild, a retired ACLU death penalty expert, speculates that California would have responded by quickly joining the national trend toward lethal injection.

Michael Kroll of the Death Penalty Information Center objects to televising executions for exactly this reason. He argues that a video camera would capture only a "very antiseptic moment at the end of a very septic process." With the advent of death by the needle, execution itself is becoming so denatured and mechanistic as to be unshocking even to most live witnesses. This throws death penalty opponents back upon a less vivid, but more compelling case: that it is punishing people with death, not the manner in which they are killed, that is the true issue here; that capital punishment is to be opposed not simply because it is cruel, but because it is wrong.

37 Death Penalty Sentiment in the United States

Hans Zeisel and Alec M. Gallup

HANS ZEISEL was professor of law and sociology at the University of Chicago. ALEC GALLUP is co-chairman of the Gallup Organization in Princeton, New Jersey. In this article, based on national public opinion polling data, Zeisel and Gallup present a very well reasoned analysis of sentiment about the death penalty and changes in that sentiment over the 50-year period from 1936 to 1986. They explore the intensity of sentiment on this issue, the reasons people either favor or oppose the death penalty, the extent to which people believe it is a deterrent, and what kinds of factual information would change their views on the issue. They also present data with respect to death penalty sentiment broken down by background variables such as gender, income, education, ethnicity, and region.

1. HISTORY

For half a century now, the Gallup Poll has been recording the country's sentiment about the death penalty. In 1936, Gallup asked for the first time the question that would be repeated periodically: "Do you favor the death penalty for a person convicted of murder?" In the 1986 poll, the question elicited the responses shown in Table 1.

Figure 1 shows the trend of death penalty sentiment over the last 50 years in percentages of adult Americans who favor the death penalty. The complementary fraction opposes the death penalty, except for the "uncertain" ones, who have been fluctuating between 7 and 13%.

From a peak of 68% in 1953, support for the death penalty steadily declined until 1966, when it reached its low point of 42%. Since then, pro-death penalty sentiment shows an almost uninterrupted growth to its present all-time high of 71 or 72%.

A critical observer could argue that the question is slightly leading and not very precise. Any simple, single question would be open to this criticism. For

TABLE 1   1986 Public Sentiment About the
Death Penalty

	Percentage
Favor the death penalty	71
Do not favor it	21
Uncertain	8
Total	100
N	(3091)

the purpose of charting a trend over time, it is sufficient that the question re-main unchanged. Although a different question might have produced a higher or lower level at any given point, the curve over time would in all likelihood have run parallel to the curve in Figure 1.

2. THE IMPORTANCE OF POPULAR SENTIMENT

The law of the land, as it now stands, leaves it largely to the state legislatures to decide whether to keep, abolish, or reintroduce the death penalty. At present, 37 of our states have the death penalty, and 13 states do not have it. Three of the death penalty states, New Hampshire, Vermont, and South Dakota, did not sentence anybody to death in the past fifty years. In these circumstances, the electorate's sentiments are a crucial factor. In any legislative debate on the death penalty, one is bound to hear that the great majority of the voters want it. Such a reference is not always dispositive of a legislator's actions. Both the British and the German legislatures abolished the death penalty at a time when the ma-jority of their voters favored it. But American legislators apparently do not have the moral independence of their European counterparts. Favoring the death penalty, moreover, is usually seen in this country as revealing a legisla-tor's general law-and-order spirit and his or her attitude toward crime in general.

The country's sentiment about the death penalty is important in still an-other respect. The leading U.S. Supreme Court decisions imply the possibility that the death penalty might become unconstitutional if prevailing standards of decency condemned it unmistakably.[1] A radical change in popular sentiment could thus affect the Court's position.

Last, but by no means least, our sentiments about the death penalty are of awesome importance when we are asked to serve as jurors in capital trials and

[1]See Furman v. Georgia, 408 U.S. 238 (1972) and Gregg v. Georgia 428 U.S. 153 (1976).

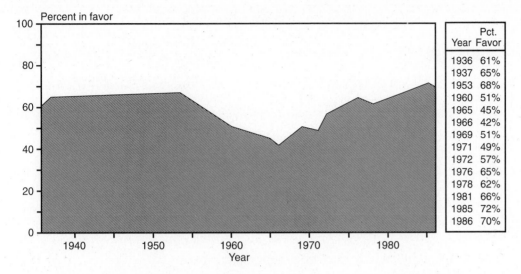

Year	Pct. Favor
1936	61%
1937	65%
1953	68%
1960	51%
1965	45%
1966	42%
1969	51%
1971	49%
1972	57%
1976	65%
1978	62%
1981	66%
1985	72%
1986	70%

FIGURE 1   Percentage of U.S. adults responding "yes" to the question, "Do you favor the death penalty for a person convicted of murder?"

must decide whether a death sentence should be imposed. In making that decision jurors have uncommonly wide latitude; hence, their sentiments about the death penalty are bound to affect their vote.

For all these reasons, it would seem important to analyze the electorate's feelings about the death penalty in some detail.

3. THE STRENGTH OF THE SENTIMENT

The standard Gallup question yields only three basic response groups: those who favor the death penalty, those who oppose it, and the small group who have not made up their mind. Since it is likely that there are shades of pro-and-con sentiments, the authors of this paper decided to explore the intensity with which these basic positions are held, by adding to the 1985 and 1986 poll a number of probing questions.

The first question was whether the respondents favored or opposed the death penalty "very strongly" or "not so strongly." Table 2 presents the answers.

On both sides of the fence, the "very strong" feelings outweigh the "not so strong" ones. This is more noticeable among those who favor the death penalty than among its opponents. Overall, roughly two-thirds of the respondents feel "very strongly" about their respective positions.

TABLE 2 Strength of the Death Penalty Sentiment

	Percentage
Favor the death penalty	71
Very strongly	56
Not strongly	15
Undecided	8
Oppose the death penalty	21
Not too strongly	8
Very strongly	13
Total	100

4. REASONS FOR FAVORING OR OPPOSING THE DEATH PENALTY

Next we asked, "Why are you for (against) the death penalty?" The simple question "why?" is not a penetrating probing device in a polling context, because it seldom elicits more than one reason and not necessarily the most salient one. Still, the question is likely to produce what is called the "top of the mind" reason (Zeisel, 1985).

Table 3 shows that there are two types of reasons for favoring or opposing the death penalty; one type is utilitarian, e.g., it will deter murder. The other and strongly dominant type is moralistic, e.g., a life for a life. The situation is similar among the opponents of the death penalty: a majority opposes it for moralistic reasons; a minority for utilitarian ones.

5. THE BELIEF IN DETERRENCE

Next we probed specifically the public's belief or disbelief in the deterrent power of the death penalty: "Do you feel that the death penalty acts as a deterrent to murder?"[2] Table 4 shows the answers.

Almost two-thirds of the respondents believe in the deterrent power of the death penalty. Only about one-third do not share their belief. As one might expect, the belief in the penalty's deterrent efficacy is greater among those who favor the death penalty (77% of whom consider it a deterrent) than among

[2]The question is somewhat ambiguous because it leaves it to each respondent to choose the sentence to which the death penalty is compared: life without parole, life sentence with the possibility of parole, or a sentence of less than life. We believe that such specification would not have yielded a very different result.

TABLE 3 Reasons for Favoring or Opposing the Death Penalty

Favor the Death Penalty	Percentage	Oppose the Death Penalty	Percentage
A life for a life	50	Wrong to take a life	40
Is a deterrent	22	Punishment should be left to God	15
Keeps them from killing again	16	Persons may be wrongly convicted	15
Costly to keep them in prison	11	Does not deter	5
Judicial system too lenient	3	Possibility of rehabilitation	5
		Unfair application of penalty	3
Miscellaneous	9	Miscellaneous	7
Do not know	2	Do not know	16
Total	113[a]	Total	106[a]

[a] Adds to more than 100% because some respondents gave more than one reason.

opponents of the death penalty (only 20% of whom believe in its deterrent power).

6. WHAT WOULD CHANGE OPINIONS?

We learned from Table 3 that, among the utilitarian reasons people give for favoring the death penalty, two reasons stand out: that it deters and thereby reduces murder and that it is the only way to keep the worst murderers from returning to the street.

To gauge the saliency of the deterrence argument we asked those who favor the death penalty, "Suppose that new evidence showed that the death penalty does *not* act as a deterrent to murder, would you then favor or oppose the death penalty?" We also asked them whether they would favor the death penalty if a life sentence without parole were available. Opponents of the death penalty were asked correspondingly, "Suppose that new evidence showed that the death penalty acts as a deterrent to murder, would that make you change your position?" Table 5 shows the answers to these questions.

If people were convinced that the death penalty is no deterrent to murder,

TABLE 4 Is the Death Penalty a Deterrent?

	Percentage
Yes	62
No	31
Not sure	7
Total	100

the present 71% pro-death penalty majority would shrink to (71 – 16 =)55%. If life without parole were available, pro-death penalty sentiment would shrink to (71 – 19 =)52%. If both conditions—life without parole and proof of no deterrence—were present, the reduction would be to the 43% level. Of the 21% who oppose the death penalty, 3% would be in favor of it if they became convinced that it deters murder.

Among both supporters and opponents of the death penalty, the majority cannot be moved by these utilitarian considerations. This is essentially the same picture we obtained in rough outline in Table 3, in response to the simple "Why?" question.

7. ANALYSIS BY SUBGROUPS

So far we have considered only the average level of the pro-death sentiment in the adult U.S. population. We now turn to subgroups of that population, many of which deviate significantly from the average. We made an effort to learn which demographic characteristics are associated with these deviations. Preliminary examination identified several such potential characteristics: ethnic background, sex, political affiliation, region of the country, income, schooling, and religion.

Table 6 presents the pro-death penalty scores for the subgroups examined. Most of these subgroups were structured as dichotomies, some natural (such as male and female) and some defined so as to preserve a numerical balance that would allow further statistical analysis such as grouping the major racial minorities—Blacks and Hispanics—against the remainder of the predominantly Anglo population.

Table 6 shows major differences between the various subgroups. But none of these differences reflects with precision the degree of association between a demographic characteristic and the death penalty sentiment, because most of the characteristics are interrelated. The ethnic minorities are also poorer, the Republicans on the whole are more affluent, the regions differ in their use of the

Table 5 Conditional Strength of the Pro-and-Con Death Penalty Sentiment

	Percentage
Those who favor the death penalty	71
Would oppose it if they were convinced that it was no deterrent	16[a]
Would oppose it if life sentence without parole were available	19[a]
Would *not* oppose it even if it did not deter and life without parole were available	43
Those who oppose the death penalty	21
Would favor it if they were convinced that it is a deterrent	4
Would not favor it even if convinced that it is a deterrent	12

[a] Seven percent of the 16 or 19 in these two groups would give up the death penalty if one *or* the other of the two conditions were realized.

death penalty, and so forth. Therefore, we used logistic regression to isolate the net association of each demographic factor.[3]

By holding all but one demographic factor constant for purposes of analysis, logistic regression removes the effects of the interrelations between the factors. The results appear in Table 7.

As this table shows, five of the seven factors were found to be significantly associated with the death penalty sentiment and thus are good predictors of the death penalty sentiment in any subgroup of the population: ethnic background, political leaning, sex, region of the country, and income.

The strength of these sentiments—that is, the difference between "strongly" and "not so strongly"—are not shown in Table 7. The computation shows that the sentiments that give the Midwest a pro-death penalty position are held with below average strength. The same statement holds for males vs. females and Anglo vs. minority ethnicity. The Republicans who favor the death penalty do it more strongly than the Democrats who favor it, and conversely, the Democrats who oppose the death penalty do it more strongly than the Republicans who oppose it.

Table 7, it can be seen, records certain numbers, not for *all* demographic characteristics but only for that half of the dichotomies that showed the higher level of pro-death penalty sentiment—for Anglos (not for Blacks and Hispanics), for Republicans (not for Democrats and Independents), and so forth. We

[3]We want to thank Richard Chappell of the Statistics Department of the University of Chicago for his help.

TABLE 6 Pro-Death Penalty Sentiments in Various Subgroups
of the U.S. Population

	Percentage Pro-death Penalty in Group	Percentage Share of Sample
Total U.S. population	71	(100)
Political affiliation		
Republican	82	(33)
Democratic-Independent	66	(67)
Sex		
Male	77	(47)
Female	67	(53)
Income		
$20,000 or more	76	(54)
Less than $20,000	66	(46)
Ethnicity		
Anglo	75	(83)
Black and Hispanic	53	(17)
Schooling		
High-school graduate or more	74	(76)
Less than high-school graduate	64	(24)
Region		
West	77	(20)
South	70	(29)
Midwest	72	(25)
East	64	(26)

use this approach because logistic regression analysis computes the deviations from a particular group chosen as baseline. In the present case we selected as baseline the population subgroup that has the lowest level of pro-death penalty sentiment: female persons of Black or Hispanic origin who are part of the lower-income bracket in the Eastern region of the country and who do not consider themselves Republicans.

Table 7 has still another peculiarity; the listed numbers, the end products of the logistic repression, are what is called "odds multipliers." They indicate for each of the groups the odds of finding a member who favors the death penalty for every one member who does not favor it.

TABLE 7 Predictors of Pro-Death Penalty Sentiment
Ranked According to their Relative Strength

	Odds Multiplier[a]
Anglo	2.55
Republican	2.28
Male	1.67
West	1.74
Midwest	1.58
South	1.24
Upper income	1.12
Baseline population	0.69

[a] The first three predictors are significant at the 0.01 level.
So are, jointly, the three geographic regions. Upper income
is significant at the 0.03 level.

These odds allow us to determine the pro-death penalty level for any particular subgroup by the following simple operation.

The computation begins by transforming the baseline odds into the pro-
death penalty level in that group:

$$\frac{0.69}{1.0+0.69} = 43\%$$

Suppose now that we wanted to compute the level for the group that has all
characteristics of the baseline group except that we replace the women by the
men. In that case we proceed as follows:

$$\frac{0.69\times1.67}{1.0+(0.69\times1.67)} = \frac{1.15}{1.0+1.15} = 53\%$$

If we wanted to change both the sex and the political affiliation of the respondents in the baseline group, we would compute

$$\frac{0.69\times1.67\times2.28}{1.0+(0.69\times1.67\times2.55)} = \frac{2.62}{3.62} = 72\%$$

and so forth.

If we want to replace all low-pro-death penalty characteristics by their opposites, we obtain the value for the group with the highest death penalty
score—male Anglos living in the West in the upper economic strata who consider themselves Republican. It is reassuring to see in Table 8 how the com-

TABLE 8 Comparing Computed with Actual Pro-Death
Penalty Level in the Two Extreme Subgroups

	Lowest Pro-death Penalty Percentage	Highest Pro-death Penalty Percentage
Computed	43[a]	93[b]
Actual	42	94

[a] Baseline group.

[b] $\dfrac{0.69 \times 2.55 \times 2.28 \times 1.67 \times 1.74 \times 1.12}{1.0 + (0.69 \times 2.55 \times 2.28 \times 1.67 \times 1.74 \times 1.12)} = \dfrac{13.06}{14.06} = 93\%.$

puted and actual pro-death penalty values compare for the two extreme groups.

There are other demographic characteristics that may be associated with the sentiment toward the death penalty, such as religion, age, and education. The present sample did not allow us to pursue these possibilities to a definite conclusion. Later studies may be able to do this.

8. CONCLUSION

What has this analysis of the death penalty sentiment taught us?

First, pro-death penalty sentiment in the United States for the last 25 years has kept rising almost without interruption. Second, most people have a position on the issue: the proportion of undecided persons is now constantly below 10%. Third, not everybody who takes a position feels equally strong about it. About one-seventh of all persons who favor the death penalty would change their minds if a life sentence without parole were the available alternative. About one-fifth say that they might change if they could be persuaded that the death penalty fails to reduce murder.

Together, those who might change their position under proper conditions are roughly equal to those (about one-third) who say that they do not feel very strongly in favor of the death penalty. Two-thirds of those favoring the death penalty do feel strongly about it.

In addition, this study yields insights into the relationships between death penalty sentiment and the various demographic characteristics of our population.

Blacks and Hispanics show a significantly lower pro-death penalty sentiment than Anglos, women show a significantly lower pro-death penalty sentiment than men, poorer people favor the death penalty significantly less frequently than persons in the higher economic brackets, and persons who consider themselves Democrats or Independents have significantly less sympathy for the death penalty than those who consider themselves Republicans.

This study, then, has shown us that wide deviations exist from the national level of pro-death penalty sentiment and that these deviations hinge on the demographic characteristics of the various subgroups of the population. It tells us less about what changed the average level of pro-death penalty sentiment from 42 to 71% during the 20 years between 1966 and 1986. This means that a goodly number of millions of people must have changed their position toward favoring the death penalty for murder. This number must include many who now describe their views in terms which seem to admit of little or no possibility for change. The phenomenon is puzzling and bespeaks the probable influence of factors that are more emotional than rational. These factors may have much to do with the widely observed increase in personal fears, dissatisfaction with society in general, and feelings of helplessness. What moved them is not easy to say. The present study merely points up the relative weakness of utilitarian arguments. The pursuit of these arguments for or against the death penalty does not penetrate far into the core of the problem. Debates over the death penalty soon reach an impasse that argument cannot easily break. Two centuries ago, the great philosopher Kant argued that the moral law required that every convicted murderer be executed. Had Jesus Christ or Gandhi been asked about their view of the death penalty, they might have answered that the moral law required that nobody be killed in cold blood. Arguments over such basic value positions have little power to change minds. Whoever has attempted it knows how frustrating it is. Moral positions are seldom changed by persuasion; they are changed, as a rule, only by the more complex and more mysterious process of conversion.

This is the more so because there is evidence that sentiments about the death penalty are part of a more general network of attitudes that split roughly along the liberal-conservative syndrome. This suggestion came first from an early analysis of Gallup poll data (Zeisel, 1968; Neapolitan, 1983). Hugo Bedau, in his careful monitoring efforts, has bolstered this insight (1982).

As this paper goes through the last stages of preparation, the results of a new Gallup poll on the death penalty are being released. Interviewing took place during the last week of the 1988 presidential campaign. Also at that time, the Ted Bundy case was moving to its widely noted climax (see Fox, 1989). The pro-death penalty vote for murder rose from its 1986 level of 71% to a new high of 79%. Inspection of the level among the various population subgroups suggests that, on the whole, no major changes have occurred in the relative position of the various subgroups: just that each of them now has a higher pro-death penalty level.

The one exception is a shift in the regional scores. President Bush's challenge of Governor Dukakis for his opposition to the death penalty, in connection with the Willie Horton incident, may well have been the cause of the extraordinary rise in the pro-death penalty sentiment in the East by 15 percentage points.

The more fundamental question of why this campaign strategy could fall on such fertile ground goes to the context of which death penalty sentiment is likely to be a part.

As we pointed out, that sentiment is part of a broader view which sees the criminal law as an important instrument for curing societal ills. That view is not unrelated to the voters' political alignment. Both in 1986 and in 1988, the Gallup Poll release recorded that the subgroup with the highest death penalty ratings—83% in 1986 and 90% in 1988—was the Republicans. Perhaps President Bush's promise to lead us to a kinder and gentler America may both hint at the reason for the rise in the pro-death penalty sentiment and raise hope for the trend's reversal.

References

Bedau, H. A. (ed.) (1982). *The Death Penalty in America*, Oxford University Press, Oxford.

Ellsworth, P. C., and Ross, L. (1938). Public opinion and capital punishment: A close examination of the views of abolitionists and retentionists. *Crime Delinq.* 29.

Fox, J. A. (1989). Don't turn a death sentence into an orgy of vengeance. *Newsday* Jan. 27.

Neapolitan, J. (1983). Support for and opposition to capital punishment: Some associated social-psychological factors. *Crim. Just. Behav.* 2: 145.

Zeisel, H. (1968). Some data on juror attitudes towards capital punishment. Center for Studies in Criminal Justice, University of Chicago Law School, Chicago.

Zeisel, H. (1982). The verdict of 5 out of 6 civil jurors: Constitutional problems. *Am. Bar Found. Res. J.* 141.

Zeisel, H. (1985). In *Say It with Figures*, 6th ed., Harper and Row, 1985, Chap. 11.

38 Loss of Communality at Buffalo Creek

Kai T. Erikson

KAI ERIKSON is Professor Emeritus of sociology at Yale University and a past president of the American Sociological Association. He is particularly known for two of his books, *Wayward Puritans* and *Everything in Its Path*, winner of the American Sociological Association's Sorokin Award for an outstanding contribution to the progress of sociology. The present article presents a brief overview of a number of the major points made in *Everything in Its Path*. On February 26, 1972, a dam burst and the debris-filled muddy water roared through Buffalo Creek, a narrow mountain hollow in West Virginia. The survivors of the Buffalo Creek disaster suffered both individual and collective trauma, the latter being reflected in their loss of what Erikson refers to as communality. The article and the book present a study of how a disaster affects the sense of community and the consequences of a loss of this communality.

THE TRAUMA EXPERIENCED BY THE SURVIVORS of the Buffalo Creek disaster can be conceptualized as having two related but distinguishable facets—the individual trauma and the collective trauma.

By individual trauma, I mean a blow to the psyche that breaks through one's defenses so suddenly and with such force that one cannot respond effectively. As the other papers in this section make abundantly clear, the Buffalo Creek survivors experienced just such a blow. They suffered deep shock as a result of their exposure to so much death and destruction, and they withdrew into themselves, feeling numbed, afraid, vulnerable, and very alone.

By collective trauma, I mean a blow to the tissues of social life that damages the bonds linking people together and impairs the prevailing sense of communality. The collective trauma works its way slowly and even insidiously into the awareness of those who suffer from it; thus it does not have the quality of suddenness usually associated with the word "trauma." It is, however, a form of shock—a gradual realization that the community no longer exists as a source of nurturance and that a part of the self has disappeared. "I" continue to exist,

From *American Journal of Psychiatry*, Vol. 133, pp. 302–304. Copyright © 1976, the American Psychiatric Association. Reprinted by permission.

although damaged and maybe even permanently changed. "You" continue to exist, though distant and hard to relate to. But "we" no longer exist as a connected pair or as linked cells in a larger communal body.

The two traumas are closely related, of course, but they are distinct in the sense that either of them can take place in the absence of the other. For instance, a person who suffers deep psychic wounds as the result of an automobile accident, but who never loses contact with his community, can be said to suffer from individual trauma. A person whose feelings of well-being begin to wither because the surrounding community is stripped away and no longer offers a base of support (as is known to have happened in certain slum clearance projects) can be said to suffer from collective trauma. In most large-scale human disasters, of course, the two traumas occur jointly and are experienced as two halves of a continuous whole. For the purposes of this paper, however, it is worthwhile to insist on the distinction at least briefly, partly because it alerts us to look for the degree to which the psychic impairment observed in settings like Buffalo Creek can be attributed to loss of communality, and partly because it underscores the point that it is difficult for people to recover from the effects of individual trauma when the community on which they have depended remains fragmented.

I am proposing, then, that many of the traumatic symptoms experienced by the people of Buffalo Creek are as much a reaction to the shock of being separated from a meaningful community base as to the actual disaster itself.

It should be noted that "community" means much more in Buffalo Creek than it does in most other parts of the United States. Much has been said in the literature on Appalachia about the importance of kinship and neighborliness in mountain society. Although it is true that coal camps like the ones along Buffalo Creek differ in many ways from the typical Appalachian community, the people of Buffalo Creek were nonetheless joined together in the close and intimate bonds that sociologists call *gemeinschaft*. The rhythms of everyday life were largely set by the community in general and governed by long-standing traditions, and the social linkages by which people were connected were very strong. In Buffalo Creek, tightly knit communal groups were considered the natural order of things, the envelope in which people live.

Long stories must be made short in a presentation like this, so I will simply summarize my theme by stating that the human communities along Buffalo Creek were essentially destroyed by the disaster and its aftermath. The flood itself forced the residents of the hollow into a number of nearby refugee camps from which they were, for a variety of reasons, unable to escape. The result was that the majority of the Buffalo Creek survivors remained in the general vicinity of their old homes, working in familiar mines, traveling along familiar roads, trading in familiar stores, attending familiar schools, and sometimes worshipping in familiar churches. However, the people were scattered more or less at random throughout the vicinity—virtually stranded in the spots to which they had been washed by the flood—and this meant that old bonds of kinship and neighborhood, which had always depended on physical proximity, were effectively severed. People no longer related to one another in old and accustomed ways. The threads of the social fabric had snapped.

A year after the disaster (which is roughly when most of the authors represented in this section first encountered these people) visitors to Buffalo Creek were struck by a number of behavioral manifestations that seemed to be exhibited by almost everyone in the valley and, for that matter, continue to this day. Several of these manifestations are discussed elsewhere in this section. I would like to mention three by way of illustrating a larger point.

DEMORALIZATION

First, the survivors clearly suffer from a state of severe demoralization, both in the sense that they have lost much personal morale and in the sense that they have lost (or so they fear) most of their moral anchors.

The lack of morale is reflected in a profound apathy, a feeling that the world has more or less come to an end and that there are no longer any sound reasons for doing anything. People are drained of energy and conviction, not just because they are still stunned by the savagery of the flood but because activity of any kind seems to have lost much of its direction and purpose in the absence of a confirming community surround. They feel that the ground has been pulled out from under them, that the context in which they had worked, played, and cared for others has more or less disappeared. One survivor said,

> I don't know. I just got to the point where I just more or less don't care. I don't have no ambition to do the things I used to do. I used to try to keep things up. But anymore I just don't. It seems I just do enough to get by, to make it last one more day. It seems like I just lost everything at once, like the bottom just dropped out of everything.

I suppose the clinical term for this state of mind would be depression, but one can hardly escape the impression that it is, at least in part, a reaction to the ambiguities of postdisaster life in the valley. The survivors are literally out of place and uprooted. They had never realized the extent to which they relied on the rest of the community to reflect a sense of security and well-being, or how much they depended on others to supply them with a point of reference.

The people of Buffalo Creek are also haunted by a suspicion that moral standards are beginning to collapse all over the valley, and in some ways it would appear that they are right. As is so often the case, the forms of misbehavior people find cropping up in their midst are exactly those about which they are most sensitive. The use of alcohol, always a sensitive problem in Appalachian society, has apparently increased, and there are rumors everywhere that drugs have found their way into the valley. The theft rate has also gone up, and theft has always been viewed in the mountains as a sure index of social disorganization. The cruelest cut of all, however, is that younger people seem to be slipping away from parental control and are becoming involved in nameless delinquencies. This is an extremely disturbing development in a culture so devoted to the family and so concerned about generational continuity.

This apparent collapse of conventional morality has a number of curious aspects. For one thing, observers generally feel that there is much less deviation from community norms than the local people seem to fear. Moreover, there is an interesting incongruity in these reports of immorality—one gets the impression that virtually everyone is coming into contact now with persons of lower moral stature than they did formerly. This, of and by itself, does not make very much logistical sense. One survivor said flatly,

> The people of Buffalo Creek tended to group themselves together; therefore the breaking up of the old communities threw all kinds of different people together. At the risk of sounding superior, I feel we are living amidst people with lower moral values than us.

Perhaps this is true—but where did all these sordid people come from? Whatever else people may say about their new neighbors in the refugee camps, they are also from Buffalo Creek, and it is hard to avoid the suspicion that their perceived immorality has as much to do with their newness as with their actual behavior. It may be that relative strangers are almost by definition less "moral" than familiar neighbors. To live within a tightly knit community is to make allowances for behavior that might otherwise look deviant. New neighbors do not qualify for this clemency—not yet, at least—and to that extent, their very unfamiliarity may seem to hint at vice all by itself.

The collapse of morality in Buffalo Creek thus seems to have two edges. We have sufficient evidence to believe that certain forms of deviation are actually on the increase, although this is a difficult thing to measure accurately. However, we also have reason to believe that the breakdown of accustomed neighborhood patterns and the scattering of people into unfamiliar new groupings has increased the level of suspicion people feel toward one another.

DISORIENTATION

The people of Buffalo Creek are also clearly suffering from a prolonged sense of disorientation. It has often been noted that the survivors of a disaster are likely to be dazed and stunned, unable to locate themselves meaningfully in time and space. Time seems to stop for them; places and objects suddenly seem transitory. They have trouble finding stable points of reference in the surrounding terrain, both physical and human, to help fix their position and orient their behavior. All of this can be understood as a natural consequence of shock, but the people of Buffalo Creek seem to have continued to experience this sense of dislocation for months and even years after the crisis. "We find ourselves standing, not knowing exactly which way to go or where to turn," said one individual. Another survivor noted, "We feel like we're living in a strange and different place, even though it is just a few miles up Buffalo Creek from where we were."

Professional observers who have gone into the valley on medical or research errands have noted repeatedly how frequently the survivors seem to forget simple bits of everyday information—the names of close friends, their own telephone numbers, etc. People are often unable to locate themselves spatially, even when they are staring at fixed landmarks they have known all their lives. It is not at all uncommon for them to answer factual questions about time— their own age or their children's grade in school—as if history had indeed stopped on the date of the disaster. In general, people all over the valley live with a lasting sense of being out of place, disconnected, and torn loose from their moorings, and this feeling has far outlasted the initial trauma of the catastrophe itself.

People normally learn who they are and where they are by taking soundings from their fellows. As if employing a subtle form of radar, we probe other people in our immediate environment with looks, gestures, and words, hoping to learn something about ourselves from the signals we get in return. But when there are no reliable objects off of whom to bounce those exploratory probes, people have a hard time calculating where they stand in relation to the rest of the world. In a very real sense, they come to feel that they are not whole persons, not entirely human, because they do not know how to position themselves in a larger communal setting.

Well, I just don't feel like the same person. I feel like I live in a different world. I don't have no home no more. I don't feel normal anymore. I mean, sometimes I just wonder if I'm a human being. I just feel like I don't have no friends in the world, nobody cares for me, nobody knows I even exist.

LOSS OF CONNECTION

A third manifestation of the disaster's psychosocial effects is a condition that might be described as loss of connection—a sense of separation from other people. For better or worse, the people of the hollow were deeply enmeshed in the tissues of their community; they drew their very being from them. When those tissues were stripped away by the disaster, people found themselves exposed and alone, suddenly dependent on their personal resources. The cruel fact is that many of the survivors proved to have few resources—not because they lacked the heart or the competence, but because they had spent so many years placing their abilities in the service of the larger community that they did not really know how to mobilize them for their own purposes.

Many people feel that they have lost meaningful connection with themselves. Much of their apparent former strength was actually the reflected strength of the community, and they are learning—to their very great discomfort—that they cannot maintain an enduring sense of self when separated from that larger tissue. They find that they are not very good at making individual decisions, getting along with others, or establishing themselves as separate persons in the absence of a supportive surround. "Lonesome" is a word many of them use, and they do not use it to mean the lack of human company. One woman who has moved to the center of a large neighboring town said of her new home: "It is like being all alone in the middle of a desert." A man who continued to live in his damaged home on Buffalo Creek said,

> *Well, there is a difference in my condition. Like somebody being in a strange world with nobody around. You don't know nobody. You walk the floor or look for somebody you know to talk to, and you don't have nobody.*

In addition, the inability of people to come to terms with their own individual isolation is counterpointed by an inability to relate to others on a one-to-one basis. Human relations along Buffalo Creek took their shape from the expectations that pressed in on them from all sides like a mold: they were regulated by the customs of the neighborhood, the ways of the community, and the traditions of the family. When that mold was stripped away, long-standing relationships seemed to disintegrate. This is true of everyday acquaintances, but it is doubly—and painfully—true of marriages. Wives and husbands discovered that they did not know how to nourish one another, make decisions, or even to engage in satisfactory conversations when the community was no longer there to provide a context and set a rhythm. There has been a sharp increase in the divorce rate, but that statistical index does not begin to express the difficulties the survivors have relating to their spouses. It is almost as if communal forces of one sort or another had knit family groups together by holding them in a kind of gravitational field, but when the forces of that field began to dissipate, family members became scattered like aimless individual particles. Each individual nurses his or her own hurts and tends to his or her business. They do not know how to care for one another or to coordinate emotionally, because the context that lent substance and meaning to their relationships has disappeared. Two survivors put it this way:

> *Each person in the family is a loner now, a person alone. Each of us is fighting his own battles. We just don't seem to care for each other anymore.*

The family is not what they was. They're not the same people. I don't know how
you'd put this, but before there was love in the home. But now it seems like each one is
a different person, an individual by himself or herself, and there's just nothing there.

Finally, the difficulty people experience in sustaining warm relationships extends beyond marriages and families, out into the rest of the valley. In places like Buffalo Creek, relationships are part of the natural order—being inherited by birth or acquired by physical proximity—and the very idea of "making" friends or "forming" relationships is hard for these people to understand and harder still for them to achieve.

One result of all the problems I have described is that the community (what remains of it) seems to have lost its most significant quality—the power it gave people to care for one another in moments of need, to console one another in moments of distress, and to protect one another in moments of danger. In retrospect, it is apparent that the community was indeed stronger than the sum of its parts in this regard. When the people of Buffalo Creek were clustered together in the embrace of a community, they were capable of remarkable acts of generosity; when they tried to relate to one another as separate individuals, they found that they could no longer mobilize the energy to care. One woman summed it up in a phrase: "It seems like the caring part of our lives is gone."

CONCLUSIONS

To end with an oversimplified metaphor, I would suggest that the people of Buffalo Creek were accustomed to placing their individual energies and resources at the disposal of the larger collectivity—the communal store, as it were—and then drawing on those reserves when the demands of everyday life made this necessary. When the community more or less disappeared, as it did after the disaster, people found that they could not take advantage of the energies they once invested in that communal store. They found themselves almost empty of feeling, devoid of affection, and lacking all confidence and assurance. It is as if the cells had supplied raw energy to the whole body but did not have the means to convert that energy into usable personal resources once the body was no longer there to process it.

❧ 39 Night

Elie Wiesel

ELIE WIESEL, professor in the humanities at Boston University, has received
a number of awards over the years, among them the Nobel Peace Prize in
1986. As a child he was thrown into the nightmare world of the Nazi concentration camps. The story of this experience is told in his searing book,
Night. The final three sections of that book are reproduced here. The tenderness between the boy and his father is the human counterpoint to the inhuman environment in which they tried to survive.

PRESSED UP AGAINST THE OTHERS in an effort to keep out the cold, head empty
and heavy at the same time, brain a whirlpool of decaying memories. Indifference deadened the spirit. Here or elsewhere—what difference did it make? To
die today or tomorrow, or later? The night was long and never ending.

When at last a gray glimmer of light appeared on the horizon, it revealed a
tangle of human shapes, head sunk upon shoulders, crouched, piled one on top
of the other, like a field of dust-covered tombstones in the first light of the
dawn. I tried to distinguish those who were still alive from those who had
gone. But there was no difference. My gaze was held for a long time by one
who lay with his eyes open, staring into the void. His livid face was covered
with a layer of frost and snow.

My father was huddled near me, wrapped in his blanket, his shoulders covered with snow. And was he dead, too? I called him. No answer. I would have
cried out if I could have done so. He did not move.

My mind was invaded suddenly by this realization—there was no more
reason to live, no more reason to struggle.

The train stopped in the middle of a deserted field. The suddenness of the
halt woke some of those who were asleep. They straightened themselves up,
throwing startled looks around them.

Outside, the SS went by, shouting:

"Throw out all the dead! All corpses outside!"

The living rejoiced. There would be more room. Volunteers set to work. They felt those who were still crouching.

"Here's one! Take him!"

They undressed him, the survivors avidly sharing out his clothes, then two "gravediggers" took him one by the head and one by the feet, and threw him out of the wagon like a sack of flour.

From all directions came cries:

"Come on! Here's one! This man next to me. He doesn't move."

I woke from my apathy just at the moment when two men came up to my father. I threw myself on top of his body. He was cold. I slapped him. I rubbed his hands, crying:

"Father! Father! Wake up. They're trying to throw you out of the carriage. . . ."

His body remained inert.

The two gravediggers seized me by the collar.

"Leave him. You can see perfectly well that he's dead."

"No!" I cried. "He isn't dead! Not yet!"

I set to work to slap him as hard as I could. After a moment my father's eyelids moved slightly over his glazed eyes. He was breathing weakly.

"You see," I cried.

The two men moved away.

Twenty bodies were thrown out of our wagon. Then the train resumed its journey, leaving behind it a few hundred naked dead, deprived of burial, in the deep snow of a field in Poland.

We were given no food. We lived on snow; it took the place of bread. The days were like nights, and the nights left the dregs of their darkness in our souls. The train was traveling slowly, often stopping for several hours and then setting off again. It never ceased snowing. All through these days and nights we stayed crouching, one on top of the other, never speaking a word. We were no more than frozen bodies. Our eyes closed, we waited merely for the next stop, so that we could unload our dead.

Ten days, ten nights of traveling. Sometimes we would pass through German townships. Very early in the morning usually. The workmen were going to work. They stopped and stared after us, but otherwise showed no surprise.

One day when we had stopped, a workman took a piece of bread out of his bag and threw it into a wagon. There was a stampede. Dozens of starving men fought each other to the death for a few crumbs. The German workmen took a lively interest in this spectacle.

Some years later, I watched the same kind of scene at Aden. The passengers on our boat were amusing themselves by throwing coins to the "natives," who were diving in to get them. An attractive, aristocratic Parisienne was deriving special pleasure from the game. I suddenly noticed that two children were engaged in a death struggle, trying to strangle each other. I turned to the lady.

"Please," I begged, "don't throw any more money in!"

"Why not?" she said. "I like to give charity. . . ."

In the wagon where the bread had fallen, a real battle had broken out. Men threw themselves on top of each other, stamping on each other, tearing at each other, biting each other. Wild beasts of prey, with animal hatred in their eyes; an extraordinary vitality had seized them, sharpening their teeth and nails.

A crowd of workmen and curious spectators had collected along the train. They had probably never seen a train with such a cargo. Soon, nearly everywhere, pieces of bread were being dropped into the wagons. The audience stared at these skeletons of men, fighting one another to the death for a mouthful.

A piece fell into our wagon. I decided that I would not move. Anyway, I knew that I would never have the strength to fight with a dozen savage men! Not far away I noticed an old man dragging himself along on all fours. He was trying to disengage himself from the struggle. He held one hand to his heart. I thought at first he had received a blow in the chest. Then I understood; he had a bit of bread under his shirt. With remarkable speed he drew it out and put it to his mouth. His eyes gleamed; a smile, like a grimace, lit up his dead face. And was immediately extinguished. A shadow had just loomed up near him. The shadow threw itself upon him. Felled to the ground, stunned with blows, the old man cried:

"Meir. Meir, my boy! Don't you recognize me? I'm your father . . . you're hurting me . . . you're killing your father! I've got some bread . . . for you too . . . for you too. . . ."

He collapsed. His fist was still clenched around a small piece. He tried to carry it to his mouth. But the other one threw himself upon him and snatched it. The old man again whispered something, let out a rattle, and died amid the general indifference. His son searched him, took the bread, and began to devour it. He was not able to get very far. Two men had seen and hurled themselves upon him. Others joined in. When they withdrew, next to me were two corpses, side by side, the father and the son.

I was fifteen years old.

In our wagon, there was a friend of my father's called Meir Katz. He had worked as a gardener at Buna and used to bring us a few green vegetables occasionally. Being less undernourished than the rest of us, he had stood up to imprisonment better. Because he was relatively more vigorous, he had been put in charge of the wagon.

On the third night of our journey I woke up suddenly and felt two hands on my throat, trying to strangle me. I just had the time to shout, "Father!"

Nothing but this word. I felt myself suffocating. But my father had woken

up and seized my attacker. Too weak to overcome him, he had the idea of calling Meir Katz.

"Come here! Come quickly! There's someone strangling my son."

A few moments later I was free. I still do not know why the man wanted to
strangle me.

After a few days, Meir Katz spoke to my father:

"Chlomo, I'm getting weak. I'm losing my strength. I can't hold on. . . ."

"Don't let yourself go under," my father said, trying to encourage him.
"You must resist. Don't lose faith in yourself."

But Meir Katz groaned heavily in reply.

"I can't go on any longer, Chlomo! What can I do? I can't carry on. . . ."

My father took his arm. And Meir Katz, the strong man, the most robust
of us all, wept. His son had been taken from him at the time of the first selection, but it was now that he wept. It was now that he cracked up. He was finished, at the end of his tether.

On the last day of our journey a terrible wind arose; it snowed without
ceasing. We felt that the end was near—the real end. We could never hold out
in this icy wind, in these gusts.

Someone got up and shouted:

"We mustn't stay sitting down at a time like this. We shall freeze to death!
Let's all get up and move a bit. . . ."

We all got up. We held our damp blankets more tightly around us. And we
forced ourselves to move a few steps, to turn around where we were.

Suddenly a cry rose up from the wagon, the cry of a wounded animal.
Someone had just died.

Others, feeling that they too were about to die, imitated his cry. And their
cries seemed to come from beyond the grave. Soon everyone was crying out.
Wailing, groaning, cries of distress hurled into the wind and the snow.

The contagion spread to the other carriages. Hundred of cries rose up simultaneously. Not knowing against whom we cried. Not knowing why. The
death rattle of a whole convoy who felt the end upon them. We were all going
to die here. All limits had been passed. No one had any strength left. And again
the night would be long.

Meir Katz groaned:

"Why don't they shoot us all right away?"

That same evening, we reached our destination.

It was late at night. The guards came to unload us. The dead were abandoned in the train. Only those who could still stand were able to get out.

Meir Katz stayed in the train. The last day had been the most murderous.
A hundred of us had got into the wagon. A dozen of us got out—among them,
my father and I.

We had arrived at Buchenwald.

At the gate of the camp, SS officers were waiting for us. They counted us. Then we were directed to the assembly place. Orders were given us through loudspeakers:

"Form fives!" "Form groups of a hundred!" "Five paces forward!"

I held onto my father's hand—the old, familiar fear: not to lose him.

Right next to us the high chimney of the crematory oven rose up. It no longer made any impression on us. It scarcely attracted our attention.

An established inmate of Buchenwald told us that we should have a shower and then we could go into the blocks. The idea of having a hot bath fascinated me. My father was silent. He was breathing heavily beside me.

"Father," I said. "Only another moment more. Soon we can lie down—in a bed. You can rest. . . ."

He did not answer. I was so exhausted myself that his silence left me indifferent. My only wish was to take a bath as quickly as possible and lie down in a bed.

But it was not easy to reach the showers. Hundred of prisoners were crowding there. The guards were unable to keep any order. They struck out right and left with no apparent result. Others, without the strength to push or even to stand up, had sat down in the snow. My father wanted to do the same. He groaned.

"I can't go on. . . . This is the end. . . . I'm going to die here. . . ."

He dragged me toward a hillock of snow from which emerged human shapes and ragged pieces of blanket.

"Leave me," he said to me. "I can't go on. . . . Have mercy on me. . . . I'll wait here until we can get into the baths. . . . You can come and find me."

I could have wept with rage. Having lived through so much, suffered so much, could I leave my father to die now? Now, when we could have a good hot bath and lie down?

"Father!" I screamed. "Father! Get up from here! Immediately! You're killing yourself. . . ."

I seized him by the arm. He continued to groan.

"Don't shout, son. . . . Take pity on your old father. . . . Leave me to rest here. . . . Just for a bit, I'm so tired . . . at the end of my strength. . . ."

He had become like a child, weak, timid, vulnerable.

"Father," I said. "You can't stay here."

I showed him the corpses all around him; they too had wanted to rest here.

"I can see them, son. I can see them all right. Let them sleep. It's so long since they closed their eyes. . . . They are exhausted . . . exhausted. . . ."

His voice was tender.

I yelled against the wind:

"They'll never wake again! Never! Don't you understand?"

For a long time this argument went on. I felt that I was not arguing with him, but with death itself, with the death that he had already chosen.

The sirens began to wail. An alert. The lights went out throughout the camp. The guards drove us toward the blocks. In a flash, there was no one left on the assembly place. We were only too glad not to have had to stay outside longer in the icy wind. We let ourselves sink down onto the planks. The beds were in several tiers. The cauldrons of soup at the entrance attracted no one. To sleep, that was all that mattered.

It was daytime when I awoke. And then I remembered that I had a father. Since the alert, I had followed the crowd without troubling about him. I had known that he was at the end, on the brink of death, and yet I had abandoned him.

I went to look for him.

But at the same moment this thought came into my mind: "Don't let me find him! If only I could get rid of this dead weight, so that I could use all my strength to struggle for my own survival, and only worry about myself." Immediately I felt ashamed of myself, ashamed forever.

I walked for hours without finding him. Then I came to the block where they were giving out black "coffee." The men were lining up and fighting.

A plaintive, beseeching voice caught me in the spine:

"Eliezer . . . my son . . . bring me . . . a drop of coffee. . . ."

I ran to him.

"Father! I've been looking for you for so long. . . . Where were you? Did you sleep? . . . How do you feel?"

He was burning with fever. Like a wild beast, I cleared a way for myself to the coffee cauldron. And I managed to carry back a cupful. I had a sip. The rest was for him. I can't forget the light of thankfulness in his eyes while he gulped it down—an animal gratitude. With those few gulps of hot water, I probably brought him more satisfaction than I had done during my whole childhood.

He was lying on a plank, livid, his lips pale and dried up, shaken by tremors. I could not stay by him for long. Orders had been given to clear the place for cleaning. Only the sick could stay.

We stayed outside for five hours. Soup was given out. As soon as we were allowed to go back to the blocks, I ran to my father.

"Have you had anything to eat?"

"No."

"Why not?"

"They didn't give us anything . . . they said that if we were ill we should die soon anyway and it would be a pity to waste the food. I can't go on any more. . . ."

I gave him what was left of my soup. But it was with a heavy heart. I felt that I was giving it up to him against my will. No better than Rabbi Eliahou's son had I withstood the test.

He grew weaker day by day, his gaze veiled, his face the color of dead leaves. On the third day after our arrival at Buchenwald, everyone had to go to the showers. Even the sick, who had to go through last.

On the way back from the baths, we had to wait outside for a long time. They had not yet finished cleaning the blocks.

Seeing my father in the distance, I ran to meet him. He went by me like a ghost, passed me without stopping, without looking at me. I called to him. He did not come back. I ran after him:

"Father, where are you running to?"

He looked at me for a moment, and his gaze was distant, visionary; it was the face of someone else. A moment only and on he ran again.

Struck down with dysentery, my father lay in his bunk, five other invalids with him. I sat by his side, watching him, not daring to believe that he could escape death again. Nevertheless, I did all I could to give him hope.

Suddenly, he raised himself on his bunk and put his feverish lips to my ear:

"Eliezer . . . I must tell you where to find the gold and the money I buried . . . in the cellar. . . . You know. . . ."

He began to talk faster and faster, as though he were afraid he would not have time to tell me. I tried to explain to him that this was not the end, that we would go back to the house together, but he would not listen to me. He could no longer listen to me. He was exhausted. A trickle of saliva, mingled with blood, was running from between his lips. He had closed his eyes. His breath was coming in gasps.

For a ration of bread, I managed to change beds with a prisoner in my father's bunk. In the afternoon the doctor came. I went and told him that my father was very ill.

"Bring him here!"

I explained that he could not stand up. But the doctor refused to listen to anything. Somehow, I brought my father to him. He stared at him, then questioned him in a clipped voice:

"What do you want?"

"My father's ill," I answered for him. "Dysentery . . ."

"Dysentery? That's not my business. I'm a surgeon. Go on! Make room for the others."

Protests did no good.

"I can't go on, son. . . . Take me back to my bunk. . . ."

I took him back and helped him to lie down. He was shivering.

"Try and sleep a bit, father. Try to go to sleep. . . ."

His breathing was labored, thick. He kept his eyes shut. Yet I was convinced that he could see everything, that now he could see the truth in all things.

Another doctor came to the block. But my father would not get up. He knew that it was useless.

Besides, this doctor had only come to finish off the sick. I could hear him shouting at them that they were lazy and just wanted to stay in bed. I felt like leaping at his throat, strangling him. But I no longer had the courage or the strength. I was riveted to my father's deathbed. My hands hurt, I was clenching them so hard. Oh, to strangle the doctor and the others! To burn the whole world! My father's murderers! But the cry stayed in my throat.

When I came back from the bread distribution, I found my father weeping like a child:
"Son, they keep hitting me!"
"Who?"
I thought he was delirious.
"Him, the Frenchman . . . and the Pole . . . they were hitting me."
Another wound to the heart, another hate, another reason for living lost.
"Eliezer . . . Eliezer . . . tell them not to hit me. . . . I haven't done anything . . . Why do they keep hitting me?"
I began to abuse his neighbors. They laughed at me. I promised them bread, soup. They laughed. Then they got angry; they could not stand my father any longer, they said, because he was now unable to drag himself outside to relieve himself.
The following day he complained that they had taken his ration of bread.
"While you were asleep?"
"No. I wasn't asleep. They jumped on top of me. They snatched my bread . . . and they hit me . . . again. . . . I can't stand any more, son . . . a drop of water. . . ."
I knew that he must not drink. But he pleaded with me for so long that I gave in. Water was the worst poison he could have, but what else could I do for him? With water, without water, it would all be over soon anyway. . . .
"You, at least, have some mercy on me. . . ."
Have mercy on him! I, his only son!

A week went by like this.
"This is your father, isn't it?" asked the head of the block.
"Yes."
"He's very ill."
"The doctor won't do anything for him."
"The doctor *can't* do anything for him, now. And neither can you."
He put his great hairy hand on my shoulder and added:
"Listen to me, boy. Don't forget that you're in a concentration camp. Here, every man has to fight for himself and not think of anyone else. Even of his father. Here, there are no fathers, no brothers, no friends. Everyone lives and dies for himself alone. I'll give you a sound piece of advice—don't give your ration of bread and soup to your old father. There's nothing you can do

for him. And you're killing yourself. Instead, you ought to be having his ration."

I listened to him without interrupting. He was right, I thought in the most secret region of my heart, but I dared not admit it. It's too late to save your old father, I said to myself. You ought to be having two rations of bread, two rations of soup. . . .

Only a fraction of a second, but I felt guilty. I ran to find a little soup to give my father. But he did not want it. All he wanted was water.

"Don't drink water . . . have some soup. . . ."

"I'm burning . . . why are you being so unkind to me, my son? Some water. . . ."

I brought him some water. Then I left the block for roll call. But I turned around and came back again. I lay down on the top bunk. Invalids were allowed to stay in the block. So I would be an invalid myself. I would not leave my father.

There was silence all around now, broken only by groans. In front of the block, the SS were giving orders. An officer passed by the beds. My father begged me:

"My son, some water. . . . I'm burning. . . . My stomach. . . ."

"Quiet, over there!" yelled the officer.

"Eliezer," went on my father, "some water. . . ."

The officer came up to him and shouted at him to be quiet. But my father did not hear him. He went on calling me. The officer dealt him a violent blow on the head with his truncheon.

I did not move. I was afraid. My body was afraid of also receiving a blow.

Then my father made a rattling noise and it was my name: "Eliezer."

I could see that he was still breathing—spasmodically.

I did not move.

When I got down after roll call, I could see his lips trembling as he murmured something. Bending over him, I stayed gazing at him for over an hour, engraving into myself the picture of his blood-stained face, his shattered skull.

Then I had to go to bed. I climbed into my bunk, above my father, who was still alive. It was January 28, 1945.

I awoke on January 29 at dawn. In my father's place lay another invalid. They must have taken him away before dawn and carried him to the crematory. He may still have been breathing.

There were no prayers at his grave. No candles were lit to his memory. His last word was my name. A summons, to which I did not respond.

I did not weep, and it pained me that I could not weep. But I had no more tears. And, in the depths of my being, in the recesses of my weakened conscience, could I have searched it, I might perhaps have found something like— free at last!

I had to stay at Buchenwald until April eleventh. I have nothing to say of my life during this period. It no longer mattered. After my father's death, nothing could touch me any more.

I was transferred to the children's block, where there were six hundred of us.

The front was drawing nearer.

I spent my days in a state of total idleness. And I had but one desire—to eat. I no longer thought of my father or of my mother.

From time to time I would dream of a drop of soup, of an extra ration of soup. . . .

On April fifth, the wheel of history turned.

It was late in the afternoon. We were standing in the block, waiting for an SS man to come and count us. He was late in coming. Such a delay was unknown till then in the history of Buchenwald. Something must have happened.

Two hours later the loudspeakers sent out an order from the head of the camp: all the Jews must come to the assembly place.

This was the end! Hitler was going to keep his promise.

The children in our block went toward the place. There was nothing else we could do. Gustav, the head of the block, made this clear to us with his truncheon. But on the way we met some prisoners who whispered to us:

"Go back to your block. The Germans are going to shoot you. Go back to your block, and don't move."

We went back to our block. We learned on the way that the camp resistance organization had decided not to abandon the Jews and was going to prevent their being liquidated.

As it was late and there was great upheaval—innumerable Jews had passed themselves off as non-Jews—the head of the camp decided that a general roll call would take place the following day. Everybody would have to be present.

The roll call took place. The head of the camp announced that Buchenwald was to be liquidated. Ten blocks of deportees would be evacuated each day. From this moment, there would be no further distribution of bread and soup. And the evacuation began. Every day, several thousand prisoners went through the camp gate and never came back.

On April tenth, there were still about twenty thousand of us in the camp, including several hundred children. They decided to evacuate us all at once, right on until the evening. Afterward, they were going to blow up the camp.

So we were massed in the huge assembly square, in rows of five, waiting to see the gate open. Suddenly, the sirens began to wail. An alert! We went back to the blocks. It was too late to evacuate us that evening. The evacuation was postponed again to the following day.

We were tormented with hunger. We had eaten nothing for six days, except a bit of grass or some potato peelings found near the kitchens.

At ten o'clock in the morning the SS scattered through the camp, moving the last victims toward the assembly place.

Then the resistance movement decided to act. Armed men suddenly rose up everywhere. Bursts of firing. Grenades exploding. We children stayed flat on the ground in the block.

The battle did not last long. Toward noon everything was quiet again. The SS had fled and the resistance had taken charge of the running of the camp.

At about six o'clock in the evening, the first American tank stood at the gates of Buchenwald.

Our first act as free men was to throw ourselves onto the provisions. We thought only of that. Not of revenge, not of our families. Nothing but bread.

And even when we were no longer hungry, there was still no one who thought of revenge. On the following day, some of the young men went to Weimar to get some potatoes and clothes—and to sleep with girls. But of revenge, not a sign.

Three days after the liberation of Buchenwald I became very ill with food poisoning. I was transferred to the hospital and spent two weeks between life and death.

One day I was able to get up, after gathering all my strength. I wanted to see myself in the mirror hanging on the opposite wall. I had not seen myself since the ghetto.

From the depths of the mirror, a corpse gazed back at me.

The look in his eyes, as they stared into mine, has never left me.

40 Megamurders ✍

R. J. Rummel

R. J. RUMMEL is professor of political science at the University of Hawaii at Manoa. He is author of *Lethal Politics: Soviet Genocide and Mass Murder Since 1917, China's Bloody Century, Genocide and Mass Murder Since 1900,* and *Nazi Genocide and Mass Murder.* In this selection, Rummel uses the term "democide" to refer to genocide, politicide, and mass murder. He argues that eleven megamurderers of the twentieth century (states that have killed more than 1 million people, not including those killed fighting in wars against other states) have murdered over 140 million people. This includes not only Nazi Germany, but also the Soviet Union, Communist China, Khmer Rouge in Cambodia, Vietnam, and Yugoslavia, among others. He also discusses what he refers to as the "kilomurderers" (state that have killed tens or hundreds of thousands). In this group he includes such states as Argentina, Iran, Uganda, and many other authoritarian states. He argues that mass killing is much less common in democratic societies than in authoritarian societies, but he argues that it does take place even in democratic societies under some circumstances.

POWER KILLS, ABSOLUTE POWER KILLS ABSOLUTELY. This power principle—a variant of Lord Acton's dictum "Power tends to corrupt; absolute power corrupts absolutely"—is the message of my work on the causes of war and current, comparative study of genocide, politicide, and mass murder—what I call democide—in this century. The more power a government has, the more it can act arbitrarily according to the whims and desires of the elite, the more likely will it make war on others and murder its foreign and domestic subjects. As Edmund Burke said in *Vindication of Natural Society,* "Power gradually extirpates for the mind every humane and gentle virtue." The poet Percy Shelley described power as "a desolating pestilence" that "pollutes whate'er it touches."

Power in the sense used here encompasses political power and its holders, as well as the agencies (government departments and bureaucracies) and the instruments (armies, concentration camps, and propaganda) at their disposal. Therefore, the more constrained the Power of governments, the more diffused, checked, and balanced it is, the less will it aggress against others and commit democide. At the extremes of Power, totalitarian communist governments have slaughtered their people by the tens of millions, while many democracies can barely bring themselves to execute even serial murderers.

These assertions may be extreme and categorical, but so is the evidence. Consider first war. There is no case of war involving violent military action between stable democracies, although democracies have fought nondemocracies. The exception may be democratic Finland which joined Nazi Germany in its war against the Soviet Union during the Second World War. Although Great Britain declared war on Finland as a result, no military action took place between the two countries. Most wars have been fought between nondemocracies. This general principle is gaining acceptance among students of international relations and war: democracies do not make war on each other. The less democratic two states are, the more likely they will fight each other.

This belligerence of unrestrained Power is not an artifact of either a small number of democracies nor of our era. The number of democracies in the world now number around sixty-five containing about 39 percent of the world's population. Yet we have had no war among them. Nor is there any threat of war. Democracies create an oasis of peace.

This is true historically as well. If one relaxes the definition of democracy to mean simply the restraint on Power by the participation of middle and lower classes in the determinations of Power holders and policy making, then there have been many democracies throughout history. Whether one considers the classical Greek democracies, the democratic forest states of Switzerland, or modern democracies since 1787, one will find that they have not fought each other—depending on how war and democracy is defined, some might prefer to say that they rarely fought each other. Once states that had been mortal enemies and had frequently gone to war (as have France and Germany in recent centuries) became democratic, war ceased between them. Paradigmatic of this is Western Europe since 1945. The cauldron of our most disastrous wars for many centuries, in 1945 one would not find an expert so foolhardy as to predict not only forty-five years of peace, but that at the end of that time there would be a European community with central government institutions, moves toward a joint European military force by France and Germany, and no expectation of violence between any of these formerly hostile states. Yet such has happened. All because they are all democracies. Even among primitive tribes, it seems, where Power is divided and limited, war is less likely.

Were all that could be said absolute and arbitrary Power that it causes war and the attendant slaughter of the young and most capable of our species, this would be enough. But much worse is that even in the absence of combat, Power massacres in cold blood the helpless people it controls. Several times more of them. The eleven megamurderers of the twentieth century—states that have killed in cold blood, aside from warfare, 1,000,000 or more men, women, and children—have wiped out 142,583,000 people between them. This is almost four times the battle dead in all of this century's international and civil wars. States with absolute Power, that is the former Soviet Union, Communist China, Nazi Germany, Khmer Rouge Cambodia, Communist Vietnam, and Communist Yugoslavia account for 122,535,000 or 86 percent.

Among these megamurderers, by their annual percent democide rates [=100 x democide/population/(the number of years that the type of regime was in Power)], none comes even close to the lethality of the communist Khmer Rouge in Cambodia during 1975 to 1978. They exterminated near 28 percent of the country's men, women, and children; the odds of any Cambodian surviving these four long years was only 2.5 to 1.

Then there are the kilomurderers, or states that have killed innocent citizens by the tens or hundreds of thousands, such as Communist Afghanistan, Angola, Laos, Ethiopia, North Korea, and Rumania, as well as authoritarian Argentina, Burundi, Chile, Croatia (1941 to 1944), Czechoslovakia (1945 to 1946), Indonesia, Iran, Rwanda, Spain, Sudan, and Uganda. All these and other kilomurderers add another 8,361,000 people killed to the democide for this century. The total global democide from 1900 to 1987 probably amounts, to 150,944,000 people killed. This figure is the most reasonable and prudent mid-estimates within a low to high range. The overall, absolute highest estimate of democide may be around an almost inconceivable 335,000,000 killed; the absolute low near a hardly less horrible 70,000,000 killed. None of the conclusions would change, however, if we only dealt with the rock bottom total.

Putting the human cost of war and democide together Power has killed some 187,797,100 people in this century. If this many people came in one door of a room, walking at three miles per hour across the room with three feet between them, and exit an opposite door, it would take over four years for all to pass, twenty-four hours a day, 365 days a year. If all the dead were lined up they would reach from Honolulu in Hawaii, across the Pacific and then the continental United States to Washington D.C., and then back again.

Democracies too are responsible for some of these democides. Preliminary estimates show that some 1,000,000 foreigners have been killed in cold blood by democracies. This includes those killed in indiscriminate or civilian targeted city bombings, like Germany and Japan in the Second World War. (Deliberate targeting of civilians with explosive and incendiary bombs simply because they happen to be under the command and control of an enemy Power is no better than lining them up and machine gunning them—a clear atrocity.) It also includes large scale massacres of Filipinos during the American colonization of the Philippines at the beginning of this century, deaths in British concentration camps in South Africa during the Boer War, civilian deaths due to starvation during the British blockade of Germany in and after the First World War, the rape and murder of Chinese in and around Peking in 1900, the atrocities committed by Americans in Vietnam, the murder of Algerians by the French, and the deaths of German prisoners of war in French and American prisoner of war camps after the Second World War.

All these acts of killing by democracies may seem to violate the Power principle, but actually they underline it. For in each case, the killing was carried out in secret, behind a conscious cover of lies and deceit by those agencies and Power holders involved. All were shielded by tight censorship of the press and control of journalists. Even the indiscriminate bombing of German cities was disguised before the British House of Commons and in press releases as attacks on German military targets. That the general strategic bombing policy was to attack workingmen's homes was kept secret still long after the war.

The upshot is that even democracies, where Power can take root in particular institutions, remain unchecked and undisciplined, and hide its activities, are capable of murder en masse. Such Power usually flourishes during wartime, for then the military are often given their head, democratic controls over civilian leaders are weak, and the press labors under strict reigns. Democracies too then become garrison states, Power is freed from any institutional restraints (note how easy it was to put tens of thousands of Japanese Americans in concentration camps during the Second World War for nothing more than their Japanese ancestry), and where it can become absolute, as in the military, it may kill absolutely. Witness Hiroshima and Nagasaki.

Strategic reasons for killing innocent civilians in wartime have been used throughout history. The Japanese bombing of Chinese cities during the Sino-Japanese War was justified as a method to shorten the war. The killing of all inhabitants of a city by the Mongols once its defenses were breached was justified by the terror it would cause among inhabitants of other cities, who would then surrender rather than suffer the same fate. Even the Nazi reprisal murders of tens of thousands of civilians in occupied countries was justified as a way of gaining compliance and protecting German lives.

So Power kills and absolute Power kills absolutely. What then can be said of those alleged causes or factors of war, genocide, and mass murder? What about cultural-ethnic differences, out-group conflict, misperceptions, frustrations and aggression, relative deprivation, ideological imperatives, dehumanization, resource competition, and so on? At one time or another, for one state or another, one or more of these factors play an important role in democide. Some are essential for understanding some genocides, as of the Jews or Armenians; some politicide, as of enemies of the people, bourgeoisie, and clergy; some massacres, as of competing religious-ethnic groups; or some atrocities, as of those committed against poor and helpless villagers by victorious soldiers. But then neighbors in the service of Power have killed neighbors, fathers have killed their sons, faceless and unknown people have been killed by quota. One is hard put to find a race, religion, culture, or distinct ethnic group that has not murdered its own or others.

These factors accelerate the likelihood of war or of democide once some trigger event occurs and absolute or near absolute Power is present. That is to say that Power is a necessary factor for war or democide. When the elite have absolute Power, war or democide follows a common process, which I have called "the conflict helix."

In any society, including the international one, relations between individuals and groups are structured by social contracts determined by previous conflicts, accommodations, and adjustments among them. Social contracts define a structure of expectations that guide and regulate the social order, including Power. This structure is based on a particular balance of Powers (understood as an equation of interests, capabilities, and wills) among individuals and groups. Previous conflict, and possibly violence, determines a balance of Power between competing individuals and groups and a congruent structure of expectations, as for example, war or revolution ends in a new balance of Powers between nations or groups and an associated peace treaty or constitution. This structure of expectations often consists of new laws and norms defining a social order more consistent with the underlying distribution of relative Power.

However, relative Power never remains constant. It shifts as the interests, capabilities, and will of the parties change. The death of a charismatic leader, the outrage of significant groups, the loss of foreign support by out-groups, the entry into war and the resulting freedom of the elite to use force under the guise of war-time necessity, and so on, can significantly alter the balance of Power between groups. Where such a shift in Power is in favor of the governing elite, Power can achieve its potential. Where elites have built up frustrations regarding those who have lost Power but nonetheless continue to be perceived as a threat, where they see them as outside the moral universe, where they have dehumanized them, where the out-group is culturally or ethnically distinct and the elite perceive them as inferior, or where any other such factors are present, Power will achieve its murderous potential. It simply waits for an excuse, an event of some sort, an assassination, a massacre in a neighboring country, an attempted coup, a famine, or a natural disaster, that will justify beginning the murder en masse.

The result of such violence will be a new balance of Power and attendant social contract. In some cases this may end the democide by the elimination of the "inferior" group—as of the Armenians by the Turks. In many cases, the survivors will be subdued and cowered—like the Ukrainians who lived through Stalin's collectivization campaign and intentional famine. In some cases this establishes a new balance of Power so skewed toward the elite that they may throughout their reign continue to murder at will. Murder as public policy becomes part of the new structure of expectations, of the new social order. Consider the social orders of Hitler, Stalin, Mao, Pol Pot, and their henchmen.

War and democide can be understood within a common framework as part of a social process, a balancing of Powers, where Power is supreme. It is not clear, however, why among states in which Power is limited and accountable, war and significant democide do not take place. Two concepts explain this: cross pressures and the associated political culture. Where Power is diffuse, checked, and made to be accountable, society is riven by myriad independent groups, disparate institutions, and multiple interests. These forces overlap and contend with each other; they section loyalties and divide desires and wants. Churches, unions, corporations, government bureaucracies, political parties, the media, special interest groups, and such, fight for and protect their interests.

Individuals and elites are pushed and pulled by their membership in several groups and institutions making it difficult for any one driving interest to form. They are divided, weak, ambivalent; they are cross-pressured. For elites to coalesce sufficiently to commit itself to murdering its own citizens, there must be a near fanatical, driving interest. But even if such an interest were present among a few, the diversity of interests across the political elite and associated bureaucracies, the freedom of the media to uncover what is being planned or done, and the ever-present potential leaks and fear of such leaks of disaffected members of the elite to the media brake such tendencies.

As for the possibility of war between democracies, diversity and resulting cross-pressures operate as well. Not only is it very difficult for the elite to unify public interests and opinion sufficiently to make war, but the diverse, economic, social, and political bonds between democracies that tie them together usually prevent the outbreak of violence.

Cross pressures are a social force that operates wherever individual and group freedom predominates. It is natural to a spontaneous social field. But human behavior is not only a matter of social forces, it also depends on meanings, values and norms—that is, a democratic culture is also essential. When Power is checked and accountable, when cross pressures limit the operation of Power, a particular democratic culture develops. This culture involves debate, demonstrations, protests, but also negotiation, compromise, and tolerance. It involves the art of conflict resolution and the acceptance of democratic procedures at all levels of society. The ballot replaces the bullet, and particularly, people and groups come to accept a loss on this or that interest as only an unfortunate outcome of the way the legitimate game is played. "Lose today, win tomorrow."

That democratic political elites should kill opponents or commit genocide for some public policy is unthinkable—although such may occur in the isolated and secret corners of government where Power can still lurk. Even in modern democracies, public defining and dehumanizing of out-groups has become a social and political evil. Witness the current potency of such allegations as "racism" or "sexism." Of course, the culture of democracy operates between democracies as well. Diplomacy, negotiating a middle way, seeking common interests, is part of the operating medium among democracies. A detailed political history of the growth of the European Community would well display this. Since each democracy takes the legitimacy of the other and their interests for granted, conflict is only a process of nonviolent learning and adjustment. Conferences, not war, should be the instrumentality for settling disputes.

Where absolute Power exists, interests are polarized, a culture of violence develops, and war and democide follow. In this century alone, by current count, Power has killed near 187,797,000 people. Where among states Power is limited and accountable, interests are cross-pressured and a culture of nonviolence develops. No wars have occurred and comparatively very few citizens have been murdered by the governing elite—perhaps no more than one-hundred or so in this century.

This picture of Power and its human costs is new. Few are aware of the democide that has been inflicted on our fellow human beings. That Hitler murdered millions of Jews is common knowledge. That he murdered overall some 20,946,000 Jews, Slavs, Gypsies, homosexuals, Frenchmen, Balts, Czechs, and others, is virtually unknown. Similarly, that Stalin murdered tens of millions is becoming generally appreciated; but that Stalin, Lenin, and their successors murdered some 61,911,000 Soviet citizens and foreigners is little comprehended by the outside world. Then there is Mao Tse-tung's China, Chiang Kai-shek's China, the militarist's Japan, Yahya Khan's Pakistan, Pol Pot's Cambodia, and others who have murdered in the millions. Tabulations of the toll around the world have been grossly underestimated. The best, most recent such accounting came up with no more than 16,000,000 killed in genocide and politicide since the Second World War. But this estimate does not even cover half of the likely 35,236,000 murdered alone by the communists in China between 1949 and 1987.

Even the toll of war is not well understood. Many experts estimate that in the Second World War, for example, 40,000,000 to 60,000,000 people were killed. The problem with these figures is that they include tens of millions killed in democide. Many war-time governments massacred civilians and foreigners, committed atrocities or genocide against them, executed them, and subjected them to reprisals. Aside from those killed in battle or military engagements, the Nazis murdered around 20,000,000 civilians and prisoners of war, the Japanese 5,890,000, the Chinese Nationalists 5,907,000, the Chinese communists 250,000, the Croatians 655,000, the Tito partisans 600,000, and Stalin 13,053,000 (above the 20,000,000 war dead and democide by the Nazis of Soviet Jews and Slavs), not to mention the Allied bombings that killed hundreds of thousands of civilians.

Most of these are usually included among the war dead. Those killed in battle versus in democide form distinct conceptual and theoretical categories and should not be confused. That they have been consistently and sometimes intentionally confounded helps raise the toll during this war to some

60,000,000 people, way above the estimated 15,000,000 killed in battle and military action. The almost universally accepted count of genocide during this period as no more than 6 million Jews, around 13 percent of the total war-time democide, has further confused our research and thought.

The Soviets committed genocide among at least nine of their ethnic-linguistic sub-nations, including ethnic Germans, ethnic Greeks, Crimean Tatars, and Balkans. Genocides by others include those of Germans against Slavs, Gypsies, and homosexuals; Croatians against the Serbs, Jews, and Gypsies; the Serbs against Croatians and Moslems; the Hungarians against their Jews; the Serbs, Poles, and Czechs against their ethnic Germans.

Our appreciation of the incredible scale of this century's genocide, politicide, and mass murder has been stultified by a lack of concepts. Democide is committed by absolute Power, its agency is government. The discipline for studying and analyzing Power and government and associated genocide and mass murder is political science. But except for a few specific cases, such as the Holocaust and Armenian genocide, and a precious few more general works, one is hard put to find political science research specifically on this subject.

The concepts and views promoted in political science text books are grossly unrealistic. They just do not fit in or explain, and are even contradictory to, the existence of a hell state like Pol Pot's Cambodia, a Gulag state like Stalin's Soviet Union, or a genocide state like Hitler's Germany. One textbook, for instance, spends a chapter on describing the functions of government as law and order, individual security, cultural maintenance, and social welfare. Political scientists are still writing this stuff, when we have numerous examples of governments that kill millions of their own citizens, enslave the rest, and abolish traditional culture. It took only about a year for the Khmer Rouge to completely uproot and extinguish Buddhism, which had been the heart and soul of Cambodian culture.

A systems approach to politics still dominates the field. Seen through this lens, politics is a matter of inputs and outputs, of citizen inputs, aggregation by political parties, government determining policy, and bureaucracies implementing it. Then there is the common and fundamental justification of government that it exists to protect citizens against the anarchic jungle that would otherwise threaten their lives and property. Such archaic, sterile views show no appreciation of democide and related horrors and suffering. They are inconsistent with a regime that stands astride society like a gang of thugs over hikers they have captured in the woods, robbing all, raping some, torturing others for fun, murdering those they do not like, and terrorizing the rest into servile obedience. This characterization of many past and present governments, such as Idi Amin's Uganda, hardly squares with conventional political science.

Consider also that library stacks have been filled on the possible nature and consequences of nuclear war and how it might be avoided. Yet, the toll from democide (and related destruction and misery among the survivors) is equivalent to a nuclear war, especially at the high 300 million end of the estimates. It is as though one had already occurred! Yet to my knowledge, there is only one book dealing with the human cost of this "nuclear war"—Gil Elliot's *Twentieth Century Book of the Dead*. And to my knowledge he is not a political scientist.

What is needed is a reconceptualization of government and politics consistent with what we now know about democide and related misery. New concepts have to be invented, old ones realigned to correct our perception of Power. We need to invent concepts for governments that turn their states into concentration camps, purposely starve millions of their citizens, set up quotas for those who should be killed. Although murder by quota was carried out by the Soviets, Chinese communists, and Vietnamese, the general political science literature does not give recognition to this incredible inhumaneness of certain governments. We have no concept for murder as an aim of public policy, determined by discussion among the governing elite in the highest councils and imposed through government bureaucracy. There is virtually no index in any general book on politics and government that makes reference to official genocide and murder, to the number of those killed, executed, or massacred, not even in books on the Soviet Union or China. Most indexes omit references to concentration or labor camps or gulags, even if a book contains a paragraph or two on the subject.

The preeminent fact about government is that some murder millions in cold blood. This is where absolute Power reigns. The second fact is that some, usually the same governments, murder tens of thousands more through foreign aggressions and intervention. Absolute Power again. These two facts alone must be the basis of a reconceptualization and of taxonomies of states. These must be based, not only on whether a state is developed or not, third world or not, powerful or not, large or not, but also and more importantly, on whether Power in a state is absolute and has engaged in genocide, politicide, and mass murder.

The empirical and theoretical conclusion—still more work on comparative democide in this century remains to be done—is this: the way to end war and virtually eliminate the conditions for democide appears to be through restricting and checking Power. This means the fostering of democratic freedom.

BEYOND DEATH

Contents

THE SELECTION BY KASTENBAUM PRESENTS THE EVIDENCE on both sides of the debate about near-death experiences (NDEs). The contemporary debate about NDEs began with the publication of *Life After Life*, by Raymond A. Moody, Jr., in 1975. That book was based on accounts given to Moody by those who had suffered cardiac arrest, been in an auto accident, or who had had some other such experience in which they came close to death but ended up recovering. Many of the reported NDEs shared similar elements, such as a sense of serenity, an out-of-body experience, seeing a brilliant white light, etc. Kastenbaum presents the evidence from Moody's book as well as similar reports by clinical researchers and historians. After offering material that supports the notion that NDEs do, in fact, provide evidence for survival after death, he reviews the arguments by those who claim that NDEs do not provide such evidence.

The selection by philosopher Bertrand Russell also deals with the question as to whether we survive death. Russell takes issue with the concept of the soul. He argues that what we describe as a person is merely a series of experiences connected by memory, and that we are not the same person today that we were yesterday; we are in a constant state of flux. He argues that our memory and what we describe as the self are bound up with the structure of the brain. When we die, our brains will dissolve and with it our memories (and thus our selves). In his opinion, it is emotions (particularly our fear of death), and not rational arguments, that are behind the belief in survival after death.

In "The Postself," Shneidman discusses life after death in a sense that differs from the traditional religious conception. He argues that everyone will survive death at least for a period of time, to the extent that the person remains in the memory of his or her survivors. While we are alive, we all spend a certain amount of time thinking about what our reputation and influence will be after we are dead and gone. Shneidman refers to this reputation and influence that survives one's death as the "postself." Shneidman mentions a number of respects in which we can live on after death, including in the memories of others, through our creative work, through organ transplantation, and through the genes of our children.

Sociologists may want to use this essay as a starting point to explore the concept of social immortality, the different forms that social immortality takes, and differences between population subgroups with respect to access to social immortality. It may be of interest to analyze the gender, race, ethnicity, occupation, and social class of those depicted in statues and on the facades of buildings. Today, such forms of social immortality stretch all the way from having a city named in one's honor to having a seat in a college auditorium constructed in one's name. It may also be of interest to explore the extent to which some people have attained social immortality in the general society (e.g., major political and religious figures) and those who have gained this rank in a much more narrow segment of society (such as those who hold an athletic record for one of the less-popular athletic events).

41 Near Death Experiences: ❧
New Evidence for Survival?

Robert Kastenbaum

This selection is drawn from ROBERT KASTENBAUM's book, *Death, Society, and Human Experience*. In this article, he evaluates the evidence in connection with the near-death experiences reported by Raymond A. Moody, Jr. (in his book, *Life After Life*), Kenneth Ring, and others. After reviewing the reports presented by those who claim that near-death experiences provide evidence of survival after death, he goes on to present a detailed summary of the logic and evidence against this conclusion. See the introduction to Chapter 1 for a biographical comment about Robert Kastenbaum.

THE PRIMARY, OR MOODY-TYPE, NEAR-DEATH EXPERIENCE

Renewed attention has been given to the survival question since the publication of a book entitled *Life After Life* in 1975. Author Raymond A. Moody, Jr. listened to the experiences of men and women who had recovered after coming close to death. Some of these people had suffered cardiac arrest; all had been in serious peril. Moody's report and discussion of these near-death experiences (NDEs) became a surprise best seller. Almost immediately, additional NDE reports appeared from many sources. Some people had had such experiences years before but were reluctant to speak about them until Moody's book brought the phenomenon into the open. The same was true for some physicians and other allied health workers who had encountered occasional NDEs in their practice and now felt more comfortable about sharing them. Although Moody's NDE collection was not based on a controlled research effort (nor did he claim it be), it did stimulate studies by a variety of medical and sociobehavioral scientists.

Moody selected 50 cases from his collection for analysis. Some of these people were said to have been pronounced dead by a physician; all appeared to have been close to the end. Examining his interview notes, Moody found 15 elements that occurred frequently (but not necessarily all elements occurred in each interview). A typical experience follows:

> *I was hospitalized for a severe kidney condition, and I was in a coma for approximately a week. My doctors were extremely uncertain as to whether I would live. During this period when I was unconscious, I felt as though I were lifted right up, just as though I didn't have a physical body at all. A brilliant white light appeared to me. The light was so bright that I could not see through it, but going into its presence was so calming and so wonderful. There is just no experience on earth like it. In the presence of the light, the thoughts or words came into my mind: "Do you want to die?" And I replied that I didn't know since I knew nothing about death. Then the white light said, "Come over this line and you will learn." I felt that I knew where the line was in front of me, although I could not actually see it. As I went across the line, the most wonderful feelings came over me—feelings of peace, tranquility, a vanishing of all worries. (p. 56)*

This report illustrates some of the major features of the primary NDE. Instead of panic or despair there is a sense of serenity and well-being. The sensation of being "lifted right up" is also one of the most striking characteristics. Known popularly as the "out-of-body experience," this state has a more technical name as well: the *autoscopic* experience. (This scholarly term, however, does not really add anything to the explanation.) Rising and floating are also common experiences reported, as well as a sense of journey, a going toward something. A "brilliant white light" may be discovered as the journey continues. Furthermore, there is often a turning-point encounter. The individual reports feeling as though he or she had a choice about death at this time. Moody comments:

> *The most common feelings reported in the first few moments following death are a desperate desire to get back into the body and an intense regret over one's demise. However, once the dying person reaches a certain depth in his experience, he does not want to come back, and he may even resist the return to the body. This is especially the case for those who have gotten so far as to encounter the being of light. As one man put it most emphatically, "I never wanted to leave the presence of this being." (p. 11)*

Soon clinical researchers came up with additional cases of NDE (Sabom & Kreutziger, 1977). Historians pointed out ancient examples from religious experiences, especially in the Eastern tradition (Holck, 1978). The type of experience confided to Moody was not limited to the survivors who had happened to come his way.

The question now arose: How is this remarkable experience to be explained? It is here that we enter the realm of continuing controversy. Does the primary NDE constitute proof for survival of death?

Evidence favoring the NDE
as proof of survival

Moody at first did not claim that the reports he had collected were evidence for survival. "In my opinion anyone who claims that near death experiences prove or give scientific evidence of an afterlife is only betraying his ignorance of what terms like evidence or proof mean" (Moody, 1980). More recently, however, Moody (1988) has reversed this position. He now supports the survival hypothesis.

What has been learned from systematic research? Psychologist Kenneth Ring took the lead in establishing research procedures for the study of NDEs (1978; 1980; 1984). He developed a scale to assess the depth of intensity of an NDE and therefore made it possible to study the phenomenon in more adequate detail. . . . A very intense NDE would include all these possible components, some of which are also rated according to their vividness or depth.

Ring found that age, sex, economic status, and the type of near-death experience (e.g., automobile accident, surgery, etc.) did not seem to make a difference. The NDE occurs in many types of situations and among many kinds of people. In a recent summary of all available research in the field, Ring now (1989) estimates that the NDE occurs in about one of every three cases that have been studied. Although this means that two of every three people who have survived a brush with death did *not* report an NDE, the number of those now on record is in the thousands. How many have had NDEs without coming to the attention of researchers? "It seems reasonable to assume that there must be many millions who have and, because of modern cardiopulmonary resuscitation measures, many more who will" (Ring, p. 194).

According to Ring's studies, the NDE seems to have a powerful effect on many survivors. After a brush with death, people often have a renewed sense of purpose in life. Daily life also becomes more precious to them. And what about the fear of death? Many survivors report that they have become much less concerned about dying and death; there was something very comforting and reassuring about their close encounter. These changes in perception and attitude were seldom found among people who had near-death episodes without near-death experiences. The differences were greatest between people who had deep or intense NDEs and those who reported no NDE at all. People who could recall intense NDEs were much more likely to think of these as spiritual experiences that had changed their lives, whether or not religion had played an important role for them before these experiences. It would appear, then, that the renewed purpose, appreciation of life and sense of spirituality are closely associated with the *experience* rather than simply the fact of a life-threatening encounter.

In Ring's opinion the NDE does provide evidence for survival. He believes that the individual has attained an altered state in which the mind is free—temporarily—from the limitations imposed by the physical body. No longer bound by physical make-up, the individual is granted a direct perception of the universe. The perception of some form of radiant light at the end of a tunnel might represent a glimpse of astral reality, according to Ring. In attempting to provide a scientific rationale for this view, Ring refers to Karl Pribham's (1977) neurobiological theory, which suggests that the human brain functions in a holographic manner: We are biologically equipped to interpret the complex frequencies that comprise the universe and to translate these into usable sensory experience.

As a behavioral scientist, Ring attempts to keep his conclusions within the limits of his data, so he does not make the flat statement that the NDE proves survival of death. Nevertheless, he marshals his evidence and speculations in this direction and appears to be personally convinced of survival himself.

Cardiologist Michael B. Sabom (1982) was among the earliest contributors to NDE research and has now reported his investigations in some detail. His findings for the most part are consistent with those of Ring and other researchers. The NDE is frequently reported as a beautiful experience, accompanied by a sense of serenity and freedom rather than anxiety or depression. Again, no relationship was found between the NDE and characteristics of the individual or of the life-threatening condition. Among Sabom's many useful examples are several that illustrate the individual's attempt to make contact with others while in the NDE state. A Vietnam veteran, for example, immediately experienced the split-self state when a mine explosion left him close to death. He continued to watch his body and what was happening to it all the way to the surgical table in the field hospital:

> SUBJECT: I'm trying to stop them (the doctors). I really did try to grab a hold of them and stop them, because I really felt happy where I was . . . I actually remember grabbing the doctor. . . .
>
> AUTHOR: What happened?
>
> SUBJECT: Nothing. Absolutely nothing. It was almost like he wasn't there. I grabbed and he wasn't there or either I just went through him or whatever. (p. 33)

The sense of being separate from your own body comes across strongly in many of Sabom's cases, whether drawn from the battlefield, domestic accidents, or critical illness.

What gives the work of Sabom and his colleagues particular distinction is the effort to compare the survivor's subjective reports with the information available in hospital records and retrievable from staff members. This is important because it provides an opportunity to determine whether or not the person in the midst of an NDE actually does make observations that could not have been possible if trapped within a horizontal, impaired, and endangered body. Sabom is aware that people who have not been adequately anesthetized occasionally show a memory for events that happened during their surgery. Could the NDE be the same sort of occurrence? He concludes it is not likely. The NDE bears "no resemblance to the nightmarish experiences reported by inadequately anesthetized patients. *Visual* details of an operation are not later retrievable by hypnosis from the subconscious minds of patients who had been anesthetized, although *spoken* words can sometimes be recalled" (p. 80).

Furthermore, Sabom at times was able to establish a positive correspondence between what the patient "saw" and what did in fact take place during a life-and-death medical procedure (in his study this was usually the emergency procedure for reversing cardiac arrest). In a preliminary study he was able to establish what kind of educated guesses people tend to make about cardiopulmonary resuscitation (CPR) so that he would not credit a survivor with a specific and accurate description unless it was well justified by the evidence. Sabom eventually had a set of 32 people whose NDEs included visual impressions of what had taken place during the peak of their crisis. Most of their descriptions included statements that correspond to what had actually happened but were not highly specific. The key information was derived from a smaller set of six survivors who had recalled specific details of their near-death crisis. In each of these cases the individual recalled having seen one or more specific events and developments that could not have been obtained through guesswork or prior knowledge of CPR. In other words, there was objective evidence that some individuals who reported an NDE did in fact gain information consistent with out-of-the-body status.

Sabom does not rush to the conclusion that his findings constitute evidence for survival of death. Nevertheless, after considering several alternative hypotheses, he judges that the autoscopic phenomenon may be authentic, that some type of split between mind and body can occur during points of crisis, and that during this altered state a person can make accurate observations of immediate reality as well as enter into the mystical state of being often reported for NDEs. Sabom's work is highly recommended for further reading on all counts: as a human document, as an application of careful methodology in a difficult situation, and as a thoughtful assessment of alternative explanations.

Another research approach lends some indirect support to the claim that the NDE should be considered as evidence for survival. Why accept the survival interpretation if there are simpler explanations available? Scientists usually prefer explanations that stick closely to the observed facts and do not require bringing in additional assumptions and speculations. If only certain kinds of people or certain kinds of situations produced NDEs, then the survival interpretation could be criticized as an extravagant flight of fancy. We have seen that Ring's early studies found otherwise; the NDE seemed to occur to many different people in many different situations. A number of questions were left unanswered by these studies, however, and have since been examined carefully by Glen Gabbard and Stuart Twemlow (1984). Here are some of their most important findings:

1. NDEs are not caused by nor are they necessarily symptoms of mental illness. Very few people who reported NDEs showed signs of psychopathology.
2. NDEs are not related to level of education. Therefore, it cannot be said that NDE is either something that is "imagined" by people with little formal education, or "created" by people with perhaps too much education.
3. There is no evidence that NDEs occur mostly among people who had already been fascinated by mystic or other unusual phenomena. (*After* the NDE, however, people often did become more interested in spiritual phenomena.)
4. The NDE does not have much similarity to dreams. In comparing their NDE reports with studies of normal dreams, Gabbard and Twemlow observed more differences than similarities. There, it cannot be said that the survivors "dreamed" their experiences, if we are to use the term "dream" in its usual sense.

As we will see, there are other Gabbard and Twemlow findings that are not so favorable to the survival interpretation. Nevertheless, the results that have just been reviewed do suggest that some of the more conservative interpretations (e.g., mental illness, dreaming) are not well supported. However, the poor showing of these alternative interpretations does not prove the survival hypothesis. There are other alternative hypotheses still to consider, as well as some problems with the data and logic of the survival interpretation.

EVIDENCE AND LOGIC AGAINST THE NEAR-DEATH EXPERIENCE AS EVIDENCE FOR SURVIVAL

There are a number of logical as well as empirical objections to interpreting NDEs as evidence for survival:

1. Some people who return from a close encounter with death do *not* have experiences of the primary NDE (Pelletier & Garfield, 1976). They have no memories at all or only vague and dreamlike fragments to recall. This argues against the universality of the NDE and therefore weakens the NDE. Since death is universal, how could the NDE be otherwise if it is truly a visit to the other side?

2. Some survivors return with nightmarish experiences that neither in-

crease their spirituality nor decrease their fear of death. Although Sabom apparently did not come across such examples, the equally careful research of Garfield (1979) did, and I have collect both positive and negative reports myself. . . .

3. The primary, or Moody-type, NDE occurs sometimes in situations in which the individual is in no bodily peril of death, there it should not be considered as distinctively related to death (LaBarre, 1972). The out-of-the-body component of the NDE has also been reported frequently—and sometimes even created experimentally—apart from any death peril (Brent, 1979; Myers, 1975).

4. Careful research of medical records shows that many people who report NDEs actually had *not* come close to death. The most recent such study found only about half of the NDE reporters had survived a life-threatening illness or injury. Nevertheless, it was common for people to believe they had been dead or very near death even if they had not been in serious danger. Some patients had decided for themselves that they had been "dead" or "clinically dead." Others (mis)interpreted what they had been told by doctors or nurses. The researchers comment that "having had the NDE itself may have led some people to believe retrospectively that their condition must have been worse than it otherwise seemed" (Stevenson, et al., 1989–1990, p. 52).

5. The fact that many kinds of people report NDEs in many kinds of situations has weakened such alternative explanations as mental illness or a strong predisposition toward fantasy. However, there are also findings that do suggest relationships between the specific circumstances and the specific nature of the NDE. Gabbard and Twemlow, for example, found that people who had been in severe pain were more likely than others to experience a sense of distance from their bodies. They note that, "In hypnotic pain experiments, it is a common suggestion to dissociate the painful part from the body so that it is treated as 'not self'" (Gabbard & Twemlow, 1984). Furthermore, patients who had been under anesthesia were especially likely to see brilliant lights and hear unusual sounds. These effects are known to occur with many people who have been anesthesized, whether or not their conditions were life-threatening. Results such as these indicate that the overall picture is not that simple. The specific type of NDE that one experiences seems to be influenced by a number of circumstances, even though NDEs, as a class of phenomena, may occur to many kinds of people under many kinds of stress.

6. We hear NDEs only from the survivors. There is no evidence that what happens when a person really dies "and stays dead" has any relationship to the experiences reported by those who have recovered from a life-threatening episode. In fact, it is difficult to imagine how there could ever be such evidence; the very fact that a person recovered disqualifies their report of "permanent death." There is always an observing self that categorizes the observed self as

inert or dead. This split consciousness may result in the opinion that "I was dead," but there was always another "I" lively and perceptive enough to make that judgment.

Several explanations have been offered as alternatives to the conclusion that NDE survivors have actually returned from the dead. These explanations do not deny the experiences as such, nor the emotional significance and meanings that might be drawn from them. The alternative explanations, however, do attempt to provide interpretations that are plausible and that remain within the framework of basic clinical and research knowledge.

What are these alternative explanations? Psychiatrist Russell Noyes, Jr. and his colleagues conducted a series of studies (Noyes & Kletti, 1976; 1976; 1977) with people who survived a variety of life-threatening crises. He and his colleagues found a set of common features in these reports. Three major factors emerged from the statistical analyses: mystical, depersonalization, and hyperalertness.

The *mystical* dimension of experiences close to death includes:

Feeling of great understanding
Images sharp or vivid
Revival of memories
Sense of harmony, unity
Feeling of joy
Revelation
Feeling of being controlled by outside force
Colors or visions
Strange bodily sensations

The *depersonalization* dimension includes:

Loss of emotion
Body apart from self
Self strange or unreal
Objects small, far away
Detachment from body
World strange or unreal
Wall between self and emotions
Detachment from world
Body changed in shape or size
Strange sounds
Altered passage of time

The *hyperalertness* dimension includes:

Thoughts sharp or vivid
Thoughts speeded up
Vision and hearing sharper
Thoughts blurred or dull
Altered passage of time
Thoughts and movements mechanical

With these findings Noyes attempts to explain the primary NDE. He believes it is important to consider both physiological and psychological levels. Hyperalterness and depersonalization are interpreted as part of the same neural mechanism. The function of this hypothetical mechanism is to help the human organism react to dangerous circumstances. Drawing upon earlier observations of Roth and Harper (1962), Noyes suggests that this is an adaptive mechanism that combines opposing reaction tendencies, "the one serving to intensify alertness and the other to dampen potentially disorganizing emotion" (Noyes, 1979, p. 78). When this mechanism is working properly, a person is able to cope exceptionally well (coolly, calmly, objectively) in the midst of a crisis. Noyes writes:

> On a psychological *level depersonalization may be interpreted as a defense against the threat of death. Not only did people in the studies . . . find themselves calm in otherwise frightening situations but they also felt detached from what was happening. . . . The depersonalized state is one that mimics death [emphasis added]. In it a person experiences himself as empty, lifeless, and unfamiliar. In a sense he creates psychologically the very situation that environmental circumstances threaten to impose. In so doing he escapes death, for what has already happened cannot happen again; he cannot die, because he is already dead. (p. 79)*

This is a cogent and powerful explanation because it is in contact with NDE data and with the broader realm of psychobiological dynamics.

The dimension of mystical consciousness is seen by Noyes as being somewhat apart from the depersonalization-hyperalertness mechanism. This feature occurs most often with people who are dying from physical disease. Noyes suggests that the physiological changes associated with terminal illness may induce altered states of consciousness in which experiences of a mystical type are more likely to appear. Noyes' theoretical analysis, with many points of reference to clinical data, is richer than what can be presented here. (If you have a serious interest in this topic, you should become familiar with Noyes' work in more detail.)

I have suggested a related possible explanation with two components (Kastenbaum, 1981). First, you might expect that those who are closest to death—

in the most perilous physical condition—should be the most likely to have intense NDEs. The available evidence, however, finds just the opposite (Greyson, 1981). Survivors who had been very close to death reported fewer experiences of any kind than those who had been less jeopardized. This weakens the assumed connection between the NDE and death. It also highlights a question that has been somewhat neglected: Precisely when does the NDE occur? There is no firm answer. Quite possibly, the NDE is a memory created *on the way back*. In other words, it is not necessarily what the person experiences at the peak of the crisis but rather represents an attempt to make sense of the profound and confusing events that have transpired. The greatly impaired physical function close to the point of death does not allow much in the way of either perception or thought. On the way back, however, some people may be able to integrate their extraordinary but chaotic experiences through a memory story whose content and texture is drawn from the psychobiological response itself as well as individual and cultural factors.

A second component of the NDE might arise from the specific nature of the life-threatening condition. It is true that several studies have failed to find a relationship between the nature of the death threat and the production of an NDE. Such a relationship is more likely to be observed, however, if you attend to the individual's role in the crisis. A driver faced with an impending collision is much more like to make an emergency maneuver than to split off into an autoscopic experience. In general, we engage in instrumental actions—we do something—when the circumstances permit. This is a survival mechanism: action to avoid catastrophe. The NDE is more likely to occur when the jeopardized person has no instrumental action available. In such a situation the NDE serves a quieting, energy-conserving function. The sense of serenity implies the activation of self-produced brain opiates (endorphins). This altered state enables body functions to continue at a basic level with minimum expenditure of energy and is represented at the psychic level by comforting imagery. The imagery becomes more coherent as the individual recovers, although in retrospect it is attributed to an earlier phase of the crisis.

Still another explanation has been offered by psychologist Ronald K. Siegel (1980). He emphasizes the hallucinatory nature of NDEs (and the deathbed visions described later), drawing in particular upon the work of Grof and Halifax (1977):

> The specific content of complex hallucinatory imagery is determined largely by set (expectations and attitudes) and setting (physical and psychological environments). For many dying and near-death experiences, the sets (fear of approaching death, changes in body and mental functioning, etc.) and settings (hospital wards, accident scenes, etc.) can influence specific eschatological thoughts and images. Grof and Halifax suggest that the universal themes of this imagery may be related to stored memories of biological events which are activated in the brain. Accordingly . . . the feelings of peace

and quiet may be related to the original state of intrauterine existence when there is complete biological equilibrium with the environment. The experience of moving down a dark tunnel may be associated with the clinical stage of delivery in which the cervix is open and there is a gradual propulsion through the birth canal . . . the dying or near-death experience triggers a flashback or retrieval of an equally dramatic and emotional memory of the birth experience. . . . To the extent that this reasoning is correct, the experience of dying and rebirth in the afterlife may be a special case of state-dependent recall of birth itself. (Siegel, 1980, p. 920)

Why the hallucinations in the first place? Siegel suggests (as others have) that the sensory world of the terminally ill person is likely to be drastically reduced. Not much of sensory input is getting through from the outside. This lack of external stimulation encourages the release or escape of stored memories. These memories reenter conscious awareness as though they were perceptions. The result is that experiential state known as the hallucination.

There is one more way of looking at NDEs that deserves our attention. Carol Zaleski, an expert in religious studies, examines what she calls *Otherworld Journeys* (1987) that have been reported from ancient times to the present. Here is one of her examples:

Four days ago, I died and was taken by two angels to the height of heaven. And it was just as though I rose above not only this squalid earth, but even the sun and moon, the clouds and stars. Then I went through a gate that was brighter than normal daylight, into a place where the entire floor shone like gold and silver. The light was indescribable, and I can't tell you how vast it was. (p. 58)

This quotation is from a deeply religious man by the name of Salvius who had been left for dead one evening on a funeral bier. He was said to have revived and, inspired by his vision, became a bishop. Zaleski's perceptive review of "otherworldly journeys" offers some interesting comments along with the wealth of examples. She concludes that there is "a fundamental kinship" between these visions (or NDEs) and the imaginative powers that we use in everyday life:

. . . we are all, in a sense, otherworld travelers. Otherworld visions are products of the same imaginative power that is active in our ordinary ways of visualizing death; our tendency to portray ideas in concrete, embodied, and dramatic forms; the capacity of our inner states to transfigure our perception of outer landscapes; our need to internalize the cultural map of the physical universe, and our drive to experience that universe as a moral and spiritual cosmos in which we belong and have a purpose . . . we are able to grant the validity of near-death testimony as one way in which the religious imagination mediates the search for ultimate truth. (p. 205)

On this view, then, the NDE is one particularly interesting form that has been taken by the human mind in attempting to explain itself *to* itself. Science takes one path; imagination and intuition take another. Why choose only one path and dismiss the other? Zaleski's approach does not necessarily reduce the fascination and significance of NDEs, but it does attempt to show their continuity with the quest for meaning and purpose that many people have undertaken from ancient times to the present. Nevertheless, in common with the other alternative explanations that have been presented here, Zaleski's does not support the interpretation of the NDE as the report of a literal return from the dead.

The NDE clearly is of interest as a remarkable human experience. But were the survivors really dead? Do such reports provide evidence for survival of death? These questions remain controversial. In my judgment the case for the NDE as proof of survival has too many logical and empirical flaws to accept, despite the fact that some worthwhile research has been done. But what are we to make of Sabom's six survivors with demonstrably specific and accurate recollections? There may yet be important new developments in this field.

References

Brent, S. (1979). Deliberately induced, premortem out-of-the-body experiences: An experimental and theoretical approach. In R. Kastenbaum (Ed.), *Between life and death* (pp. 89–123). New York: Springer Publishing Co., Inc.

Gabbard, G. O., & Twemlow, S. W. (1984). *With the eyes of the mind.* New York: Praeger.

Garfield, C. (1979). The dying patient's concern with "life after death." In R. Kastenbaum (Ed.), *Between life and death* (pp. 45–60). New York: Springer Publishing Co., Inc.

Greyson, B. (1981). Empirical evidence bearing on the interpretation of NDE among suicide attempters. Paper presented at the annual meeting of the American Psychological Association, Los Angeles.

Grof, S., & Halifax, J. (1977). *The human encounter with death.* New York: Dutton.

Holck, F. H. (1978). Life revisited (parallels in death experiences). *Omega, Journal of Death and Dying, 9,* 1–12.

Kastenbaum, R. (1981). Recent studies of the NDE: A critical appraisal. Paper presented at the annual meeting of the American Psychological Association, Los Angeles.

La Barre, W. (1972). *The ghost dance: The origins of religion.* New York: Dell Publishing Co., Inc.

Lee, J. R. (1974). *Death and beyond in the Eastern perspective.* New York: Gordon & Brezch, Science Publishers, Inc.

Moody, R. A., Jr. (1975). *Life after life.* Atlanta: Mockingbird Books.

Moody, R. A., Jr. (1980). Commentary on "The reality of death experiences: A personal perspective" by Ernest Rodin. *Journal of Nervous and Mental Disease, 168,* 265.

Moody, R. A., Jr. (1988). *The light beyond.* New York: Bantam.

Myers, F. W. H. (1975). *Human personality and its survival of bodily death* (Vols. 1–2). New York: Arno Press. (Original work published 1903)

Noyes, R., Jr. (1979). Near-death experiences: Their interpretation. In R. Kastenbaum (Ed.), *Between life and death* (pp. 73–88). New York: Springer Publishing Co., Inc.

Noyes, R., Jr., & Kletti, R. (1976). Depersonalization in the face of life-threatening danger: A description. *Psychiatry*, *39*, 19–27.

Noyes, R., Jr., & Kletti, R. (1976). Depersonalization in the face of life-threatening danger: An interpretation. *Omega, Journal of Death and Dying*, 7, 103–114.

Noyes, R., Jr., & Kletti, R. (1977). Panoramic memory: A response to the threat of death. *Omega, Journal of Death and Dying*, 8, 181–194.

Pelletier, K., & Garfield, C. (1976). *Consciousness: East and West*. New York: Harper & Row, Publishers, Inc.

Pribham, K. H. (1977). Holonomy and structure in the organization of perception. In U.M. Nicholas (Ed.), *Images, perception and knowledge* (pp. 19–35). Dordrecht: D. Reidel.

Ring, K. (1978). Some determinants of the prototypic near death experience. Paper presented at the annual meeting of the American Psychological Association, Los Angeles.

Ring, K. (1980). *Life at death*. New York: Coward, McCann & Geoghegan.

Ring, K. (1984). *Heading toward Omega*. New York: William Morrow & Co.

Ring, K. (1989). Near-death experiences. In R. Kastenbaum & B. K. Kastenbaum (eds.), *Encyclopedia of death* (pp. 193–196). Phoenix: Oryx Press.

Roth, M., & Harper, M. (1962). Temporal lobe epilepsy and the phobic anxiety-depersonalization syndrome. Part II: Practical and theoretical considerations. *Comprehensive Psychiatry*, 3, 215–225.

Sabom, M. B. (1982). *Recollection of death*. New York: Simon & Schuster.

Sabom, M. B., & Kreutziger, S. (1977). The experience of near death. *Death Education*, 2, 195–204.

Siegel, R. K. (1980). The psychology of life after death. *American Psychologist*, 35, 911–931.

Stevenson, I., Cook, C. W., & McClean-Rice, N. (1989–1990). Are persons reporting "near-death experiences" really near death? A study of medical records. *Omega*, 20, 45–54.

Zaleski, C. (1987). *Otherworld journeys*. New York: Oxford Press.

42 Do We Survive Death?

Bertrand Russell

BERTRAND RUSSELL (1872–1970), British philosopher, mathematician, and essayist, was one of the most intellectually gifted individuals of our century. His many works, characterized by wit, clarity, and vivid metaphor, are known throughout the world. In this selection, taken from his book, *Why I Am Not a Christian*, Russell, in his typical no-nonsense pungent prose, attacks the notion of survival after death.

BEFORE WE CAN PROFITABLY DISCUSS whether we shall continue to exist after death, it is well to be clear as to the sense in which a man is the same person as he was yesterday. Philosophers used to think that there were definite substances, the soul and the body, that each lasted on from day to day, that a soul, once created, continued to exist throughout all future time, whereas a body ceased temporarily from death till the resurrection of the body.

The part of this doctrine which concerns the present life is pretty certainly false. The matter of the body is continually changing by processes of nutriment and wastage. Even if it were not, atoms in physics are no longer supposed to have continuous existence; there is no sense in saying: this is the same atom as the one that existed a few minutes ago. The continuity of a human body is a matter of appearance and behavior, not of substance.

The same thing applies to the mind. We think and feel and act, but there is not, in addition to thoughts and feelings and actions, a bare entity, the mind or the soul, which does or suffers these occurrences. The mental continuity of a person is a continuity of habit and memory: there was yesterday one person whose feelings I can remember, and that person I regard as myself of yesterday; but, in fact, myself of yesterday was only certain mental occurrences which are now remembered and are regarded as part of the person who now recollects them. All that constitutes a person is a series of experiences connected by memory and by certain similarities of the sort we call habit.

If, therefore, we are to believe that a person survives death, we must believe that the memories and habits which constitute the person will continue to be exhibited in a new set of occurrences.

No one can prove that this will not happen. But it is easy to see that it is very unlikely. Our memories and habits are bound up with the structure of the brain, in much the same way a river is connected with the riverbed. The water in the river is always changing, but it keeps to the same course because previous rains have worn a channel. In like manner, previous events have worn a channel in the brain, and our thoughts flow along this channel. This is the cause of memory and mental habits. But the brain, as a structure, is dissolved at death, and memory therefore may be expected to be also dissolved. There is no more reason to think otherwise than to expect a river to persist in its old course after an earthquake has raised a mountain where a valley used to be.

All memory, and therefore (one may say) all minds, depend upon a property which is very noticeable in certain kinds of material structures but exists little if at all in other kinds. This is the property of forming habits as a result of frequent similar occurrences. For example: a bright light makes the pupils of the eyes contract: and if you repeatedly flash a light in a man's eyes and beat a gong at the same time, the gong alone will, in the end, cause his pupils to contract. This is a fact about the brain and nervous system—that is to say, about a certain material structure. It will be found that exactly similar facts explain our response to language and our use of it, our memories and the emotions they arouse, our moral or immoral habits of behavior, and indeed everything that constitutes our mental personality, except the part determined by heredity. The part determined by heredity is handed on to our posterity but cannot, in the individual, survive the disintegration of the body. Thus both the hereditary and the acquired parts of a personality are, so far as our experience goes, bound up with the characteristics of certain bodily structures. We all know that memory may be obliterated by an injury to the brain, that a virtuous person may be rendered vicious by encephalitis lethargica, and that a clever child can be turned into an idiot by lack of iodine. In view of such familiar facts, it seems scarcely probable that the mind survives the total destruction of brain structure which occurs at death.

It is not rational arguments but emotions that cause belief in a future life.

The most important of these emotions is fear of death, which is instinctive and biologically useful. If we genuinely and wholeheartedly believed in the future life, we should cease completely to fear death. The effects would be curious, and probably such as most of us would deplore. But our human and subhuman ancestors have fought and exterminated their enemies throughout many geological ages and have profited by courage; it is therefore an advantage to the victors in the struggle for life to be able, on occasion, to overcome the natural fear of death. Among animals and savages, instinctive pugnacity suffices for this purpose; but at a certain stage of development, as the Mohammedans first proved, belief in Paradise has considerable military value as reinforcing natural pugnacity. We should therefore admit that militarists are wise in encouraging the belief in immortality, always supposing that this belief does not become so profound as to produce indifference to the affairs of the world.

Another emotion which encourages the belief in survival is admiration of the excellence of man. As the Bishop of Birmingham says, "His mind is a far finer instrument than anything that had appeared earlier—he knows right and wrong. He can build Westminster Abbey. He can make an airplane. He can calculate the distance of the sun . . . Shall, then, man at death perish utterly? Does that incomparable instrument, his mind, vanish when life ceases?"

The bishop proceed to argue that "the universe has been shaped and is governed by an intelligent purpose," and that it would have been unintelligent, having made man, to let him perish.

To this argument there are many answers. In the first place, it has been found, in the scientific investigation of nature, that the intrusion of moral or aesthetic values has always been an obstacle to discovery. It used to be thought that the heavenly bodies must move in circles because the circle is the most perfect curve, that species must be immutable because God would only create what was perfect and what therefore stood in no need of improvement, that it was useless to combat epidemics except by repentance because they were sent as punishment for sin, and so on. It has been found, however, that, so far as we can discover, nature is indifferent to our values and can only be understood by ignoring our notions of good and bad. The universe may have a purpose, but nothing that we know suggests that, if so, this purpose has any similarity to ours.

Nor is there in this anything surprising. Dr. Barnes tells us that man "knows right and wrong." But, in fact, as anthropology shows, men's views of right and wrong have varied to such an extent that no single item has been permanent. We cannot say, therefore, that man knows right and wrong, but only that some men do. Which men? Nietzsche argued in favor of an ethic profoundly different from Christ's, and some powerful governments have accepted his teaching. If knowledge of right and wrong is to be an argument for immortality, we must first settle whether to believe Christ or Nietzsche, and then argue that Christians are immortal, but Hitler and Mussolini are not, or vice versa. The decision will obviously be made on the battlefield, not in the study. Those who have the best poison gas will have the ethic of the future and will therefore be the immortal ones.

Our feelings and beliefs on the subject of good and evil are, like everything else about us, natural facts, developed in the struggle for existence and not having any divine or supernatural origin. In one of Aesop's fables, a lion is shown pictures of huntsmen catching lions and remarks that, if he had painted them, they would have shown lions catching huntsmen. Man, says Dr. Barnes, is a fine fellow because he can make airplanes. A little while ago there was a popular song about the cleverness of flies in walking upside down on the ceiling, with the chorus: "Could Lloyd George do it? Could Mr. Baldwin do it? Could Ramsay Mac do it? Why, NO." On this basis a very telling argument could be constructed by a theologically minded fly, which no doubt the other flies would find most convincing.

Moreover, it is only when we think abstractly that we have such a high opinion of man. Of men in the concrete, most of us think the vast majority very bad. Civilized states can spend more than half their revenue on killing each other's citizens. Consider the long history of the activities inspired by moral fervor: human sacrifices, persecutions of heretics, witch-hunts, pogroms leading up to wholesale extermination by poison gases, which one at least of Dr. Barnes's episcopal colleagues must be supposed to favor, since he holds pacifism to be un–Christian. Are these abominations, and the ethical doctrines by which they are prompted, really evidence of an intelligent creator? And can we really wish that the men who practiced them should live forever? The world in which we live can be understood as a result of muddle and accident: but if it is the outcome of deliberate purpose, the purpose must have been that of a fiend. For my part, I find accident a less painful and more plausible hypothesis.

༈ 43 The Postself

Edwin S. Shneidman

In this essay, drawn from his book, *Deaths of Man*, EDWIN SHNEIDMAN discusses what he refers to as the "postself," the reputation and influence we have after death. He points out that most of us survive our deaths—at least for a period of time, and often for a generation or two—in the minds of those who personally knew us when we were alive. There are several other forms that the postself takes, including the impact of one's work such as art, music, and books; or the remembrances and genetic inheritance of one's children. See the introduction to Chapter 34 for a biographical comment about Edwin Shneidman.

THERE IS A WAY in which we can experience a form of death in life, a way that is seldom damaging to the psyche and is in most instances beneficial: we can examine our fears and hopes about our reputation and influence after death—about what we may call our "postselves." This sort of introspection is, of course, a popular pastime among children ("They'll be sorry after I'm dead!"), and at one time or another all of us have entertained fantasies, varying from the sentimental to the hardheaded, of witnessing our own funerals. Few of us utterly abandon thoughts of survival in some form or other. They are our fragile hopes of escape from total annihilation.

And since our death is an experience for others if not for us, almost everyone does "survive" his own cessation for *some* period of time in *some* minds—for perhaps two generations in about a score of minds. The topic of survival after death is enormous and interesting, covering a wide range of emotionally held positions and beliefs. Of the respondents to a national death survey (Shneidman, 1971), 43 percent tended to believe in a life after death. I imagine it is obvious by now that I do not share their belief in any possibility of survival after death, except in accordance with my own special definition of "survival" as the postself. (The reader who wishes to pursue the notion of actual survival after death as it is conventionally understood can turn to Ducasse's *The Belief in a Life After Death* [1961]; Henderson and Oakes's *The Wisdom of the Serpent* [1963]; or the chapters on "Frontiers of Speculation" in Toynbee's *Man's Concern with Death* [1969].)

The concept of the postself is of an entirely different character from that of survival after death. It simply asserts that the individual who is going to die can, in the present moment, actively entertain notions (fantasies, thoughts, yearnings, dreams) about what the world will be like when he is absent from it. It is nothing more than what William Saroyan describes in *How It Is to Be*: "We talked of the dead as if they were not dead."

One can, in the present, savor his imaginings of what will transpire after he is gone, and these thoughts and images can influence important aspects of his behavior: the provision of life insurance for his potential survivors, his psychological investment in work that will not only survive him but continue to be identified with him, his preference for having children over remaining childless, for sons who will bear his name over daughters who will adopt the names of others—in short, his concern with his continued "existence" in the minds of others.

All this relates to fame, reputation, impact, "holding on." One asks oneself, "How long will my words and actions be remembered after my death? In what way? By how many people, and by whom in particular? Will they be influenced by them at all? If so, how?"

The postself needs to be distinguished from what Toynbee (1969) has called a "bonus life," what Maslow (1970) labeled a "post-mortem life," and what Keats, earlier, had called a "posthumous existence." These phrases were meant to convey the notion of added years of living after an episode that took one close to death, such as a severe coronary attack. Maslow (1970) wrote:

> After my heart attack my attitude toward life changed. The word I use for it now is the post-mortem life. I could just as easily have died, so my living constitutes a kind of extra, a bonus. One very important aspect of the post-mortem life is that everything gets doubly precious, gets piercingly important. You get stabbed by things, by flowers and by babies and by beautiful things—just the very act of living, of walking and breathing and eating and having friends and chatting. Everything seems to look more beautiful rather than less, and one gets the much-intensified sense of miracles.

The period of survival after an episode that could have been fatal is often referred to as "borrowed time." I have known half a dozen people who earlier had seriously attempted suicide (one cannot doubt that a man who shoots himself in the chest or into the skull is serious) and fortuitously survived; most of them were greatly improved psychologically after this severest kind of trial by fire, at least for a while. They had done penance, sought death, and magically survived. But alas, they were unable to maintain that sense of wonder and special appreciation that Toynbee and Maslow glowingly described when they wrote of their own post-mortem lives—largely because they were bedeviled by the possibility of a return to the mental state in which they had tried to end their lives.

Unlike the post-mortem life, the postself relates to the concerns of living individuals with their own reputation, impact, influence after death—those personal aspects that still live when the person himself does not. These thoughts seem to give many people the comfortable illusion of escape from total annihilation. Maslow (1970) wrote: "Sometimes I get the feeling of my writing being a communication to my great-great-grandchildren, who, of course, are not yet born. It's a kind of expression of love for them, leaving them not money but in effect affectionate notes, bits of counsel, lessons I have learned that might help them." And Susanne Langer dedicated her book *Mind: An Essay in Human Feeling* "to them in whom I hope to live even to the great World Peace—my children and their children." Tom Farber simply entitled a recent book *Notes to My Unborn Son's Children*.

There is, of course, a broad range in the intensity of investment in the post-self. At one extreme is the Nobel biologist James Watson's remark in the *New York Times Magazine* of August 18, 1968: "I believe in now—to hell with being discovered when you're dead." And Simone de Beauvoir, writing of her mother's death in *A Very Easy Death*, stated: "Religion could do no more for my mother than the hope of posthumous success could do for me. Whether you think of it as heavenly or as earthly, if you love life, immortality is no consolation for death." At the other extreme is the tragic hunger for immortality of Unamuno, the Spanish philosopher and writer (1954): "For the sake of a name man is ready to sacrifice not only life but happiness—life as a matter of course. 'Let me die, but let my fame live! death is bitter, but fame is eternal.'" Unamuno was obsessed with immortality. "If we all die utterly," he wrote, "wherefore does everything exist?" And "If there is no immortality, of what use is God?"

It is interesting to note the parallel between Unamuno's statement and one of Freud's. Unamuno (1954), as far from the psychoanalytic orientation as a twentieth-century thinker can be, said, "It is impossible for us, in effect, to conceive of ourselves as not existing, and no effort is capable of enabling consciousness to realize absolute unconsciousness, its own annihilation." Freud's (1915) often quoted statement reads: "Our own death is indeed unimaginable, and whenever we make the attempt to imagine it we can perceive that we really survive as spectators. Hence the psychoanalytic school could venture on the assertion that at bottom no one believes in his own death, or to put the thing in another way, in the unconscious every one of us is convinced of his own immortality."

There are a number of ways in which an individual can continue to "live on" after his death:

1. In the memories of others. "We can make our actions count and endow our days on earth with a scope and meaning that the finality of death cannot defeat." (Lamont 1950)
2. By the active stimulation of others through one's works, e.g., art, mu-

sic, books. "As with men, it always seemed to me that books have their peculiar destinies. They go towards the people who are waiting for them and reach them at the right moment. They are made of living material and continue to cast light through the darkness long after the death of their authors." (Serrano 1966)

3. In the bodies of others, through organ transplantation. Malcolm Muggeridge (1970) has a sardonic bit to say on this score:

There is even a hope, turning into an assumption, that "Science" will somehow provide a remedy; from steadily expanding our expectation of life, find the means to prevent its termination ever. Keeping us on the road indefinitely, like vintage cars, by replacing our worn-out parts—new hearts, new lungs, new kidneys, new brains even, and above all, new genitals as and when required. The everlasting life promised so dubiously by the Christians will then become an actuality. We shall, at last, be immortal. Or rather, some of us will. The supply of spare parts and the availability of skilled fitters is unlikely to stretch, initially at any rate, to more than a favored few, selected, presumably, among the richest, cleverest and most successful, with the retardataires furnishing the requisite organs.

4. In the genes of one's children. Hinton (1967) puts it this way:

There is some biological immortality. It is more lasting than the short-lived remembrance of the deceased in the society to which he belonged. For a while personal memories and influences may linger and perhaps a lifetime's achievements will endure rather longer, but firmer assurance that personal life does not utterly perish depends on the individual's children. The elderly get comfort when they see their children and perhaps their children's children continuing in this life. They are links in a potentially immortal chain. Within the living bodies are the chromosomes, inherited from parents and ancestors and capable of infinite replication. Once the individual has safely passed on this genetic endowment he has contributed to his immortality. In accordance with much that goes on in nature, however, he himself need survive no longer. It is egocentric to hope otherwise.

Hinton would seem rather severe on spinsters, bachelors, and childless couples. But this feeling, the sense of what Erikson has called "generativity," is a very deep one, perhaps one of the most influential of human motives. In Volume 2 of his autobiography Bertrand Russell (1967) addresses himself to thoughts of this nature:

Parental feeling, as I have experienced it, is very complex. There is, first and foremost, sheer animal affection, and delight in watching what is charming in the ways of the young. Next, there is the sense of inescapable responsibility, providing a purpose for daily activities which skepticism does not easily question. Then there is an egoistic element, which is very dangerous: the hope that one's children may succeed where one has failed, that they may carry on one's work when death or senility puts an end to one's efforts, and, in any case, that they will supply a biological escape from death, making one's own life part of the whole stream, and not a mere stagnant puddle without any overflow into the future.

5. And, philosophically, in the cosmos. Serrano, speaking of Hesse, says (1966):

I sat on the grass across from the grave and thought of my friend, trying to recall his features, and to fix them in my mind as they had been before he had been carried down that immense river which vanishes completely in the sea and which disperses everything beyond the recall of memory. And then I remembered his words. "To die is to go into the Collective Unconscious, to lose oneself in order to be transformed into form, pure form."

In one's investment in his postself two orientations can generally be distinguished: self-orientation, the wish to be recognized for one's contributions, made up of such elements as narcissism, pride, vainglory, and egocentricity, not to mention "proper self-respect"; and service orientation, the wish to contribute to humanity, made up of selflessness, humility, compassion, and sacrifice. In most of us these two skeins intertwine; we have threads of both. We are givers and takers, selfish and selfless. R. D. Laing (1967) asks:

Who is not engaged in trying to impress, to leave a mark, to engrave his image on others and on the world—graven images held more dear than life itself? We wish to die leaving our imprints burned into the hearts of others. What would life be if there were no one left to remember us, to think of us when we are absent, to keep us alive when we are dead? And when we are dead, suddenly or gradually, our presence, scattered in ten or ten thousand hearts, will fade and disappear. How many candles in how many hearts? Of such stuff is our hope and our despair. . . .

Perhaps it is the poet, after all, who expresses this sentiment most pointedly. When W. H. Auden received the 1967 National Medal for Literature, he said in his acceptance speech:

To believe in the value of art is to believe that it is possible to make an object, be it an epic or a two-line epigram, which will remain permanently on hand in the world. The probabilities of success are against him, but an artist must not attempt anything less. In the meantime, and whatever is going to happen, we must try to live as E. M. Forster recommends that we should: "The people I respect must behave as if they were immortal and as if society were eternal. Both assumptions are false. But both must be accepted as true if we are to go on working and eating and loving, and are able to keep open a few breathing holes for the human spirit."

I turn to Herman Melville's convoluted life as an example and note that many of his more profound identity-seeking and death-focused labors—

Mardi, *Moby-Dick*, *Redburn*, *Pierre*, *Clarel*, *Billy Budd*, those words that sprang out of his deeper shaping and crushing concerns—expressed the concept that I have labeled the postself: . . . .

> *[In* Moby-Dick*]: It may seem strange that of all men sailors should be tinkering at their last wills and testaments. . . . After the ceremony was concluded upon the present occasion, I felt all the easier; a stone was rolled away from my heart. Besides, all the days I should now live would be as good as the days that Lazarus lived after his resurrection; a supplementary clean gain of so many months or weeks as the case might be. I survived myself. . . .*
>   *Immortality is but ubiquity in time.*

And from his letters:

To Evert Duyckinck, April 5, 1849: "All ambitious authors should have ghosts capable of revisiting the world, to snuff up the steam of adulation, which begins to rise straightway as the Sexton throws his last shovelfull on him.—Down goes his body and up flies his name."

To Lemuel Shaw, April 23, 1849: "These attacks are matters of course, and are essential to the building up of any permanent reputation—if such should ever prove to be mine."

To Hawthorne, June 1, 1851: "What 'reputation' H. M. has is horrible. Think of it! To go down to posterity is bad enough, any way; but to go down as a 'man who lived among the cannibals'!" . . . .

The concept of the postself is, of course, directly related to the notion of annihilation. Without these "breathing holes for the human spirit" we suffocate. And without the belief or the wistful hope that we shall survive—some part of us, in some way—our lives tend to lose whatever meaning we can manage to find in them. Not unexpectedly, Melville had a few things to say on these issues:

Israel Potter: "Few things remain. . . . He was repulsed in efforts after a pension by certain caprices of law. His scars provided his only medals. He dictated a little book, the records of his fortunes. But long ago it faded out of print—himself out of being—his name out of memory."

Redburn: "But all is now lost; I know not who he was; and this estimable author must need share the oblivious fate of all literary incognitos."

White-Jacket: "It is a good joke, for instance, and one often perpetrated on board ship, to stand talking to a man in a dark nightwatch, and all the while be cutting the buttons from his coat. But once off, those buttons never grow on again. There is no spontaneous vegetation in buttons." . . .

From his letter to Hawthorne, June 1, 1851: "Though I wrote the Gospels in this Century, I should die in the gutter."

To cease as though one had never been, to exit life with no hope of living on in the memory of another, to be obliterated, to be expunged from history's record—that is a fate literally far worse than death.

References

Freud, Sigmund. (1915/1957). "Thoughts for the Times on War and Death," in *The Standard Edition of the Complete Psychological Works*. London: Hogarth Press.

Hinton, John (1967). *Dying*. Baltimore: Penguin Books.

Laing, R. D. (1967). *The Politics of Experience*. New York: Pantheon Books.

Lamont, Corliss. (1950). *The Illusion of Immortality*. 2nd ed. New York: Philosophical Library.

Maslow, Abraham. (1970). Editorial in *Psychology Today*, August.

Melville, Herman. *Redburn* (1849); *White-Jacket* (1850); *Moby-Dick* (1851); *Pierre* (1852); *Israel Potter* (1855); *Letters* (1849–1862).

Muggeridge, Malcolm (1970). *The Observer*, February 20.

Russell, Bertrand. (1967). *The Autobiography of Bertrand Russell, 1872–1914*, 2 vols. Boston: Little, Brown.

Serrano, Miguel. (1966). *C. G. Jung and Herman Hesse: A Record of Two Friendships*. New York: Schocken Books.

Shneidman, Edwin. (1971). "You and Death" in *Psychology Today*, June. Pp. 43–45, 74–80.

Toynbee, Arnold. (1969). "Why and How I Work," in *Saturday Review*, April 5.

Unamuno, Miguel de. (1954). *The Tragic Sense of Life*. New York: Dover Publications. Originally published in 1921.

Annotated Bibliography ❧

A FEW YEARS AGO, the British–South African psychiatrist Michael A. Simpson published *Dying, Death and Grief: A Critically Annotated Bibliography and Source Book of Thanatology and Terminal Care.*[1] The main part of the book consists of several hundred annotated references on death and dying. Simpson has evaluated each of these by awarding them from one to five stars, where five stars means "highly recommended; buy and read." He evaluated more than 700 books. Below you will find an annotated bibliography that includes 50 items; of these, 29 describe books published prior to 1980. For these 29 items, the citations and comments are taken directly from Simpson's 1979 book.[2] They are all from his highly recommended category (five stars). To bring that list up to date, we have added citations for 21 books published since 1980.

★James Agee. *A death in the family*. Bantam, New York, 1985, paperbound.
Pulitzer Prize–winning novel dealing with the effects of the sudden death of a young father on a close-knit family.

★Lisa Alther. *Kinflicks*. Chatto & Windus, London, 1976. Penguin, 1977, paperbound. A. A. Knopf, New York (Random House Canada), 1975. Signet, New York, 1977. Also 'Haut-Kontakte' Ullstein Verlag, Berlin, 1977.
"My family has always been into death," it begins. At long last someone who had something new to say about death in America and a sparkling style to say it in. The story of Ginny Babcock is not merely brilliantly funny and poignant as a novel (it's a cliché for a reviewer to admit to laughing aloud, but the occurrence is still rare enough to be worth recording). It is also a fine account of varying responses to death, and of the dying, from idiopathic thrombocytopenic purpura, of Ginny's mother, for whom death was a demon lover for whose assignation one must be ready. "The trick was in being both willing to die and able to do so at the same time. Dying properly was like achieving simultaneous orgasm."

★A. Alvarez. *The savage god*. Weidenfeld & Nicolson, London, 1972, 250 pp. Bantam, New York, paperbound.

---

[1]The items marked with a star have been excerpted from *Dying, Death and Grief: A Critically Annotated Bibliography and Source Book of Thanatology and Terminal Care* by Michael A. Simpson © 1979 Plenum Publishing Corporation. Reprinted with permission of the publisher.

[2]An update of Simpson's bibliography was published in 1987 by the University of Pittsburgh Press. Most of the more than 1,700 books reviewed in that excellent volume were published between 1979 and 1986. We have decided to do our own update.

A study of attitudes toward suicide and death through history and literature, and the fascination this theme has had for writers at all times. Includes an account of his relations with Sylvia Plath, and her suicide and his own suicide attempt.

Phillipe Ariès. *The hour of our death.* (Translated from the French by Helen Weaver.) Vintage Books, New York, 1982. Alfred A. Knopf, 1981, 651 pp., paperbound.

Phillipe Ariès—who was a French civil service botanist—was that rare creature, a true European amateur scholar-historian. As one aspect of his research effort, Ariès checked virtually all records in France pertaining to death for the past several hundred years. He shows how "death" changes over the centuries and does this in an absolutely captivating and convincing way, with careful documentation and lively anecdote. One reviewer called the book "a feast for the imagination"; another said that it was "an absolutely magnificent thousand-year panorama . . . the masterwork of a masterful writer of history." An hour spent browsing through this book is like an afternoon in an imaginary thanatological section of the Louvre.

★Howard Brodie. *Ethical decisions in medicine.* Little, Brown & Co., Boston, 1976, 340 pp.

Probably the best available book on medical ethics. Soundly organized with clearly stated objectives and self-evaluation components. Proposes a concise method for dealing with ethical problems and provides many lucid examples of its use. It examines key issues, including informed consent, determination of the quality of life, ethical participation, allocation of scarce resources, euthanasia, and allowing to die. As some recent thanatology research has breached some of the principles of ethical research on human beings, everyone involved in this area could benefit from reading this book, which will also provide a valuable basis for teaching the subject.

George Howe Colt. *The enigma of suicide.* Summit Books, New York, 1991, 575 pp.

This is the best available layman's book on suicide. George Howe Colt, who is a working journalist and poet, is an alumnus of Harvard College with postgraduate work at Johns Hopkins. This long and full book is an amalgam of what is known about suicide and what is useful in suicide prevention. The book includes some wonderfully written case histories. The hallmark of this book is its readability; the secret of the book is that— even with its easy digestibility—it contains so much interesting information. It is the best introduction to the technical literature in suicidology. There are separate sections on adolescent suicide, the right to die, and survivors.

★Diana Crane. *The sanctity of social life: Physicians' treatment of critically ill patients.* Russell Sage Foundation, New York, 1975, 286 pp.

A uniquely valuable study based on extensive interviews, observations, hospital record audits, and detailed questionnaires. Rather than pontificating on what ought to be done, Crane describes what doctors actually do for the critically ill. She shows that while withdrawal of treatment is widespread in some types of cases, positive euthanasia is rare. Both adults and children seem to be regarded as "treatable" while they retain the potential for interacting in some meaningful way with others. A much-needed antidote to the usually speculative literature on this subject, with commendable detail and objectivity.

★Simone de Beauvoir. *A very easy death.* Penguin Books, Harmondsworth, 1969,

92 pp. Celo Press, Burnsville, N.C., 1965, 139 pp. Warner, New York, 1973, paperbound.

> *Unreservedly recommended. A brilliant and unforgettable account of her mother's death in France, a death that was anything but easy. Deeply moving description of a proud woman's humiliation and the conflicting love and hostility her famous daughter experienced in confronting her mother's death.*

Lynne Ann De Spelder and Albert Lee Strickland. *The last dance: Encountering death and dying* (3rd ed.). Mayfield Publishing Company, Mountain View, Calif., 1992, 656 pp.

> *This book is a comprehensive core textbook for interdisciplinary undergraduate courses on death and dying. It is well-suited for courses taught in a variety of different academic departments. The graphics and boxed inserts are well done and the writing is clear. It is particularly useful for first and second year students.*

★Herman Feifel, ed. *New meanings of death.* McGraw–Hill, New York, 1977.

> *A splendid volume—even more interesting and accessible than Feifel's 1959 classic. Includes Feifel on death in contemporary America; Kastenbaum on death and development through the life span; Bluebond-Langer on meanings of death to children; Shneidman on death and the college student; Weisman on the psychiatrist and the inexorable; Garfield on the personal impact of death on the clinician; Saunders on St. Christopher's Hospice, Kelly on Make Today Count; Kalish on death and the family; Levition on death education; Lifton on immortality; Simpson on death and poetry; Gutman on death and power; Shaffer and Rodes on death and the law.*

★Robert Fulton, compiler, with others. *Death, grief & bereavement: A bibliography 1845–1975.* Arno Press, New York, 1976, 253 pp.

> *The most comprehensive and reliable bibliography of the literature on death, grief, and bereavement in print. Some 4,000 entries, mainly journal articles, indexed by subject, with nearly eighty classifications.*

★E. A. Grollman. *Talking about death.* Beacon Press, Boston, 1970, 30 pp., paperbound.

> *Strongly recommended. A beautiful book, probably the best available for use in discussing death with children. Well-illustrated and well-constructed; simple, direct, honest.*

★Earl A. Grollman. *Talking about death: A dialogue between parent & child.* Beacon Press, Boston, 1976, 98 pp.

> *Simply excellent. A new edition of the fine earlier version with a greatly expanded guide to parents on how to use the book and how to discuss death with children. Lists some resources such as organizations, cassettes, films, books. Explicit and observant.*

★John Hinton. *Dying.* Pelican Books, Harmondsworth, Baltimore, 1967. 2nd edition, 1972, 220 pp.

> *Succinct and highly capable review of existing knowledge on attitudes toward death, what dying is like, terminal care, and mourning based on a thorough review of the literature up to the 1960s and the author's own experience. Compact.*

★Mark and Dan Jury. *Gramp.* Grossman Publishers (Viking Press), New York, 1976, 152 pp., illustrated, paperbound.

> *Simply superb. A moving, honest, and direct account of the dying of Frank Tugend, as*

recorded in photographs and words, by a family who made his death an act of love. Arteriosclerotic dementia led to a grueling three-year deterioration. On February 11, 1974, aged 81, he removed his false teeth and announced that he was no longer going to eat or drink. The family decided to respect his wishes and not hospitalize him. Three weeks later, he died at home. Death with dignity? Perhaps, though not how most people would picture it. An invaluable, unromanticized corrective to the stickily sentimental nature of too much death literature.

Robert J. Kastenbaum. *Death, society, and human experience* (4th ed). Merrill, New York, 1991, 347 pp., paperbound.

This book is a text suitable for use in courses on death and dying taught in a variety of different departments, but it does not attempt to be as comprehensive as a text such as The Last Dance. *Of particular note are chapter-length treatments of such topics as AIDS, hospice care, ethical issues linked to the right-to-die debate, and death education. This edition also gives more attention than earlier editions to murder and terrorism. It contains an excellent chapter that presents a critical assessment of the evidence with respect to near-death experiences.*

Robert Kastenbaum. *The psychology of death* (2nd ed.). Springer Publishing Co., New York, 1992, 280 pp.

This superlative book is, if anything, even better than the first-rate book that it supplants. It is certainly one of the finest texts in thanatology. It is a book about the psychology of death, "the death that is in our minds," our construction of death from a developmental perspective. It includes the topics of suicide, murder, and longevity. If a book on death can be a pleasure to read, Kastenbaum's book is the one.

Robert Kastenbaum and Beatrice Kastenbaum, eds. *Encyclopedia of death.* Oryx Press, Phoenix, Arizona, 1989, 295 pp., illustrated.

This encyclopedia includes approximately 150 entries on a very wide range of topics related to thanatology. For those who want a more extended treatment on various topics, a few key sources are given. It includes entries under major events (such as Jonestown), names of organizations (such as the Make-A-Wish Foundation), and a number of historical terms (such as Ars Moriendi). Many of the entries are excellent essays. It is a particularly useful resource for undergraduates starting term papers.

★Jay Katz and Alexander Morgan Capron. *Catastrophic diseases: Who decides what? A psychosocial and legal analysis of the problems posed by hemodialysis and organ transplantation.* Russell Sage Foundation, New York, 1975, 295 pp.

*A highly able explanation of important issues, extending and complementing both Katz's earlier work (*Experimentation with Human Beings, *1972) and Fox and Swazey's recent book (*The Courage to Fail*). The authors explore the nature and effects of catastrophic illness and such goals and values as the preservation of life, reduction of suffering, personal integrity and dignity, pursuit of knowledge, economy, and the public interest. There's a cogent account of the development and present status of the technical procedures and a study of the characteristics, authority and capacity of the physician-investigators and patient-subjects, and the functions and limitations of informed consent. The stages of decision making are reviewed; the activities of professional and public institutions involved are scrutinized and proposals are made for the formulation of policy regarding the allocation of resources and selection of donors and the* *administration of such major medical interventions at local and national levels, with a review of decisions and consequences. Lucid, readable, fascinating, and challenging.*

Michael C. Kearl. *Endings: A sociology of death and dying.* Oxford University Press, New York, 1989, 521 pp.

This is a core textbook particularly well suited for sociology courses on death and dying. It differs from The Last Dance *in that it is much more focused on themes and issues that are likely to be emphasized in a sociology course on death and dying, but it does make extensive use of materials from psychology, religion, philosophy, anthropology, and political science as well. It is more conceptual than* The Last Dance *and is written at a level more suitable for third- and fourth-year undergraduates who have some background in sociology.*

★Elisabeth Kübler-Ross. *On death and dying.* Macmillan, New York, 1968, 250 pp. Tavistock, London, 1973, paperbound.

Strongly recommended. A classic and highly influential work in which Dr. Ross advanced her model of the "five stages" in the progress of the dying patient. Interesting and humane, with sound practical advice and transcripts of some interviews.

★C. S. Lewis. *A grief observed.* Faber and Faber, London. 1961/1973, 60 pp., paperbound. Seabury Press, New York.

"No one ever told me that grief felt so much like fear. . . ." An outstandingly honest, naked observation of a widower's grief. Begun, without plans for publication, as a means of self-therapy, written informally in odd notebooks, during his first weeks alone. Unique, moving, memorable.

Heather G. Miller, Charles F. Turner, and Lincoln E. Moses, eds. *AIDS: The second decade.* National Academy Press, Washington, D.C., 1990, 495 pp.

This book is based on a report prepared by a very distinguished committee organized by the National Research Council. It describes the shifting patterns of the AIDS epidemic and makes proposals about what should be done to deal with this epidemic over the next ten years. The authors point out that gay men and intravenous drug users will continue to comprise the majority of those with the HIV virus, but they also note that the proportion of cases due to heterosexual transmission is increasing. Considerable attention is given to such issues as HIV among women (particularly female prostitutes) and sexual risk-taking among adolescents.

★Jessica Mitford. *The American way of death.* Simon and Schuster, New York, 1963, 280 pp. Fawcett/Crest, paperbound.

Justly famous, witty, well-documented and merciless exposure of the multimillion-dollar death industry and American funeral practices.

Sherwin B. Nuland. *How we die: Reflections on life's final chapter.* New York: Alfred A. Knopf, 1994, 278 pp.

Dr. Nuland—a surgeon at Yale—writes about the biological and clinical realities of the six main contemporary avenues leading to the Arc de Mort: cancer, heart attack, AIDS, Alzheimer's disease, trauma, and old age. And what a Baedeker he has provided us! Perhaps the best guide-book currently available. It is beautifully written, marvelously insightful, and eloquently instructive. It elevates the field of thanatology. A must read. As an example, consider his thoughts about that key word, hope (p. 257): "Hope lies not only in an expectation of cure or even of the remission of present distress.

For dying patients, the hope of cure will always be shown to be ultimately false, and even the hope of relief often turns to ashes. When my time comes, I will seek hope in the knowledge that insofar as possible I will not be allowed to suffer or to be subjected to needless attempts to maintain life; I will seek it in the certainty that I will not be abandoned to die alone; I am seeking it now, in the way that I try to live my life, so that those who value what I am will have profited by my time on earth and be left with comforting recollections of what we have meant to one another."

Marian Osterweis, Frederic Solomon, and Morris Green, eds. *Bereavement: Reactions, consequences, and care.* (Prepared under the auspices of the Institute of Medicine). National Academy Press, Washington, D.C., 1984, 312 pp., paperbound.

This book represents that rare case in which a committee labored and brought forth not a camel but a marvelously sensitive catalogue of a whole Noah's Ark of well-groomed conceptual beasts, a veritable zoological garden relating to bereavement. The 21 contributors to this excellent volume represent the country's clinical (and conceptual) experts on grief and mourning, both in its normal and pathological forms. It is both a scholarly book and a "how to" book. Its quality is first-rate. The volume is highly recommended, not so much to actual mourners, but to students of this topic.

★Lily Pincus. *Death and the family: The importance of mourning.* Pantheon Books, New York, 1974, 278 pp. Vintage, paperbound, New York, 1976.

Written by a social worker with great experience in marital and family therapy; a brilliant book, sensitive and well written, always readable, wise, and human. A genuine, fresh, and substantial contribution to the understanding and therapy of bereavement and the dying family. Highly recommended.

★Sylvia Plath. *The bell jar.* Bantam, New York, 1972, 216 pp., paperbound.

A brilliant novel, autobiographical in many respects, about a nineteen-year-old girl who attempts suicide, finding life difficult to bear. One of the best evocations of suicidal thinking in literature.

Timothy E. Quill. *Death and dignity: Making choices and taking charge.* W. W. Norton, New York, 1993, 255 pp.

This book is written for physicians and their terminally ill patients. It makes the case for an open discussion of all options at the end stage. He emphasizes the active role the patient should play in deciding how aggressively to fight illness toward the end of life. He makes the case for physician-assisted suicide under some circumstances.

Terese A. Rando. *Treatment of complicated mourning.* Research Press, Champaign, Illinois, 1993, 751 pp.

This unusually comprehensive volume is particularly well-suited for clinicians and caregivers who are doing or will be doing grief therapy. The focus is patients who are resistant to the standard techniques of therapeutic facilitation.

Beverley Raphael. *When disaster strikes: How individuals and communities cope with catastrophe.* Basic Books, New York, 1986, 342 pp.

This book pulls together the literature on the psychological response to disaster. It is aimed at those who will be responsible for helping the survivors of disasters. Loss and grief are major themes, as are the psychological consequences of dislocation and relocation. In Chapter 1 Raphael presents several useful models for analyzing the impact of a disaster. For example, one describes the stages of disaster: warning, threat, impact, inventory, rescue, remedy, and recovery.

★Jack Riemer. *Jewish reflections on death.* Schocken Books, New York, 1974, 184 pp.
An eloquent anthology of great interest and value to Jews and non-Jews alike. The laws of Judaism, especially with regard to bereavement, show great psychological and spiritual wisdom, giving a structure to grief that relates to death firmly and realistically as a normal part of life. These essays give a clear account of the beauty and insight of the traditional procedures for the business of mourning and also explore the modern problems relating to death, from the Jewish experience, of suffering and solace. An unusually interesting book. A short glossary of Hebrew terms used would aid the comprehension of non-Jewish readers.

★B. Schoenberg, A. C. Carr, D. Peretz, and A. H. Kutscher, eds. *Loss and grief: Psychological management in medical practice.* Columbia University Press, New York, 1970, 400 pp., paperbound.
Strongly recommended. Deals with the broader issues of reactions to loss of different kinds, including loss of limb, organ, sensory loss, or loss of sexual function; also with the reactions to death in the patient, family, and the health care team. A very high standard of contributions from a distinguished group of authors. Includes a 45-item annotated bibliography.

Richard Selzer. *Raising the dead.* Whittle/Viking, New York, 1994, 118 pp.
Dr. Selzer, a former surgeon and current best-selling author, has written an extraordinary book about his own life-threatening illness (from Legionnaire's disease) and his near-death experience. He describes—from notes of his own case and his experiences with many patients—the course of his 23-day coma and its dicey life-and-death conclusion. The joy of the book lies in its clinical detail and its sumptuous (albeit sometimes baroque) autobiographical writing. One reviewer described the prose as "gorgeous descriptive writing." There is also a special bonus for women in this strong book: Dr. Selzer tells the story of Fanny Burney, a prolific eighteenth- and nineteenth-century English novelist, who endured a mastectomy (the third on record) without anesthesia in 1811 and of the platonic relationship that developed between her and her sympathetic surgeon.

Randy Shilts. *And the band played on: Politics, people, and the AIDS epidemic.* St. Martin's Press, 1987, 630 pp.
A major thesis of this searing critique is that the AIDS epidemic did not just happen; it was allowed to happen by a variety of institutions that failed to respond adequately at the early stages of the epidemic. He is critical of the medical establishment, of various public health organizations, of federal and private scientific research organizations, the mass media, and the leaders of the gay movement. He traces the epidemic to its origins in Africa, but the emphasis is on what did and what did not happen during the period between the early and mid-1980s in the United States. It is one of the most influential books on AIDS to date.

Edwin Shneidman. *Suicide as psychache: A clinical approach to self-destructive behavior.* Jason Aronson Inc., Northvale, New Jersey, 1993, 259 pp., paperbound.
This book contains a number of papers by Shneidman. The volume takes its title from Chapter 4, "Suicide as Psychache," one of the shortest, but also one of the most impor-

tant, essays. The stated purpose for preparing this book is to bring together in one place a number of his papers written between 1971 and 1993, papers of potential use to a broad range of mental health clinicians who treat suicidal patients. These essays are not just reprints of prior work; most represent a refinement of the ideas presented in his earlier papers on these topics.

★Michael A. Simpson. *The facts of death.* Spectrum/Prentice-Hall, 1979, 250 pp.
An eloquent and warm practical book for families and helpers. Reviews succinctly what we know about the nature of death and dying, patients' rights, how to manage one's own death and to cope with the dying of another, death and children, suicide, how to cope with a suicidal person and with one's own suicidal impulses, bereavement and grief, funerals, and how to plan one's estate and funeral and avoid the Terminal R.I.P.-off. Maybe they told you the facts of life: this is what they left out.

Michael A. Simpson. *Dying, death, and grief: A critical bibliography.* University of Pittsburgh Press, Pittsburgh, 1987, 259 pp.
This is a revised edition of Simpson's 1979 bibliography. This excellent volume reviews approximately 1,700 books on topics relating to death and dying published between 1979 and 1986. It uses the same five-star rating system used in the 1979 edition. He does not include items published during the time period covered by the first version.

★A. Solzhenitsyn. *Cancer ward.* Bantam, New York, 1969, 560 pp.
A great novel, that defies any brief review, about life in the cancer ward of a Russian hospital.

Samuel Southard. *Death and dying: A bibliographical survey.* Greenwood Press, New York, 1991, 514 pp.
This book will be very useful as a reference volume. If you cannot find what you want from among the more than 8,000 books and articles that are included, you may want to take a close look at Chapter 8, in which he reviews 54 items—many of which are annotated bibliographies dealing with topics relevant to thanatology.

★P. Steinfels and R. M. Veatch, eds. *Death inside out.* Hastings Center Report, Harper Forum Books, Harper and Row, New York. Fitzhenry and Whiteside, Canada, 1975, 150 pp., paperbound.
One of the more refreshing books on death. Elegant, clear thinking, critical, thoughtful and stimulating. Principally concerned with philosophical, ethical, and historical issues rather than practical and personal problems. One of the comparatively few books of genuine intellectual interest in the field. Includes Ariès's "Death Inside Out" again, and Ivan Illich on the political uses of natural death; Eric Cassell on dying in a technological society; William May on the metaphysical plight of the family (the great family secret: God is dead); Robert Morison on death (process or event?), Paul Ramsey on the indignity of "death with dignity"; David Smith on letting some babies die; and other works by Leon Kass and Tristram Engelhardt.

Judith M. Stillion. *Suicide across the life span—premature exits.* Eugene E. McDowell and Jacque H. May. Hemisphere Publishing Corporation, New York, 1989, 287 pp., paperbound.
This text synthesizes the literature on suicide with an emphasis on life span perspectives. This life span perspective is reflected in the attention given to differences among different ages groups with respect to the causes of suicide. It is also reflected in the model

of the suicide trajectory presented in Chapter 8. In Chapter 2, the authors review seven different perspectives on suicide: five are psychological (the psychoanalytic perspective, the psychosocial perspective, the behavioral perspective, the cognitive perspective, the humanistic perspective), one is sociological, and one is biological. This book is most appropriate for advanced undergraduate students and beginning graduate students in the helping professions.

★David Sudnow. *Passing on: The social organization of dying.* Prentice-Hall, Englewood Cliffs, N.J., 1967, 176 pp., paperbound.
  Excellent sociological study of death in a county hospital and its management by the staff, including counting of deaths and their visibility, social death, preparing and moving bodies, how we announce death and bad news, uses of a corpse, etc. Fascinating reading, introducing a new way of looking at what we do. Strongly recommended.

★Leo Tolstoy. *The death of Ivan Ilyich.* New American Library, New York, paperbound, and other editions.
  Strongly recommended. Brilliant account of the death of a bourgeois Russian judge, with probably more insight into the psychology of death than any other 19th-century author.

★Arnold Toynbee, et al. *Man's concern with death.* Hodder and Stoughton, London, 1968, 280 pp.
  One of the early and persisting classics of death literature. Among its competent chapters are several by Ninian Smart on philosophical and religious concepts, Keith Mant on the medical definition of death, Simon Yudkin on death and the young, and Eric Rhode on death in twentieth-century fiction. But best of all are the splendid chapters by Arnold Toynbee, erudite and elegant and superbly literate. The epilogue, a moving account of Toynbee's personal experience and his feelings about the imminent prospect of death, is especially poignant reading.

★Dalton Trumbo. *Johnny got his gun.* Bantam, New York, 1982, paperbound.
  A powerful antiwar novel; a nineteen-year-old World War I veteran has been left, after multiple injuries, blind, speechless, and limbless. He beats out messages on his pillow with his head, begging to be taken out of his hospital room, to show the world a survivor of Every War.

★Alan Watts. *The book (on the taboo against knowing who you are).* Vintage Books, New York, 1972, 146 pp., paperbound.
  A classic, elegantly, lucidly, and wittily written book dealing with the delusion of the lonely separate ego alienated from the universe, with his usual skillful understanding of Eastern and Western religions and philosophies. Offers a coherent philosophical style that genuinely deals with fear of death and a manner of coming to terms with life. Highly recommended.

★Avery Weisman. *On dying and denying.* Behavioral Publ., New York, 1972.
  A very significant study of "terminality," concentrating on the central role of denial. Very competent and illustrated with many clinical examples. Of the highest quality both intellectually and practically.

Avery D. Weisman. *The vulnerable self: Confronting the ultimate questions.* Insight Books, New York, 1993, 253 pp.
  Avery Weisman is Professor of Psychiatry Emeritus at Harvard Medical School; for

years he was the director of Project Omega (relating to dying patients) at the Massachu-setts General Hospital. His early training was in philosophy. The book is a must for someone dying of cancer, or someone who wants to help someone dying of cancer. In a masterfully humanistic and secular way, Weisman spins a solid web of conceptions of the human life course as a pilgrimage best done when it relates to making sense (finding meanings) and to mustering courage. Undeniably, death makes people vulnerable. Weisman's gift to us is his almost poetic explication of "vulnerability," his explanations grounded in a lifetime of intense clinical practice and research. One reviewer said: "The author enriches us with his distilled wisdom from a half century of thoughtful and philo-sophically illuminated clinical practice. The book is a gem."

Anna M. Wolf. *Helping your children to understand death.* Revised edition, 1973. Child Study Press, New York, 64 pp., paperbound.

Possibly the best book available to help parents and children talk about death. Simple but not simplistic, wise but not know-all, and soundly practical. Well grounded in child development and family dynamics, it deals sensibly with the common questions of chil-dren and parents. Issues of faith, inescapable in this area, are considered from the view-point of the major faiths; other matters covered include suicide, assassination and war, and hypocrisy. Very highly recommended to all who deal with children.